United Health Foundation℠

Fall 2008

Dear Colleague,

We at the United Health Foundation recognize and support your commitment to provide the best possible evidence-based clinical care to achieve optimal health outcomes for your patients. That is why we are once again pleased to provide you with this newest edition of *BMJ Clinical Evidence Handbook*.

Clinical Evidence remains the gold standard in evidence-based synopses on the effectiveness of common clinical interventions. It provides systematic reviews of evidence for over 3,100 interventions and provides answers to more than 600 clinical questions. It is currently used by more than one million clinicians worldwide, including 500,000 physicians in the U.S.

In addition to this Handbook, I strongly encourage you to take advantage of **free internet access** which we make available to you at no cost. To take advantage of the internet access, go to www.clinicalevidence.bmj.com/uhf, and enter the password: **United Health Foundation 2008**.

All of us at the United Health Foundation are pleased to support you and your patients in achieving optimal health outcomes by providing internet access to the best scientific-based evidence available.

Sincerely,

Reed V. Tuckson, M.D., FACP
United Health Foundation

BMJ

clinical
evidence
handbook

The international source of
the best available evidence
for effective health care

FALL
2008

Editorial office
BMJ Publishing Group Limited (BMJ Group), BMA House, Tavistock Square, London, WC1H 9JR, United
Kingdom. Tel: +44 (0)20 7387 4410 ● Fax: +44 (0)20 7383 6242 ● www.bmjgroup.bmj.com

Subscription prices for *BMJ Clinical Evidence*
The *BMJ Clinical Evidence Handbook* is published six monthly (June/December) by the BMJ Group. The
annual subscription rates are:

Online format
Personal: £137 ● €203 ● US$260
Student/nurse: £69 ● €102 ● US$131
Online and print format
Personal: £200 ● €296 ● US$380
Student/nurse: £100 ● €148 ● US$190

Print format
Personal: £114 ● €169 ● US$217
Institutional: £240 ● €355 ● US$456
Student/nurse: £56 ● €83 ● US$106

Institutional subscriptions are for print editions only. Institutions may purchase online site licenses
separately. For further information, or to purchase *BMJ Clinical Evidence*, please visit our website
www.clinicalevidence.bmj.com or email us at subscriptions@bmjgroup.com (UK and ROW) or
bmj-clinicalevidence@ebsco.com (Americas). You may also telephone us or fax us on the following
numbers:
UK and ROW Tel: +44 (0)20 7383 6270 ● Fax: +44 (0)20 7383 6402
Americas Tel: +1 800 373 2897/240 646 7000 ● Fax: +1 205 995 1588

Bulk subscriptions for societies and organisations
The BMJ Group offers discounts for any society or organisation buying bulk quantities for their
members/specific groups. Please contact us at consortiasales@bmjgroup.com

Institutional site license (online)
The BMJ Group offers institutions the opportunity to purchase online access to clinicalevidence.bmj.com.
To discuss your institutional needs further please contact us at bmj-clinical
evidence@subscriptionsoffice.com.

Rights and permission to reproduce
For information on translation rights, please contact Caroline Gomm at cgomm@bmjgroup.com.
To request permission to reprint all or part of any contribution in *BMJ Clinical Evidence* please contact
Jennie Wilkinson on Jwilkinson@bmjgroup.com.

British Library Cataloguing in Publication Data. A catalogue record for this book is available from the
British Library. ISSN 1475–9225, ISBN 978-1-905545-29-2..

Typeset in the UK by Letterpart Ltd, Reigate, Surrey, UK.
Printed in the USA by Quebecor World Taunton.

Designed by Paragraphics Ltd, London, UK.

Acknowledgements

The BMJ Publishing Group would like to thank United Health Foundation for their leadership, advice and support in advancing evidence based medicine and clinical practice. We would also like to thank the following people and organisations for their advice and support: The Cochrane Collaboration, and especially Iain Chalmers, Mike Clarke, Phil Alderson, and Carol Lefebvre; Tom Mann, Ron Stamp, Ben Toth, Veronica Fraser, and Nick Rosen; the British National Formulary, and especially Dinesh Mehta, Eric Connor, and John Martin; Martindale: The Complete Drug Reference, and especially Sean Sweetman; the Health Information Research Unit at McMaster University, and especially Brian Haynes and Ann McKibbon; previous staff who have contributed to this issue, and the clinicians, epidemiologists, and members of patient groups who have acted as contributors, advisors, and peer reviewers.

The BMJ Publishing Group values the ongoing support it has received from the global medical community for *BMJ Clinical Evidence*. The BMJ Publishing Group wishes to thank United Health Foundation for its efforts in providing educational funding which has allowed the wide dissemination of this valuable resource to millions of physicians and health professionals in the USA. We are grateful to the clinicians and patients who have taken part in focus groups, which are crucial to the development of *BMJ Clinical Evidence*. Finally, we would like to acknowledge the readers who have taken the time to send us their comments and suggestions.

Contents

Contents

Contents

SUPPORTING CLINICAL DECISION MAKING

BMJ Clinical Evidence helps healthcare professionals find answers to important clinical questions. We provide systematic reviews of the most important conditions that practices and hospitals have to deal with every day. The evidence is supplemented by clinical interpretation and links to validated guidelines, drug safety alerts, and prescribing advice. In all, we systematically review the evidence on over 3100 interventions, and provide answers to 650 clinical questions.

BMJ CLINICAL EVIDENCE IS A UNIQUE RESOURCE

We focus on the evidence that matters the most, concentrating our efforts around the clinical questions that are the highest priority for clinicians and patients.

Our expert team of information specialists searches the world's literature for important new findings, selecting studies and systematic reviews that report the outcomes that matter most to clinicians and patients.

Leading medical experts check and summarise the evidence, and together with our specialist editors provide summaries describing what is known about the benefits and harms associated with particular interventions.

We place new evidence in the context of what is already known and regularly completely reappraise each systematic review.

We support patient–doctor partnerships by ensuring that professionals have easy access to the answers to patients' questions, and are best placed to promote realistic expectations of the effects of interventions.

We make it easy to find and use the evidence.

BMJ CLINICAL EVIDENCE SUPPORTS EBM AT THE POINT OF CARE

Evidence-based medicine (EBM) is well into its third decade, and yet worldwide the challenges of bringing EBM into clinical practice are a constant cause for debate. In a systematic review published in the *BMJ*, Kawamoto, Houlihan, Balas, and Lobach identified four features that, where present, improved the likelihood of clinical decision support systems improving practice:

- automatic provision of decision support as part of clinician workflow
- provision of recommendations rather than just assessments
- provision of decision support at the time and location of decision making
- computer-based decision support.

Of 32 systems possessing all four features, 30 (94%) significantly improved clinical practice. This review provides a guide to where evidence-based resources should be positioning themselves in the future. We are very pleased that not only has *BMJ Clinical Evidence* been successfully integrated into clinical record systems, but we have also undertaken experimental work in which our content underpins different decision support applications.

The *BMJ Clinical Evidence Handbook*, which is updated every 6 months, provides an instant overview of the current evidence, easily accessible at the point of care.

The full edition of *BMJ Clinical Evidence* is available online — easily searchable, with up-to-the-minute coverage of the evidence, and structured to help you get straight to the information you need.

BMJ Clinical Evidence can now also be delivered to PDAs (Personal Digital Assistants), providing access to evidence wherever it's needed.

For more information on other formats of *BMJ Clinical Evidence,* please visit: www.clinicalevidence.bmj.com

BMJ CLINICAL EVIDENCE IS KNOWN AND TRUSTED ALL OVER THE WORLD

BMJ Clinical Evidence has an international circulation, reaching more than a million clinicians worldwide in several languages, including Spanish, Russian, German,

Hungarian, and Portuguese. *BMJ Clinical Evidence* is also available free online to people in resource-poor countries as part of the HINARI initiative spearheaded by the WHO and the BMJ Group. Details of those countries that qualify are available from the *BMJ Clinical Evidence* website (www.clinicalevidence.bmj.com).

FEEDBACK

We encourage and appreciate all feedback via our website. You can contact us at CEfeedback@bmjgroup.com or use the 'Contact Us' button on every page. Alternatively, you can send a response for publication by clicking on the button on the left hand side of every webpage marked 'Your Response'. Responses are screened before publication and may not be posted if they do not meet the requirements described in the guidance provided to potential correspondents. Users who do not have access to email or the website can contact the Editor of *BMJ Clinical Evidence*, Dr Charles Young, on +44 (0)20 7383 6257. We are particularly interested to know the clinical question that led you to consult *BMJ Clinical Evidence* and the extent to which this was answered. If you have comments on any of our content, or think that important evidence might have been missed, or have suggestions for new reviews or questions, please let us know.

Readers who would like to be involved, either as contributors or peer reviewers, are also invited to send a letter and a brief resumé to Jennie Wilkinson at jwilkinson@bmjgroup.com.

The *BMJ Clinical Evidence* website (www.clinicalevidence.bmj.com) summarises the current state of knowledge and uncertainty about interventions used for prevention and treatment of important clinical conditions. To achieve this, we systematically search and appraise the world literature to provide rigorous systematic reviews of evidence on the benefits and harms of clinical interventions.

Making summaries involves discarding detail, and users of *BMJ Clinical Evidence* need to be aware of the limitations of the evidence presented. It is not possible to make global statements that are both useful and apply to every patient or clinical context that occurs in practice. For example, when stating that we found evidence that a drug is beneficial, we mean that there is evidence that the drug has been shown to deliver more benefits than harms when assessed in at least one group of people, using at least one outcome at a particular point in time. It does not mean that the drug will be effective in all people given that treatment or that other outcomes will be improved, or even that the same outcome will be improved at a different time after the treatment.

OUR CATEGORISATION OF INTERVENTIONS

Each systematic review contains a page that lists key clinical questions and interventions and describes whether they have been found to be effective or not.

We have developed these categories of effectiveness from one of the Cochrane Collaboration's first and most popular products, *A guide to effective care in pregnancy and childbirth*. The categories are explained in the table below.

Intervention	Description
Beneficial	for which effectiveness has been demonstrated by clear evidence from systematic reviews, RCTs, or the best alternative source of information, and for which expectation of harms is small compared with the benefits.
Likely to be beneficial	for which effectiveness is less well established than for those listed under "beneficial".
Trade-off between benefits and harms	for which clinicians and patients should weigh up the beneficial and harmful effects according to individual circumstances and priorities.
Unknown effectiveness	for which there are currently insufficient data or data of inadequate quality.
Unlikely to be beneficial	for which lack of effectiveness is less well established than for those listed under "likely to be ineffective or harmful".
Likely to be ineffective or harmful	for which ineffectiveness or associated harm has been demonstrated by clear evidence.

Fitting interventions into these categories is not always straightforward. For one thing, the categories represent a mix of several hierarchies: the size of benefit (or harm), the strength of evidence (RCT or observational data), and the degree of certainty around the finding (represented by the confidence interval). Another problem is that much of the evidence most relevant to clinical decisions relates to comparisons between different interventions rather than to comparison with placebo or no intervention. Where necessary, we have indicated the comparisons. A third problem is that interventions may have been tested, or found to be effective, in only one group of people, such as those at high risk of an outcome. Again, we have indicated this where possible. But perhaps most difficult of all is trying to maintain consistency across different systematic reviews. We continue to work on refining the criteria for categorising interventions. Interventions that cannot be tested in an RCT for ethical or practical reasons are sometimes included in the categorisation table and are identified with an asterisk.

HOW MUCH DO WE KNOW?

So, what can *BMJ Clinical Evidence* tell us about the state of our current knowledge from our evidence categories? Figure 1 illustrates the percentage of treatments falling into each category.

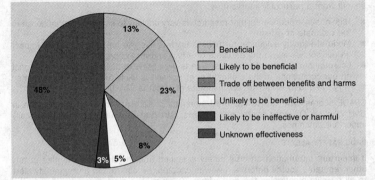

Figure 1.

Dividing treatments into categories is never easy. It always involves a degree of subjective judgement and is sometimes controversial. Why do we do it? Because users tell us it is helpful, but in the knowledge that clinical decisions must always be informed by more than simply the evidence, and in particular informed by individual circumstances and patient's preferences. However, as Figure 1 shows, the research community still has a large task ahead. Even this assessment underestimates the extent of what is 'unknown' since within many of the treatments categorised as beneficial or potentially harmful, this may reflect only one comparison. So, for example, treatment A might be 'likely to be beneficial' because of demonstrated benefit in comparison with placebo, but whether it is better or worse than treatment B may be unproven.

We are continuing to make use of what is 'unknown' in *BMJ Clinical Evidence* by feeding back to the UK NHS Health Technology Assessment Programme (HTA) with a view to help inform the commissioning of primary research. Every six months we evaluate *BMJ Clinical Evidence* interventions categorised as 'unknown effectiveness' and submit those fitting the appropriate criteria to the HTA via their website http://www.ncchta.org/.

ADDITIONAL FEATURES AVAILABLE ON *BMJ CLINICAL EVIDENCE* ONLINE

A detailed exploration of the evidence will require looking up the detail on *BMJ Clinical Evidence* online (www.clinicalevidence.bmj.com). Detailed quantitative results are presented online, where we are able to discuss their interpretation in more detail. Your suggestions on improvements are welcome.

The electronic versions of each review on the *BMJ Clinical Evidence* website link, whenever possible, to abstracts of the original research in *PubMed* or published online versions. In this way, *BMJ Clinical Evidence* is also designed to act as a pointer, connecting the clinician rapidly to the relevant original evidence.

ADDING VALUE TO THE CORE EVIDENCE

GRADE SCORES

GRADE is an internationally used system to evaluate the quality of evidence for a specific treatment comparison and a specific outcome. It takes into account methodological flaws within the component studies, issues about consistency of results across different studies, how generalisable the research results are to all patients who have the condition, and how effective the treatments have been shown to be. All treatment comparisons are given one of four GRADE scores reflecting the quality of the evidence: high-, moderate-, low-, or very low-quality evidence. When taken with our existing intervention categorisations, we believe that this will give clinicians a clearer idea about how certain they can be that their patient is likely to benefit from a particular intervention.

- High-quality evidence: further research is very unlikely to change our confidence in the estimate of effect
- Moderate-quality evidence: further research is likely to have an important impact on our confidence in the estimate of effect and may change the estimate
- Low-quality evidence: further research is very likely to have an important impact on our confidence in the estimate of effect and is likely to change the estimate
- Very low-quality evidence: any estimate of effect is very uncertain

GRADE scores have led to improved summary statements for each intervention in *BMJ Clinical Evidence* systematic reviews, structured around the most clinically important outcomes.

DRUG SAFETY ALERTS

If important information on drug safety is issued from regulatory authorities or any other reputable source before a review is updated, we aim to add a drug safety alert to all reviews mentioning the drug within 72 hours. The alert contains a link to the source of the drug safety alert for more information. The information prompting a drug safety alert is processed together with any new evidence we may find for the next update of the review.

GUIDELINES

To assist clinicians put evidence into practice, *BMJ Clinical Evidence* reviews now have links to the full text of major guidelines relevant to the review's clinical area. All linked guidelines have been produced by national or international government sources, professional medical organisations or medical speciality societies, and have met predetermined quality requirements. New guidelines are added regularly, and old guidelines are replaced by their revised versions as these are published.

FOREIGN LANGUAGE NAVIGATION

Control tabs are written in a variety of languages: Spanish, Chinese, Turkish, Japanese, and Thai.

PATIENT INFORMATION LEAFLETS

These are based on *BMJ Clinical Evidence* systematic reviews: summarising important condition information in plain English in an easily downloadable format to be given to patients at the point of care.

UPDATES

We aim to update *BMJ Clinical Evidence* reviews annually. In addition to this cycle, details of clinically important studies are added to the relevant reviews throughout the year using the *BMJ Updates* service. *BMJ Updates* is produced by collaboration between the BMJ Group and the internationally acclaimed McMaster University's Health Information Research Unit to provide clinicians with access to current best evidence from research. All citations (from over 110 premier clinical journals) are rated by trained researchers for quality, and then rated for clinical relevance, importance and interest by at least three members of a worldwide panel of practising physicians. The final content is indexed by health professionals to allow news of studies to be added to all relevant *BMJ Clinical Evidence* reviews.

'YOUR RESPONSES'

The *BMJ Clinical Evidence* website also has a 'Your Responses' facility which appears in every systematic review and for every intervention. Users are encouraged to both post comments and to read and respond. All 'Responses' are screened before publication on the website. This service is very similar to the *BMJ*'s successful 'Rapid

Responses' service and we have adopted the same publication policy for the responses that we receive. Examples received since the service opened include suggestions for research questions not yet covered within *BMJ Clinical Evidence*, and comments on how the research evidence relates to clinical practice. We hope that this will become a valued and well-used feature as the number of responses grows.

REFERENCES

1 Enkin M, Keirse M, Renfrew M, et al. A guide to effective care in pregnancy and childbirth. Oxford: Oxford University Press, 1998.

Evangelos Terpos and Amin Rahemtulla

KEY POINTS

- People with Hodgkin's lymphoma usually present with a lump in the neck or upper chest, but a quarter of people also have fever, sweating, weight loss, fatigue, and itch.

  Almost all people with localised disease can be cured, and, even among people with relapsed advanced disease, almost 80% survive event free for 4 years or longer.

- In people with localised Hodgkin's lymphoma, consensus is that ABVD plus radiotherapy is the 'gold-standard' treatment, with ABVD preferred to MOPP as single-regimen chemotherapy. However, we don't know for certain if this is the most effective regimen.

  ABVD seems less likely than MOPP to cause infertility and secondary leukaemia. However, ABVD increases the risk of cardiotoxicity and pulmonary adverse effects, especially if given with radiotherapy.

  Adding MOPP or VBM regimens to radiotherapy has not been shown to improve overall survival compared with radiotherapy alone in people with localised Hodgkin's lymphoma, and increases the risk of adverse effects.

  Adding radiotherapy to CVPP or to ABVD has not been shown to improve survival compared with the chemotherapy regimen alone.

  EBVP plus radiotherapy seems to have similar efficacy to MOPP/ABV plus radiotherapy in increasing overall survival.

- In people with localised Hodgkin's lymphoma, involved-field radiotherapy is as effective as extended-field radiotherapy in increasing overall survival, but is less likely to cause adverse effects. We don't know which radiotherapy dose regimen is most likely to improve survival.

- In people with advanced Hodgkin's lymphoma, ABVD is as effective as other chemotherapy regimens such as MOPP, MEC and Stanford V at improving long-term survival, with a more favourable adverse-effect profile.

  Intensified chemotherapy with Ch1VPP/EVA may improve 5-year survival compared with VAPEC-B, and escalating-dose BEACOPP may be more effective than COPP/ABVD, but has greater toxicity.

- In people with advanced disease, adding radiotherapy to MOPP or to MOPP/ABV does not improve survival, and adding radiotherapy to ABVPP may worsen survival, compared with the chemotherapy regimen alone.

(i) **Please visit www.clinicalevidence.bmj.com for full text and references**

What are the effects of single-regimen chemotherapy treatments for first presentation stage 1 or 2 non-bulky disease?	
Beneficial	• ABVD (as effective as combined regimens with radiotherapy but with fewer adverse effects)
Trade-off Between Benefits And Harms	• MOPP

What are the effects of combined chemotherapy and radiotherapy treatments compared with radiotherapy alone for first-presentation stage 1 or 2 non-bulky disease?

Trade-off Between Benefits And Harms	• MOPP plus radiotherapy
Unlikely To Be Beneficial	• VBM plus radiotherapy

What are the effects of combined chemotherapy and radiotherapy treatments compared with the same chemotherapy agent alone for first-presentation stage 1 or 2 non-bulky disease?

Beneficial	• ABVD plus radiotherapy*
Unlikely To Be Beneficial	• CVPP plus radiotherapy

What are the effects of specific combined chemotherapy and radiotherapy treatments versus each other in stage 1 or 2 non-bulky disease?

Beneficial	• ABVD plus radiotherapy (improved progression-free survival compared with MOPP plus radiotherapy and less gonadal toxicity)
Unlikely To Be Beneficial	• EBPV plus radiotherapy (reduced failure-free survival compared with MOPP-ABV plus radiotherapy)

What are the effects of different radiotherapy treatment strategies in stage 1 or 2 non-bulky disease?

Beneficial	• Involved-field radiotherapy (as effective as extended field radiotherapy with fewer adverse effects)
Unknown Effectiveness	• Increased-dose regimens

What are the effects of single-regimen chemotherapy treatments for first-presentation stage 2 bulky disease, stage 3, or stage 4 disease?

Beneficial	• ABVD
Trade-off Between Benefits And Harms	• MOPP

What are the effects of dose-intensified chemotherapy treatments for first-presentation stage 2 bulky disease, stage 3, or stage 4 disease?

Trade-off Between Benefits And Harms	• Escalating-dose BEACOPP (more effective than COPP-ABVD but increased adverse effects)
Unknown Effectiveness	• ChlVPP-EVA (more effective than VAPEC-B)

What are the effects of combined chemotherapy plus radiotherapy treatments compared with chemotherapy alone for first presentation stage 2 bulky disease, stage 3, or stage 4 disease?

Unlikely To Be Beneficial	• ABVPP plus radiotherapy
	• COPP-ABVD plus radiotherapy
	• MOPP-ABV plus radiotherapy
	• MOPP plus radiotherapy

Search date May 2005

*Categorisation based on consensus.

DEFINITION Hodgkin's lymphoma, also known as Hodgkin's disease, is a malignancy of the lymph nodes and lymphatic system. The majority of people present with an enlarged but otherwise asymptomatic lump, most often in the lower neck or supraclavicular region. Mediastinal masses are frequent and are revealed after routine chest x rays. About a quarter of people present systemic symptoms at diagnosis, such as unexplained fever, profuse sweating, fatigue, itchy skin, and unexplained weight loss. Hepatosplenomegaly, anaemia, lymphocytopenia, and eosinophilia are also non-specific manifestations of the disease. Hodgkin's lymphoma is categorised according to appearance under the microscope (histology) and extent of disease (stage). **Histology:** Diagnosis is based on the recognition of Reed–Stenberg cells and/or Hodgkin cells in an appropriate cellular background in tissue sections from a lymph node or another organ, such as the bone marrow, lung, or bone. Fine needle aspiration biopsy is not adequate for diagnosis of Hodgkin's lymphoma; an open biopsy is always required. Reed–Stenberg cells are typically multinucleated giant cells, which, in 98% of cases, are thought to be derived from the germinal centre of peripheral B cells. The WHO classification is based on histological subtype. The distribution of histological subtypes varies between age groups, with young adults reportedly showing a greater proportion of nodular sclerosis compared with older adults. Nodular lymphocyte-predominant (LP) Hodgkin's lymphoma is a rare subtype which usually has a more indolent natural history, and is often treated differently. This subtype has been excluded in the trials in this review. **Stage:** There are several different staging classification systems for Hodgkin's lymphoma. Computerised tomography scanning is the major method of staging both intra-thoracic and intra-abdominal disease, while bone marrow trephine biopsy is used for the detection of marrow infiltration by malignant cells. Magnetic resonance imaging (MRI) scanning and fluorodeoxyglucose positron emission tomography (FDG-PET) scanning may also have a role in Hodgkin's lymphoma staging, mainly by revealing disease in sites difficult to discover by computerised tomography imaging. Classification systems include the Ann Arbor classification and the Cotswolds. Staging methods have changed substantially over the last 20 years. Staging laparotomy with splenectomy is no longer routine practice owing to a number of possible complications (including post-splenectomy sepsis, small-bowel obstruction, and even mortality), delay to the start of treatment, similar survival rates between people with or without a staging

(continued over)

(from previous page)

laparotomy, and the introduction of combined modality treatment for all stages. **Population:** For the purposes of this review, we considered adults with a first presentation of Hodgkin's lymphoma. We considered treatments separately in two groups of people: stage I or II non-bulky disease, and II (bulky), III, or IV disease; most studies used the Ann Arbor classification system.

INCIDENCE/PREVALENCE The annual incidence of Hodgkin's lymphoma is about 3/100,000 in the UK, without any large variations in incidence or in nature between countries or population groups. However, the age distribution of Hodgkin's lymphoma differs across geographical areas as well as across ethnic groups. In resource-rich countries, there is a bimodal age distribution with peaks at 15–34 years and over 60 years, with nodular sclerosis being the most common subtype. Early-stage nodular sclerosis Hodgkin's lymphoma is the most common form in children living in resource-rich countries, but advanced mixed cellularity and lymphocyte-rich subtypes are seen most commonly in resource-poor countries. In children in Europe and the USA, incidence in men is double that of incidence in women, but in adolescents there is an equal distribution between sexes. The incidence rate of Hodgkin's lymphoma in general increases with the level of economic development.

AETIOLOGY/RISK FACTORS The exact cause of Hodgkin's lymphoma remains unclear. However, it is accepted that Hodgkin's lymphoma is a heterogeneous condition that probably consists of more than one aetiological entity. The Epstein–Barr virus has been implicated in the development of Hodgkin's lymphoma, but this association varies with age, with positivity being most prominent in children and the elderly. Epstein–Barr-virus positivity is high in childhood Hodgkin's lymphoma worldwide, but low in adolescents in resource-rich countries with nodular sclerosis Hodgkin's lymphoma. Histological subtype, age, sex, socioeconomic status, and ethnic background have all been shown to influence the association between the Epstein–Barr virus and Hodgkin's lymphoma. Although the pathogenesis of Hodgkin's disease is not yet fully understood, the nature of the Hodgkin/Reed–Stenberg (H/RS) cell has been recognised. The H/RS cell is derived from a B lymphocyte with clonal rearrangements in the V, D, and J segments of the IgH chain locus. Regulation of Fas-mediated apoptosis, and the nuclear factor-kappa B pathway seem to be strongly implicated in the pathogenesis of Hodgkin's lymphoma.

PROGNOSIS Overall survival: The outcome in both localised and advanced Hodgkin's lymphoma has improved greatly over the last 20 years. The disease is now considered curable in the majority of cases. Even if first-line treatment fails, the person may be cured later. Therefore, doctors confront the dilemma of whether to use more intensive therapy initially to cure the maximum number of people possible, or whether to use less-aggressive therapy initially and rely on more-intensive salvage therapy in a greater proportion of people. The overall survival differs in terms of disease extent. People with localised disease (stage I/II) have a 6-year overall survival of more than 90% even in poor-risk groups. People with advanced disease (stage III/IV) have a 5-year overall survival of almost 85%. **Relapse:** The event-free survival at 4 years is near 99% for people with localised disease and almost 80% in people with advanced disease. **Prognostic indicators:** Despite an enormous effort to define clinically relevant and generally acceptable prognostic factors, stage and systemic B cell symptoms are still the two major determinants for stratifying people with Hodgkin's lymphoma. Bulky disease (more than 10 cm nodal mass) has recently emerged as a third prognostic factor that meets general acceptance. In the USA, most centres treat people according to the traditional classifications of early stages (I–IIA or B) and advanced stages (III–IVA or B; I–IIB with bulky disease), which is the classification used for the purposes of this review. The International Prognostic Score (IPS) has been used by several study groups currently tailoring treatment strategies at first diagnosis depending on the risk for treatment failure (IPS 0–2 and 3–7), but stratifying people on the basis of the IPS is still an experimental approach. Another group looked at prognostic factors specifically for children and young adults with Hodgkin's disease treated with combined modality treatment. They analysed 328 people aged 2–20 years old (48% were aged over 14 years), and multivariate analysis identified five pretreatment factors that correlated with inferior disease-free survival: male sex; stage IIB, IIIB, or IV disease; bulky mediastinal disease; white blood count of more than 13.5×10^9 /L; and haemoglobin less than 11.0 g/dL. In the study, age was not a significant prognostic factor (14 years and under compared with over 14 years old). Using this prognostic score, people with Hodgkin's lymphoma could be stratified into four groups with significantly different 5-year disease-free survivals. Response to initial chemotherapy was also shown to be a predictor of outcome. Other paediatric studies found that nodular sclerosis histology and B symptoms also correlated with inferior outcome.

Myeloma (multiple)

Ambuj Kumar and Benjamin Djulbegovic

KEY POINTS

- Multiple myeloma is a neoplastic proliferation of plasma cells, mainly within the bone marrow, causing anaemia, renal dysfunction, infections, and bone lesions. Monoclonal protein is found in serum and/or urine in 97% of people.

- Early chemotherapy plus corticosteroids have not been shown to improve survival in people with asymptomatic, early-stage multiple myeloma.

- In people with advanced multiple myeloma, combination chemotherapy or single-agent chemotherapy plus prednisolone improves survival more effectively than single-agent chemotherapy alone, and adding corticosteroids to combination chemotherapy is more effective still.

  High- or intermediate-dose chemotherapy with bone marrow or peripheral blood stem cell rescue improves progression-free and overall survival compared with conventional-dose chemotherapy.

  Syngeneic (from a twin) or autologous stem-cell transplantation may increase event-free, but not overall, survival if given early rather than late.

  An optimum priming regimen with stem cell factor may increase the yield of CD34+ cells for transplantation, but increases the risk of adverse effects.

  Very high-dose melphalan may increase overall survival and have fewer adverse effects compared with high-dose melphalan plus total body irradiation.

- Adding interferon to chemotherapy increases response rates and progression free, but not overall, survival, but increases toxicity.

  We don't know which are the most effective salvage regimens, or if thalidomide increases survival, but bortezomib may increase response rates and overall short-term survival.

- In people with advanced disease, bisphosphonates reduce skeletal fractures and pain, epoetin alpha may improve anaemia, prophylactic treatment with antibiotics and immunoglobulin may reduce infections, and plasmapheresis may improve renal function when added to forced diuresis plus chemotherapy.

  However, we don't know whether any of these treatments improve survival, and they may increase adverse effects.

 Please visit www.clinicalevidence.bmj.com for full text and references

What are the effects of treatment in people with asymptomatic early-stage multiple myeloma (stage I)?	
Unlikely To Be Beneficial	• Early chemotherapy plus corticosteroids in stage I disease (no benefit over deferred treatment)

What are the effects of first-line treatments in people with advanced-stage multiple myeloma (stages II and III)?	
Beneficial	• Adding prednisolone to single-agent chemotherapy (increased survival compared with melphalan alone) • Combination chemotherapy (increased survival compared with melphalan) • Combination chemotherapy plus corticosteroids (similar survival with different regimens, no survival benefit compared with melphalan plus prednisolone or cyclophosphamide)

	• High-dose chemotherapy plus stem cell rescue (increased survival compared with conventional-dose chemotherapy)
	• High-dose melphalan conditioning regimen before autologous stem-cell transplantation (increased overall survival compared with melphalan plus total-body irradiation)
	• Intermediate-dose chemotherapy plus stem-cell rescue (increased survival compared with conventional-dose chemotherapy)
	• Relative effectiveness of different single-agent chemotherapy plus corticosteroid regimens (similar survival with bendamustine plus prednisolone, melphalan plus prednisolone, or melphalan plus dexamethasone)
	• Relative effectiveness of different single-agent chemotherapy regimens (similar survival with melphalan, cyclophosphamide, lomustine, and carmustine)
	• Single-agent chemotherapy (more effective than placebo)
Likely To Be Beneficial	• Autologous stem-cell transplant (increased survival compared with allogeneic transplant)
	• Peripheral blood stem cells (similar survival, reduces duration of neutropenia and thrombocytopenia compared with bone-marrow stem cells)
	• Syngeneic transplantation (increased survival compared with autologous transplant if a twin donor was available)
	• Timing of autologous stem cell transplant (increased event-free survival compared with late transplantation)
Trade-off Between Benefits And Harms	• Interferon
	• Optimum priming regimen
Unknown Effectiveness	• Bortezomib
	• Double versus single autologous transplant
	• Non-myeloablative allogeneic stem-cell transplant (reduced intensity conditioning, mini-transplant)
	• Thalidomide and thalidomide derivatives
Unlikely To Be Beneficial	• Purging of autologous stem cells
Likely To Be Ineffective Or Harmful	• Allogeneic stem-cell transplant (increased treatment-related mortality compared with autologous transplant)

What are the effects of salvage treatments in people with advanced-stage multiple myeloma (stages II and III)?

Beneficial	• Bortezomib
Unlikely To Be Beneficial	• Salvage therapy regimens

What are the effects of treatments (supportive therapy) in people with advanced-stage multiple myeloma (stages II and III)?

Beneficial	• Bisphosphonates
Likely To Be Beneficial	• Epoetin alpha
Trade-off Between Benefits And Harms	• Infection prophylaxis
Unknown Effectiveness	• Plasmapheresis

Search date November 2004

DEFINITION Multiple myeloma is characterised by neoplastic proliferation of plasma cells, mainly contained within the bone marrow. It is a debilitating malignancy that is part of a spectrum of diseases ranging from monoclonal gammopathy of unknown significance (MGUS) to plasma cell leukaemia. Multiple myeloma can present outside the bone marrow as solitary plasmacytoma or extramedullary plasmacytoma. However, this review does not currently deal with these forms. The most common symptoms of multiple myeloma are those relating to anaemia, renal dysfunction, infections, or bone lesions. Multiple myeloma is most common in people aged over 40 years. A diagnosis of symptomatic myeloma requires the presence of monoclonal protein (M-protein) in serum, urine, or both; bone marrow clonal plasma cells (more than 10%) or plasmacytoma; and related organ or tissue impairment (ROTI). Ninety-seven per cent of people with multiple myeloma have a presence of M-protein in serum, urine, or both. A diagnosis of asymptomatic myeloma (also known as smouldering myeloma) requires the presence of M-protein in serum of 30 g/L or more, bone marrow clonal plasma cells of 10% or more, or both; and no ROTI or symptoms. The most common differential diagnoses of symptomatic multiple myeloma are MGUS and asymptomatic (smouldering) multiple myeloma. Other less common differential diagnoses include non-secretory myeloma, solitary and extramedullary plasmacytoma, plasma cell leukaemia, primary systemic amyloidosis, and Waldenstorm's macroglobulinaemia, and other non-Hodgkin's lymphoma. Durie and Salmon proposed the initial clinical staging system for multiple myeloma in 1975. People with Durie Salmon stage I disease are usually asymptomatic. In addition to the WHO classification, a new international staging system for multiple myeloma was recently proposed, based on clinical and laboratory data from 10,750 people with previously untreated symptomatic myeloma.

INCIDENCE/PREVALENCE Multiple myeloma is the most common primary cancer of the bones in adults, representing about 1% of all cancers diagnosed in the US in 2004, and 14% of all haematological malignancies. The annual incidence of multiple myeloma in the US is three or four cases per 100,000 population and prevalence is 43 cases per 100,000. In the UK, multiple myeloma accounts for 1% of all new cases of cancer diagnosed each year. In 2001, the incidence of multiple myeloma in the UK was 6.1 cases per 100,000 population.

AETIOLOGY/RISK FACTORS The exact aetiology of multiple myeloma remains unclear. Genetic and environmental factors have been associated with the occurrence of multiple myeloma. However, evidence linking the genetic or environmental factors has not been substantiated.

PROGNOSIS Currently, no cure is available for multiple myeloma. The recently proposed new international staging system for multiple myeloma found median survival to be 29–62 months, based on clinical and laboratory data from 10,750 people with previously untreated symptomatic myeloma.

Ellen R Copson and J. Paul Kerr

KEY POINTS

- NHL is the sixth most common cancer in the UK, with a 10% increase in incidence between 1993 and 2002.

  Risk factors include immunosuppression, certain viral and bacterial infections, and exposure to drugs and other chemicals.

  Overall 5-year survival is around 55%. The main risk factors for a poor prognosis are older age, elevated serum lactate dehydrogenase levels, and severity of disease.

- CHOP 21 has been shown to be superior or equivalent to all other combination chemotherapy regimens in terms of overall survival or toxicity in adults older or younger than 60 years.

  Adding radiotherapy to a short CHOP 21 schedule (3 cycles) increases 5-year survival, while reducing the risks of congestive heart failure, compared with longer schedules of CHOP 21 alone.

  Adding rituximab to CHOP 21 increases response rates and 5-year survival compared with CHOP 21 alone.

  CHOP 14 may increase 5-year survival compared with CHOP 21 in adults aged over 60 years, but remains unproven in younger adults. Toxicity is similar for the two regimens.

- Consensus is that conventional-dose salvage chemotherapy should be used in people with relapsed NHL. Phase II studies report similar response rates with a number of different chemotherapy regimens.

  Adding rituximab to salvage chemotherapy may improve initial response rates but no more than 10% of people remain disease free after 3–5 years.

- High-dose salvage chemotherapy plus autologous bone marrow transplantation may increase 5-year event-free survival compared with conventional-dose chemotherapy in people with relapsed, chemotherapy-sensitive disease, but it increases the risk of severe adverse effects.

  We don't know if allogenic bone-marrow transplantation improves survival. Retrospective studies suggest that it increases the risk of graft-versus-host disease and complications of immunosuppression.

(i) **Please visit www.clinicalevidence.bmj.com for full text and references**

What are the effects of first-line treatments for aggressive NHL (diffuse large B cell lymphoma)?	
Beneficial	• CHOP 21 (no alternative regimen [MACOP-B, m-BACOD, ProMACE-CytaBOM, PACEBOM] shown to be superior)
	• CHOP 21 plus radiotherapy (increases disease-free survival compared with CHOP 21 alone)
	• CHOP 21 plus rituximab (increases survival compared with CHOP 21 alone)
Likely To Be Beneficial	• CHOP 14

What are the effects of treatments for relapsed aggressive non-Hodgkin's lymphoma (diffuse large B cell lymphoma)?

Likely To Be Beneficial	• Conventional-dose salvage chemotherapy (consensus that treatment should be given but relative benefits of different regimens unclear)*
	• High-dose chemotherapy plus autologous transplant stem-cell support (increases survival compared with conventional-dose chemotherapy in people with chemosensitive disease)
Unknown Effectiveness	• Allongeneic stem-cell support

Search date April 2006

*Based on consensus

DEFINITION NHL consists of a complex group of cancers arising mainly from B lymphocytes (85% of cases) and occasionally from T lymphocytes. NHL usually develops in lymph nodes (nodal lymphoma) but can arise in other tissues almost anywhere in the body (extranodal lymphoma). NHL is categorised according to its appearance under the microscope (histology) and the extent of the disease (stage). **Histology:** Since 1966, four major different methods of classifying NHLs according to their histological appearance have been published. At present, the WHO system is accepted as the gold standard of classification. The WHO system is based on the underlying principles of the REAL classification system. Historically, NHLs have been divided into slow-growing "low-grade" lymphomas and fast-growing "aggressive" lymphomas. This review deals only with the most common aggressive NHL — diffuse B cell lymphoma (WHO classification). Interpretation of older studies is complicated by histological methods have changed and there is no direct correlation between lymphoma types in the WHO and other classification systems. Attempts to generalise results must therefore be treated with caution. We have, however, included some older studies referring to alternative classification methods if they included people with the following types of aggressive lymphomas, which overlap substantially with the WHO classification of interest: Working Formulation classification — primarily intermediate grades (grades E–H); Kiel classification — centroblastic, immunoblastic, and anaplastic; and Rappaport classification — diffuse histiocytic, diffuse lymphocytic, poorly differentiated, and diffuse mixed (lymphocytic and histiocytic). **Stage:** NHL has traditionally been staged according to extent of disease spread using the Ann Arbor system. The term "early disease" is used to describe disease that falls within Ann Arbor stage I or II, whereas "advanced disease" refers to Ann Arbor stage III or IV disease. However, all people with bulky disease, usually defined as having a disease site larger than 10 cm in diameter, are treated as having advanced disease, regardless of their Ann Arbor staging. **Relapsed disease:** Relapsed disease refers to the recurrence of active disease in a person who has previously achieved a complete response to initial treatment for NHL. Most studies of treatments in relapsed disease require a minimum duration of complete response of 1 month before relapse.

INCIDENCE/PREVALENCE NHL is the sixth most common cancer in the UK; 9443 new cases were diagnosed in the UK in 2002 and it caused 4418 UK deaths in 2003. Incidence rates show distinct geographical variation, with age-standardised incidence rates ranging from 17 per 100,000 in Northern America to 4 per 100,000 in South-central Asia. NHL occurs more commonly in males than in females, and the age-standardised UK incidence increased by 10.3% between 1993 and 2002.

AETIOLOGY/RISK FACTORS The aetiology of most NHLs is unknown. Incidence is higher in individuals who are immunosuppressed (congenital or acquired). Other risk factors include viral infection (human T cell leukaemia virus type-1, Epstein–Barr virus, HIV), bacterial

(continued over)

(from previous page)

infection (e.g. *Helicobacter pylori*), previous treatment with phenytoin or antineoplastic drugs, and exposure to pesticides or organic solvents.

PROGNOSIS Overall survival: Untreated aggressive NHLs would generally result in death in a matter of months. High-grade lymphomas, particularly diffuse large B cell lymphomas and Burkitt's lymphomas, have a high cure rate with both initial and salvage chemotherapy. The 5-year relative age-standardised survival for people diagnosed with and treated for NHL between 2000 and 2001 was 55% for men and 56% for women. **Relapse:** About 50% of people with NHL will be cured by initial treatment. Of the rest, about 30% will fail to respond to initial treatment (so called "chemotherapy-refractory disease") and about 20–30% will relapse. Most relapses occur within 2 years of completion of initial treatment. Up to 50% of these have chemotherapy-sensitive disease; the remainder tend to have chemotherapy-resistant disease. **Prognostic indicators:** Prognosis depends on histological type, stage, age, performance status, and lactate dehydrogenase levels. Prognosis varies substantially within each Ann Arbor stage, and further information regarding prognosis can be obtained from applying the International Prognostic Index (IPI). The IPI model stratifies prognosis according to the presence or absence of five risk factors: age (less than 60 years *v* more than 60 years), serum lactate dehydrogenase (normal *v* elevated), performance status (0 or 1 *v* 2–4), Ann Arbor stage (I or II *v* III or IV), and number of extranodal sites involved (0 or 1 *v* 2–4). People with two or more high-risk factors have a less than 50% chance of relapse-free and overall survival at 5 years. IPI staging is currently the most important system used to define disease stage and treatment options. However, most studies identified by our search predate the IPI staging system.

Martin M Meremikwu

KEY POINTS

- In sub-Saharan Africa, up to a third of adults are carriers of the defective sickle cell gene, and 1–2% of babies are born with the disease.

  Sickle cell disease causes chronic haemolytic anaemia, dactylitis, and painful acute crises, and increases the risk of stroke, organ damage, bacterial infections, and complications of blood transfusion.

- We don't know whether avoidance of cold environments or physical exercise, or dehydration can prevent crises or complications in people with sickle cell disease.

  Penicillin prophylaxis in children under 5 years of age reduces invasive pneumococcal infections regardless of pneumococcal vaccination status. We don't know whether penicillin prophylaxis is beneficial in older children.

  Malaria chemoprophylaxis is considered useful to prevent malaria-induced crises, but very few studies have been found that evaluated its benefit.

- Hydroxyurea, piracetam, and zinc sulphate may reduce some complications of sickle cell disease, such as painful crises, compared with placebo, but their long-term effects and safety are unknown.

- Morphine is widely used to treat severe pain, but we found no RCT evidence comparing it with placebo in people with sickle cell crises.

  Controlled-release oral morphine and patient-controlled analgesia may be as effective as repeated intravenous doses of morphine. Oral morphine increases the risk of acute chest syndrome compared with intravenous administration.

  High-dose corticosteroids may reduce the need for analgesia when added to intravenous morphine in people with a sickle cell crisis, but may increase the risks of adverse effects such as infections, hypertension, and metabolic problems.

- It is still unclear whether acupuncture, blood transfusion, hydration, oxygen, aspirin, codeine, diflunisal, ibuprofen, ketorolac, or paracetamol reduce pain during a sickle cell crisis.

Please visit www.clinicalevidence.bmj.com for full text and references

What are the effects of non-pharmaceutical interventions to prevent sickle cell crisis and other acute complications in people with sickle cell disease?	
Unknown Effectiveness	• Avoidance of cold environment
	• Limiting physical exercise
	• Rehydration

What are the effects of pharmaceutical interventions to prevent sickle cell crisis and other acute complications in people with sickle cell disease?	
Beneficial	• Antibiotic prophylaxis in children under 5 years of age
Likely To Be Beneficial	• Hydroxyurea
	• Malaria chemoprophylaxis
	• Piracetam

	• Zinc sulphate
Unknown Effectiveness	• Penicillin prophylaxis in children over 5 years of age • Pneumococcal vaccines

What are the effects of non-pharmaceutical interventions to treat pain in people with sickle cell crisis?

Unknown Effectiveness	• Acupuncture • Blood transfusion • Hydration • Oxygen

What are the effects of pharmaceutical interventions to treat pain in people with sickle cell crisis?

Likely To Be Beneficial	• Patient-controlled analgesia
Trade-off Between Benefits And Harms	• Controlled-release oral morphine given after an initial intravenous bolus dose of morphine versus repeated doses of intravenous morphine • Corticosteroid as adjunct to narcotic analgesics
Unknown Effectiveness	• Aspirin • Codeine • Diflunisal • Ibuprofen • Ketorolac • Paracetamol

Search date August 2006

DEFINITION Sickle cell disease refers to a group of disorders caused by inheritance of a pair of abnormal haemoglobin genes, including the sickle cell gene. It is characterised by chronic haemolytic anaemia, dactylitis, and acute episodic clinical events called "crises". Vaso-occlusive (painful) crises are the most common, and occur when abnormal red cells clog small vessels, causing tissue ischaemia. The others are hyper-haemolytic crisis (excessive haemolysis), acute chest syndrome, sequestration crisis, and aplastic crisis. A common variant of sickle cell disease, also characterised by haemolytic anaemia, occurs in people with one sickle and one thalassaemia gene. **Sickle cell trait** occurs in people with one sickle gene and one normal gene. People with sickle cell trait do not have any clinical manifestation of illness. This review covers people with sickle cell disease with or without thalassaemia.

INCIDENCE/PREVALENCE Sickle cell disease is most common among people living in or originating from sub-Saharan Africa. The disorder also affects people of Mediterranean, Caribbean, Middle Eastern, and Asian origin. The sickle cell gene is most common in areas where malaria is endemic — sickle cell trait affects about 10–30% of Africa's tropical populations. Sickle cell disease affects an estimated 1–2% (120,000) of newborns in Africa annually. About 178 babies (0.28/1000 conceptions) are affected by sickle cell disease in England annually. About 60,000 people in the USA and 10,000 in the UK suffer from the disease.

AETIOLOGY/RISK FACTORS Sickle cell disease is inherited as an autosomal recessive disorder. For a baby to be affected, both parents must have the sickle cell gene. In parents with sickle cell trait, the risk of having an affected baby is one in four for each pregnancy. Painful (vaso-occlusive) crisis is the most common feature of the disease, and these episodes start in infancy and early childhood. Factors that precipitate or modulate the occurrence of sickle cell crisis are not fully understood, but infections, hypoxia, dehydration, acidosis, stress (such as major surgery or childbirth), and cold are believed to play some role. In tropical Africa, malaria is the most common cause of anaemic and vaso-occlusive crisis. High levels of fetal haemoglobin are known to ameliorate the severity and incidence of sickle cell crisis and other complications of the disease.

PROGNOSIS People affected by sickle cell disease are predisposed to bacterial infections, especially those caused by encapsulated organisms such as *Pneumococcus*, *Haemophilus influenzae*, *Meningococcus*, and *Salmonella* species. Severe bacterial infections such as pneumonia, meningitis, and septicaemia are common causes of morbidity and mortality, especially among young children. About 10% of children with sickle cell anaemia may develop a stroke, and more than 50% of these may suffer recurrent strokes. Abnormal features of cerebral blood vessels shown by transcranial Doppler scan predict a high risk of stroke in children with sickle cell disease. Frequent episodes of crisis, infections, and organ damage reduce the quality of life of people with sickle cell disease. A high rate of vaso-occlusive (painful) crisis is an index of clinical severity that correlates with early death. Life expectancy remains low, especially in communities with poor access to health services. In some parts of Africa, about 50% of children with sickle cell disease die before their first birthday. The average life expectancy with sickle cell disease in the USA is about 42 years for men, and about 48 years for women. Frequent blood transfusions could increase the risk of immune reactions and infections, such as HIV and hepatitis B or C viruses, and Chagas' disease. The need for repeated blood transfusions in people with sickle cell disease predisposes them to the risk of iron overload.

Nicholas Danchin and Eric Durand

KEY POINTS

- About a quarter of people having an acute MI in the USA will die of it, half of them within 1 hour of the onset of symptoms.

  Cardiogenic shock develops in over 5% of people surviving the first hour after an acute MI, with a mortality of 50–80% in the first 48 hours.

- Aspirin reduces mortality, reinfarction, and stroke at 1 month in people with an acute MI compared with placebo.

  Thrombolysis within 6 hours reduces mortality in people with an acute MI, but increases the risk of stroke or major bleeding, with different agents seeming to have similar efficacy.

  Adding low molecular weight heparin or glycoprotein IIb/IIIa inhibitors to thrombolytics may reduce the risk of further cardiovascular events, but these treatments have not been shown to improve survival.

- Beta-blockers and ACE inhibitors reduce mortality in people with acute MI compared with placebo.

  Nitrates reduce mortality and improve symptoms in people not receiving thrombolysis, but may not be beneficial in people after thrombolysis.

  Calcium channel blockers have not been shown to reduce mortality after an acute MI, and early treatment with nifedipine may increase mortality.

- Primary PTCA within 12 hours of onset of chest pain reduces the risk of death, reinfarction, and stroke, compared with thrombolysis.

- In people with cardiogenic shock, invasive cardiac revascularisation within 48 hours of acute MI reduces mortality at 12 months compared with medical treatment alone, but people aged over 75 years may not benefit.

  We don't know whether thrombolysis, vasodilators, intra-aortic balloon counterpulsation, ventricular assistance devices and cardiac transplantation, or early cardiac surgery improve survival in people with cardiogenic shock.

  There is consensus that positive inotropes and pulmonary artery catheterisation are beneficial, but we found no studies that confirmed this.

ⓘ **Please visit www.clinicalevidence.bmj.com for full text and references**

Which treatments improve outcomes in acute MI?	
Beneficial	• ACE inhibitors
	• Aspirin
	• Beta-blockers
	• Primary PTCA versus thrombolysis (performed in specialist centres)
	• Thrombolysis
Likely To Be Beneficial	• Adding low molecular weight heparin (enoxaparin) to thrombolytics (reduces acute MI rates)

	• Nitrates (in the absence of thrombolysis)
Trade-off Between Benefits And Harms	• Glycoprotein IIb/IIIa inhibitors
Unlikely To Be Beneficial	• Adding unfractionated heparin to thrombolytics • Nitrates (in addition to thrombolysis)
Likely To Be Ineffective Or Harmful	• Calcium channel blockers

Which treatments improve outcomes for cardiogenic shock after acute MI?	
Beneficial	• Early invasive cardiac revascularisation
Unknown Effectiveness	• Early cardiac surgery • Intra-aortic balloon counterpulsation • Positive inotropes • Pulmonary artery catheterisation • Thrombolysis • Vasodilators • Ventricular assistance devices and cardiac transplantation

Search date August 2004

DEFINITION Acute MI: The sudden occlusion of a coronary artery leading to myocardial cell death. **Cardiogenic shock:** Defined clinically as a poor cardiac output plus evidence of tissue hypoxia that is not improved by correcting reduced intravascular volume. When a pulmonary artery catheter is used, cardiogenic shock may be defined as a cardiac index below 2.2 L/minute/m^2 despite an elevated pulmonary capillary wedge pressure (at least 15 mm Hg).

INCIDENCE/PREVALENCE Acute MI: Acute MI is one of the most common causes of mortality worldwide. In 1990, ischaemic heart disease was the world's leading cause of death, accounting for about 6.3 million deaths. The age-standardised incidence varies among and within countries. Each year, about 900,000 people in the USA experience MI, about 225,000 of whom die. About half of these people die within 1 hour of symptoms and before reaching a hospital emergency room. Event rates increase with age for both sexes, and are higher in men than in women, and in poorer than richer people at all ages. The incidence of death from MI has fallen in many Western countries over the past 20 years. **Cardiogenic shock:** Cardiogenic shock occurs in about 7% of people admitted to hospital with MI. Of these, about half have established cardiogenic shock at the time of admission to hospital, and most of the others develop it during the first 24–48 hours after their admission.

AETIOLOGY/RISK FACTORS Acute MI: Identified major risk factors for CVD include increasing age, male sex, raised low density lipoprotein cholesterol, reduced high density lipoprotein cholesterol, raised blood pressure, smoking, diabetes, family history of CVD, obesity, and sedentary lifestyle. For many of these risk factors, observational studies show a continuous gradient of increasing risk of CVD with increasing levels of the risk factor, with

(continued over)

(from previous page)

no obvious threshold level. The immediate mechanism of MI is rupture or erosion of an atheromatous plaque causing thrombosis and occlusion of coronary arteries and myocardial cell death. Factors that may convert a stable plaque to an unstable plaque (the "active plaque") have yet to be fully elucidated. Shear stresses, inflammation, and autoimmunity have been proposed. The changing rates of CHD in different populations are only partly explained by changes in the standard risk factors for ischaemic heart disease (particularly a fall in blood pressure and smoking). **Cardiogenic shock:** Cardiogenic shock after MI usually follows a reduction in functional ventricular myocardium, and is caused by left ventricular infarction (79% of people with cardiogenic shock) more often than by right ventricular infarction (3% of people with cardiogenic shock). Cardiogenic shock after MI may also be caused by cardiac structural defects, such as mitral valve regurgitation due to papillary muscle dysfunction (7% of people with cardiogenic shock), ventricular septal rupture (4% of people with cardiogenic shock), or cardiac tamponade after free cardiac wall rupture (1% of people with cardiogenic shock). Major risk factors for cardiogenic shock after MI are previous MI, diabetes mellitus, advanced age, hypotension, tachycardia or bradycardia, congestive heart failure with Killip class II–III, and low left ventricular ejection fraction (ejection fraction less than 35%).

PROGNOSIS Acute MI: May lead to a host of mechanical and cardiac electrical complications, including death, ventricular dysfunction, congestive heart failure, fatal and non-fatal arrhythmias, valvular dysfunction, myocardial rupture, and cardiogenic shock. **Cardiogenic shock:** Mortality rates for people in hospital with cardiogenic shock after MI vary between 50–80%. Most deaths occur within 48 hours of the onset of shock. People surviving until discharge from hospital have a reasonable long-term prognosis (88% survival at 1 year).

Laurence O'Toole

KEY POINTS

- Stable angina is a sensation of discomfort or pain in the chest, arm, or jaw brought on predictably by factors that increase myocardial oxygen demand, such as exertion, and relieved by rest or nitroglycerin.

  Stable angina is usually caused by coronary atherosclerosis, and affects up to 16% of men and 10% of women aged 65–74 years in the UK. Risk factors include hypertension, elevated serum cholesterol levels, smoking, physical inactivity, and overweight.

  People with angina are at increased risk of other cardiovascular events and mortality compared with people without angina.

  Among people not thought to need coronary artery revascularisation, annual mortality is 1–2%, and annual non-fatal MI rates are 2–3%.

- There is consensus that beta-blockers, calcium channel blockers, nitrates, and potassium channel openers are effective for treating the symptoms of stable angina in the long term, although few studies have been done to confirm this.

  Beta-blockers seem to be as effective as calcium channel blockers at reducing angina attacks, cardiovascular events, and mortality, and are equally well tolerated in the long term.

  Nitrates may be as effective as calcium channel blockers at reducing angina attacks and improving quality of life.

  We found no RCTs on the effects of long-term monotherapy with potassium channel openers in people with stable angina.

(i) **Please visit www.clinicalevidence.bmj.com for full text and references**

What are effects of long-term single-drug treatment for stable angina?	
Likely To Be Beneficial	• Beta-blockers*
	• Calcium channel blockers*
	• Nitrates*
	• Potassium channel openers*

Search date December 2005

*Based on consensus.

DEFINITION Angina pectoris, often simply known as angina, is a clinical syndrome characterised by discomfort in the chest, shoulder, back, arm, or jaw. Angina is usually caused by coronary artery atherosclerotic disease. Rarer causes include valvular heart disease, hypertrophic cardiomyopathy, uncontrolled hypertension, or vasospasm or endothelial dysfunction not related to atherosclerosis. The differential diagnosis of angina includes non-cardiac conditions affecting the chest wall, oesophagus, and lungs. Angina may be classified as stable or unstable. **Stable angina** is defined as regular or predictable angina symptoms that have been occurring for over 2 months. Symptoms are transient and are typically provoked by exertion, and alleviated by rest or nitroglycerin. Other precipitants include cold weather, eating, or emotional distress. This review deals specifically with stable angina caused by coronary artery atherosclerotic disease. For management of **unstable angina**, see separate review on unstable angina, p 21.

INCIDENCE/PREVALENCE The prevalence of stable angina remains unclear. Epidemiological studies in the UK estimate that 6–16% of men and 3–10% of women aged 65–74 years

(continued over)

(from previous page)

have experienced angina. Annually, about 1% of the population visit their general practitioner with symptoms of angina, and 23,000 people with new anginal symptoms present to their general practitioner each year in the UK. These studies did not distinguish between stable and unstable angina.

AETIOLOGY/RISK FACTORS Stable angina resulting from CHD is characterised by focal atherosclerotic plaques in the intimal layer of the epicardial coronary artery. The plaques encroach on the coronary lumen and may limit blood flow to the myocardium, especially during periods of increased myocardial oxygen demand. The major risk factors that lead to the development of stable angina are similar to those that predispose to CHD. These risk factors include increasing age, male sex, overweight, hypertension, elevated serum cholesterol level, smoking, and relative physical inactivity.

PROGNOSIS Stable angina is a marker of underlying CHD, which accounts for 1 in 4 deaths in the UK. People with angina are 2–5 times more likely to develop other manifestations of coronary heart disease than people who do not have angina. One population-based study (7100 men aged 51–59 years at entry) found that people with angina had higher mortality than people with no history of coronary artery disease at baseline (16-year survival rate: 53% with angina *v* 72% without coronary artery disease *v* 34% with a history of MI). Clinical trials in people with stable angina have tended to recruit participants who were not felt to be in need of coronary revascularisation and in these people prognosis is better, with an annual mortality of 1–2%, and an annual rate of non-fatal MI of 2–3%. Features that indicate a poorer prognosis include: more severe symptoms, male sex, abnormal resting ECG (present in about 50% of people with angina), previous MI, left ventricular dysfunction, easily provoked or widespread coronary ischaemia on stress testing (present in about a third of people referred to hospital with stable angina), and significant stenosis of all three major coronary arteries or the left main coronary artery. In addition, the standard coronary risk factors continue to exert a detrimental and additive effect on prognosis in people with stable angina. Control of these risk factors is dealt with in the review on secondary prevention of ischaemic cardiac events, p 45.

Madhu Natarajan

KEY POINTS

- Unstable angina is characterised by episodes of chest pain at rest or coming on increasingly rapidly with exertion, which are increasing in frequency or severity, in the absence of persistent ECG changes.

    Up to 10% of people with unstable angina die or have an MI within 7 days, and up to 14% are dead within 1 year.

- Aspirin at doses up to 325 mg daily reduces the risk of death, MI, and stroke compared with placebo in people with unstable angina.

    Higher doses of aspirin are not more effective, and increase the risk of complications.

    Adding clopidogrel or ticlodipine to aspirin or standard therapy may reduce mortality and MI rates, but increases the risk of bleeding or other adverse effects.

- Intravenous glycoprotein IIb/IIIa platelet receptor inhibitors reduce death and MI after 6 months in people with unstable angina, but increase the risk of bleeding, and longer-term benefits are unclear.

    Oral glycoprotein IIb/IIIa platelet receptor inhibitors have not been shown to improve outcomes, but increase the risk of bleeding.

    Unfractionated or low molecular weight heparin plus aspirin may reduce death and MI at 1 week, but longer-term benefits are unclear.

    Direct thrombin inhibitors may reduce death and MI compared with heparin, but warfarin has not been shown to be beneficial and increases the risk of major bleeding.

- We don't know whether intravenous nitrates, beta-blockers or calcium channel blockers reduce the risk of myocardial infarction or death, although they may reduce the frequency and severity of chest pain.

- CAUTION: Short-acting dihydropyridine calcium channel blockers may increase mortality in people with CHD.

- We don't know whether routine early cardiac catheterisation and revascularisation reduces death and other cardiac events in people with unstable angina.

Please visit www.clinicalevidence.bmj.com for full text and references

What are the effects of antiplatelet treatments?	
Beneficial	• Aspirin
Likely To Be Beneficial	• Clopidogrel/ticlopidine
	• Intravenous glycoprotein IIb/IIIa inhibitors
Likely To Be Ineffective Or Harmful	• Oral glycoprotein IIb/IIIa inhibitors

What are the effects of antithrombin treatments?	
Likely To Be Beneficial	• Direct thrombin inhibitors
	• Low molecular weight heparin

	• Unfractionated heparin
Unlikely To Be Beneficial	• Warfarin

What are the effects of anti-ischaemic treatments?

Unknown Effectiveness	• Beta-blockers (for MI or death) • Nitrates (for MI or death)
Unlikely To Be Beneficial	• Calcium channel blockers

What are the effects of invasive treatments?

Unknown Effectiveness	• Routine early cardiac catheterisation and revascularisation

Search date March 2004

DEFINITION Unstable angina is distinguished from stable angina, acute MI, and non-cardiac pain by the pattern of symptoms (characteristic pain present at rest or on lower levels of activity), the severity of symptoms (recently increasing intensity, frequency, or duration), and the absence of persistent ST segment elevation on a resting ECG. Unstable angina includes a variety of different clinical patterns: angina at rest of up to 1 week of duration; angina increasing in severity to moderate or severe pain; non-Q wave MI; and post-MI angina continuing for longer than 24 hours. Unstable angina and non-ST segment elevation MI (non-STEMI) are clinically overlapping entities in terms of diagnosis and treatment strategies. Unstable angina, broadly defined as new or persistent chest pain, becomes classified as non-STEMI if, in addition to chest pain, there is elevation of cardiac enzymes, such as troponin, or persistent ST depression on ECG. Many trials include people with either unstable angina or non-STEMI. We have included RCTs in a mixed population of people with unstable angina or non-STEMI, as well as RCTs solely in people with unstable angina.

INCIDENCE/PREVALENCE In industrialised countries, the annual incidence of unstable angina is about 6/10,000 people in the general population.

AETIOLOGY/RISK FACTORS Risk factors are the same as for other manifestations of ischaemic heart disease: older age, previous atheromatous cardiovascular disease, diabetes mellitus, smoking cigarettes, hypertension, hypercholesterolaemia, male sex, and a family history of ischaemic heart disease. Unstable angina can also occur in association with other disorders of the circulation, including heart valve disease, arrhythmia, and cardiomyopathy.

PROGNOSIS In people with unstable angina taking aspirin, the incidence of serious adverse outcomes (such as death, acute MI, or refractory angina requiring emergency revascularisation) is 5–10% within the first 7 days and about 15% at 30 days. Between 5%–14% of people with unstable angina die in the year after diagnosis, with about half of these deaths occurring within 4 weeks of diagnosis. No single factor identifies people at higher risk of an adverse event. Risk factors include severity of presentation (e.g. duration of pain, speed of progression, evidence of heart failure), medical history (e.g. previous unstable angina, acute MI, left ventricular dysfunction), other clinical parameters (e.g. age, diabetes), ECG changes (e.g. severity of ST segment depression, deep T wave inversion, transient ST segment elevation), biochemical parameters (e.g. troponin concentration), and change in clinical status (e.g. recurrent chest pain, silent ischaemia, haemodynamic instability).

Atrial fibrillation (acute onset) | 23

Gregory YH Lip and Timothy Watson

KEY POINTS

- Acute atrial fibrillation is rapid, irregular, and chaotic atrial activity of less than 48 hours' duration. It resolves spontaneously within 24–48 hours in over 50% of people.

    Risk factors for acute atrial fibrillation include increasing age, CVD, alcohol abuse, diabetes, and lung disease.

    Acute atrial fibrillation increases the risk of stroke and heart failure.

- The consensus is that people with haemodynamically unstable atrial fibrillation should have immediate direct current cardioversion. In people who are haemodynamically stable, we found no studies of adequate quality to show whether direct current cardioversion increases reversion to sinus rhythm.

    There is consensus that antithrombotic treatment with heparin should be given before cardioversion to reduce the risk of embolism in people who are haemodynamically stable, but we found no studies to show whether this is beneficial.

- Oral or intravenous flecainide or propafenone increase the likelihood of reversion to sinus rhythm compared with placebo in people with haemodynamically stable acute atrial fibrillation.

- CAUTION: Flecainide and propafenone should not be used in people with ischaemic heart disease as they can cause (life-threatening) arrhythmias.

- Intravenous bolus amiodarone improves likelihood of conversion to sinus rhythm compared with digoxin.

- We don't know whether quinidine or sotalol increase reversion to sinus rhythm in people with haemodynamically stable atrial fibrillation, as results from studies have been inconclusive.

    Digoxin and verapamil do not seem to increase reversion to sinus rhythm compared with placebo.

- Treatment with digoxin, diltiazem, timolol, and verapamil may control heart rate in people with haemodynamically stable atrial fibrillation despite being unlikely to restore sinus rhythm.

    No one drug has been shown to be more effective than all the others at controlling heart rate. However, intravenous bolus amiodarone is more effective than digoxin. Verapamil may cause hypotension. We don't know whether sotalol can control heart rate in people with acute atrial fibrillation who are haemodynamically stable.

(i) **Please visit www.clinicalevidence.bmj.com for full text and references**

What are the effects of interventions to prevent embolism in people with recent-onset atrial fibrillation who are haemodynamically stable?

Unknown Effectiveness	• Antithrombotic treatment before cardioversion

What are the effects of interventions for conversion to sinus rhythm in people with recent onset atrial fibrillation who are haemodynamically stable?

Trade-off Between Benefits And Harms	• Flecainide for rhythm control • Propafenone for rhythm control
Unknown Effectiveness	• Amiodarone for rhythm control • Direct-current cardioversion for rhythm control

	• Quinidine for rhythm control
	• Sotalol for rhythm control
Unlikely To Be Beneficial	• Digoxin for rhythm control
	• Verapamil for rhythm control

What are the effects of interventions to control heart rate in people with recent-onset atrial fibrillation who are haemodynamically stable?

Likely To Be Beneficial	• Amiodarone for rate control
	• Digoxin for rate control
	• Diltiazem for rate control
	• Timolol for rate control
	• Verapamil for rate control
Unknown Effectiveness	• Sotalol for rate control

Search date October 2006

DEFINITION Acute atrial fibrillation is rapid, irregular, and chaotic atrial activity of less than 48 hours' duration. It includes both the first symptomatic onset of chronic or persistent atrial fibrillation, and episodes of paroxysmal atrial fibrillation. It is sometimes difficult to distinguish new onset atrial fibrillation from previously undiagnosed long-standing atrial fibrillation. Atrial fibrillation within 72 hours of onset is sometimes called recent-onset atrial fibrillation. By contrast, chronic atrial fibrillation is more sustained and can be described as paroxysmal (with spontaneous termination and sinus rhythm between recurrences), persistent, or permanent atrial fibrillation. This review deals with people with acute and recent atrial fibrillation who are haemodynamically stable. The consensus is that people who are not haemodynamically stable should be treated with immediate direct-current cardioversion. We have excluded studies in people with atrial fibrillation arising during or soon after cardiac surgery. **Diagnosis:** Acute atrial fibrillation should be suspected in people presenting with dizziness, syncope, dyspnoea, or palpitations. Moreover, atrial fibrillation can contribute to a large number of other non-specific symptoms. Palpation of an irregular pulse is generally considered sufficient only to raise suspicion of atrial fibrillation. The diagnosis requires confirmation with an ECG. However, in those with paroxysmal atrial fibrillation, ambulatory monitoring may be required.

INCIDENCE/PREVALENCE We found limited evidence of the incidence or prevalence of acute atrial fibrillation. Extrapolation from the Framingham study suggests an incidence in men of 3/1000 person-years at age 55 years, rising to 38/1000 person-years at 94 years. In women, the incidence was 2/1000 person-years at age 55 years and 32.5/1000 person-years at 94 years. The prevalence of atrial fibrillation ranged from 0.5% for people aged 50–59 years to 9% in people aged 80–89 years. Among acute emergency medical admissions in the UK, 3–6% had atrial fibrillation, and about 40% were newly diagnosed. Among acute hospital admissions in New Zealand, 10% (95% CI 9% to 12%) had documented atrial fibrillation.

AETIOLOGY/RISK FACTORS Common precipitants of acute atrial fibrillation are acute MI and the acute effects of alcohol. Age increases the risk of developing acute atrial fibrillation. Men are more likely than women to develop atrial fibrillation (38 years' follow-up from the Framingham Study, RR after adjustment for age and known predisposing conditions 1.5). Atrial fibrillation can occur in association with underlying disease (both cardiac and non-cardiac) or can arise in the absence of any other condition. Epidemiological surveys found that risk factors for the development of acute atrial fibrillation include ischaemic heart disease, hypertension, heart failure, valve disease, diabetes, alcohol abuse, thyroid disorders, and disorders of the lung and pleura. In a British survey of acute hospital admissions of people with atrial fibrillation, a history of ischaemic heart disease was present in 33%, heart failure in 24%, hypertension in 26%, and rheumatic heart disease in 7%. In some populations, the acute effects of alcohol explain a large proportion of the incidence of acute atrial fibrillation. Paroxysms of atrial fibrillation are more common in athletes.

PROGNOSIS Spontaneous reversion: Observational studies and placebo arms of RCTs found that more than 50% of people with acute atrial fibrillation revert spontaneously within 24–48 hours, especially if atrial fibrillation was associated with an identifiable precipitant such as alcohol or MI. **Progression to chronic atrial fibrillation:** We found no evidence about the proportion of people with acute atrial fibrillation who develop more chronic forms of atrial fibrillation (e.g. paroxysmal, persistent, or permanent atrial fibrillation). **Mortality:** We found little evidence about the effects on mortality of acute atrial fibrillation where no underlying cause is found. Acute atrial fibrillation during MI is an independent predictor of both short-term and long-term mortality. **Heart failure:** Onset of atrial fibrillation reduces cardiac output by 10–20%, irrespective of the underlying ventricular rate, and can contribute to heart failure. People with acute atrial fibrillation who present with heart failure have worse prognoses. **Stroke:** Acute atrial fibrillation is associated with a risk of imminent stroke. One case series used transoesophageal echocardiography in people who had developed acute atrial fibrillation within the preceding 48 hours; 15% had atrial thrombi. An ischaemic stroke associated with atrial fibrillation is more likely to be fatal, have a recurrence, and leave a serious functional deficit among survivors compared with a stroke not associated with atrial fibrillation.

Christopher J Boos, Deirdre A Lane, and Gregory YH Lip

KEY POINTS

- Atrial fibrillation is a supraventricular tachyarrhythmia, which is characterised by the presence of uncoordinated atrial activation and deteriorating atrial mechanical function of over 7 days' duration.

  Risk factors for chronic atrial fibrillation are increasing age, male sex, coexisting cardiac disease, thyroid disease, pyrexial illness, electrolyte imbalance, cancer, and acute infections.

- Consensus is that beta-blockers are more effective than digoxin for controlling symptoms of chronic atrial fibrillation, but very few studies have been found. When a beta-blocker alone is ineffective, the addition of digoxin is likely to be beneficial.

- Current consensus is that calcium channel blockers are more effective than digoxin for controlling heart rate, but very few studies have been found. When a calcium channel blocker alone is ineffective, the addition of digoxin is likely to be beneficial.

- The choice between using a beta-blocker or a calcium channel blocker is dependent on individual risk factors and co-existing morbidities.

- We found inconclusive evidence comparing rhythm- versus rate-control strategies. Current consensus supports the use of either strategy depending on individual risk factors and co-existing morbidities.

  Adverse effects are likely to be more common with rhythm-control strategies.

(i) **Please visit www.clinicalevidence.bmj.com for full text and references**

What are the effects of oral medical treatments to control heart rate in people with chronic (longer than 1 week) non-valvular atrial fibrillation?

Likely To Be Beneficial	• Beta-blockers plus digoxin versus beta-blockers alone (beta-blockers plus digoxin more effective than beta-blockers alone)*
	• Beta-blockers versus digoxin (beta-blockers more effective than digoxin in controlling symptoms) *
	• Calcium channel blocker (rate-limiting) plus digoxin versus calcium channel blocker (rate limiting) alone (calcium channel blocker plus digoxin more effective than calcium channel blocker alone)
	• Calcium channel blockers (rate-limiting) versus digoxin (calcium channel blockers more effective than digoxin for controlling heart rate)*
Trade-off Between Benefits And Harms	• Beta-blockers versus rate limiting calcium channel blockers (selection is dependent on individual risk factors and co-existing morbidities)

What is the effect of different treatment strategies for people with persistent non-valvular atrial fibrillation?

Trade-off Between Benefits And Harms	• Rhythm control versus rate control (selection dependent on individual risk factors and co-existing morbidities)

Search date June 2006

*Categorisation based on consensus.

DEFINITION Atrial fibrillation is the most frequently encountered and sustained cardiac arrhythmia in clinical practice. It is a supraventricular tachyarrhythmia, which is characterised by the presence of uncoordinated atrial activation and deteriorating atrial mechanical function. On the surface ECG P waves are absent and are replaced by rapid fibrillatory waves which vary in size, shape, and timing, leading to an irregular ventricular response when atrioventricular conduction is intact. **Classification:** Chronic atrial fibrillation is most commonly classified according to its temporal pattern. Faced with a first detected episode of atrial fibrillation, three recognised patterns of chronic disease may develop: (1) "persistent atrial fibrillation" describes an episode of sustained atrial fibrillation (usually more than 7 days) that does not convert to sinus rhythm without medical intervention, with the achievement of sinus rhythm either by pharmacological or electrical cardioversion; (2) "paroxysmal atrial fibrillation" refers to self-terminating episodes of atrial fibrillation, usually lasting less than 48 hours (both paroxysmal and persistent atrial fibrillation may be recurrent); (3) "permanent atrial fibrillation" where episodes of persistent (usually more than 1 year) atrial fibrillation, in which cardioversion is not attempted or is unsuccessful, with atrial fibrillation accepted as the long-term rhythm for that person. "Lone atrial fibrillation" is largely a diagnosis of exclusion and refers to atrial fibrillation occurring in the absence of concomitant CVD (e.g. hypertension), structural heart disease (normal ECG), with a normal ECG and chest x ray. This review covers only chronic atrial fibrillation (persistent and permanent). Acute atrial fibrillation is covered in a separate review (see atrial fibrillation (recent onset), p 23. **Diagnosis:** In most cases of suspected atrial fibrillation, a 12-lead ECG is sufficient for diagnosis confirmation. However, where diagnostic uncertainty remains, such as in chronic permanent atrial fibrillation, the use of 24-hour (or even 7-day) Holter monitoring or event recorder (e.g. Cardiomemo) may also be required. The most common presenting symptoms of chronic atrial fibrillation are palpitations, shortness of breath, fatigue, chest pain, dizziness, and stroke.

INCIDENCE/PREVALENCE Atrial fibrillation carries an overall population prevalence of 0.5–1.0% and an incidence of 0.54 cases per 1000 person-years. The prevalence of atrial fibrillation is highly age dependent, and increases markedly with each advancing decade of age, from 0.5% at age 50–59 years to almost 9% at age 80–90 years. The incidence of atrial fibrillation has a male predisposition, affecting men 1.5 times more commonly than women. The Screening for Atrial Fibrillation in the Elderly (SAFE) project reported that the baseline prevalence of atrial fibrillation in subjects aged over 65 years was 7.2%, with a higher prevalence in men (7.8%) and in people aged 75 years or more, with an incidence of 0.69–1.64% a year, depending on screening method. These incidence data refer to cross-sectional study data whereby most people would have atrial fibrillation of over 7 days' duration (persistent, paroxysmal, or permanent atrial fibrillation), and not to acute atrial fibrillation.

AETIOLOGY/RISK FACTORS Atrial fibrillation is linked to all types of cardiac disease, including cardiothoracic surgery, as well as to a large number of non-cardiac conditions such as thyroid disease, any pyrexial illness, electrolyte imbalance, cancer, and acute infections.

PROGNOSIS Chronic atrial fibrillation confers an enormous and significant clinical burden. It is an independent predictor of mortality and is associated with an odds ratio for death of 1.5 for men and 1.9 in women, independent of other risk factors. It increases the risk of ischaemic stroke and thromboembolism by, on average, fivefold. Furthermore, the presence of chronic atrial fibrillation is linked to far more severe strokes, with greater disability and

(continued over)

(from previous page)

lower discharge rate to home. Chronic atrial fibrillation is frequent (3–6% of all medical admissions) and results in longer hospital stay. In addition, chronic atrial fibrillation increases the development of heart failure and adversely affects quality of life, including cognitive function.

Robert McKelvie

KEY POINTS

- Heart failure occurs in 3–4% of adults aged over 65 years, usually as a consequence of coronary artery disease or hypertension, and causes breathlessness, effort intolerance, fluid retention, and increased mortality.

  The 5-year mortality in people with systolic heart failure ranges from 25–75%, often because of sudden death following ventricular arrhythmia. Risks of cardiovascular events are increased in people with left ventricular systolic dysfunction (LVSD) or heart failure.

- Multidisciplinary interventions and exercise may reduce admissions to hospital and mortality in people with heart failure compared with usual care, although long-term benefits remain unclear.

- ACE inhibitors, angiotensin II receptor blockers, and beta-blockers reduce hospitalisations and mortality from heart failure compared with placebo, with greater absolute benefits seen in people with more-severe heart failure.

  Combined treatment with angiotensin II receptor blockers and ACE inhibitors may lead to a greater reduction in cardiovascular deaths and admission for heart failure than with ACE inhibitor treatment alone.

- The aldosterone receptor antagonists spirinolactone and eplerenone may reduce mortality in people with heart failure already on other medical treatments, but increase the risk of hyperkalaemia.

- Digoxin slows the progression of heart failure compared with placebo, but may not reduce mortality.

- Implantable cardiac defibrillators and cardiac resynchronisation therapy can reduce mortality in people with heart failure who are at high risk of ventricular arrhythmias. However, studies evaluating cardiac resynchronisation therapy were performed in centres with considerable experience which may have overestimated the benefits.

- Hydralazine plus isosorbide dinitrate may improve survivial and quality-of-life scores compared with placebo in people with chronic congestive heart failure.

- ACE inhibitors delay the onset of symptomatic heart failure, reduce cardiovascular events, and improve long-term survival in people with asymptomatic LVSD compared with placebo.

- We don't know whether any treatment is beneficial in reducing mortality in people with diastolic heart failure.

- CAUTION: Positive inotropic agents (other than digoxin), calcium channel blockers, and antiarrhythmic drugs (other than amiodarone and beta-blockers) may all increase mortality and should be used with caution, if at all, in people with heart failure.

Please visit www.clinicalevidence.bmj.com for full text and references

What are the effects of non-drug treatments for heart failure?

Beneficial	• Multidisciplinary interventions
Likely To Be Beneficial	• Exercise

What are the effects of drug and invasive treatments for heart failure?

Beneficial	• ACE inhibitors • Angiotensin II receptor blockers • Beta-blockers • Digoxin (improves morbidity in people already receiving diuretics and ACE inhibitors) • Implantable cardiac defibrillators in people at high risk of arrhythmia
Likely To Be Beneficial	• Cardiac resynchronisation therapy • Eplerenone (in people with MI complicated by left ventricular dysfunction and heart failure already on medical treatment) • Hydralazine plus isosorbide dinitrate • Spironolactone in people with severe heart failure
Unknown Effectiveness	• Amiodarone • Anticoagulation • Antiplatelet agents
Likely To Be Ineffective Or Harmful	• Antiarrhythmics other than amiodarone • Calcium channel blockers • Positive inotropes other than digoxin

What are the effects of ACE inhibitors in people at high risk of heart failure?

Beneficial	• ACE inhibitors in people with asymptomatic left ventricular dysfunction or other risk factors

What are the effects of treatments for diastolic heart failure?

Likely To Be Beneficial	• Angiotensin II receptor blockers
Unknown Effectiveness	• Treatments other than angiotensin II receptor blockers for diastolic heart failure

Search date January 2007

DEFINITION Heart failure occurs when abnormal cardiac function causes failure of the heart to pump blood at a rate sufficient for metabolic requirements under normal filling pressure. It is characterised clinically by breathlessness, effort intolerance, fluid retention, and poor survival. Fluid retention and the congestion related to this can often be relieved with diuretic therapy. However, diuretic therapy should generally not be used alone and, if required, should be combined with the pharmacological therapies outlined in this review. Heart failure can be caused by systolic or diastolic dysfunction, and is associated with neurohormonal changes. Left ventricular systolic dysfunction (LVSD) is defined as a left ventricular ejection fraction below 0.40. It may be symptomatic or asymptomatic. Defining and diagnosing diastolic heart failure can be difficult. Recently proposed criteria include: (1) clinical evidence of heart failure; (2) normal or mildly abnormal left ventricular systolic function; and (3) evidence of abnormal left ventricular relaxation, filling, diastolic distensibility, or diastolic stiffness. However, assessment of some of these criteria is not standardised.

INCIDENCE/PREVALENCE Both the incidence and prevalence of heart failure increase with age. Studies of heart failure in the USA and Europe found that the annual incidence in people under 65 years of age is 1/1000 for men and 0.4/1000 for women. Over 65 years of age, the annual incidence is 11/1000 for men and 5/1000 for women. Under 65 years of age, the prevalence of heart failure is 1/1000 for men and 1/1000 for women; over age 65 years the prevalence is 40/1000 for men and 30/1000 for women. The prevalence of asymptomatic LVSD is 3% in the general population. The mean age of people with asymptomatic LVSD is lower than that for symptomatic individuals. Both heart failure and asymptomatic LVSD are more common in men. The prevalence of diastolic heart failure in the community is unknown. The prevalence of heart failure with preserved systolic function in people in hospital with clinical heart failure varies from 13–74%. Less than 15% of people with heart failure under 65 years of age have normal systolic function, whereas the prevalence is about 40% in people over 65 years of age.

AETIOLOGY/RISK FACTORS Coronary artery disease is the most common cause of heart failure. Other common causes include hypertension, and idiopathic dilated congestive cardiomyopathy. After adjustment for hypertension, the presence of left ventricular hypertrophy remains a risk factor for the development of heart failure. Other risk factors include cigarette smoking, hyperlipidaemia, and diabetes mellitus. The common causes of left ventricular diastolic dysfunction are coronary artery disease and systemic hypertension. Other causes are hypertrophic cardiomyopathy, restrictive or infiltrative cardiomyopathies, and valvular heart disease.

PROGNOSIS The prognosis for heart failure is poor, with 5-year mortality ranging from 26–75%. Up to 16% of people are re-admitted with heart failure within 6 months of first admission. In the USA, heart failure is the leading cause of hospital admission among people over 65 years of age. In people with heart failure, a new MI increases the risk of death (RR 7.8, 95% CI 6.9 to 8.8). About a third of all deaths in people with heart failure are preceded by a major ischaemic event. Sudden death, mainly caused by ventricular arrhythmia, is responsible for 25–50% of all deaths, and is the most common cause of death in people with heart failure. The presence of asymptomatic LVSD increases an individual's risk of having a cardiovascular event. One large prevention trial found that the risk of heart failure, admission for heart failure, and death increased linearly as ejection fraction fell (for each 5% reduction in ejection fraction: RR for mortality 1.20, 95% CI 1.13 to 1.29; RR for hospital admission 1.28, 95% CI 1.18 to 1.38; RR for heart failure 1.20, 95% CI 1.13 to 1.26). The annual mortality for people with diastolic heart failure varies in observational studies (1–18%). Reasons for this variation include age, presence of coronary artery disease, and variation in the partition value used to define abnormal ventricular systolic function. The annual mortality for left ventricular diastolic dysfunction is lower than that found in people with systolic dysfunction.

Kevin Cassar

KEY POINTS

- Up to 20% of adults aged over 55 years have detectable peripheral arterial disease of the legs, but this may cause symptoms of intermittent claudication in only a small proportion of affected people.

  The main risk factors are smoking and diabetes mellitus, but other risk factors for CVD are also associated with peripheral arterial disease.

  Overall mortality is about 30% 5 years after diagnosis of peripheral arterial disease, and 70% after 15 years.

- Antiplatelet agents reduce major cardiovascular events, arterial occlusion, and revascularisation compared with placebo, with the overall balance of benefits and harms supporting treatment of people with peripheral arterial disease.

- Regular exercise increases maximal walking distance compared with no exercise.

  Stopping smoking and taking vitamin E may also increase walking distance when combined with exercise.

- Statins have been shown to reduce cardiovascular events in studies that included people with peripheral vascular disease, and may increase walking distance and time to claudication compared with placebo.

  Cilostazol may improve walking distance compared with placebo, but adverse effects are common.

  We don't know whether pentoxifylline improves symptoms compared with placebo, and it may be less effective than cilostazol.

- PTCA may improve walking distance compared with no intervention, but the benefit may not last beyond 6 months.

- Bypass surgery may improve arterial patency for 12–24 months compared with PTA, but there seems to be no longer term benefit.

- Prostaglandins may improve amputation-free survival in critical ischaemia at 6 months when surgical revascularisation is not an option.

  Prostaglandins are unlikely to be of benefit in intermittent claudication.

(i) **Please visit www.clinicalevidence.bmj.com for full text and references**

What are the effects of treatments for people with chronic peripheral arterial disease?

Beneficial	• Antiplatelet agents • Exercise
Likely To Be Beneficial	• Bypass surgery (compared with PTCA) • HMG-CoA reductase inhibitors (statins) • PTCA (transient benefit only) • Smoking cessation*
Trade-off Between Benefits And Harms	• Cilostazol • Prostaglandins
Unknown Effectiveness	• Pentoxifylline

Search date December 2006

*Based on observational evidence and consensus.

DEFINITION Peripheral arterial disease arises when there is significant narrowing of arteries distal to the arch of the aorta. Narrowing can arise from atheroma, arteritis, local thrombus formation, or embolisation from the heart, or more central arteries. This review includes treatment options for people with symptoms of reduced blood flow to the leg that are likely to arise from atheroma. These symptoms range from calf pain on exercise (intermittent claudication) to rest pain, skin ulceration, or symptoms of ischaemic necrosis (gangrene) in people with critical limb ischaemia.

INCIDENCE/PREVALENCE Peripheral arterial disease is more common in people aged over 50 years than in younger people, and is more common in men than in women. The prevalence of peripheral arterial disease of the legs (assessed by non-invasive tests) is about 13.9–16.9% in men and 11.4–20.5% in women over 55 years of age. The overall annual incidence of intermittent claudication is 4.1–12.9/1000 in men and 3.3–8.2/1000 in women.

AETIOLOGY/RISK FACTORS Factors associated with the development of peripheral arterial disease include age, gender, cigarette smoking, diabetes mellitus, hypertension, hyperlipidaemia, obesity, and physical inactivity. The strongest associations are with smoking (RR 2.0–4.0) and diabetes (RR 2.0–3.0).

PROGNOSIS The symptoms of intermittent claudication can resolve spontaneously, remain stable over many years, or progress rapidly to critical limb ischaemia. About 15% of people with intermittent claudication eventually develop critical limb ischaemia, which endangers the viability of the limb. The annual incidence of critical limb ischaemia in Denmark and Italy in 1990 was 0.25–0.45/1000 people. CHD is the major cause of death in people with peripheral arterial disease of the legs. Over 5 years, about 20% of people with intermittent claudication have a non-fatal cardiovascular event (MI or stroke). The mortality rate of people with peripheral arterial disease is two to three times higher than that of age- and sex-matched controls. Overall mortality after the diagnosis of peripheral arterial disease is about 30% after 5 years and 70% after 15 years.

Primary prevention of CVD: diet and weight loss

Lee Hooper

KEY POINTS

- Diet is an important cause of many chronic diseases.

   Individual change in behaviour has the potential to decrease the burden of chronic disease, particularly CVD.

   This review focuses on the evidence that specific interventions to improve diet and increase weight loss lead to changed behaviour, and that these changes may prevent CVD.

- Intensive advice to healthy people to reduce sodium intake reduces sodium intake, as measured by sodium excretion.

- Reducing sodium intake reduces blood pressure, even in people without hypertension.

- Advice to reduce saturated fat intake may reduce the saturated fat intake, and multiple advice components reduce saturated fat intake more.

- Reducing saturated fat intake can reduce mortality in the longer term.

- Complex combined interventions to lose weight (physical plus dietary plus behavioural) are effective in helping people lose weight. Simpler interventions are less effective.

   We don't know what lifestyle interventions can maintain weight loss or what lifestyle interventions prevent weight gain, or if training health professionals is effective in promoting weight loss.

   We don't know whether diets and behavioural interventions to lose weight reduce the risk of CVD.

- Increasing fruit and vegetable intake may decrease the risk of CVD.

   We don't know whether advising people to increase their fruit and vegetable intake will actually increase their intake.

- Taking a high dose of antioxidant supplements (vitamin E and beta carotene) does not reduce mortality or cardiovascular events.

- We don't know whether omega 3 oil supplementation or advice to increase omega 3 intake can reduce mortality.

- We also don't know how effective a Mediterranean diet is at reducing cardiovascular events or deaths in the general population.

(i) Please visit www.clinicalevidence.bmj.com for full text and references

What are the effects of interventions in the general population to reduce sodium intake?	
Beneficial	• Advice to reduce sodium intake: reduction in CVD risk
Likely To Be Beneficial	• Advice to reduce sodium intake: reduction in sodium intake

What are the effects of a cholesterol-lowering diet in the general population?	
Likely To Be Beneficial	• Advice to reduce saturated fat intake: reduction in CVD risk
	• Advice to reduce saturated fat intake: reduction in fat intake

What are the effects of interventions to increase or maintain weight loss?

Beneficial	• Diets and behavioural interventions to lose weight: weight loss (effective in combination but not alone)
Unknown Effectiveness	• Diets and behavioural interventions: reduction in CVD risk • Lifestyle interventions: maintainance of weight loss • Lifestyle interventions: preventing weight gain • Training health professionals in promoting weight loss: weight loss

What are the effects on reducing CVD risk in the general population of eating more fruit and vegetables?

Likely To Be Beneficial	• Increase fruit and vegetable intake: reduction in CVD risk
Unknown Effectiveness	• Behavioural and counselling interventions: increase in fruit and vegetable intake

What are the effects on reducing CVD risk of antioxidants in the general population?

Unlikely To Be Beneficial	• High-dose antioxidant supplements: reduction in CVD risk

What are the effects on reduction of CVD risk of omega 3 fatty acids in the general population?

Unknown Effectiveness	• Omega 3 fatty acids: reduction in CVD risk

What are the effects on reduction of CVD risk of a Mediterranean diet in the general population?

Unknown Effectiveness	• Mediterranean diet: reduction in CVD risk

Search date August 2006

DEFINITION Diet is important in the cause of many chronic diseases. Individual change in behaviour has the potential to decrease the burden of chronic disease, particularly CVD. This review focuses on the evidence that specific interventions to improve diet and increase weight loss lead to changed behaviour, and that these changes may prevent CVD. Primary prevention in this context is the long-term management of people at increased risk but with no evidence of CVD. Clinically overt ischaemic vascular disease includes acute MI, angina, stroke, and peripheral vascular disease. Many adults have no symptoms or obvious signs of vascular disease, even though they have atheroma and are at increased risk of ischaemic

(continued over)

(from previous page)

vascular events because of one or more risk factors. In this review, we have taken primary prevention to apply to people who have not had clinically overt CVD, or people at low risk of ischaemic cardiovascular events. Prevention of cerebrovascular events is discussed in detail elsewhere in *BMJ Clinical Evidence* (see review on stroke prevention, p 50).

INCIDENCE/PREVALENCE CVD was responsible for 39% of UK deaths in 2002. Half of these were from CHD, and a quarter from stroke. CVD is also a major cause of death before 75 years of age, causing 34% of early deaths in men and 25% of deaths before 75 years of age in women. CHD deaths rose dramatically in the UK during the 20th century, peaked in the 1970s, and have fallen since then. Numbers of people living with CVD are not falling, and the British Heart Foundation estimates that there are about 1.5 million men and 1.2 million women who have or have had an MI or angina. Worldwide, it is estimated that 17 million people die of CVDs every year, and more than 60% of the global burden of CHD is found in resource-poor countries (10% of DALYs lost in low- and middle-income countries and 18% in high-income countries). The USA has a similar burden of heart disease to the UK; in 2002, 18% of deaths in the USA were from heart disease, compared with 20% in the UK. The USA lost 8 DALYs per 1000 population to heart disease and a further 4 DALYs per 1000 population to stroke, and the UK lost 7 DALYs per 1000 population to heart disease and 4 DALYs per 1000 population to stroke. Afghanistan has the highest rate of DALYs lost to heart disease (36 DALYs per 1000 population), and France, Andorra, Monaco, Japan, Korea, Dominica, and Kiribati have the lowest (1–3 DALYs per 1000 population). Mongolia has the highest rate for stroke (25 DALYs per 1000 population lost) and Switzerland the lowest (2 DALYs per 1000 population lost).

AETIOLOGY/RISK FACTORS Deaths from CHD are not evenly distributed across the population. They are more common in men than in women; 67% more common in men from Scotland and the north of England than in men from the south of England; 58% more common in male manual workers than in male non-manual workers; twice as common in female manual workers than female non-manual workers; and about 50% higher in South Asian people living in the UK than in the average UK population. In the UK there are 14% more CHD deaths in the winter months than in the rest of the year. CVD in the UK generally results from the slow build-up of atherosclerosis over many decades, with or without thrombosis. The long development time of atherosclerosis means that small changes in lifestyle may have profound effects on risk of CVD over decades. However, while there is strong evidence from epidemiological studies of the importance of lifestyle factors — such as smoking, physical activity, and diet — in the process of development of CVD, adjusting for confounding can be difficult, and the long timescales involved make proving the effectiveness of preventive interventions in trials difficult. In practice, risk factors — rather than disease outcomes — are often the only practical outcomes for intervention studies in low-risk people. Such risk factors include blood pressure, BMI, serum lipids, and development of diabetes.

PROGNOSIS Improvements in diet and reduction in weight may lower the risk of CVD by exerting favourable changes on CVD risk factors (obesity, high blood pressure, elevated serum lipids, diabetes).

Michael Pignone

KEY POINTS

- Dyslipidaemia, defined as elevated total or low density lipoprotein (LDL) cholesterol levels or low levels of high density lipoprotein (HDL) cholesterol, is an important risk factor for CHD and stroke.

    The incidence of dyslipidaemia is high: in 2000, approximately 25% of adults in the US had total cholesterol greater than 6.2 mmol/L or were taking lipid-lowering medication.

    Primary prevention in this context is defined as long-term management of people at increased risk but with no clinically overt evidence of CVD, such as acute MI, angina, stroke, and PVD, and who have not undergone revascularisation.

- We found no evidence that examined the effects of lipid-lowering therapies on people at low risk of CHD (less than 0.6% annual CHD risk).

- In people at medium risk of CHD (0.6%–1.4% annually), fibrates have been shown to effectively reduce the rate of CHD, but not of overall mortality, compared with placebo.

    Resins and statins may also be beneficial in reducing non-fatal MI and CHD death in this group, but we found no evidence relating to the effectiveness of niacin.

- Statins have been shown to be highly effective in treating people at high risk of CHD (more than 1.5% annually), although it appears that the size of benefit is related to the individual's baseline risk of CHD events and to the degree of cholesterol lowering, rather than to the initial cholesterol concentration.

    We found no evidence that examined the efficacy of niacin, fibrates, or resins in people at high risk of CHD.

- The effectiveness of reduced-fat diets to reduce cardiovascular events in primary prevention is unclear.

(i) **Please visit www.clinicalevidence.bmj.com for full text and references**

What are the effects of pharmacological cholesterol-lowering interventions in people at low risk (less than 0.6% annual CHD risk)?	
Unknown Effectiveness	• Fibrates
	• Niacin
	• Resins
	• Statins

What are the effects of pharmacological cholesterol-lowering interventions in people at medium risk (0.6–1.4% annual CHD risk)?	
Beneficial	• Fibrates
Likely To Be Beneficial	• Resins
	• Statins
Unknown Effectiveness	• Niacin

What are the effects of pharmacological cholesterol-lowering interventions in people at high risk (at least 1.5% annual CHD risk)?

Beneficial	• Statins
Unknown Effectiveness	• Fibrates
	• Niacin
	• Resins

What are the effects of reduced- or modified-fat diet?

Likely To Be Beneficial	• Reduced- or modified-fat diet

Search date March 2006

DEFINITION Dyslipidaemia, defined as elevated total or low density lipoprotein (LDL) cholesterol levels or low levels of high density lipoprotein (HDL) cholesterol, is an important risk factor for CDH and stroke (cerebrovascular disease). This review examines the evidence for treatment of dyslipidaemia for primary prevention of CHD. Primary prevention in this context is defined as long-term management of people at increased risk but with no clinically overt evidence of CVD, such as acute MI, angina, stroke, and PVD, and who have not undergone revascularisation. Most adults at increased risk of CVD have no symptoms or obvious signs, but they may be identified by assessment of their risk factors (see aetiology/risk factors below). We have divided people with no known CVD into three groups: low risk (less than 0.6% annual CHD risk), medium risk (0.6–1.4% annual CHD risk), and high risk (at least 1.5% annual CHD risk). Prevention of cerebrovascular events is discussed in detail elsewhere in *BMJ Clinical Evidence* (see review on stroke prevention, p 50). In the USA the preferred method to calculate CVD risk would be to use the Framingham risk equations, the best validated method from a US population.

INCIDENCE/PREVALENCE Dyslipidaemia, defined as elevated total or LDL cholesterol, or low HDL cholesterol, is common. Data from the US NHANES survey conducted in 1999–2000 found that 25% of adults had total cholesterol greater than 6.2 mmol/L or were taking a lipid-lowering medication. According to the World Health Report 1999, ischaemic heart disease was the leading single cause of death in the world, the leading single cause of death in high-income countries, and second only to lower respiratory tract infections in low- and middle-income countries. In 1998 it was still the leading cause of death, with nearly 7.4 million estimated deaths a year in member states of the WHO and causing the eighth highest burden of disease in the low- and middle-income countries (30.7 million disability-adjusted life years).

AETIOLOGY/RISK FACTORS Major risk factors for ischaemic vascular disease include increased age, male sex, raised LDL cholesterol, reduced HDL cholesterol, raised blood pressure, smoking, diabetes, family history of CVD, obesity, and sedentary lifestyle. For many of these risk factors, including elevated LDL cholesterol, observational studies show a continuous gradient of increasing risk of cardiovascular disease with increasing levels of the risk factor, with no obvious threshold level. Although by definition event rates are higher in high-risk people, most ischaemic vascular events are in people with intermediate levels of absolute risk because there are many more of them than there are people at high risk.

PROGNOSIS One Scottish study found that about half of people who suffer an MI die within 28 days, and two thirds of MIs occur before the person reaches hospital. People with known CVD are at high risk for future ischaemic heart disease events (see review on secondary prevention of ischaemic cardiac events, p 45) as are people with diabetes (see review on Diabetes: prevention of cardiovascular events, p 139). For people without known CVD, the absolute risk of ischaemic vascular events is generally lower, but varies widely. Estimates of absolute risk can be based on simple risk equations or tables. Such information may be helpful in making treatment decisions.

Stacey Sheridan

KEY POINTS

- Hypertension (persistent diastolic blood pressure of 90 mm Hg or higher and systolic blood pressure 140 mm Hg or higher) affects 20% of the world's adult population, and increases the risk of CVD, end-stage renal disease, and retinopathy.

  Risk factors for hypertension include age, sex, race/ethnicity, genetic predisposition, diet, physical inactivity, obesity, and psychological and social characteristics.

- No antihypertensive drug has been found to be more effective than the others at reducing total mortality, cardiovascular mortality, or MI.

  Apparent differences in outcomes with different antihypertensive drugs may be due to different levels of blood pressure reduction.

  Diuretics may be more effective than ACE inhibitors and alpha-blockers at reducing stroke and combined cardiovascular events, and more effective than ACE inhibitors, calcium channel blockers, and alpha-blockers at reducing heart failure.

  Beta-blockers may be as effective as diuretics at reducing stroke, but calcium channel blockers may be even more effective than beta-blockers or diuretics.

  ACE inhibitors may be more effective than calcium channel blockers at reducing heart failure.

  Choice of second-line antihypertensive agent should be based on other morbidity and likely adverse effects, as we don't know which is the most likely to reduce cardiovascular events.

- We found no RCT evidence assessing whether dietary modification reduces morbidity or mortality from hypertension compared with a normal diet.

  Advice to reduce dietary intake of salt to below 50 mmol/day, fish-oil supplementation, potassium supplementation, and calcium supplementation may all reduce systolic blood pressure by approximately 1–5 mm Hg and reduce diastolic blood pressure by 1–3 mm Hg in people with hypertension.

  Potassium supplementation should not be used in people with kidney failure, or in people taking drugs that can increase potassium levels.

  Magnesium supplementation has not been shown to be beneficial at reducing blood pressure.

 Please visit www.clinicalevidence.bmj.com for full text and references

What are the effects of different antihypertensive drugs for people with hypertension?	
Unknown Effectiveness	• Antihypertensive drugs (unclear which antihypertensive drug is more effective)

What are the effects of dietary modification for people with hypertension?	
Likely To Be Beneficial	• Fish-oil supplementation • Low-salt diet • Potassium supplementation
Unknown Effectiveness	• Calcium supplementation

• Magnesium supplementation

Search date March 2006

DEFINITION Hypertension, a clinically important elevation in blood pressure, is usually defined in adults as a diastolic blood pressure of 90 mm Hg or higher, or a systolic blood pressure of 140 mm Hg or higher. The WHO defines grade 1 hypertension as office blood pressures ranging from 140–159 mm Hg systolic or 90–99 mm Hg diastolic, grade 2 hypertension as pressures of 160–179 mm Hg systolic or 100–109 mm Hg diastolic, and grade 3 hypertension as pressures at least 180 mm Hg systolic and 110 mm Hg diastolic. Systematic reviews have consistently shown that treating essential hypertension (namely the elevation of systolic and diastolic blood pressures, in isolation or combination, with no secondary underlying cause) with antihypertensive drugs reduces fatal and non-fatal stroke, cardiac events, and total mortality compared with placebo in those with severe hypertension or high cardiovascular risk owing to age or other co-morbid risk factors. This review therefore focuses on the effects of treating essential hypertension with different pharmacological agents, and also examines the effect of treating hypertension with non-pharmacological agents compared with placebo. **Diagnosis:** It is usually recommended that clinicians diagnose hypertension only after obtaining two or more elevated blood pressure readings at each of two or more separate visits over a period of one or more weeks. This recommendation follows the pattern of blood pressure measurement in the RCTs of antihypertensive treatment, and represents a compromise between reliable detection of elevated blood pressure and clinical practicality.

INCIDENCE/PREVALENCE CHD is a major cause of morbidity and mortality throughout the world. It is a leading cause of disability and rising healthcare costs, and it is responsible for 13% of deaths worldwide. Most of this burden of heart disease can be linked to several "traditional" risk factors, including age, sex, increasing blood pressure, increasing cholesterol, smoking, diabetes, and left ventricular hypertrophy. Of these, hypertension is most common, affecting 20% of the world adult population. The relative risk of adverse events associated with hypertension is continuous and graded. The absolute risk of adverse outcomes from hypertension depends on the presence of other cardiovascular risk factors, including smoking, diabetes, and abnormal blood lipid levels, as well as the degree of blood pressure elevation. Even modest elevations in blood pressure in young adulthood are associated with increased risk of cardiovascular events in middle age.

AETIOLOGY/RISK FACTORS Identified risk factors for hypertension include age, sex, genetic predisposition, diet, physical inactivity, obesity, and psychological and social characteristics. In addition, certain ethnic groups, such as non-hispanic black people, are at higher risk of hypertension.

PROGNOSIS People with hypertension have a two- to fourfold increased risk of stroke, MI, heart failure, and PVD than those without hypertension. Additionally, they have an increased risk of end stage renal disease, retinopathy, and aortic aneurysm. The absolute risk of adverse outcomes from hypertension depends on other cardiovascular risk factors and the degree of blood pressure elevation (see incidence/prevalence section).

Primary prevention of CVD: physical activity

David Stensel

KEY POINTS

- Increasing physical activity has been associated with reduced risk of mortality and CVD.

  The proportion of people doing no physical activity in a week varies between countries, but can reach nearly 25% in Europe and the Americas.

- Counselling people to increase physical activity increases people's activity levels over 12 months if accompanied by written materials and telephone follow-up.

  Counselling people to do higher-intensity exercise may increase activity levels more than counselling people to do lower-intensity exercise.

  People counselled to perform a higher-intensity exercise programme were also found to adhere to it better than those given a more moderate-intensity programme.

- We don't know whether counselling people to increase physical activity or to do higher-intensity exercise can reduce CVD, although it may reduce BMI and blood pressure.

(i) **Please visit www.clinicalevidence.bmj.com for full text and references**

Does counselling people in the general population to increase physical activity lead to increased physical activity?	
Likely To Be Beneficial	• Counselling people to increase physical activity versus no advice
	• Counselling people to perform higher- compared with lower-intensity exercise programmes

What are the health benefits of increasing physical activity in relation to cardiovascular outcomes in the general population?	
Unknown Effectiveness	• Counselling people to increase physical activity versus no advice
	• Counselling people to perform higher- compared with lower-intensity exercise programmes

Search date June 2006

DEFINITION There are no internationally agreed definitions of physical activity. It has been defined as "any bodily movement produced by contraction of skeletal muscle that substantially increases energy expenditure". Activities include formal exercise programmes as well as walking, hiking, gardening, sport, and dance. The common element is that these activities result in substantial energy expenditure, although the intensity and duration can vary considerably. Exercise is considered a subcategory of physical activity and may be defined as planned, structured, and repetitive bodily movements performed to improve or maintain one or more components of physical fitness. Level of physical activity is important in the causes of many chronic diseases. Individual change in behaviour has the potential to decrease the burden of chronic disease, particularly CVD. This review focuses on the evidence that specific interventions may lead to increases in physical activity, and that these changes may prevent CVD. The relationship between physical activity and physical fitness is complex. There is consensus that increasing levels of both activity and fitness may reduce CVD. However, it is unclear whether activity or fitness is more important for health. There are many types of physical fitness — cardiovascular fitness, muscular strength, muscular endurance, flexibility, coordination, speed, and power. The most common descriptor of physical fitness is cardiovascular fitness, which is usually determined using either prediction or direct measurement of maximum oxygen uptake. It is important to note that moderate-intensity physical activity may not necessarily lead to an increase in physical fitness (as defined by maximum oxygen uptake), but studies suggest that there will still be benefits from such activity in terms of lowering disease risk. We have therefore, in this review, assessed as outcomes both increases in intensity, frequency, and duration of physical activity, and increases in physical fitness. Primary prevention in this context is the long-term management of people at increased risk of CVD, but with no evidence of overt ischaemic CVD. We have only included studies in adults aged over 18 years who are free-living and healthy, excluding studies if more than 10% of participants had a reported diagnosis such as obesity, diabetes, or hypertension. Prevention of cerebrovascular events is discussed in detail elsewhere in *BMJ Clinical Evidence* (see review on stroke prevention, p 50).

INCIDENCE/PREVALENCE For general health benefits it is recommended in government guidelines that adults achieve a total of at least 30 minutes a day of at least moderate-intensity physical activity on five or more days of the week. The recommended levels of activity can be achieved either by doing all the daily activity in one session, or through several shorter bouts of 10 minutes or more. The activity can be lifestyle activity, or structured exercise or sport, or a combination of these. Activity levels in England are low. About two thirds of men and three quarters of women report less than 30 minutes of moderate-intensity physical activity a day on at least five days a week. Levels of physical activity in the UK fall just below the EU average. In a survey of 15 EU countries, the percentage of adults reporting no moderate physical activity (e.g. "carrying light loads, cycling at a normal pace, doubles tennis") ranged from 8% to 53%. International comparisons of physical activity/inactivity are difficult, because there are no internationally agreed definitions. Some data are available from the WHO, however, and these indicate that the prevalence of complete inactivity ("doing no or very little physical activity at work, home, for transport or in discretionary [leisure] time") is: 11–12% in Africa, 20–23% in the Americas, 18–19% in the Eastern Mediterranean, 17–24% in Europe, 15–17% in South East Asia, and 16–17% in the Western Pacific region.

AETIOLOGY/RISK FACTORS Low levels of physical activity and lack of physical fitness are strong risk factors for CHD. Both confer an increased risk similar to that associated with smoking, hypertension, and high blood cholesterol. The most frequently cited reasons for inactivity in the general population are increased urbanisation and mechanisation. Most occupations now involve little physical activity, while television viewing and computer use compete with more active pursuits in leisure time. Greater use of cars along with an increase in the use of labour-saving devices has also reduced the need for physical activity. There has been a decline in walking and cycling as modes of transport — a 2001 survey in the UK reported that the number of miles travelled by each person a year on foot and on bicycle declined by about a quarter between 1975–1976 and 1999–2001. One proposed reason for the decline in walking is increased fears over personal safety. Barriers to physical activity include physical barriers such as an injury, emotional barriers such as embarrassment, motivational barriers such as a perceived lack of energy, time barriers, and availability barriers such as lack of facilities.

PROGNOSIS Increases in physical activity may lower the risk of CVD by exerting favourable changes on CVD risk factors (lowering blood pressure, triglyceride concentrations, and blood cholesterol concentrations, and raising high-density lipoprotein cholesterol concentrations) and by exerting direct effects on the heart (reduced heart rate, increased stroke volume) and on blood vessels (improved endothelial function which increases the ability of blood vessels to vasodilate and enhance blood supply when necessary). In the Harvard Alumni Health study (10,269 men aged 45–84 years), men who reported changing their lifestyles after baseline to include moderately vigorous activity (4 METs or more) had a 23% lower risk of all-cause mortality at follow-up after about 20 years compared with men who continued not to engage in such activity (RR 0.77, 95% CI 0.58 to 0.96; P less than 0.02). The main cause of death was CVD. In the Aerobics Centre Longitudinal Study (9777 men aged 20–82 years), men classified as unfit on their first examination but fit on their second (mean of 4.9 years between examinations) had a 52% lower risk of CVD mortality during follow-up (RR 0.48, 95% CI 0.31 to 0.74) than men classified as unfit on both

(continued over)

(from previous page)

examinations. Fitness was assessed by a treadmill test, and the 20% of people with lowest treadmill times were classed as "unfit". The Nurses' Health Study (72,488 female nurses aged 40–65 years) assessed physical activity using a questionnaire. It found that women reporting higher levels of energy expenditure had lower rates of coronary events over 6 years. Women who walked the equivalent of 3 hours or more a week at a brisk pace (5 km an hour or more [3 miles an hour]) had significantly lower rates of coronary events compared with women who walked infrequently (RR 0.65, 95% CI 0.47 to 0.91). Similar results were found in the Women's Health Initiative prospective cohort study of 73,743 postmenopausal women.

Apoor Gami

KEY POINTS

- Coronary artery disease is the leading cause of mortality in resource-rich countries, and is becoming a major cause of morbidity and mortality in resource-poor countries.

  Secondary prevention in this context is long-term treatment to prevent recurrent cardiac morbidity and mortality in people who have either had a prior acute MI or are at high risk owing to severe coronary artery stenoses, angina, or prior coronary surgical procedures.

- Of the antithrombotic treatments, there is good evidence that aspirin (especially when combined with clopidogrel), thienopyridines (more effective than aspirin) and oral anticoagulants all effectively reduce the risk of cardiovascular events.

  Oral anticoagulants substantially increase the risk of haemorrhage and, when combined with antiplatelet treatments, these risks outweigh the benefits.

  Oral glycoprotein IIb/IIIa receptor inhibitors appear to increase the risk of mortality when combined with aspirin.

- Other effective drug treatments include beta-blockers (after MI), ACE inhibitors (in people at high risk or after MI), angiotensin II receptor blockers (in people with coronary artery disease) and amiodarone (in people with MI and high risk of death from cardiac arrhythmia).

  Calcium channel blockers, class I antiarrhythmic agents and sotalol all appear to increase mortality compared with placebo in people who have had an MI.

  Contrary to decades of large observational studies, multiple RCTs show no cardiac benefit from HRT in postmenopausal women.

- Lipid-lowering treatments effectively reduce the risk of cardiovascular mortality and non-fatal cardiovascular events in people with CHD.

- There is good evidence that statins reduce the risk of mortality and cardiac events in people at high risk, but the evidence is less clear for fibrates.

- The magnitude of cardiovascular risk reduction in people with coronary artery disease correlates directly with the magnitude of blood pressure reduction.

- Cardiac rehabilitation (including exercise), pyschosocial treatments and smoking cessation all reduce the risk of cardiac events in people with CHD.

  Antioxidant vitamins (such as vitamin E, beta-carotene or vitamin C) do not appear to have any effect on cardiovascular events in high-risk people, and in some cases may actually increase risk of cardiac mortality.

  We don't know whether changing diet alters the risk of cardiac episodes, although a Mediterranean diet may have some survival benefit over a Western diet.

- CABG and PTCA plus stenting are both more effective than medical treatment, although PTCA leads to increased revascularisation and recurrent angina compared with CABG.

(i) **Please visit www.clinicalevidence.bmj.com for full text and references**

What are the effects of antithrombotic treatment?

Beneficial	• Aspirin
	• Oral anticoagulants in the absence of antiplatelet treatment

	• Thienopyridines
Likely To Be Beneficial	• Combinations of antiplatelets
Likely To Be Ineffective Or Harmful	• Oral anticoagulants in addition to antiplatelet treatment • Oral glycoprotein IIb/IIIa receptor inhibitors

What are the effects of other drug treatments?

Beneficial	• ACE inhibitors (in people with and without left ventricular dysfunction) • Amiodarone • Angiotensin II receptor blockers • Beta-blockers
Unknown Effectiveness	• Angiotensin II receptor blockers added to ACE inhibitors
Likely To Be Ineffective Or Harmful	• Calcium channel blockers • Class I antiarrhythmic agents (quinidine, procainamide, disopyramide, encainide, flecainide, and moracizine) • HRT • Sotalol

What are the effects of cholesterol reduction?

Beneficial	• Non-specific cholesterol reduction • Statins
Likely To Be Beneficial	• Fibrates

What are the effects of blood pressure reduction?

Beneficial	• Blood pressure reduction

What are the effects of non-drug treatments?

Beneficial	• Cardiac rehabilitation (including exercise)
Likely To Be Beneficial	• Advice to eat a Mediterranean diet • Psychological and stress management • Smoking cessation
Unknown Effectiveness	• Advice to eat less fat • Advice to eat more fibre

**For more information on
United Health Foundation
Go to: www.unitedhealthfoundation.com**

**Or email
ce@unitedhealthfoundation.org**

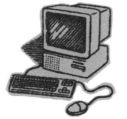

To receive future free information on evidence-based medicine from
United Health Foundation, please provide the information requested below.

Name

Address

City

State

Zip

United Health Foundation has provided you with a free, 12-month online subscription to *BMJ Clinical Evidence.*

FREE Online Access

To take full advantage of this go to www.clinicalevidence.bmj.com/uhf and type in the password: United Health Foundation 2008
To comment or change your information regarding this mailing, send an email to ce@unitedhealthfoundation.org

FREE Online Access
www.clinicalevidence.bmj.com/uhf
Password: United Health Foundation 2008

Why access *BMJ Clinical Evidence* online?
- Just-in-time information for your clinical decision making
- Summarizes scientific evidence for over 250 conditions
- Reviews are updated continuously
- New reviews added monthly
- Useful site tools available
- Register for e-mail alerts
- Evidence-Based Medicine training resources available

Please add postage for mailing

United Health Foundation™
MN008-T800
PO Box 1459
Minneapolis, MN 55440-1459

United Health Foundation
Clinical Evidence
MN008-T800
PO Box 1459
Minneapolis, MN 55440-1459

clinical.
evidence
handbook

BMJ

	• Advice to increase fish-oil consumption (from oily fish or capsules)
Unlikely To Be Beneficial	• Antioxidant vitamin combinations • Multivitamins • Vitamin C
Likely To Be Ineffective Or Harmful	• Beta-carotene • Vitamin E

What are the effects of revascularisation procedures?

Beneficial	• CABG versus medical treatment alone • Intracoronary stents (versus PTCA alone)
Likely To Be Beneficial	• CABG (versus PTCA with or without stenting for multivessel disease) • PTCA versus medical treatment

Search date July 2004

DEFINITION Secondary prevention in this context is the long-term treatment to prevent recurrent cardiac morbidity and mortality and to improve quality of life in people who either had a prior acute MI or are at high risk of ischaemic cardiac events for other reasons, such as severe coronary artery stenoses, angina, or prior coronary surgical procedures.

INCIDENCE/PREVALENCE Coronary artery disease is the leading cause of mortality in resource-rich countries and is becoming a major cause of morbidity and mortality in resource-poor countries. There are international, regional, and temporal differences in incidence, prevalence, and death rates. In the USA, the prevalence of coronary artery disease is over 6%, and the annual incidence is over 0.33%.

AETIOLOGY/RISK FACTORS Most ischaemic cardiac events are associated with atheromatous plaques that can lead to acute obstruction of coronary arteries. Coronary artery disease is more likely in people who are older or who have risk factors, such as smoking, hypertension, high cholesterol, and diabetes mellitus.

PROGNOSIS Within 1 year of having a first MI, 25% of men and 38% of women will die. Within 6 years of having a first MI, 18% of men and 35% of women will have another MI, 22% of men and 46% of women will have heart failure, and 7% of men and 6% of women will die suddenly.

Stroke management

Elizabeth Warburton

KEY POINTS

- Stroke is characterised by rapidly developing clinical symptoms and signs of focal, and at times global, loss of cerebral function lasting more than 24 hours or leading to death, with no apparent cause other than that of vascular origin.

    Ischaemic stroke (which accounts for about 80% of all acute strokes) is caused by vascular insufficiency (such as cerebrovascular thromboembolism) rather than haemorrhage.

    It is the third most common cause of death in most resource-rich countries, with approximately 4.5 million people worldwide dying from stroke each year.

    About 10% of all people with acute ischaemic strokes will die within 30 days of onset, and of those who survive the acute event, about 50% will still experience some level of disability after 6 months.

- Specialised stroke rehabilitation seems more effective than conventional care at reducing death and dependency after 1 year.

- Aspirin effectively reduces death or dependency at 6 months when given within 48 hours of ischaemic stroke.

    It has a similar effectiveness as anticoagulants, but has a lower risk of intra- and extracranial haemorrhage.

- Thrombolysis (given within 3 hours of symptom onset) reduces dependency at 6 months in people with confirmed ischaemic stroke, but increases the risk of symptomatic haemorrhage.

    The reduction in dependency may not to apply to streptokinase treatment.

- While there does seem to be a direct link between blood pressure and risk of recurrent stroke, acute blood pressure lowering in acute ischaemic stroke may actually lead to increased cerebral ischaemia.

- Neuroprotective drugs do not appear to significantly reduce the risk of poor outcome (including death) or improve outcome in people with ischaemic stroke.

- In people with supratentorial haematomas, surgical evacuation does not appear an effective treatment for the majority, but may still be indicated in a few specific clinical situations.

    We found no evidence examining the effects of evacuation in people with infratentorial haematoma whose consciousness level is declining.

(i) **Please visit www.clinicalevidence.bmj.com for full text and references**

What are the effects of specialised care in people with acute stroke?

Beneficial	• Specialised care (specialist stroke rehabilitation)

What are the effects of medical treatment in people with acute ischaemic stroke?

Beneficial	• Aspirin
Trade-off Between Benefits And Harms	• Systemic anticoagulation (unfractionated heparin, low molecular weight heparin, heparinoids, oral anticoagulants, or specific thrombin inhibitors)

	• Thrombolysis (increased overall mortality and fatal haemorrhages but reduced dependency in survivors; beneficial effects on dependency do not extend to streptokinase)
Unlikely To Be Beneficial	• Neuroprotective agents (calcium channel antagonists, citicoline, GABA agonists, glycine antagonists, lubeluzole, magnesium, N-methyl-D-aspartate antagonists, tirilazad)
Likely To Be Ineffective Or Harmful	• Acute reduction in blood pressure

What are the effects of surgical treatment for intracerebral haematomas?

Unlikely To Be Beneficial	• Evacuation (evidence early surgical evacuation unlikely to be beneficial compared with conservative treatment in supratentoral haematomas; insufficient evidence in infratentoral haematomas)

Search date May 2006

DEFINITION Stroke is characterised by rapidly developing clinical symptoms and signs of focal, and at times global, loss of cerebral function lasting more than 24 hours or leading to death, with no apparent cause other than that of vascular origin. Ischaemic stroke is stroke caused by vascular insufficiency (such as cerebrovascular thromboembolism) rather than by haemorrhage.

INCIDENCE/PREVALENCE Stroke is the third most common cause of death in most resource-rich countries. It is a worldwide problem; about 4.5 million people die from stroke each year. Stroke can occur at any age, but half of all strokes occur in people over 70 years old.

AETIOLOGY/RISK FACTORS About 80% of all acute strokes are ischaemic, usually resulting from thrombotic or embolic occlusion of a cerebral artery. The remainder are caused either by intracerebral or subarachnoid haemorrhage.

PROGNOSIS About 10% of all people with acute ischaemic strokes will die within 30 days of stroke onset. Of those who survive the acute event, about 50% will experience some level of disability after 6 months.

50 | Stroke prevention

Gregory YH Lip, Peter Rothwell, and Cathie Sudlow

KEY POINTS

- **Prevention in this context is the long-term management of people with previous stroke or transient ischaemic attack, and of people at high risk of stroke for other reasons, such as atrial fibrillation.**

  Risk factors for stroke include previous stroke or transient ischaemic attack, increasing age, hypertension, diabetes, cigarette smoking, and emboli associated with atrial fibrillation, artificial heart valves, or MI.

- **Antiplatelet treatment effectively reduces the risk of stroke in people with previous stroke or transient ischaemic attack.**

  We found no evidence showing whether alternative antiplatelet regimens to aspirin were any more or less effective than aspirin alone.

  High-dose aspirin (500–1500 mg/day) does not appear to be any more beneficial compared with low-dose aspirin (75–150 mg/day), although it may increase adverse gastrointestinal effects.

- **Blood pressure reduction treatments are effective for reducing the risk of serious vascular events in people with previous stroke or transient ischaemic attack.**

  Blood pressure reduction seems beneficial irrespective of the type of qualifying cerebrovascular event (ischaemic or haemorrhagic), or even whether people are hypertensive.

  Aggressive blood pressure lowering should probably not be considered in people with acute stenosis of the carotid or vertebral arteries, because of the possibility of precipitating a stroke.

- **Carotid endartectomy effectively reduces the risk of stroke in people with greater than 50% carotid stenosis, is not effective in people with 30–49% carotid stenosis, and increases the risk of stroke in people with less than 30% stenosis. However, it does not appear to be beneficial in people with near occlusion.**

- **Cholesterol reduction using statins seems to reduce the risk of stroke irrespective of baseline cholesterol or coronary artery disease.**

  Non-statin cholesterol reduction does not appear to reduce the risk of stroke.

- **We found no sufficient evidence to judge the efficacy of carotid and vertebral PTCA in people with recent carotid or vertebral transient ischaemic attack or stenosis.**

- **Anticoagulation does not appear beneficial in reducing stroke in people with previous ischaemic stroke and normal sinus rhythm, but does increase the risk of intra- and extracranial haemorrhage.**

- **In people with atrial fibrillation, oral anticoagulants reduce the risk of stroke regardless of whether they have previously had a stroke or transient ischaemic attack.**

  Aspirin may be effective in people with atrial fibrillation but no previous stroke when there are contraindications to anticoagulants, but we don't know whether it is effective in people with previous stroke or transient ischaemic attack.

(i) **Please visit www.clinicalevidence.bmj.com for full text and references**

What are the effects of preventive interventions in people with previous stroke or transient ischaemic attack?

| Beneficial | • Antiplatelet treatment |
| | • Blood pressure reduction |

	• Carotid endarterectomy in people with moderately severe (50–69%) symptomatic carotid artery stenosis • Carotid endarterectomy in people with severe (greater than 70%) symptomatic carotid artery stenosis • Cholesterol reduction
Likely To Be Beneficial	• Carotid endarterectomy in people with asymptomatic but severe carotid artery stenosis
Unknown Effectiveness	• Alternative antiplatelet regimens to aspirin (no evidence that any regimen is more or less effective than aspirin alone) • Carotid and vertebral PTCA • Different blood pressure-lowering regimens (no evidence that any regimen is more or less effective than any other)
Unlikely To Be Beneficial	• Carotid endarterectomy in people with moderate (30–49%) symptomatic carotid artery stenosis • Carotid endarterectomy in people with symptomatic near occlusion of the carotid artery • High-dose versus low-dose aspirin (no additional benefit but may increase harms)
Likely To Be Ineffective Or Harmful	• Anticoagulation in people in sinus rhythm • Carotid endarterectomy in people with less than 30% symptomatic carotid artery stenosis

What are the effects of preventive anticoagulant and antiplatelet treatments in people with atrial fibrillation and previous stroke or transient ischaemic attack?

Beneficial	• Oral anticoagulants
Unknown Effectiveness	• Aspirin

What are the effects of preventive anticoagulant and antiplatelet treatment in people with atrial fibrillation and without previous stroke or transient ischaemic attack?

Likely To Be Beneficial	• Aspirin in people with contraindications to anticoagulants • Oral anticoagulation

Search date September 2005

DEFINITION Prevention in this context is the long-term management of people with previous stroke or transient ischaemic attack, and of people at high risk of stroke for other reasons such as atrial fibrillation. **Stroke:** See definition under review on stroke management, p 48. **Transient ischaemic attack:** This is similar to a mild ischaemic stroke, except that symptoms last for less than 24 hours.

INCIDENCE/PREVALENCE See incidence/prevalence under stroke management, p 48.

AETIOLOGY/RISK FACTORS See aetiology under stroke management, p 48. Risk factors for stroke include previous stroke or transient ischaemic attack, increasing age, hypertension, diabetes, cigarette smoking, and emboli associated with atrial fibrillation, artificial heart valves, or MI. The relationship with cholesterol is less clear. Overviews of prospective studies of healthy middle-aged people found no association between total cholesterol and overall stroke risk. However, two of the overviews found that increased cholesterol increased the risk of ischaemic stroke but reduced the risk of haemorrhagic stroke.

PROGNOSIS People with a history of stroke or transient ischaemic attack are at high risk of all vascular events, such as MI, but are at particular risk of subsequent stroke (about 10% in the first year and about 5% each year thereafter). People with intermittent atrial fibrillation treated with aspirin should be considered at similar risk of stroke compared with people with sustained atrial fibrillation treated with aspirin (rate of ischaemic stroke/year: 3.2% with intermittent *v* 3.3% with sustained).

KEY POINTS

- DVT or pulmonary embolism may occur in almost 2% of people each year, with up to 25% of people having a recurrence.

  About 5–15% of people with untreated DVT may die from pulmonary embolism.

  The risk of recurrence of thromboembolism falls over time, but the risk of bleeding from anticoagulation remains constant.

- Oral anticoagulants are considered effective in people with proximal DVT, although few studies have been found that confirm this.

  In people with proximal DVT or pulmonary embolism, long-term anticoagulation reduces the risk of recurrence, but high-intensity treatment has not been shown to be beneficial. Both approaches increase the risk of major bleeding.

  Low molecular weight heparin is more effective than unfractionated heparin, and may be as effective as oral anticoagulants, although both are associated with some adverse effects.

  There are insufficient data to support the tapering off of oral anticoagulant agents.

  We don't know whether once-daily low molecular weight heparin is as effective as twice-daily administration, or whether home treatment is as effective as hospital-based treatment at preventing recurrence.

  Venae cavae filters reduce the short-term rate of pulmonary embolism, but may increase the long-term risk of recurrent DVT.

  Elastic compression stockings reduce the incidence of post-thrombotic syndrome after a DVT.

- In people with isolated calf DVT, anticoagulation with warfarin may reduce the risk of proximal extension, although prolonged treatment does not appear to be any more beneficial than short-term treatment.

- Anticoagulation may reduce mortality compared with no anticoagulation in people with a pulmonary embolus, but increases the risk of bleeding. Few studies have been found that evaluate treatments for pulmonary embolism.

  Low molecular weight heparin may be as effective and safe as unfractionated heparin.

  Thrombolysis seems as effective as heparin in treating people with major pulmonary embolism, but is also associated with adverse effects.

  Use of computerised decision support may increase the time spent adequately anticoagulated, but has not been shown to reduce death or major haemorrhage.

(i) **Please visit www.clinicalevidence.bmj.com for full text and references**

What are the effects of treatments for proximal DVT?

Beneficial	• Compression stockings

	• Low molecular weight heparin (reduced mortality, recurrence, and risk of major haemorrhage compared with unfractionated heparin)
Likely To Be Beneficial	• Oral anticoagulants*
Trade-off Between Benefits And Harms	• Long-term low molecular weight heparin versus long-term oral anticoagulation (both showed similar levels of benefits but with important adverse effects)
	• Long-term oral anticoagulation versus short-term oral anticoagulation
	• Venae cavae filters
Unknown Effectiveness	• Abrupt discontinuation of oral anticoagulation
	• Home treatment with short-term low molecular weight heparin
	• Once-daily versus twice-daily low molecular weight heparin
Unlikely To Be Beneficial	• High-intensity oral anticoagulation

What are the effects of treatments for isolated calf DVT?

Likely To Be Beneficial	• Warfarin (reduced rate of proximal extension compared with no further treatment in people who had received initial heparin and wore compression stockings)
Unlikely To Be Beneficial	• Prolonged duration of anticoagulation

What are the effects of treatments for pulmonary embolism?

Trade-off Between Benefits And Harms	• Anticoagulation*
	• Prolonged duration of anticoagulation
	• Thrombolysis
Unknown Effectiveness	• Low molecular weight heparin (no clear evidence of a difference in mortality or new episodes of thromboembolism or a difference in risk of major haemorrhage compared with unfractionated heparin)
Unlikely To Be Beneficial	• High-intensity anticoagulation (based on extrapolated data from people with proximal DVT)

What are the effects of computerised decision support on oral anticoagulation management?

Unknown Effectiveness	• Computerised decision support in oral anticoagulation (increased time spent in target international normalised range, but effect on clinical outcomes unknown)

Search date September 2006

*Clinical consensus based on observational data.

DEFINITION Venous thromboembolism is any thromboembolic event occurring within the venous system, including DVT and pulmonary embolism. **DVT** is a radiologically confirmed partial or total thrombotic occlusion of the deep venous system of the legs sufficient to produce symptoms of pain or swelling. **Proximal DVT** affects the veins above the knee (popliteal, superficial femoral, common femoral, and iliac veins). **Isolated calf DVT** is confined to the deep veins of the calf and does not affect the veins above the knee. **Pulmonary embolism** is radiologically confirmed partial or total thromboembolic occlusion of pulmonary arteries, sufficient to cause symptoms of breathlessness, chest pain, or both. **Post-thrombotic syndrome** is oedema, ulceration, and impaired viability of the subcutaneous tissues of the leg occurring after DVT. **Recurrence** refers to symptomatic deterioration owing to a further (radiologically confirmed) thrombosis, after a previously confirmed thromboembolic event, where there had been an initial partial or total symptomatic improvement. **Extension** refers to a radiologically confirmed, new, constant, symptomatic intraluminal filling defect extending from an existing thrombosis.

INCIDENCE/PREVALENCE We found no reliable study of the incidence or prevalence of DVT or pulmonary embolism in the UK. A prospective Scandinavian study found an annual incidence of 1.6–1.8/1000 people in the general population. One postmortem study estimated that 600,000 people develop pulmonary embolism each year in the USA, of whom 60,000 die as a result.

AETIOLOGY/RISK FACTORS Risk factors for DVT include immobility, surgery (particularly orthopaedic), malignancy, pregnancy, older age, and inherited or acquired prothrombotic clotting disorders. The oral contraceptive pill is associated with increased risk of death from venous thromboembolism (ARI with any combined oral contraception: 1–3 deaths/million women/year). The principal cause of pulmonary embolism is a DVT.

PROGNOSIS The annual recurrence rate of symptomatic calf DVT in people without recent surgery is over 25%. Proximal extension develops in 40–50% of people with symptomatic calf DVT. Proximal DVT may cause fatal or non-fatal pulmonary embolism, recurrent venous thrombosis, and post-thrombotic syndrome. One case series (462 people) published in 1946 found 5.8% mortality from pulmonary emboli in people in a maternity hospital with untreated DVT. More recent cohorts of treated people have reported mortality of 4.4% at 15 days and 10% at 30 days. One non-systematic review of observational studies found that, in people after recent surgery who have an asymptomatic deep calf vein thrombosis, the rate of fatal pulmonary embolism was 13–15%. The incidence of other complications without treatment is not known. The risk of recurrent venous thrombosis and complications is increased by thrombotic risk factors.

Paul Tisi

KEY POINTS

- Varicose veins are considered to be enlarged tortuous superficial veins of the leg.

  Varicose veins are caused by poorly functioning valves in the veins, and decreased elasticity of the vein wall, allowing pooling of blood within the veins, and their subsequent enlargement.

  Varicose veins affect up to 40% of adults and are more common in obese people, and in women who have had more than two pregnancies.

- Compression stockings are often used as first-line treatment for varicose veins, but we don't know whether they reduce symptoms compared with no treatment.

- Injection sclerotherapy may be more effective than compression stockings, but less effective than surgery, at improving symptoms and cosmetic appearance.

  We don't know which sclerotherapy agent is the best to use.

- Surgery (saphenofemoral ligation, stripping of the long saphenous vein, oravulsion) is likely to be beneficial in reducing recurrence and improving cosmetic appearance, compared with sclerotherapy alone.

  We don't know whether stripping the long saphenous vein after saphenofemoral ligation improves outcomes compared with avulsion alone after ligation, or what the best method is for vein stripping.

  Powered phlebectomy may be as effective as avulsion, but may cause pain, bruising, and discoloration.

  We don't know whether radiofrequency ablation or self-help are effective in people with varicose veins.

(i) **Please visit www.clinicalevidence.bmj.com for full text and references**

What are the effects of treatments in adults with varicose veins?	
Likely To Be Beneficial	• Surgery (avulsion)* • Surgery (stripping)*
Trade-off Between Benefits And Harms	• Surgery (powered phlebectomy)
Unknown Effectiveness	• Compression stockings • Endovenous laser • Injection sclerotherapy • Radiofrequency ablation • Self-help (exercise, diet, elevation of legs, avoidance of tight clothing, advice)

Search date May 2007

*Categorisation based on consensus.

DEFINITION Although we found no consistent definition of varicose veins, it is commonly taken to mean enlarged tortuous subcutaneous veins. Any vein may become varicose, but the term "varicose veins" conventionally applies to the superficial veins of the leg, which may appear green, dark blue, or purple in colour. The condition is caused by poorly functioning (incompetent) valves within the veins and decreased elasticity of the vein walls, which allow de-oxygenated blood to be pumped back to the heart, and to flow backward and pool in the superficial veins, causing them to enlarge and become varicose. This often occurs in the saphenofemoral and saphenopopliteal junctions, and in the perforating veins that connect the deep and superficial venous systems along the length of the leg. The presence or absence of reflux caused by venous incompetence can be determined by clinical examination, handheld Doppler, or duplex ultrasound. Symptoms of varicose veins include pain, itching, limb heaviness, cramps, and distress about cosmetic appearance, although most lower-limb symptoms may have a non-venous cause. This review focuses on uncomplicated, symptomatic varicose veins. We have excluded treatments for chronic venous ulceration and other complications. We have also excluded studies that solely examine treatments for small, dilated veins in the skin of the leg, known as thread veins, spider veins, or superficial telangiectasia.

INCIDENCE/PREVALENCE One large US cohort study found the biannual incidence of varicose veins was 3% in women and 2% in men. The prevalence of varicose veins in Western populations was estimated in one study to be about 25–30% in women and 10–20% in men. However, a recent Scottish cohort study has found a higher prevalence of varices of the saphenous trunks and their main branches in men than in women (40% men v 32% women). Other epidemiological studies have shown prevalence rates ranging from 1% to 40% in men, and 1% to 73% in women.

AETIOLOGY/RISK FACTORS One cohort study found that parity with three or more births was an independent risk factor for development of varicose veins. A further large case-control study found that women with two or more pregnancies were at increased risk of varicose veins compared with women with one or no pregnancies (RR about 1.2–1.3 after adjustment for age, height, and weight). It found that obesity was also a risk factor, although only in women (RR about 1.3). One narrative systematic review found insufficient evidence on the effects of other suggested risk factors, including genetic predisposition, prolonged sitting or standing, tight undergarments, low-fibre diet, constipation, DVT, and smoking. However, a large Danish population study found that prolonged standing or walking at work was an independent predictor of the need for varicose vein treatment.

PROGNOSIS We found no reliable data on prognosis, or on the frequency of complications, which include chronic inflammation of affected veins (phlebitis), venous ulceration, and bleeding rupture of varices.

Eddy S Lang and Marwan Al Raisi

KEY POINTS

- Pulseless ventricular tachycardia and ventricular fibrillation are the main causes of sudden cardiac death, but other ventricular tachyarrhythmias can occur without haemodynamic compromise.

  Ventricular arrhythmias occur mainly as a result of myocardial ischaemia or cardiomyopathies, so risk factors are those of CVD.

- Cardiac arrest associated with ventricular tachyarrhythmias is managed with cardiopulmonary resuscitation and electrical defibrillation, where available.

  Adrenaline is given once intravenous access is obtained or endotracheal intubation has been performed.

- Amiodarone may increase the likelihood of arriving alive at hospital in people with ventricular tachyarrhythmia that has developed outside hospital, compared with placebo or with lidocaine, but has not been shown to increase longer-term survival.

  Amiodarone is associated with hypotension and bradycardia.

- We don't know whether lidocaine or procainamide improve survival in people with ventricular tachyarrhythmias in out-of-hospital settings, as very few studies have been found.

  Procainamide is given by slow infusion, which may limit its usefulness to people with recurrent ventricular tachyarrhythmias.

- We don't know whether bretylium improves survival compared with placebo or lidocaine, and it may cause hypotension and bradycardia. It is no longer recommended for use in ventricular fibrillation or pulseless ventricular tachycardia.

(i) **Please visit www.clinicalevidence.bmj.com for full text and references**

What are the effects of antiarrhythmic drug treatments for use in out-of-hospital cardiac arrest associated with shock-resistant ventricular tachycardia or ventricular fibrillation?

Unknown Effectiveness	• Amiodarone • Lidocaine • Procainamide
Unlikely To Be Beneficial	• Bretylium

Search date May 2006

DEFINITION Ventricular tachyarrhythmias are defined as abnormal patterns of electrical activity originating within ventricular tissue. The most commonly encountered ventricular tachyarrhythmias of greatest clinical importance to clinicians, and those which will be the focus of this review are ventricular tachycardia and ventricular fibrillation. **Ventricular tachycardia** is further classified as monomorphic when occurring at a consistent rate and amplitude and polymorphic when waveforms are more variable and chaotic. **Torsades de pointes** is a specific kind of polymorphic ventricular tachycardia associated with a prolonged QT interval and a characteristic twisting pattern to the wave signal. It is often associated with drug toxicity and electrolyte disturbances and is commonly treated with intravenous magnesium. Torsades de pointes will not be specifically covered in this review. **Pulseless ventricular tachycardia** results in similar clinical manifestations, but is diagnosed by a QRS width complex of greater than 120 milliseconds and electrical rhythm of 150–200 beats a minute. Waveforms in ventricular fibrillation are characterised by an irregular rate, usually exceeding 300 beats a minute as well as amplitudes generally exceeding 0.2 mV. Ventricular fibrillation usually fades to asystole (flat line) within 15 minutes. Ventricular fibrillation and ventricular tachycardia associated with cardiac arrest and sudden cardiac death (SCD) are abrupt pulseless arrhythmias. **Non-pulseless (stable) ventricular tachycardia** has the same electrical characteristics as ventricular tachycardia but without haemodynamic compromise. The treatment of stable ventricular tachycardia is not covered in this review. **Ventricular fibrillation** is characterised by irregular and chaotic electrical activity and ventricular contraction in which the heart immediately loses its ability to function as a pump. Pulseless ventricular tachycardia and ventricular fibrillation are the primary causes of SCD. **Population:** In this review we focus on drug treatments, given generally by paramedics, for ventricular tachycardia and ventricular fibrillation associated with cardiac arrest in an out-of-hospital setting.

INCIDENCE/PREVALENCE The annual incidence of SCD is believed to approach 2/1000 population but can vary depending on the prevalence of CVD in the population. It is estimated that 300,000 SCDs are recorded annually in the US, representing 50% of all cardiovascular mortality in that country. Data from Holter monitor studies suggest that about 85% of SCDs are the result of ventricular tachycardia/ventricular fibrillation.

AETIOLOGY/RISK FACTORS Ventricular arrhythmias occur as a result of structural heart disease arising primarily from myocardial ischaemia or cardiomyopathies. In resouce-rich countries, ventricular tachycardia or ventricular fibrillation-associated cardiac arrest is believed to occur most typically in the context of myocardial ischaemia. As a result, major risk factors for SCD reflect those that lead to progressive coronary artery disease. Specific additional risk factors attributed to SCD include dilated cardiomyopathy (especially with ejection fractions of below 30%), age (peak incidence 45–75 years), and male sex.

PROGNOSIS Ventricular fibrillation and ventricular tachycardia associated with cardiac arrest results in lack of oxygen delivery and major ischaemic injury to vital organs. If untreated this condition is uniformly fatal within minutes.

KEY POINTS

- Absence seizures are characterised by sudden, brief, frequent periods of unconsciousness, which may be accompanied by automatic movements. They may occur alone, or, in a child with other epileptic syndromes, may coexist with other types of seizures.

  Absence seizures have a typical spike and wave pattern on the EEG. Atypical absence seizures have different EEG changes and clinical manifestations, and have a different natural history and response to treatment.

  Absence seizures can be differentiated from complex partial seizures by their abrupt ending and lack of a postictal phase.

  About 10% of seizures in children with epilepsy are typical absence seizures, with genetic factors considered to be the main cause. Where they are the only manifestation of epilepsy, they generally resolve spontaneously by the age of 12 years.

- Lamotrigine increases the likelihood of being seizure free compared with placebo, but it can cause serious skin reactions.

- There is consensus that ethosuximide and sodium valproate are beneficial in childhood absence seizures, although we don't know this for sure.

  Ethosuximide is associated with aplastic anaemia, skin reactions, and renal and hepatic impairment.

  Valproate is associated with behavioural and cognitive abnormalities, liver necrosis, and pancreatitis.

- We don't know whether clonazepam or gabapentin reduce the frequency of absence seizures.

(i) **Please visit www.clinicalevidence.bmj.com for full text and references**

What are the effects of treatments for typical absence seizures in children?	
Trade-off Between Benefits And Harms	• Ethosuximide
	• Lamotrigine
	• Valproate
Unknown Effectiveness	• Clonazepam
	• Gabapentin

Search date October 2007

DEFINITION Absence seizures are sudden, frequent episodes of unconsciousness lasting a few seconds, and are often accompanied by simple automatisms or clonic, atonic, or autonomic components. Typical absence seizures display a characteristic EEG showing regular symmetrical generalised spike and wave complexes with a frequency of 3 Hz, and usually occur in children with normal development and intelligence. Typical absence seizures are often confused with complex partial seizures — especially in cases of prolonged seizure with automatisms. However, the abrupt ending of typical absence seizures, without a postictal phase, is the most useful clinical feature in distinguishing the two types. Typical absence seizures should not be confused with atypical absence seizures — which differ markedly in EEG findings and ictal behaviour, and usually present with other seizure types in a child with a background of learning disability and severe epilepsy. Typical absence seizures may be the sole seizure type experienced by a child. If this is the case, and the child is of normal development and has no structural lesions, the child is said to have childhood absence epilepsy. Alternatively, typical absence seizures may coexist in children with other epileptic syndromes — such as juvenile myoclonic epilepsy or juvenile absence epilepsy, in which other seizure types are also present. This differentiation into typical versus atypical seizures is important, as the natural history and response to treatment vary between the two groups. Interventions for atypical absence seizures or for absence seizures secondary to structural lesions are not included in this review.

INCIDENCE/PREVALENCE About 10% of seizures in children with epilepsy are typical absence seizures. Annual incidence has been estimated at 0.7–4.6/100,000 people in the general population, and 6–8/100,000 in children aged 0–15 years. Prevalence is 5–50/100,000 people in the general population. Similar figures were found in the USA (Connecticut) and in Europe-based (Scandinavia, France) population studies. Age of onset ranges from 3–13 years, with a peak at 6–7 years.

AETIOLOGY/RISK FACTORS The cause of childhood absence epilepsy is presumed to be genetic. In susceptible children, seizures can be triggered by hyperventilation. Some anticonvulsants, such as phenytoin, carbamazepine, and vigabatrin are associated with an increased risk of absence seizures.

PROGNOSIS In childhood absence epilepsy, in which typical absence seizures are the only type of seizures suffered by the child, seizures generally cease spontaneously by 12 years of age or sooner. Less than 10% of children develop infrequent generalised tonic clonic seizures, and it is rare for them to continue having absence seizures. In other epileptic syndromes (in which absence seizures may coexist with other types of seizure) prognosis is varied, depending on the syndrome. Absence seizures have a significant impact on quality of life. The episode of unconsciousness may occur at any time, and usually without warning. Affected children need to take precautions to prevent injury during absences, and should refrain from activities that would put them at risk if seizures occur (e.g. climbing heights, swimming unsupervised, or cycling on busy roads). Often, school staff members are the first to notice the recurrent episodes of absence seizures, and treatment is generally initiated because of the adverse impact on learning.

Deborah Pritchard

KEY POINTS

- Core symptoms of ADHD are inattention, hyperactivity, and impulsivity, although other conditions frequently coexist with ADHD, including oppositional defiant disorder, and conduct, anxiety, and depressive disorders.

   Symptoms must be present for at least 6 months, observed in children before the age of 7 years, and clinically important impairment in social, academic or occupational functioning must be evident in more than one setting.

   Prevalence estimates among school children range from 3–5%.

- Methylphenidate improves core symptoms and school performance in children with ADHD when used alone, and may be beneficial when added to psychological/behavioural treatment.

   Dexamfetamine and atomoxetine may also reduce symptoms of ADHD, but can cause adverse effects.

   We don't know how effective any treatment for ADHD is in the long term.

- CAUTION: Atomoxetine may cause rare but serious liver injury.

- Clonidine may improve symptoms of ADHD compared with placebo, but we don't know for sure that it makes a clinically significant difference, and it may cause bradycardia.

- We don't know how effective psychological/behavioural treatments are compared with each other or with pharmacological treatments, as few high-quality studies have been done.

   The combination of methylphenidate plus behavioural treatment seems to work better than behavioural treatment alone in reducing core symptoms and improving behaviour in children with ADHD.

(i) **Please visit www.clinicalevidence.bmj.com for full text and references**

What are the effects of treatments for ADHD in children?	
Likely To Be Beneficial	• Atomoxetine • Dexamfetamine sulphate • Methylphenidate • Methylphenidate plus psychological/behavioural treatment
Unknown Effectiveness	• Clonidine • Psychological/behavioural treatment

Search date May 2005

DEFINITION ADHD is "a persistent pattern of inattention and hyperactivity and impulsivity that is more frequent and severe than is typically observed in people at a comparable level of development" (DSM-IV). Inattention, hyperactivity, and impulsivity are commonly known as the core symptoms of ADHD. Symptoms must be present for at least 6 months, observed before the age of 7 years, and "clinically important impairment in social, academic, or occupational functioning" must be evident in more than one setting. The symptoms must not be better explained by another disorder, such as an anxiety disorder, mood disorder, psychosis, or autistic disorder. The ICD-10 uses the term "hyperkinetic disorder" for a more restricted diagnosis. It differs from the DSM-IV classification in that all three problems of attention, hyperactivity, and impulsiveness must be present, more stringent criteria for "pervasiveness" across situations must be met, and the presence of another disorder is an exclusion criterion. The evidence presented in this review largely relates to children aged 5 years and above. There is a paucity of evidence of efficacy and safety of treatments in pre-school children.

INCIDENCE/PREVALENCE Prevalence estimates of ADHD vary according to the diagnostic criteria used and the population sampled. DSM-IV prevalence estimates among school children in the US are 3–5%, but other estimates vary from 1.7% to 16.0%. No objective test exists to confirm the diagnosis of ADHD, which remains a clinical diagnosis. Other conditions frequently co-exist with ADHD. Oppositional defiant disorder is present in 35% (95% CI 27% to 44%) of children with ADHD, conduct disorder in 26% (95% CI 13% to 41%), anxiety disorder in 26% (95% CI 18% to 35%), and depressive disorder in 18% (95% CI 11% to 27%).

AETIOLOGY/RISK FACTORS The underlying causes of ADHD are not known. There is limited evidence that it has a genetic component. Risk factors also include psychosocial factors. There is increased risk in boys compared with girls, with ratios varying from 3:1 to 4:1.

PROGNOSIS More than 70% of hyperactive children may continue to meet criteria for ADHD in adolescence, and up to 65% of adolescents may continue to meet criteria for ADHD in adulthood. Changes in diagnostic criteria cause difficulty with interpretation of the few outcome studies that exist. One cohort of boys followed up for an average of 16 years found a ninefold increase in antisocial personality disorder, and a fourfold increase in substance misuse disorder.

Clare Bradley-Stevenson, Paddy O'Neill, and Tony Roberts.

KEY POINTS

- AOM is characterised by sudden onset of earache with a cloudy or bulging erythematous eardrum caused by middle-ear infection.

  Middle-ear effusion without signs of infection lasting more than 3 months suggests OME (glue ear), while chronic suppurative otitis media is characterised by continuing middle-ear inflammation and discharge through a perforated eardrum. These disorders are assessed in other reviews in *BMJ Clinical Evidence*.

  The most common pathogens in AOM in the USA and UK are *Streptococcus pneumoniae*, *Haemophilus influenzae*, and *Moraxella catarhalis*.

  In the UK, about 30% of children aged under 3 years visit their GP each year with AOM, and 97% of these receive antibiotics. In the USA, AOM is the most common reason for outpatient antibiotic treatment.

- Without antibiotics, AOM resolves within 24 hours in about 60% of children, and within 3 days in about 80% of children.

  Analgesics and topical anaesthetics may reduce earache when given with antibiotics.

- Antibiotics may lead to more rapid reduction in symptoms of AOM, but increase the risk of adverse effects.

  Antibiotics seem to reduce pain at 2–7 days, and may prevent development of contralateral AOM, but increase the risks of vomiting, diarrhoea, and rashes compared with placebo.

  Immediate antibiotic use seems most beneficial in children younger than 2 years with bilateral AOM.

  We do not know whether any one antibiotic regimen should be used in preference to another.

  Longer courses of antibiotics reduce short-term treatment failure, but have no benefit over the longer term compared with shorter regimens.

  Immediate use of antibiotics may reduce some, but not all symptoms of AOM, but increases the risk of vomiting, diarrhoea, and rashes compared with delayed treatment.

- Myringotomy appears to be less effective than antibiotics in reducing symptoms. Tympanostomy with ventilation tube insertion leads to short-term reduction in the number of episodes of AOM, but increases the risk of complications.

  We found limited evidence that there was only a short-term benefit from tympanostomy with ventilation tubes, with possibly increased risks of tympanosclerosis.

- Long-term antibiotic prophylaxis may reduce recurrence rates; however, the possibility of adverse effects and antibiotic resistance should be taken into account.

  We do not know whether any one regimen should be used in preference to another to prevent recurrent attacks.

- In children aged from 2 months to 7 years, large scale pneumococcal vaccination strategies are unlikely to be effective.

(i) **Please visit www.clinicalevidence.bmj.com for full text and references**

What are the effects of treatments for AOM in children?	
Likely To Be Beneficial	• Analgesics
Trade-off Between Benefits And Harms	• Antibiotics (reduce symptoms more quickly than placebo but increase adverse effects)

	• Choice of antibiotic regimen
	• Immediate compared with delayed antibiotic treatment
	• Longer courses of antibiotics (reduce treatment failure in the short term but not the long term)
Likely To Be Ineffective Or Harmful	• Myringotomy

What are the effects of interventions to prevent recurrence of AOM in children?

Trade-off Between Benefits And Harms	• Antibiotic prophylaxis (long term)
Unlikely To Be Beneficial	• Vaccination (pneumococcal)
Likely To Be Ineffective Or Harmful	• Tympanostomy (ventilation tubes)

Search date January 2007

DEFINITION Otitis media is an inflammation in the middle ear. Subcategories include AOM, recurrent AOM, and chronic suppurative otitis media (CSOM). AOM is the presence of middle-ear effusion in conjunction with rapid onset of one or more signs or symptoms of inflammation of the middle ear. AOM presents with systemic and local signs, and has a rapid onset. The diagnosis is made on the basis of signs and symptoms, principally earache in the presence of a cloudy or bulging eardrum (and immobility of the eardrum if pneumatic otoscopy is performed). Erythema is a moderately useful sign for helping establish the diagnosis. If the eardrum has a normal colour, then risk of AOM is low. Uncomplicated AOM is limited to the middle-ear cleft. The persistence of an effusion beyond 3 months without signs of infection defines OME (also known as glue ear; see review on OME, p 115), which can arise as a consequence of AOM, but can also occur independently. CSOM is characterised by continuing inflammation in the middle ear causing discharge (otorrhoea) through a perforated tympanic membrane (see review on chronic suppurative otitis media, p 190). This review deals only with AOM in children.

INCIDENCE/PREVALENCE AOM is common, and has a high morbidity and low mortality in otherwise healthy children. In the UK, about 30% of children under 3 years visit their general practitioner with AOM each year, and 97% receive antimicrobial treatment. By 3 months, 10% of children have had an episode of AOM. It is the most common reason for outpatient antimicrobial treatment in the USA.

AETIOLOGY/RISK FACTORS The most common bacterial causes of AOM in the USA and UK are *Streptococcus pneumoniae*, *Haemophilus influenzae*, and *Moraxella catarrhalis*. Similar pathogens are found in Colombia. There is some evidence that the predominant causative pathogen in recurrent AOM is changing from *Streptococcus pneumoniae* to *Haemophilus influenzae* after the release and widespread use of pneumococcal conjugate vaccine. The established risk factors for recurrent AOM that are capable of being modified are the use of pacifiers, and care in daycare centres. Probable risk factors are privation of mother's milk, presence of siblings, craniofacial abnormalities, passive smoking, and presence of adenoids.

(continued over)

(from previous page)

PROGNOSIS Without antibiotic treatment, AOM symptoms improve in 24 hours in about 60% of children, and in about 80% of children the condition resolves in about 3 days. Suppurative complications occur in about 0.12% of children if antibiotics are withheld. Serious complications are rare in otherwise healthy children but include hearing loss, mastoiditis, meningitis, and recurrent attacks. The WHO estimates that, in resource-poor countries, 51,000 children under the age of 5 years die from complications of otitis media each year.

Duncan Keeley and Michael McKean

KEY POINTS

- Childhood asthma can be difficult to distinguish from viral wheeze and can affect up to 20% of children.

- The consensus is that oxygen, high-dose nebulised beta$_2$ agonists and systemic corticosteroids should be used to treat an acute asthma attack.

  High-dose beta$_2$ agonists may be equally effective when given intermittently or continuously via a nebuliser, or from a metered-dose inhaler using a spacer, in children with an acute asthma attack.

  Admission to hospital may be averted by adding ipratropium bromide to beta$_2$ agonists, or by using high-dose nebulised or oral corticosteroids.

- Prophylactic inhaled corticosteroids improve symptoms and lung function in children with asthma. Their effect on final adult height is unclear.

  Inhaled nedocromil, inhaled long-acting beta$_2$ agonists, oral theophylline, and oral leukotriene receptor antagonists are less effective than corticosteroids.

  Inhaled sodium cromoglycate does not seem to improve symptoms.

- CAUTION: Monotherapy with long-acting beta$_2$ agonists reduces the frequency of asthma episodes, but may increase the chance of severe asthma episodes and death when those episodes occur.

  Intravenous theophylline may improve lung function in children with severe asthma, but can cause cardiac arrhythmias and convulsions.

- We don't know whether adding higher doses of corticosteroids, long-acting beta$_2$ agonists, oral leukotriene receptor antagonists, or oral theophylline to standard treatment improves symptoms or lung function in children with uncontrolled asthma.

- In infants with acute wheeze, short-acting beta$_2$ agonists via a nebuliser or a spacer may improve symptoms, but we don't know whether high-dose inhaled or oral corticosteroids or inhaled ipratropium bromide are beneficial.

- Oral short-acting beta$_2$ agonists and inhaled high-dose corticosteroids may prevent or improve wheeze in infants, but can cause adverse effects.

  We don't know whether lower-dose inhaled or oral corticosteroids, inhaled ipratropium bromide, or inhaled short-acting beta$_2$ agonists improve wheezing episodes in infants.

(i) **Please visit www.clinicalevidence.bmj.com for full text and references**

What are the effects of treatments for acute asthma in children?

Beneficial	
	• Beta$_2$ agonists (high-dose nebulised)*
	• Corticosteroids (high-dose inhaled)
	• Corticosteroids (systemic)
	• Metered-dose inhaler plus spacer devices for delivery of beta$_2$ agonists (as effective as nebulisers)
	• Multiple-dose ipratropium bromide (inhaled) added to beta$_2$ agonists for severe acute asthma (in emergency room)

	• Oxygen*
Likely To Be Beneficial	• Theophylline (intravenous)
Unknown Effectiveness	• Ipratropium bromide (inhaled) added to salbutamol (after initial stabilisation) • Single-dose ipratropium bromide (inhaled) added to beta$_2$ agonists (in emergency room)

What are the effects of single-agent prophylaxis in children taking as-needed inhaled beta agonists for asthma?

Beneficial	• Corticosteroids (inhaled)
Likely To Be Beneficial	• Leukotriene receptor antagonists (oral montelukast in children over 2 years of age) • Nedocromil (inhaled)
Trade-off Between Benefits And Harms	• Long-acting beta$_2$ agonist (inhaled salmeterol) • Theophylline (oral)
Unlikely To Be Beneficial	• Sodium cromoglycate (inhaled)

What are the effects of additional prophylactic treatments in childhood asthma inadequately controlled by standard-dose inhaled corticosteroids?

Unknown Effectiveness	• Adding leukotriene receptor antagonists (montelukast) • Adding long-acting beta$_2$ agonist • Adding oral theophylline • Increased dose of inhaled corticosteroid (beclometasone)

What are the effects of treatments for acute wheezing in infants?

Likely To Be Beneficial	• Short-acting beta$_2$ agonists (salbutamol by nebuliser) • Short-acting beta$_2$ agonists delivered by metered-dose inhaler/spacer versus nebuliser
Unknown Effectiveness	• Corticosteroids (high-dose inhaled) • Corticosteroids (oral prednisolone) • Ipratropium bromide (inhaled)

What are the effects of prophylactic treatments for wheezing in infants?	
Likely To Be Beneficial	• Short-acting beta$_2$ agonists (oral salbutamol)
Trade-off Between Benefits And Harms	• Corticosteroids (inhaled higher dose)
Unknown Effectiveness	• Corticosteroids (inhaled lower dose) • Ipratropium bromide (inhaled) • Short-acting beta$_2$ agonists (inhaled salbutamol)

Search date October 2005

*In the absence of RCT evidence, categorisation based on observational evidence and strong consensus.

DEFINITION Differentiation between asthma and non-asthmatic viral-associated wheeze may be difficult; persisting symptoms and signs between acute attacks are suggestive of asthma, as are a personal or family history of atopic conditions such as eczema and hay fever. **Childhood asthma** is characterised by chronic or recurrent cough and wheeze. The diagnosis is confirmed by demonstrating reversible airway obstruction, preferably on several occasions over time, in children old enough to perform peak flow measurements or spirometry. Diagnosing asthma in children requires exclusion of other causes of recurrent respiratory symptoms. Acute asthma is a term used to describe a severe exacerbation of asthma symptoms accompanied by tachycardia and tachypnoea. The aim of prophylactic treatments in asthma is to minimise persistent symptoms and prevent acute exacerbations. **Wheezing in infants** is characterised by a high-pitched purring or whistling sound produced mainly on the out-breath, and is commonly associated with an acute viral infection such as bronchiolitis (see bronchiolitis, p 77) or asthma. These are not easy to distinguish clinically.

INCIDENCE/PREVALENCE Childhood asthma: Surveys have found an increase in the proportion of children diagnosed with asthma. The increase is higher than can be explained by an increased readiness to diagnose asthma. One questionnaire study from Aberdeen, Scotland, surveyed 2510 children aged 8–13 years in 1964 and 3403 children in 1989. Over the 25 years, the diagnosis of asthma rose from 4% to 10%. The increase in the prevalence of childhood asthma from the 1960s to 1980s was accompanied by an increase in hospital admissions over the same period. In England and Wales, this was a sixfold increase. **Wheezing in infants** is common and seems to be increasing, although the magnitude of any increase is not clear. One Scottish cross-sectional study (2510 children aged 8–13 years in 1964 and 3403 children in 1989) found that the prevalence of wheeze rose from 10% in 1964 to 20% in 1989, and episodes of shortness of breath rose from 5% to 10% over the same period. Difficulties in defining clear groups (phenotypes) and the transient nature of the symptoms, which often resolve spontaneously, have confounded many studies.

AETIOLOGY/RISK FACTORS Childhood asthma: Asthma is more common in children with a personal or family history of atopy, increased severity and frequency of wheezing episodes, and presence of variable airway obstruction or bronchial hyperresponsiveness. Precipitating factors for symptoms and acute episodes include infection, house dust mites, allergens from pet animals, exposure to tobacco smoke, and anxiety. **Wheezing in infants:** Most wheezing episodes in infancy are precipitated by viral respiratory infections.

PROGNOSIS Childhood asthma: A British longitudinal study of children born in 1970 found that 29% of 5-year-olds wheezing in the past year were still wheezing at the age of 10 years. Another study followed a group of children in Melbourne, Australia from the age of 7 years (in 1964) into adulthood. The study found that a large proportion (73%) of 14-year-olds with infrequent symptoms had few or no symptoms by the age of 28 years, whereas two thirds

(continued over)

(from previous page)

of those 14-year-olds with frequent wheezing still had recurrent attacks at the age of 28 years. **Wheezing in infants:** One cohort study (826 infants followed from birth to 6 years) suggests that there may be at least three prognostic categories for wheezing in infants: "persistent wheezers" (14% of total, with risk factors for atopic asthma such as elevated immunoglobulin E levels and a maternal history of asthma), who initially suffered wheeze during viral infections and in whom the wheezing persisted into school age; "transient wheezers" (20% of total, with reduced lung function as infants but no early markers of atopy), who also suffered wheeze during viral infections but stopped wheezing after the first 3 years of life; and "late-onset wheezers" (15% of total), who did not wheeze when aged under 3 years but had developed wheeze by school age. Another retrospective cohort study found that 14% of children with one attack and 23% of children with four or more attacks in the first year of life had experienced at least one wheezing illness in the past year at the age of 10 years. Administering inhaled treatments to young children can be difficult. Inconsistencies in results could reflect the effects of the differences in the drugs used, delivery devices used, dosages used, and the differences in the pattern of wheezing illnesses and treatment responses among young children.

Jeremy Parr

KEY POINTS

- Autism is one of a group of pervasive developmental disorders, and is characterised by qualitative impairments in communication and social interaction, and by repetitive and stereotyped behaviours and interests.

  Abnormal development is present before the age of 3 years. A quarter of affected children show developmental regression, with loss of previously acquired skills.

  A third of children with autism have epilepsy, and three quarters have mental retardation. Only 15% of adults with autism will lead independent lives.

  Twin and family studies suggest that most cases of autism occur because of a combination of genetic factors. Autism is not caused by perinatal factors or by the MMR vaccine.

- It may be difficult to apply the results of research in practice, as improvements in outcomes assessed in RCTs using standardised assessment tools may not correlate with improvements in function in a particular child with autism.

- Some interventions are administered by (or in conjunction with) parents, and may be carried out in the home. Consideration of the direct financial costs, indirect costs (through possible lost earnings), and the impact on relationships within the family (to siblings or spouse) must be balanced against likely and possible improvements in outcome for the child with autism.

- There is a lack of good-quality evidence on the effectiveness of early multidisciplinary intervention programmes, or for other treatments for children with autism.

  There is consensus, supported by a small RCT, that applied behavioural analysis is likely to be beneficial in children with autism.

  Attendance at a "More Than Words" training course for parents may improve communication between parents and children, as may participation in Child's Talk.

  There is consensus that the Autism Pre-school Programme and TEACCH may be effective, although no RCTs or cohort studies evaluating these interventions have been found.

  We don't know whether early intervention using the Early Bird Programme, the Portage scheme, relationship development intervention, Social stories, or Son-Rise are beneficial in children with autism.

- Methylphenidate may reduce hyperactivity in children with autism.

  Methylphenidate may increase social withdrawal and irritability. Growth and blood pressure monitoring are required.

- Risperidone may improve behaviour in children with autism compared with placebo, but its use is limited by adverse effects such as weight gain, drowsiness, and tremors.

- There is consensus that SSRIs improve symptoms in children with autism, although no RCTs have been found. The adverse effects of SSRIs, including possible increases in agitation, hostility, and suicidal ideation, are well documented.

- We don't know whether auditory integration training, sensory integration training, chelation, a gluten-and-casein free diet, digestive enzymes, omega 3 fish oil, secretin, vitamin A, vitamin B6 plus magnesium, or vitamin C are beneficial for treating children with autism, as few studies have been found.

Please visit www.clinicalevidence.bmj.com for full text and references

What are the effects of early intensive multidisciplinary intervention programmes in children with autism?

Likely To Be Beneficial	• Applied behavioural analysis* • Autism Pre-school Programme* • Child's Talk* • More than words* • Picture Exchange Communication System* • TEACCH*
Unknown Effectiveness	• Early Bird Programme • Floor time • Portage scheme • Relationship development intervention • Social-skills training • Social stories • Son-Rise

What are the effects of dietary interventions in children with autism?

Unknown Effectiveness	• Digestive enzymes • Gluten-and-casein free diet • Omega 3 (fish oil) • Probiotics • Vitamin A • Vitamin B6 (pyridoxine) plus magnesium • Vitamin C

What are the effects of drug treatments in children with autism?

Likely To Be Beneficial	• Methylphenidate (for hyperactivity only)
Trade-off Between Benefits And Harms	• Risperidone • SSRIs*
Unknown Effectiveness	• Immunoglobulins • Memantine
Unlikely To Be Beneficial	• Secretin

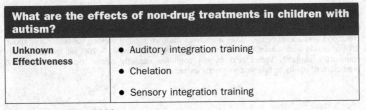

What are the effects of non-drug treatments in children with autism?

Unknown Effectiveness	• Auditory integration training
	• Chelation
	• Sensory integration training

Search date May 2006

*In the absence of robust RCT evidence in children with autism, categorisation is based on observational evidence and strong consensus that these interventions are likely to be beneficial.

DEFINITION Autism is one of the pervasive developmental disorders (PDD), a group of conditions that also includes Asperger syndrome, pervasive developmental disorder not otherwise specified (PDD-NOS), Rett syndrome, and childhood disintegrative disorder. Collectively, autism, Asperger syndrome, and PDD-NOS are often referred to as "autistic spectrum disorders" (ASD). However, Rett syndrome and childhood disintegrative disorder fall outside the autistic spectrum. Autism is characterised by qualitative impairments in communication and social interaction, and by restricted, repetitive, and stereotyped patterns of behaviours and interests. Abnormal development is present before the age of 3 years. The clinical features required for a diagnosis of autism to be made are set out in ICD-10 and DSM-IV. Individuals with autism have a history of language delay (single word or phrase speech delay), and a quarter lose previously acquired skills (regression), most commonly in the second year of life. A third of individuals develop epilepsy, and three quarters have mental retardation. Males are affected more commonly than females (3.5–4.0:1). The findings of this review apply to children and adolescents with autism, and results may not be generalisable to children with other ASDs. **Diagnosis:** The generally accepted "gold standard" assessment tools for autism are the Autism Diagnostic Interview-Revised (ADI-R), a semistructured, interviewer-based schedule administered to the primary caregiver, and the Autism Diagnostic Observational Schedule, a semistructured assessment carried out with the individuals themselves. Although these schedules are informative for the clinician, autism remains a clinical diagnosis.

INCIDENCE/PREVALENCE The detected prevalence of autism has increased in recent years, and a recent high-quality UK study found 40/10,000 children to have childhood autism. The prevalence of autism for studies published between 1977 and 1991 was 4.4/10,000, whereas that for the studies published during the period 1992–2001 was 12.7/10,000. When considering all autism spectrum disorders, findings suggest that the prevalence rises to 120/10,000; many of these people have PDD-NOS.

AETIOLOGY/RISK FACTORS Evidence from twin and family studies suggests that most cases of autism arise because of a combination of genetic factors. Family studies indicate that the rate of autism in siblings of autistic individuals is about 2.2%, and the sibling recurrence rate for all PDDs is 5–6% — significantly greater than that of the general population. Monozygotic-twin studies show 60–91% concordance for autism, and therefore it is likely that most cases arise on the basis of multiple susceptibility genes, with influence from environmental or other factors. A minority of cases of autism can be attributed to genetic disorders, including chromosomal abnormalities, fragile X syndrome, tuberose sclerosis, neurofibromatosis type 1, and a variety of other medical conditions. Although perinatal factors have been implicated, it is unlikely that they have a causal role. Research evidence suggests that autism is not caused by the MMR vaccine, or by thimerosal (mercury) in vaccines (See review on measles, mumps, and rubella: prevention, p 100). There is strong evidence supporting a neurobiological basis of autism. Ongoing research into the relationship between neurophysiology, neuroanatomy, neurochemistry, and genetic factors is likely to increase our understanding, and represents the best chance of unravelling the complex aetiology of ASD. The presence of phenotypic and genetic heterogeneity may have significant implications for studies of interventions/treatments for autism, as efficacy may vary with phenotype.

(continued over)

(from previous page)

PROGNOSIS Autism is a lifelong condition with a highly variable clinical course throughout childhood and adolescence. Many adults with autism require lifelong full-time care. About 15% of adults with autism will live independent lives, whereas 15–20% will live alone with community support. Verbal and overall cognitive capacity seem the most important predictors of ability to live independently as an adult.

Deborah Pritchard

KEY POINTS

- Blood samples are usually taken from infants via heel punctures or venepuncture.

  Both procedures are likely to be painful, especially in younger infants, but analgesia is rarely given.

  Infants who have already experienced pain during heel punctures seem more likely to show signs of pain during later blood sampling than infants new to the procedure.

- High concentrations of oral sugar solutions are likely to reduce pain when given on a pacifier or directly into the mouth before blood sampling.

  Oral 24–30% sucrose and 25–30% glucose solutions reduce signs of pain, especially crying, compared with water or no treatment, in term and preterm infants. Oral 30% dextrose solution may also be effective.

  Lower concentrations of sugars (10–12% solutions) do not seem effective at reducing pain.

  Long-term use of oral sugar solutions has theoretical risks of hyperglycaemia and necrotising enterocolitis.

- Pacifiers without sugar solutions may also reduce pain responses compared with no treatment.

  Transient choking and oxygen desaturation may occur with the use of pacifiers, or after giving oral sugar solutions directly into the mouth.

- Topical anaesthetics may reduce pain responses to blood sampling compared with placebo.

  Topical lidocaine–prilocaine cream, and tetracaine gel or patches reduced signs of pain in most studies of term and preterm infants.

  Adverse effects tend to be minor and transient, but systemic absorption may occur in young infants, which increases the risk of methaemoglobinaemia.

  We do not know whether oral sugars are more or less effective than topical anaesthetics in reducing pain from blood sampling.

(i) **Please visit www.clinicalevidence.bmj.com for full text and references**

What are the effects of interventions to reduce pain-related distress and morbidity during venepuncture in preterm or term babies under 12 months in a neonatal unit?	
Likely To Be Beneficial	• Oral sweet solutions • Pacifiers • Topical anaesthetics [lidocaine–prilocaine cream, tetracaine]

Search date May 2006

DEFINITION Methods of sampling blood in infants include heel puncture, venepuncture, and arterial puncture. **Venepuncture** involves aspirating blood through a needle from a peripheral vein. Heel puncture involves lancing of the lateral aspect of the infant's heel, squeezing the heel, and collecting the pooled capillary blood. Heel puncture and arterial blood sampling are not discussed in this review. For this review, we included premature and term infants up to 12 months in a hospital setting.

(continued over)

(from previous page)

INCIDENCE/PREVALENCE Preterm or ill neonates may undergo 1–21 heel punctures or venepunctures per day. These punctures are likely to be painful. Heel punctures comprise 61–87% and venepunctures comprise 8–13% of the invasive procedures performed on ill infants. Analgesics are rarely given specifically for blood sampling procedures, but 5–19% of infants receive analgesia for other indications. In one study, comfort measures were provided during 63% of venepunctures and 75% of heel punctures.

AETIOLOGY/RISK FACTORS Blood sampling in infants can be difficult to perform, particularly in preterm or ill infants. Young infants may have increased sensitivity and prolonged response to pain compared with older age groups. Factors that may affect the infant's pain responses include postconceptional age, previous pain experience, and procedural technique.

PROGNOSIS Pain caused by blood sampling is associated with acute behavioural and physiological deterioration. Experience of pain during heel puncture seems to heighten pain responses during subsequent blood sampling. Other adverse effects of blood sampling include bleeding, bruising, haematoma, and infection.

Juan Manuel Lozano

KEY POINTS

- Bronchiolitis is a virally induced acute bronchiolar inflammation that is associated with signs and symptoms of airway obstruction.

  It is the most common lower respiratory tract infection in infants. It is a common reason for attendance in the emergency department and for admission to hospital.

  Bronchiolitis is associated with increased morbidity and mortality in high-risk children (those with congenital heart disease, chronic lung disease, history of premature birth, hypoxia, immune deficiency, and age less than 6 weeks)

- In high-risk children, prophylaxis with either respiratory syncytial virus immunoglobulin or the monoclonal antibody, palivizumab, reduces hospital admissions compared with placebo.

- Nursing interventions such as cohort segregation, hand-washing and wearing gowns, masks, gloves, and goggles seem to successfully prevent spreading of the disease in hospital.

- We do not know how effective most current interventions are in treating bronchiolitis.

  Although we don't know whether inhaled or oral bronchodilators such as inhaled adrenaline or inhaled or oral salbutamol are effective in treating bronchiolitis, they do seem to improve overall clinical scores in the short term.

  We don't know whether ribavirin, respiratory syncytial virus immunoglobulin, pooled immunoglobulins or palivizumab, chest physiotherapy, montelukast, or surfactants work better than placebo or no treatment in reducing mortality, duration of hospital stay, or respiratory deterioration, although most of the studies have been too small to detect any clinically important differences.

- Corticosteroids do not seem to be a useful treatment for bronchiolitis.

(i) **Please visit www.clinicalevidence.bmj.com for full text and references**

What are the effects of prophylactic interventions for bronchiolitis in high-risk children?	
Beneficial	• Respiratory syncytial virus immunoglobulin or palivizumab (monoclonal antibody) in children at high risk

What are the effects of measures to prevent transmission of bronchiolitis in hospital?	
Likely To Be Beneficial	• Nursing interventions (cohort segregation, hand-washing, gowns, masks, gloves, and goggles) in children admitted to hospital

What are the effects of treatment for children with bronchiolitis?	
Unknown Effectiveness	• Bronchodilators (inhaled salbutamol, inhaled adrenaline [epinephrine])

- Bronchodilators (oral)

- Chest physiotherapy

- Montelukast

- Respiratory syncytial virus immunoglobulins, pooled immunoglobulins, or palivizumab (monoclonal antibody) for treating bronchiolitis

- Ribavirin

- Surfactants

Unlikely To Be Beneficial	• Corticosteroids

Search date October 2006

DEFINITION Bronchiolitis is a virally induced acute bronchiolar inflammation that is associated with signs and symptoms of airway obstruction. **Diagnosis:** The diagnosis of bronchiolitis, as well as the assessment of its severity, is based on clinical findings (history and physical examination). Bronchiolitis is characterised by a cluster of clinical manifestations in children less than 2 years of age, beginning with an upper respiratory prodrome, followed by increased respiratory effort and wheezing. Suggestive findings include rhinorrhoea, cough, wheezing, tachypnoea, and increased respiratory distress manifested as grunting, nasal flaring, and chest indrawing. There is no good evidence supporting the value of diagnostic tests (chest radiographs, acute-phase reactants, viral tests) in infants with suspected bronchiolitis. Respiratory syncytial virus-test results rarely influence management decisions. Virologic tests, however, may be useful when cohorting of infants is feasible. Given these issues, it is not surprising to find wide variation in how bronchiolitis is diagnosed and treated in different settings.

INCIDENCE/PREVALENCE Bronchiolitis is the most common lower respiratory tract infection in infants, occurring in a seasonal pattern, with highest incidence in the winter in temperate climates, and in the rainy season in warmer countries. Bronchiolitis is a common reason for attendance and admission to hospital. It accounted for around 3% (1.9 million) of emergency department visits in children below 2 years of age between 1992 and 2000 in the USA. The RSV-bronchiolitis hospitalisation rate in the USA infant population in 2000–2001 was 24.2 per 1000 births. In a retrospective cohort study carried out in the USA in 1989–1993, a third of RSV-associated hospitalisations were in infants less than 3 months old. Admission rates are even higher among infants and young children with bronchopulmonary dysplasia (BPD), CHD, prematurity, and other conditions such as chronic pulmonary diseases and immunodeficiency.

AETIOLOGY/RISK FACTORS Respiratory syncytial virus is responsible for bronchiolitis in 70% of cases. This figure reaches 80–100% in the winter months. Reinfections are common and can occur throughout life. Other causal agents include human metapneumovirus, influenza, parainfluenza, and adenovirus.

PROGNOSIS Morbidity and mortality: Disease severity is related to the size of the infant, and to the proximity and frequency of contact with infective infants. It is estimated that between 66 and 127 bronchiolitis-associated deaths occurred annually between 1979 and 1997 among US children aged under 5 years. Estimated annual RSV-attributed deaths in the UK were 8.4/100,000 in infants aged 1–12 months, and 0.9/100,000 population per year for children 1–4 years, between 1989 and 2000. Children at increased risk of morbidity and mortality include those with congenital heart disease, chronic lung disease, history of premature birth, hypoxia, immune deficiency, and age less than 6 weeks. Rates of admission to intensive-care units are higher in those with one risk factor (17.7%) compared with those with no risk factors (3.2%). Rates of needing mechanical ventilation are also higher in those with one risk factor (13.1%) compared with those with no risk factor (1.5%). The risk of death within 2 weeks is higher for children with congenital heart disease

(3.4%) or chronic lung disease (3.5%) compared with other groups combined (0.1%). The percentage of these children needing oxygen supplementation is also high (range 63–80%).
Long-term prognosis: Studies on the long-term prognosis of bronchiolitis — in particular regarding its association with asthma, allergic sensitisation, and atopy — have not produced clear answers. Possible confounding factors include variation in illness severity, smoke exposure, and being in overcrowded environments.

Hilary Writer

KEY POINTS

- Cardiorespiratory arrest outside hospital occurs in approximately 1/10,000 children a year in resource-rich countries, with two thirds of arrests occurring in children under 18 months of age.

  Approximately 40% of cases have undetermined causes, including SIDS. Of the rest, 20% are caused by trauma, 10% by chronic disease, and 6% by pneumonia.

- Overall survival for out-of-hospital cardiorespiratory arrest in children is poor.

  Overall survival for children who sustain cardiorespiratory arrest outside hospital not caused by submersion in water is about 5%.

  Of those who survive, between half and three quarters will have moderate to severe neurological sequelae.

- There is very poor evidence for any intervention in cardiorespiratory arrest in children. Placebo-controlled trials would be unethical, and few observational studies have been performed.

- Immediate airway management, ventilation, and high-quality chest compressions with minimal interruption are widely accepted to be key interventions.

  Ventilation with a bag and mask seems to be as effective as intubation. The most suitable method for the situation should be used.

- Direct-current cardiac shock is likely to be beneficial in children with ventricular fibrillation or pulseless ventricular tachycardia.

  Ventricular fibrillation or pulseless ventricular tachycardia are the underlying rhythms in 10% of cardiorespiratory arrests in children, and are associated with a better prognosis than asystole or pulseless electrical activity.

  Defibrillation within 10 minutes of the arrest may improve the outcome.

- Intravenous adrenaline is widely accepted to be the initial medication of choice in an arrest.

  The standard dose of intravenous adrenaline is 0.01 mg/kg.

  Weak evidence suggests that higher-dose adrenaline (0.1 mg/kg) is no more effective in improving survival.

  The effects of cooling a child after arrest are unknown.

(i) **Please visit www.clinicalevidence.bmj.com for full text and references**

What are the effects of treatments for non-submersion out-of-hospital cardiorespiratory arrest in children?

Likely To Be Beneficial	• Airway management and ventilation (including bag–mask ventilation and intubation)*
	• Bystander cardiopulmonary resuscitation*
	• Direct-current cardiac shock (for ventricular fibrillation or pulseless ventricular tachycardia)*
	• Intravenous adrenaline (epinephrine) at standard dose*
Unknown Effectiveness	• Hypothermia (induced in child after out-of-hospital arrest)
	• Intravenous adrenaline at high dose (compared with standard dose)

- Intravenous sodium bicarbonate
- Intubation versus bag–mask ventilation (relative benefits unclear)
- Training parents to perform cardiopulmonary resuscitation

Search date February 2007

*Although we found no direct evidence to support their use, widespread consensus holds that, on the basis of indirect evidence and extrapolation from adult data, these interventions should be universally applied to children who have arrested. Placebo-controlled trials would be considered unethical.

DEFINITION This review covers non-submersion, out-of-hospital cardiorespiratory arrest in children. The paediatric Utstein style definition is cessation of cardiac mechanical activity, determined by the inability to palpate a central pulse, unresponsiveness, and apnoea occurring outside of a medical facility and not caused by submersion in water.

INCIDENCE/PREVALENCE We found 15 observational studies (5 prospective, 10 retrospective) reporting the incidence of non-submersion out-of-hospital cardiorespiratory arrest in children. Two studies reported the incidence in both adults and children, and 13 reported the incidence in children alone. The incidence in the general population ranged from 1.3–5.7/100,000 people a year (mean 2.9, 95% CI 0.22 to 5.58). The incidence in children ranged from 6.3–18.0/100,000 children a year (mean 9.6, 95% CI 2.27 to 16.93). Two prospective studies (761 children in total) found that 40–50% of cadiorespiratory arrests in children aged under 12 months occur out of hospital. One prospective study identified that children are aged under 18 months in approximately two thirds of out-of-hospital cardiorespiratory arrests.

AETIOLOGY/RISK FACTORS We found 30 observational studies reporting the causes of non-submersion pulseless arrests in a total of 2109 children. The most common causes were undetermined (as in SIDS, 39%), trauma (21%), chronic disease (9%), and pneumonia (6%).

PROGNOSIS We found no observational studies that investigated non-submersion arrests alone. We found one systematic review (search date 2004) of 41 case series and cohort studies (9 prospective, 32 retrospective; total of 5363 children), which reported outcomes for out-of-hospital cardiopulmonary arrest of any cause, including submersion, in children up to 18 years. Studies were excluded if survival, with survival to hospital discharge as a minimum, was not reported as an outcome. The overall survival rate (to hospital discharge) for the children meeting the paediatric Utstein style definition for out-of-hospital non-submersion arrest was 5.5% (190/3475 children). Of the 190 surviving children, 43/190 (23%) had no or mild neurological disability, and 147/190 (77%) had moderate or severe neurological disability. One subsequent prospective cohort study of 503 children, including 42 children who sustained submersion events, reported a 2% survival to hospital discharge. One subsequent retrospective cohort study of 84 children with non-submersion out-of-hospital cardiac arrest reported a 4.7% survival rate to hospital discharge, with 50% of the survivors sustaining severe neurological deficits. We found one systematic review (search date 1997), which reported outcomes after cardiopulmonary resuscitation for both in-hospital and out-of-hospital arrests in children of any cause, including submersion. Studies were excluded if they did not report on survival. The review found evidence from prospective and retrospective observational studies that out-of-hospital arrest of any cause in children has a poorer prognosis than within-hospital arrest (132/1568 [8%] children survived to hospital discharge after out-of-hospital arrest v 129/544 [24%] children after in-hospital arrests). About half of the survivors were involved in studies that reported neurological outcome. Of these, survival with "good neurological outcome" (i.e. normal or mild neurological deficit) was higher in children who arrested in hospital compared with those who arrested elsewhere (60/77 [78%] surviving children in hospital v 28/68 [41%] elsewhere).

Aruna Abhyankar, Iris Carcani, Graham Clayden

KEY POINTS

- Diagnostic criteria for functional constipation in children vary but involve infrequent, possibly painful passing of large, hard stools.

  Prevalence of chronic constipation has been estimated at 1–5% of children in the UK and USA, most of whom have no obvious aetiological factors.

  A third of children with chronic constipation continue to have problems beyond puberty.

  Half of children with chronic faecal impaction and soiling have experienced an episode of painful defecation and many children with chronic constipation exhibit withholding behaviour.

  Disimpaction may be needed if spontaneous expulsion of the faecal mass is unlikely, or if it is causing discomfort or affecting normal feeding.

- Low fibre intake is associated with constipation, and limited evidence shows that fibre reduces constipation and encopresis compared with placebo.

  Increasing oral fluid intake has not been shown to be of benefit.

- Very limited evidence supports the use of osmotic or bulk-forming laxatives in children.

  No studies show a benefit from osmotic laxatives compared with placebo, and the relative benefits of different types of osmotic laxatives are unclear.

  Osmotic laxatives can cause abdominal pain and flatulence, although macrogols (e.g. PEG 3350) seem less likely to do so than lactulose.

  There is no evidence on the use of bulk-forming laxatives such as methylcellulose, ispaghula husk, or sterculia.

- Very limited evidence suggests that the stimulant laxative senna is less effective than mineral oil (liquid paraffin) or lactulose, and is more likely to cause colic, diarrhoea, or abdominal distension.

- Behavioural treatments such as biofeedback, diaries, toilet training or anorectal manometry, or anal dilatation, have not been shown to be of benefit, but the evidence is very limited.

- Macrogols may be more effective than mineral oil for clearing faecal impaction, but evidence for enemas or surgical disimpaction is very limited.

  Moderate evidence suggests that macrogols are more effective than mineral oil at bowel disimpaction, but are more likely to lead to compliance problems owing to the higher volumes required.

 Please visit www.clinicalevidence.bmj.com for full text and references

What are the effects of treatments for children with chronic constipation?

Likely To Be Beneficial	• Fibre • Osmotic laxatives
Unknown Effectiveness	• Behavioural treatments (biofeedback, diaries, or toilet training) • Bulk-forming laxatives • Faecal softeners
Unlikely To Be Beneficial	• Anal dilatation • Oral fluids

> • Stimulant laxatives

What are the effects of treatments for clearing the bowel in children with faecal impaction?

Unknown Effectiveness	• Enemas
	• Macrogols (by oral or nasogastric tube)
	• Surgical disimpaction

Search date June 2005

DEFINITION According to the **Rome II criteria**, functional childhood constipation is defined as at least 2 weeks of: scybalous, pebble-like, hard stools for most of the stools; or firm stools two or fewer times a week, and no evidence of structural endocrine or metabolic disease. These criteria are not necessarily comprehensive, and are considered restrictive by some researchers. (There are now Rome III criteria, which have yet to be responded to by the PACCT [Paris Consensus on Childhood Constipation Terminology] group.) The **PACCT group** has defined childhood constipation as the occurrence of two or more of the following six criteria in the previous 8 weeks: frequency of movements fewer than 3 a week; more than one episode of faecal incontinence a week; large stools in the rectum or palpable on abdominal examination; passing of stools so large that they may obstruct the toilet; retentive posturing and withholding behaviour; painful defecation. In selecting studies for this review, we did not use a singular definition because of lack of clear agreement over the definitions.

INCIDENCE/PREVALENCE Constipation accounts for about 3% of consultations in an average paediatric outpatient clinic in the USA. In the UK population, 5% of school children aged 4–11 years experience constipation lasting more than 6 months. The incidence of constipation has been reported as 28% in an inner-city population in Brazil, and 1–2% in healthy school children in the USA.

AETIOLOGY/RISK FACTORS No aetiological factors can be found in most children. Hirschsprung's disease, cystic fibrosis, anorectal abnormalities, and metabolic conditions such as hypothyroidism are rare organic causes of childhood constipation. An episode of painful defecation has been noted in more than 50% of people who were suffering from faecal soiling or chronic faecal impaction. **Risk factors:** One study found higher incidence of constipation among children with birth weight under 750 g associated with neurodevelopment impairment. Low fibre intake may be associated with childhood constipation. Constipation and soiling are more prevalent in obese children. We found no evidence for a difference between bottle- and breast-fed babies, although it is generally accepted that bottle-fed babies are more at risk of relative water deficiency, and breast-fed babies frequently have delays of many days between passing normal stools.

PROGNOSIS Childhood constipation continues beyond puberty in up to a third of the children followed up beyond that age. Children aged 2–4 years seem to have a higher recurrence rate and need for prolonged medication and support than younger infants. One follow-up study has noted increased risk of persistent constipation in children who developed constipation early in infancy, and who have a family history of constipation. **Faecal impaction:** Disimpaction is necessary if the amount and character of faeces in the colon is of such magnitude that spontaneous expulsion in unlikely, or if it is causing discomfort and affecting normal feeding. Some children with a large rectosigmoid faecaloma may have difficulty passing urine.

David Johnson

KEY POINTS

- Croup leads to signs of upper-airway obstruction, and must be differentiated from acute epiglottitis, bacterial tracheitis, or an inhaled foreign body.

  Croup affects about 3% of children a year, usually between the ages of 6 months and 3 years, and 75% of infections are caused by parainfluenza virus.

  Symptoms usually resolve within 48 hours, but severe infection can, rarely, lead to pneumonia, and to respiratory failure and arrest.

- A single oral dose of dexamethasone improves symptoms compared with placebo in children with mild croup.

  Although humidification and oral decongestants are often used in children with mild to moderate croup, there is no evidence to support their use in clinical practice.

  There is consensus that antibiotics do not improve symptoms in croup of any severity, as croup is usually viral in origin.

- In children with moderate to severe croup, intramuscular ororal dexamethasone, nebulised adrenaline, and nebulised budesonide reduce symptoms compared with placebo.

  Oxygen is standard treatment in children with respiratory distress. Oral dexamethasone is as effective as nebulised budesonide at reducing symptoms, and is less distressing for the child.

  A dexamethasone dose of 0.15 mg/kg may be as effective as a dose of 0.6 mg/kg. Adding nebulised budesonide to oral dexamethasone does not seem to improve efficacy compared with either drug alone.

  Nebulised adrenaline (epinephrine) has a short-term effect on symptoms of croup, but we don't know whether adding intermittent positive pressure breathing to nebulised adrenaline further improves symptoms.

  We don't know whether heliox (helium–oxygen mixture), humidification, short-acting nebulised beta$_2$ agonists, or oral decongestants are beneficial in children with moderate to severe croup, or with impending respiratory failure.

- In children with impending respiratory failure caused by severe croup, nebulised adrenaline (epinephrine) is considered likely to be beneficial. Oxygen is standard treatment.

  Nasogastric prednisolone may reduce the need for, or duration of, intubation, but sedatives and antibiotics are unlikely to be beneficial.

(i) **Please visit www.clinicalevidence.bmj.com for full text and references**

What are the effects of treatments in children with mild croup?	
Beneficial	• Dexamethasone (oral single dose; reduced need for further medical attention for ongoing symptoms compared with placebo)
Unknown Effectiveness	• Decongestants (oral) • Humidification
Unlikely To Be Beneficial	• Antibiotics*

©BMJ Publishing Group Ltd 2008

What are the effects of treatments in children with moderate to severe croup?

Beneficial	• Adrenaline (epinephrine), nebulised
	• Budesonide, nebulised (compared with placebo)
	• Dexamethasone, intramuscular or oral (compared with placebo)
Likely To Be Beneficial	• Dexamethasone, intramuscular (compared with nebulised budesonide for croup scores)
	• Dexamethasone, oral (compared with nebulised budesonide)*
	• Dexamethasone, oral (compared with oral prednisolone)
	• Oxygen*
Unknown Effectiveness	• Adrenaline (epinephrine) (nebulised) plus intermittent positive pressure breathing (compared with nebulised adrenaline alone)
	• Beta$_2$ agonists, short-acting (nebulised)
	• Decongestants (oral)
	• Dexamethasone (oral) plus budesonide (nebulised)
	• Dexamethasone (unclear which dose and route of administration is most effective)
	• Heliox (helium–oxygen mixture)
	• L-adrenaline (epinephrine) compared with racemic adrenaline
Unlikely To Be Beneficial	• Antibiotics*
	• Humidification

What are the effects of treatments in children with impending respiratory failure caused by severe croup?

Beneficial	• Adrenaline (epinephrine), nebulised*
	• Corticosteroids
Likely To Be Beneficial	• Oxygen*
Unknown Effectiveness	• Heliox (helium–oxygen mixture)
Unlikely To Be Beneficial	• Antibiotics*

● Sedatives

Search date November 2006

*Based on consensus.

DEFINITION Croup is characterised by the abrupt onset, most commonly at night, of a barking cough, inspiratory stridor, hoarseness, and respiratory distress caused by upper airway obstruction. Croup symptoms are often preceded by symptoms of upper respiratory tract infection-like symptoms. The most important diagnoses to differentiate from croup include bacterial tracheitis, epiglottitis, and the inhalation of a foreign body. Some investigators distinguish subtypes of croup; the subtypes most commonly distinguished are acute laryngotracheitis and spasmodic croup. Children with acute laryngotracheitis have an antecedent upper respiratory tract infection, are usually febrile, and are thought to have more persistent symptoms. Children with spasmodic croup do not have an antecedent upper respiratory tract infection, are afebrile, have recurrent croup, and are thought to have more transient symptoms. However, there is little empirical evidence justifying the view that spasmodic croup responds differently from acute laryngotracheitis. **Population:** In this review, we have included children up to the age of 12 years with croup; no attempt has been made to exclude spasmodic croup. We could not find definitions of clinical severity that are either widely accepted or rigorously derived. For this review, we have elected to use definitions derived by a committee consisting of a range of specialists and subspecialists during the development of a clinical practice guideline from Alberta Medical Association (Canada). The definitions of severity have been correlated with the Westley croup score, as it is the most widely used clinical score, and its validity and reliability have been well demonstrated. However, RCTs included in the review use a variety of croup scores. **Mild croup:** Occasional barking cough; no stridor at rest; and no to mild suprasternal, intercostal indrawing (retractions of the skin of the chest wall), or both corresponding to a Westley croup score of 0–2. **Moderate croup:** Frequent barking cough, easily audible stridor at rest, and suprasternal and sternal-wall retraction at rest, but no or little distress or agitation, corresponding to a Westley croup score of 3–5. **Severe croup:** Frequent barking cough, prominent inspiratory and — occasionally — expiratory stridor, marked sternal-wall retractions, decreased air entry on auscultation, and significant distress and agitation, corresponding to a Westley croup score of 6–11. **Impending respiratory failure:** Barking cough (often not prominent), audible stridor at rest (occasionally can be hard to hear), sternal-wall retractions (may not be marked), usually lethargic or decreased level of consciousness, and often dusky complexion without supplemental oxygen, corresponding to a Westley croup score of greater than 11. During severe respiratory distress, a young child's compliant chest wall "caves in" during inspiration, causing unsynchronised chest and abdominal wall expansion (paradoxical breathing). About 85% of children attending general emergency departments, by this classification scheme, have mild croup, and less than 1% have severe croup (unpublished prospective data obtained from 21 Alberta general emergency departments).

INCIDENCE/PREVALENCE Croup has an average annual incidence of 3% and accounts for 5% of emergent admissions to hospital in children under 6 years of age in North America (unpublished population-based data from Calgary Health Region, Alberta, Canada, 1996–2000). One retrospective Belgian study found that 16% of 5–8-year-old children had suffered from croup at least once, and 5% had experienced recurrent croup (at least 3 episodes). We are not aware of epidemiological studies establishing the incidence of croup in other parts of the world.

AETIOLOGY/RISK FACTORS One long-term prospective cohort study suggested that croup occurred most commonly in children between 6 months and 3 years, but can also occur in children as young as 3 months and as old as 12–15 years. Case report data suggest it is extremely rare in adults. Infections occur predominantly in late autumn, but can occur during any season, including summer. Croup is caused by a variety of viral agents and, occasionally, by *Mycoplasma pneumoniae*. Parainfluenza accounts for 75% of all cases, with the most common type being parainfluenza type 1. Prospective cohort studies suggest that the remaining proportion of cases is largely accounted for by respiratory syncytial virus, metapneumovirus, influenza A and B, adenovirus, coronavirus, and mycoplasma. Viral invasion of the laryngeal mucosa leads to inflammation, hyperaemia, and oedema. This leads to narrowing of the subglottic region. Children compensate for this narrowing by breathing more quickly and deeply. In children with more severe illness, as the narrowing progresses, their increased effort at breathing becomes counterproductive, airflow through the upper airway becomes turbulent (stridor), their compliant chest wall begins to cave in during inspiration, resulting in paradoxical breathing, and consequently the child becomes fatigued. With these events — if untreated — the child becomes hypoxic and hypercapnoeic, which eventually results in respiratory failure and arrest.

PROGNOSIS Croup symptoms resolve in most children within 48 hours. However, a small percentage of children with croup have symptoms that persist for up to 1 week. Rates of hospital admission vary significantly between communities but, on average, less than 5% of all children with croup are admitted to hospital. Of those admitted to hospital, only 1–3% are intubated. Mortality is low; in one 10-year study, less than 0.5% of intubated children died. Uncommon complications of croup include pneumonia, pulmonary oedema, and bacterial tracheitis.

Philip Hazell

KEY POINTS

- Depression in children and adolescents may have a more insidious onset than in adults, with irritability a more prominent feature than sadness.

  Depression may affect 2–6% of children and adolescents, with a peak incidence around puberty.

  It may be self-limiting, but about 40% of affected children experience a recurrent attack, a third will make a suicide attempt, and 3–4% will die from suicide.

- Fluoxetine improves symptoms and may delay relapse compared with placebo over 7–12 weeks in children and adolescents.

  Fluoxetine may be more effective at improving symptoms compared with CBT, and combined fluoxetine plus CBT treatment may be more effective than either treatment alone.

  Paroxetine, fluvoxamine, sertraline, citalopram, and venlafaxine have not been shown to be beneficial in adolescents and children with depression.

  TCAs have not been shown to reduce symptoms of depression and can be toxic in overdose, so their use is not recommended.

  We do not know whether moclobemide or St John's Wort are beneficial.

- CAUTION: SSRIs (other than fluoxetine) and venlafaxine have been associated with serious suicide-related events in people under the age of 18 years.

- Group CBT and interpersonal therapy may improve symptoms in children and adolescents with mild to moderate depression, but may not prevent relapse.

  We do not know whether other psychological treatments, guided self-help, or individual psychodynamic psychotherapy improve symptoms.

- We do not know whether electroconvulsive therapy or lithium are beneficial in children or adolescents with refractory depression.

(i) **Please visit www.clinicalevidence.bmj.com for full text and references**

What are the effects of treatments for depression in children and adolescents?

Beneficial	• Fluoxetine (prevents acute remission and relapse) in children and adolescents • Fluoxetine plus CBT in adolescents • Interpersonal therapy in adolescents with mild to moderate depression
Likely To Be Beneficial	• CBT (group) in children and adolescents with mild to moderate depression
Unknown Effectiveness	• Citalopram in children and adolescents • CBT (individual) in children and adolescents with mild to moderate depression • Fluoxetine plus cognitive therapy in children • Fluvoxamine in children and adolescents • Group therapeutic support (other than CBT) in children and adolescents • Guided self-help in children and adolescents

	• Individual psychodynamic psychotherapy in children and adolescents
	• Interpersonal therapy in children
	• Mirtazapine in children and adolescents
	• MAOIs in children and adolescents
	• Paroxetine in children
	• St John's Wort (*Hypericum perforatum*) in children and adolescents
Unlikely To Be Beneficial	• CBT (for relapse prevention) in children and adolescents
	• Family therapy in children and adolescents
	• Paroxetine in adolescents
	• Sertraline in children and adolescents
Likely To Be Ineffective Or Harmful	• TCAs (oral) in children and adolescents
	• Venlafaxine in children and adolescents

What are the effects of treatments for refractory depression in children and adolescents?

Unknown Effectiveness	• Electroconvulsive therapy in children and adolescents
	• Lithium in children and adolescents

Search date April 2006

DEFINITION Compared with adult depression (see depression in adults, p 341), depression in children (6–12 years) and adolescents (13–18 years) may have a more insidious onset, may be characterised more by irritability than sadness, and occurs more often in association with other conditions such as anxiety, conduct disorder, hyperkinesis, and learning problems. The term "major depression" is used to distinguish discrete episodes of depression from mild, chronic (1 year or longer) low mood, or irritability, which is known as "dysthymia". The severity of depression may be defined by the level of impairment and the presence or absence of psychomotor changes and somatic symptoms (see depression in adults, p 341). In some studies, severity of depression is defined according to cut-off scores on depression-rating scales. Definitions of refractory depression, also known as treatment-resistant depression, vary, but in this review will refer to depression that has failed to respond or has only partially responded to an adequate trial of at least two recognised treatments.

INCIDENCE/PREVALENCE Estimates of prevalence of depression among children and adolescents in the community range from 2–6%. Prevalence tends to increase with age, with a sharp rise at around the onset of puberty. Pre-adolescent boys and girls are affected equally by the condition, but, in adolescents, depression is more common among girls than boys.

AETIOLOGY/RISK FACTORS Depression in children usually arises from a combination of genetic vulnerability, suboptimal early developmental experiences, and exposure to stresses. However, depressive syndromes sometimes occur as sequelae to physical illness, such as viral infection, and may overlap with fatigue syndromes. The heritability of

(continued over)

(from previous page)

depression may increase with age, but findings from genetics studies are inconsistent. Recurrent depression seems to have a stronger familial association compared with single-episode depression. Depression-prone individuals have a cognitive style characterized by an overly pessimistic outlook on events. This cognitive style precedes the onset of depression and appears to be independent of recent life events and ongoing stresses. Stressful life events may trigger the first occurrence of depression, but are rarely sufficient on their own to cause depression. Lower levels of stress are needed to provoke subsequent episodes of illness. Enduring problems in the relationship with the primary caregivers is an important risk factor for depression, but such difficulties also predispose to other psychiatric disorders.

PROGNOSIS In children and adolescents, the recurrence rate after a first depressive episode is 40%. Young people experiencing a moderate to severe depressive episode may be more likely than adults to have a manic episode within the following few years. Trials of treatments for child and adolescent depression have found high rates of response to placebo (as much as two thirds of people in some inpatient studies), suggesting that episodes of depression may be self-limiting in many cases. A third of young people who experience a depressive episode will make a suicide attempt at some stage, and 3–4% of those who experience depression will die from suicide.

Leena D Mewasingh

KEY POINTS

- Febrile seizures are defined 'an event in infancy or childhood usually occurring between 3 months and 5 years of age associated with a fever, but without evidence of intracranial infection' or 'defined cause for their seizure.'

  Simple febrile seizures are generalised in onset, last less than 15 minutes, and do not occur more than once in 24 hours. Complex seizures are longer lasting, have focal symptoms, and can recur within 24 hours. This review only deals with simple febrile seizures.

  About 2–5% of children in the USA and Western Europe, and 6–9% of infants and children in Japan will have experienced at least one febrile seizure by the age of 5 years.

  Simple febrile seizures may slightly increase the risk of developing epilepsy, but have no known adverse effects on behaviour, scholastic performance, or neurocognition.

- We do not know whether antipyretics are useful in treating episodes of fever to prevent seizure recurrence in children with one or more previous simple febrile seizures.

  Intermittent anticonvulsants are associated with adverse effects including hyperactivity, irritability, and difficulties with speech, activity level, or sleep.

- Continuous anticonvulsant treatment may be effective for reducing recurrence in children with a history of simple febrile seizures, but is associated with adverse effects — for example, phenobarbital is associated with cognitive impairments and behavioural adverse effects including hyperactivity, irritability, and aggressiveness.

  Anticonvulsants do not seem to reduce the risk of epilepsy up to 12 years later in children with a history of simple febrile seizures.

(i) **Please visit www.clinicalevidence.bmj.com for full text and references**

What are the effects of treatments given during episodes of fever in children with one or more previous simple febrile seizures?	
Unknown Effectiveness	• Antipyretic treatments (physical antipyretic measures, paracetamol, ibuprofen)
Likely To Be Ineffective Or Harmful	• Anticonvulsants (intermittent)

What are the effects of long-term (daily, longer than 1 month) anticonvulsant treatment in children with a history of simple febrile seizures?	
Trade-off Between Benefits And Harms	• Anticonvulsants (continuous)

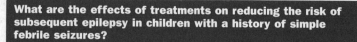

What are the effects of treatments on reducing the risk of subsequent epilepsy in children with a history of simple febrile seizures?

Unlikely To Be Beneficial	• Anticonvulsants (intermittent and continuous)

Search date July 2006

DEFINITION Febrile seizures are divided into three types: simple febrile seizures, complex febrile seizures, and febrile status epilepticus. **This review focuses on children with simple febrile seizures.** The National Institutes of Health (NIH) definition of a febrile seizure is 'an event in infancy or childhood usually occurring between 3 months and 5 years of age associated with a fever, but without evidence of intracranial infection or defined cause for their seizure', after having excluded children with previous afebrile seizures. Another definition from the International League Against Epilepsy (ILAE) is that of "a seizure occurring in childhood after 1 month of age associated with a febrile illness not caused by an infection of the central nervous system (CNS), without previous neonatal seizures or a previous unprovoked seizure, and not meeting the criteria for other acute symptomatic seizures'. In working practice the lower age limit for febrile seizures is generally taken to be 6 months, given concerns regarding the possibility of an underlying serious but treatable infection in younger infants masquerading as a febrile seizure (e.g. meningitis). A simple febrile seizure is a generalised seizure, lasting less than 15 minutes in duration, which does not occur more than once in 24 hours, and is followed by full recovery within 1 hour. Treatment for the actual seizure is generally not indicated, given the short duration. Often by the time the child presents to hospital, the seizure has already stopped. A febrile seizure may be the presenting sign of a fever episode. **This review does not include children experiencing complex febrile seizures**, which are characterised by any of the following features: greater than 15 minutes in duration, focal symptoms, recurrence within 24 hours, and not followed by full consciousness within 1 hour. Investigations including neuroimaging and lumbar puncture are often warranted. **Also excluded are children experiencing febrile status epilepticus** which lasts longer than 30 minutes and requires treatment. Addressing parental anxiety forms a key part of the management of simple febrile seizures, as often parents' (unspoken) worry with a first seizure is that their child could have died. However, there is little in the medical literature about this aspect of education and reassurance in management of simple febrile seizures.

INCIDENCE/PREVALENCE About 2–5% of children in the USA and Western Europe and 6–9% of infants and children in Japan will have experienced at least one febrile seizure, simple or complex, by the age of 5 years. Elsewhere the incidence varies, being 5–10% in India and as high as 14% in Guam. There are no specific data available for simple febrile seizures.

AETIOLOGY/RISK FACTORS The exact cause of simple febrile seizures is unknown. In some cases, there is a genetic predisposition, with febrile seizures occurring in families. However, the exact mode of inheritance is not known and seems to vary between families. A "febrile seizure susceptibility trait" has been described with an autosomal dominant pattern of inheritance with reduced penetrance. In addition, mutations in several genes have been found that account for enhanced susceptibility to febrile seizures. Febrile seizures are more frequent in children attending day-care centres and those having a first- or second-degree relative with a history of febrile seizures. The risk of another child having febrile seizures is one in five if one sibling is affected, and one in three if both parents and a previous child have had febrile seizures. Other risk factors associated with an increased rate of febrile-seizure recurrence include young age at onset (less than 12 months), history of simple or complex febrile seizures, and body temperature at onset of less than 40 °C. Among these, age at onset seems to be the most constant predictive factor, with 50% of children aged less than 12 months and 30% of children aged more than 12 months presenting with a recurrent febrile seizure. Positive family history of epilepsy is not consistently associated with increased simple febrile-seizure recurrence.

PROGNOSIS Simple febrile seizures may slightly increase the risk of developing epilepsy, but have no adverse effects on behaviour, scholastic performance, or neurocognition. The risk of developing epilepsy is increased further in children with a history of complex febrile seizures. A strong association exists between febrile status epilepticus or febrile seizures characterised by focal symptoms, and later development of temporal-lobe epilepsy.

Gastroenteritis in children

Jacqueline Dalby-Payne and Elizabeth Elliott

KEY POINTS

- Gastroenteritis in children worldwide is usually caused by rotavirus, which leads to considerable morbidity and mortality.

  Bacterial causes of gastroenteritis are more common in resource-poor countries.

- Enteral rehydration solutions containing sugar or food plus electrolytes are as effective as intravenous fluids at correcting dehydration and reducing the duration of hospital stay, and may have fewer major adverse effects.

  Experimental models have shown that clear fluids, including fruit juices and carbonated drinks, are low in electrolytes, and often high in sugar, and can worsen diarrhoea.

  Lactose-free feeds may reduce the duration of diarrhoea in children with mild to severe dehydration compared with feeds containing lactose, but studies have shown conflicting results.

- Loperamide can reduce the duration of diarrhoea in children with mild to moderate dehydration compared with placebo, but studies have shown conflicting results, and adverse effects have been reported.

(i) **Please visit www.clinicalevidence.bmj.com for full text and references**

What are the effects of treatments for acute gastroenteritis?	
Beneficial	• Enteral (oral or gastric) rehydration solutions (as effective as intravenous fluids)
Likely To Be Beneficial	• Lactose-free feeds (may reduce duration of diarrhoea) • Loperamide (reduces duration of diarrhoea, but risk of adverse effects)
Unknown Effectiveness	• Clear fluids (other than oral rehydration solutions)

Search date August 2006

DEFINITION Acute gastroenteritis results from infection of the gastrointestinal tract, most commonly with a virus. It is characterised by rapid onset of diarrhoea with or without vomiting, and by nausea, fever, and abdominal pain. In children, the symptoms and signs can be non-specific. Diarrhoea is defined as the frequent passage of unformed, liquid stools. Regardless of the cause, the mainstay of management of acute gastroenteritis is provision of adequate fluids to prevent and treat dehydration. In this review, we examine the benefits and harms of different treatments for gastroenteritis, irrespective of its cause.

INCIDENCE/PREVALENCE Worldwide, about 3–5 billion cases of acute gastroenteritis occur each year in children under 5 years, resulting in nearly 2 million deaths. In the UK, acute gastroenteritis accounts for 204/1000 general-practitioner consultations in children under 5 years. Gastroenteritis leads to hospital admission in 7/1000 children under 5 years each year in the UK, and 13/1000 in the USA. In Australia, gastroenteritis accounts for 6% of all hospital admissions in children under 15 years.

AETIOLOGY/RISK FACTORS In resource-rich countries, acute gastroenteritis is predominantly caused by viruses (87%), of which rotavirus is the most common. Bacteria, predominantly *Campylobacter*, *Salmonella*, *Shigella*, and *Escherichia coli*, cause most of the remaining cases. In resource-poor countries, where bacterial pathogens are more frequent, rotavirus is also a major cause of gastroenteritis.

PROGNOSIS Acute gastroenteritis is usually self-limiting, but if untreated it can result in morbidity and mortality secondary to water loss, and electrolyte and acid–base disturbance. Acute diarrhoea causes 4 million deaths each year in children under 5 years in Asia (excluding China), Africa, and Latin America, and more than 80% of deaths occur in children under 2 years of age. Although death is uncommon in resource-rich countries, dehydration secondary to gastroenteritis is a significant cause of morbidity and hospital admission.

Yadlapalli Kumar and Rajini Sarvananthan

KEY POINTS

- Reflux of gastric contents into the oesophagus in children causes recurrent vomiting (usually before 6 weeks of age), epigastric and abdominal pain, feeding difficulties, failure to thrive, and irritability.

  At least half of infants regurgitate feeds at least once a day, but this only causes other problems in about 20% of infants, and most cases resolve spontaneously by 12–18 months of age.

  Risk factors include lower oesophageal sphincter disorders, hiatus hernia, gastric distension, raised intra-abdominal pressure, and neurodevelopmental problems.

- Sleeping in the left lateral or prone position may improve oesophageal pH compared with sleeping supine or on the right side, but these positions may increase the risk of SIDS compared with supine sleeping, and their effect on clinically important outcomes is unknown.

  We don't know whether sleeping in the prone elevated position reduces symptoms compared with the prone horizontal position, or whether weight loss reduces symptoms.

- Thickened feeds may reduce the severity and frequency of regurgitation in the short term.

- Sodium alginate may reduce the frequency of regurgitation compared with placebo, although studies have given conflicting results.

  The high sodium content of sodium alginate may make it unsuitable for use in preterm babies.

- Metoclopramide may be effective, but studies have given conflicting results, and it may cause adverse effects.

- We don't know whether domperidone, H_2 antagonists, proton pump inhibitors, or surgery reduce symptoms in babies with GORD, and they can cause adverse effects.

(i) **Please visit www.clinicalevidence.bmj.com for full text and references**

What are the effects of treatment for symptomatic GORD?	
Likely To Be Beneficial	• Feed thickeners in infants • Sodium alginate
Trade-off Between Benefits And Harms	• Left lateral or prone sleep positioning • Metoclopramide
Unknown Effectiveness	• Domperidone • H_2 antagonists • Head elevated sleep positioning • Proton pump inhibitors • Surgery • Weight loss

Search date July 2006

DEFINITION GORD is the passive transfer of gastric contents into the oesophagus caused by transient or chronic relaxation of the lower oesophageal sphincter. A survey of 69 children (median age 16 months) with GORD attending a tertiary referral centre found that presenting symptoms were recurrent vomiting (72%), epigastric and abdominal pain (36%), feeding difficulties (29%), failure to thrive (28%), and irritability (19%). However, results may not be generalisable to younger children or to children presenting in primary care, who make up the most of the cases. Over 90% of children with GORD have vomiting before 6 weeks of age.

INCIDENCE/PREVALENCE Gastro-oesophageal regurgitation is considered a problem if it is frequent, persistent, and is associated with other symptoms such as increased crying, discomfort with regurgitation, and frequent back arching. A cross-sectional survey of parents of 948 infants attending 19 primary-care paediatric practices found that regurgitation of at least one episode a day was reported in 51% of infants aged 0–3 months. "Problematic" regurgitation occurred in significantly fewer infants (14% with problematic regurgitation v 51% with regurgitation of at least 1 episode a day; P less than 0.001). Peak regurgitation reported as "problematic" was reported in 23% of infants aged 6 months. A prospective study of 2879 infants followed up from just after birth (up to 2 weeks) to age 6 months by primary-care paediatricians found that regurgitation occurred in 23.1% of infants during the study period.

AETIOLOGY/RISK FACTORS Risk factors for GORD include immaturity of the lower oesophageal sphincter, chronic relaxation of the sphincter, increased abdominal pressure, gastric distension, hiatus hernia, and oesophageal dysmotility. Premature infants and children with severe neurodevelopmental problems or congenital oesophageal anomalies are particularly at risk.

PROGNOSIS Regurgitation is considered benign, and most cases resolve spontaneously by 12–18 months of age. In a cross-sectional survey of 948 parents, the peak age for reporting four or more episodes of regurgitation was at 5 months of age (23%), which decreased to 7% at 7 months (P less than 0.001). One cohort study found that infants with frequent spilling in the first 2 years of life (at least 90 days in the first 2 years) were more likely to have symptoms of GORD at 9 years of age than those with no spilling (RR 2.3, 95% CI 1.3 to 4.0). The prevalence of "problematic" regurgitation also reduced from 23% in infants aged 6 months to 3.25% in infants aged 10–12 months. Rare complications of GORD include oesophagitis with haematemesis and anaemia, respiratory problems (such as cough, apnoea, and recurrent wheeze), and failure to thrive. A small comparative study (40 children) suggested that, when compared with healthy children, infants with GORD had slower development of feeding skills, and had problems affecting behaviour, swallowing, food intake, and mother–child interaction.

Peter Lucassen

KEY POINTS

- Infantile colic is defined as excessive crying in an otherwise healthy and thriving baby. The crying typically starts in the first few weeks of life and ends by age 4–5 months.

  It causes one in six families with children to consult a health professional.

- We found no sufficient evidence to judge whether replacing cows milk or breast milk with casein hydrolysate milk, low-lactose milk, soya-based infant feeds, or whey hydrolysate formula is effective in reducing crying time.

  Breastfeeding mothers should generally be encouraged to continue breast feeding.

  Soya milk is associated with possible long-term harmful effects on reproductive health.

- The studies examining the effectiveness of reducing stimulation (by not patting, lifting, or jiggling the baby, or by reducing auditory stimulation), crib vibration, infant massage, focused counselling, or spinal manipulation were too small for us to draw reliable conclusions.

- We did not find any good evidence assessing cranial osteopathy or gripe water for treating infantile colic.

  Despite a lack of evidence from well-conducted trials, gripe water is commonly used by parents for their colicky infants.

- Increasing the time spent carrying the infant (by at least 3 hours) does not seem to reduce the time spent crying, and may increase anxiety and stress in the parents.

- We found no studies of sufficient quality to judge the effects of simethicone in infants with colic.

(i) **Please visit www.clinicalevidence.bmj.com for full text and references**

What are the effects of treatments for infantile colic?

Unknown Effectiveness	• Advice to increase carrying
	• Advice to reduce stimulation
	• Casein hydrolysate milk (compared with cows' milk)
	• Cranial osteopathy
	• Crib vibrator device (car-ride simulation)
	• Focused counselling
	• Gripe water
	• Infant massage
	• Low-lactose milk (compared with cow's milk or breast milk)
	• Simethicone (activated dimeticone)
	• Soya-based infant feeds (compared with cows' milk)
	• Spinal manipulation
	• Whey hydrolysate milk

Search date January 2007

DEFINITION Infantile colic is defined as excessive crying in an otherwise healthy and thriving baby. The crying typically starts in the first few weeks of life and ends by age 4–5 months. Excessive crying is defined as crying that lasts at least 3 hours a day, for 3 days a week, for at least 3 weeks. Because of the natural course of infantile colic, it can be difficult to interpret trials that do not include a placebo or have no treatment group for comparison.

INCIDENCE/PREVALENCE Infantile colic causes one in six families (17%) with children to consult a health professional. One systematic review of 15 community-based studies found a wide variation in prevalence, which depended on study design and method of recording. Two prospective studies identified by the review yielded prevalence rates of 5% and 19%. One prospective study (89 breast- and formula-fed infants) found that, at 2 weeks of age, the prevalence of crying more than 3 hours a day was 43% among formula-fed infants and 16% among breastfed infants. The prevalence at 6 weeks was 12% among formula-fed infants and 31% among breast-fed infants. A national survey of 3345 infants found that maternal smoking was potentially associated with colic (OR 1.34, 95% CI 0.88 to 2.04).

AETIOLOGY/RISK FACTORS The cause is unclear and, despite its name, infantile colic may not have an abdominal cause. It may reflect part of the normal distribution of infantile crying. Other possible explanations are painful intestinal contractions, lactose intolerance, gas, or parental misinterpretation of normal crying.

PROGNOSIS Infantile colic improves with time. One self-reporting parent questionnaire on crying patterns found that 29% of infants aged 1–3 months cried for more than 3 hours a day, but by 4–6 months of age the prevalence had fallen to 7–11%.

Measles, mumps, and rubella: prevention

David Elliman, Nitu Sengupta, Haitham El Bashir, and Helen Bedford

KEY POINTS

- Measles, mumps, and rubella are viral infections which can all be associated with serious disease in non-immune people.

    Measles virus causes an estimated 30 million infections and 770,000 deaths a year worldwide, with increased risks of neurological, respiratory, and bleeding complications in survivors.

    Mumps can cause neurological problems and hearing loss, orchitis with infertility, and pancreatitis.

    Rubella infection is usually mild, but can lead to fetal death or severe congenital abnormalities if contracted in early pregnancy.

    The incidence of all three infections has decreased significantly in countries with routine vaccination programmes targeted at these diseases, but decreased vaccination rates are associated with increased risks of infection.

- The MMR vaccine is considered to be effective in preventing measles, mumps, and rubella infection, but placebo-controlled studies have not been done and would now be considered unethical.

    The MMR vaccine can cause fever, febrile seizures, and anaphylaxis, with aseptic meningitis more likely after some strains compared with others.

    There is no evidence of an association between the MMR vaccine and risks of asthma, Guillain–Barré syndrome, autism, diabetes, gait disturbance, demyelinating disorders, or inflammatory bowel disease.

- Measles vaccination with monovalent or MMR vaccine is associated with reduced risks of measles, measles-related mortality, and subacute sclerosing panencephalitis.

    The use of MMR, rather than monovalent measles, mumps, and rubella vaccines, provides earlier protection against all three diseases, requires fewer injections over a shorter period of time, and decreases the pool of individuals susceptible to these infections in the community.

    Seroconversion rates are similar for MMR and monovalent vaccines against measles, mumps, and rubella, but use of monovalent vaccines requires more injections and so may take longer to achieve full protection.

    Both the MMR vaccine and naturally acquired measles infection may increase the risk of idiopathic thrombocytopenic purpura.

(i) **Please visit www.clinicalevidence.bmj.com for full text and references**

What are the effects of measles vaccination?	
Beneficial	• Monovalent measles vaccine or combined MMR vaccine versus placebo or no vaccine
Unknown Effectiveness	• Comparative effects of MMR versus monovalent measles vaccine

What are the effects of mumps vaccination?	
Beneficial	• Monovalent mumps vaccine or combined MMR vaccine versus placebo or no vaccine
Unknown Effectiveness	• Comparative effects of MMR versus monovalent mumps vaccine

What are the effects of rubella vaccination?

Beneficial	• Monovalent rubella vaccine or combined MMR vaccine versus placebo or no vaccine
Unknown Effectiveness	• Comparative effects of MMR versus monovalent rubella vaccine

Search date July 2006

DEFINITION Measles, mumps, and rubella are infectious diseases. **Measles** is caused by a ribonucleic acid paramyxovirus. The illness is characterised by an incubation period of 6–19 days (median 13 days), a prodromal period of 2–4 days with upper respiratory tract symptoms, conjunctivitis, Koplik's spots on mucosal membranes, and high fever, followed by a widespread maculopapular rash that persists, with fever, for 5–6 days. **Mumps** is caused by a ribonucleic acid virus classified as a rubulavirus in the *Paramyxoviridae* family. The illness is characterised by an incubation period of 15–24 days (median 19 days), with a prodromal period of non-specific flu-like symptoms preceding the development of parotitis. This swelling, which is frequently bilateral and accompanied by abdominal pain and headache, usually resolves within 7–10 days. About a third of mumps infections are subclinical or mild non-specific illnesses not recognised as mumps. **Rubella** is caused by rubivirus, a ribonucleic acid enveloped togavirus in the *Togaviridae* family. There are no animal reservoirs and only one serotype. The incubation period is 15–20 days (median 17 days). Although virus is shed from 7 days before to 6 days after the appearance of the rash, the period of infectivity with rubella is not known. The infection is frequently subclinical. In clinical infection, there are often no prodromal symptoms. A generalised lymphadenopathy is followed by a rash up to 7 days later. Babies with congenital rubella syndrome (CRS) may excrete virus for years and therefore be a source of infection.

INCIDENCE/PREVALENCE The incidence of measles, mumps, and rubella varies according to vaccination coverage. **Measles:** Worldwide, there are an estimated 30 million cases of measles each year, but the incidence is only 0–10/100,000 people in countries with widespread vaccination programmes such as the USA, UK, Mexico, India, China, Brazil, and Australia. In the USA, before licensing of effective vaccines, more than 90% of people were infected by the age of 15 years. After licensing in 1963, incidence fell by about 98%. The mean annual incidence in Finland was 366/100,000 in 1970, but declined to about zero by the late 1990s. Similarly, the annual incidence declined to about zero in Chile, the English-speaking Caribbean, and Cuba during the 1990s, when vaccination programmes were introduced. **Mumps** predominantly affects children, with 32% of reported cases worldwide in children aged 0–4 years, and 53% in children aged 5–14 years. In the prevaccine era, by 10 years of age, 87% of the population in England had serological evidence of mumps infection. Since the introduction of the MMR vaccine, there has been a decrease in the incidence of disease, such that in some countries (e.g. Finland), there is no longer any indigenous disease. Those cases that still occur are usually in older unvaccinated people. For example, in 2005, over 56,000 cases of mumps were reported in England and Wales (compared with 16,000 cases in 2004). In contrast to figures from 1989, where 12% of cases occurred in people aged 15 years or over, in 2005 over 80% of cases occurred in this age group. **Rubella:** In the prevaccine era in the UK, rubella was uncommon under the age of 5 years, with the peak incidence being at 5–10 years. Serological surveys around the world found that by late adolescence/early adulthood, 80% of women had been infected.

AETIOLOGY/RISK FACTORS Measles is highly contagious, with mumps and rubella being less so. As with most other infectious diseases, risk factors include overcrowding and low herd immunity. **Measles** spreads through airborne droplets. Newborn babies have a lower risk of measles compared with older infants, owing to protective maternal antibodies, although in recent US outbreaks, maternal antibody protection was lower than expected. Antibody levels are lower in babies born to vaccinated mothers compared with offspring of naturally infected mothers. **Mumps** spreads through respiratory droplets, saliva, and

(continued over)

(from previous page)

possibly urine. The period of infectivity extends from a few days before the salivary glands become enlarged to about 5 days after. As with measles, the risk of mumps is lower in the first 9–12 months of age, owing to the presence of maternal antibodies, although this pattern may change in a largely vaccinated maternal population. **Rubella** spreads through direct contact or airborne droplets.

PROGNOSIS Measles: The WHO estimated that measles caused 777,000 deaths and 27.5 million DALY in 2000. **Measles in healthy people:** In resource-rich countries, most prognostic data come from the prevaccination era and from subsequent outbreaks in unvaccinated populations. The overall rate of complications in the UK was 6.7% before the introduction of measles vaccination. Encephalitis affected 1.2/1000 diseased people, and respiratory complications arose in 38/1000 diseased people. Other complications before the introduction of the vaccine included seizures, with or without fever, affecting 5/1000 people with measles. Idiopathic thrombocytopenic purpura (ITP) has been reported, but the frequency is not known. Subacute sclerosing panencephalitis is an inevitably fatal, progressive degenerative disorder of the central nervous system, with a mean onset 7–10 years after measles infection. It is more common when measles occurs under the age of 1 year (18/100,000 in children below 1 year of age v 4/100,000 overall), as identified by a passive reporting system set up in England and Wales to monitor the incidence of subacute sclerosing panencephalitis. Between 1989 and 1991 in the USA, measles resurgence among young children (aged under 5 years) who had not been immunised led to 55,622 cases, with more than 11,000 hospital admissions and 166 deaths. Measles complications also include diarrhoea (9%) and pneumonia (6%). Measles during pregnancy results in a higher risk of premature labour, but no proven increase in congenital anomalies. **Measles in malnourished or immunocompromised people:** In malnourished people, particularly those with vitamin A deficiency, measles case fatality can be as high as 25%. Immunocompromised people have a higher morbidity and mortality. Children younger than 5 years, and adults older than 20 years, have a higher risk of severe complications and death. In the period 1974–1984, four UK centres reported that 15/51 (29%) deaths in children in their first remission from leukaemia resulted from measles. Another report reviewing cases from the same four UK centres between 1973 and 1986 found that 5/17 (29%) cases of measles in children with malignancies proved fatal. At least 5/36 (14%) measles associated deaths in 1991 in the USA were in HIV-infected people. Worldwide, measles is a major cause of blindness, and causes 5% of deaths in young children (aged under 5 years). **Mumps:** Deaths following mumps are uncommon, with about five registered annually in the prevaccine era in England and Wales, although only half of these were judged to be directly due to mumps. Deaths occurred mainly in people aged over 40 years. The most important complications of mumps are those relating to the central nervous system, the gonads, and the pancreas. Before the introduction of the MMR vaccine in the UK, mumps was one of the most common causes of aseptic meningitis, accounting for about 20% of cases. The outcome was usually benign. Mumps encephalitis is less common and the outcome more serious. A case series (41 children) in Finland found that 2/40 (5%) children had continuing ataxia and 7/42 (17%) had behavioural disturbances at 4 months to 2 years after mumps encephalitis. Sensorineural hearing loss, usually unilateral, occurs after mumps infection, but its prevalence is unknown, although paediatricians in Israel who had observed cases of hearing loss following a mumps epidemic in 1984 suggested that it may be as common as 1/3400 (0.03%). A large population-based study of mumps undertaken in the USA (1310 cases from 1935–1974) found orchitis in 10% of males overall, being much more common in adults. Orchitis was bilateral in 17% of men. The study found testicular atrophy in 47/132 (36%) men, of whom two developed testicular neoplasms. A smaller population-based study of mumps in a virgin population (561 Eskimos on St Lawrence Island) found that 52/205 (25%) of men with mumps had orchitis, of which 26 cases were unilateral, 19 bilateral, and seven unknown. Most cases (73%) occurred in males aged 15 years or over, of whom 37% had bilateral disease. In females who had mumps, 15% had mastitis, a third of whom were aged 15 years or over. In a community-based study in the USA (342 cases), the most frequent complication of mumps was pancreatitis, occurring in 12/342 (4%) people, whereas in a case series, 50/109 (46%) people admitted to hospital had clinical signs of pancreatitis. There is an increase in the rate of spontaneous abortion following mumps infection in the first trimester, but no increase in congenital anomalies or prematurity. **Rubella:** Complications of rubella are rare in children. In an epidemic in Japan in 1987, 8250 children under 15 years of age were estimated to have suffered rubella infection. Five children developed encephalitis (1 with adverse sequelae), three had meningitis, four had ITP, four vascular purpura, two haemolytic anaemia, and eight pneumonia. Retrospective observational data suggest that ITP may occur at a rate of about 1/3000. Rubella encephalopathy occurs, but rarely, and a case series suggested that long-term sequelae were less frequent than after measles encephalopathy. Arthralgia is rare in children, but common in adults, especially women. A review of hospital records (74 adults with rubella) in London found that most had arthralgia and 11/74 (15%) had arthritis. Arthritis may be recurrent, but is usually self-limiting. The most serious consequence of rubella infection is congenital rubella syndrome (CRS), first described by Gregg in 1941. Almost any system can be affected by CRS, depending on the stage of pregnancy at which the infection occurs. In a prospective cohort study of over 1000 pregnant women in England and Wales with confirmed rubella infection, the frequency of congenital infection after maternal rubella with a rash during the first 12 weeks of pregnancy was more than 80%, declining to 25% when the infection occurred at the end of the second trimester. Rubella defects occurred in all infants infected before the 11th week, in 35% of those infected at 13–16 weeks, and in no infants infected later in pregnancy. The earlier the infection occurs, the more serious the defects; for example, children infected before the 11th week had both congenital heart disease and deafness, whereas children with later infections only had deafness.

Nick Barnes, Guy Millman, and Elizabeth James

KEY POINTS

- Diagnosis of migraine headache in children can be difficult as it depends on subjective symptoms, and diagnostic criteria are broader than in adults.

  Migraine occurs in 3–10% of children and increases with age up to puberty.

  Migraine spontaneously remits after puberty in half of children, but if it begins during adolescence it may be more likely to persist throughout adulthood.

- We don't know whether paracetamol, NSAIDs, codeine phosphate, or $5HT_1$ antagonists (triptans) relieve the pain of migraine in children, as few studies have been found.

  Nasal sumatriptan may reduce pain at 2 hours compared with placebo in children aged 12–17 years, but results have been inconsistent, and it can cause taste disturbance.

  Rizatriptan may reduce nausea but has not been shown to reduce pain compared with placebo.

- We don't know whether antiemetics are beneficial in childhood migraine, as we found no studies.

- Pizotifen is widely used as prophylaxis in children with migraine, but we found no studies assessing its efficacy.

  Stress-management programmes may improve headache severity and frequency in the short term, compared with no stress management.

  Studies of beta-blockers as prophylaxis in children have given inconsistent results, and propranolol may increase the duration of headaches compared with placebo.

  We don't know whether dietary manipulation, thermal biofeedback, or progressive muscle relaxation can prevent recurrence of migraine in children.

Please visit www.clinicalevidence.bmj.com for full text and references

What are the effects of treatments for acute attacks of migraine headache in children?	
Unknown Effectiveness	• $5HT_1$ antagonists (e.g. triptans)
	• Antiemetics
	• Codeine phosphate
	• NSAIDs
	• Paracetamol

What are the effects of prophylaxis for migraine in children?	
Likely To Be Beneficial	• Stress management
Unknown Effectiveness	• Beta-blockers
	• Dietary manipulation
	• Pizotifen
	• Progressive muscle relaxation

● Thermal biofeedback

Search date August 2005

DEFINITION Migraine is defined by the International Headache Society (IHS) as a recurrent headache that occurs with or without aura and lasts 2–48 hours. It is usually unilateral in nature, pulsating in quality, of moderate or severe intensity, and is aggravated by routine physical activity. Nausea, vomiting, photophobia, and phonophobia are common accompanying symptoms. This review focuses on children younger than 18 years. Diagnostic criteria for children are broader than for adults, allowing for a broader range of duration and a broader localisation of the pain. Diagnosis is difficult in young children because the condition is defined by subjective symptoms. Studies that do not explicitly use criteria congruent with IHS diagnostic criteria (or revised IHS criteria in children under 15 years of age) have been excluded from this review.

INCIDENCE/PREVALENCE Migraine occurs in 3–10% of children, and currently affects 50/1000 school-age children in the UK, and an estimated 7.8 million children in the European Union. Studies in resource-rich countries suggest that migraine is the most common diagnosis among children presenting with headache to a medical practitioner. It is rarely diagnosed in children under 2 years of age because of the symptom-based definition, but increases steadily with age thereafter. It affects boys and girls similarly before puberty, but after puberty girls are more likely to suffer from migraine.

AETIOLOGY/RISK FACTORS The cause of migraine headaches is unknown. We found few reliable data identifying risk factors or measuring their effects in children. Suggested risk factors in genetically predisposed children and adolescents include stress, foods, menses, and exercise.

PROGNOSIS We found no reliable data about prognosis of childhood migraine headache diagnosed by IHS criteria. It has been suggested that more than half of children will have spontaneous remission after puberty. It is believed that migraine that develops during adolescence tends to continue in adult life, although attacks tend to be less frequent and severe in later life. We found one longitudinal study from Sweden (73 children with "pronounced" migraine and mean age of onset of 6 years) with over 40 years' follow-up, which predated the IHS criteria for migraine headache. It found that migraine headaches had ceased before the age of 25 years in 23% of people. However, by the age of 50 years, more than 50% of people continued to have migraine headaches. We found no prospective data examining long-term risks in children with migraine.

James Hanley

KEY POINTS

- Early-onset neonatal sepsis, typically caused by group B streptococcal infection, usually begins within 24 hours of birth, affects up to 8 infants per 1000 live births, and leads to death if untreated.

  One in three women carry group B streptococci vaginally, which can infect the amniotic fluid even if the membranes are intact, or infect the baby during delivery, causing sepsis, pneumonia, or meningitis.

  Very low-birthweight infants are at much higher risk of infection or mortality, with up to 3% infected, and mortality rates of up to 30%, even with immediate antibiotic treatment.

  Late-onset group B streptococcal infection begins after 7–9 days and usually causes fever or meningitis, but is less often fatal compared with early infection.

  We don't know which antibiotic regimen is most effective at preventing group B streptococcal infection in high-risk neonates.

  Routine antibiotic prophylaxis given to low-birthweight babies after birth does not seem to be beneficial in reducing neonatal infection or mortality compared with monitoring and selective antibiotics.

  Increasing peripartum antibiotic prophylaxis is associated with a shift in pathogens causing neonatal sepsis, with *Escherichia coli* becoming a more prevalent cause.

(i) **Please visit www.clinicalevidence.bmj.com for full text and references**

What are the effects of prophylactic treatment of asymptomatic neonates less than 7 days old with known risk factors for early-onset group B streptococcal infection?

Unknown Effectiveness	• Different antibiotics
Unlikely To Be Beneficial	• Routine antibiotic prophylaxis (no more effective than monitoring and selective treatment)

Search date March 2007

DEFINITION Early-onset neonatal sepsis usually occurs within the first 7 days of life, and is typically caused by infection with group B streptococcus. About 90% of cases present within 24 hours of birth. One in three women carry group B streptococcus, which exists as part of the normal bacterial flora in the vaginal and anal areas. Infection can be transmitted by aspiration of group B streptococcus-positive amniotic fluid by the fetus. Symptoms of early-onset group B streptococcal infection may be non-specific, including temperature instability, poor feeding, excessive crying or irritability, and respiratory distress. Early-onset group B streptococcal infection typically presents with sepsis (69% of cases), leukopenia (31% of cases), pneumonia (26% of cases), respiratory distress (13% of cases), and, rarely, meningitis (11% of cases). Late-onset group B streptococcus infection occurs from 7–9 days of age, through to the end of the second month of life, and differs from early-onset group B streptococcal infection in terms of group B streptococcus serotype, clinical manifestations, and outcome. Late-onset infection typically presents with fever (100% of cases) and meningitis (60% of cases). This review deals with full-term and premature asymptomatic babies born with a known risk factor for group B streptococcal infection, but in whom a specific diagnosis of group B streptococcus (either by blood, urine, or cerebrospinal fluid) has not yet been made. The antenatal or intrapartum treatment of women with known group B streptococcal colonisation or infection is outside the scope of this review.

INCIDENCE/PREVALENCE The overall incidence of neonatal bacterial infections is between one and eight infants per 1000 live births, and between 160 and 300 per 1000 in very low-birthweight infants. Group B streptococcal infection accounts for nearly 50% of serious neonatal bacterial infections. One survey conducted in 2000–2001 estimated that there were 0.72 cases of group B streptococcal infection per 1000 live births in the UK and Ireland and that, of these, 0.48 cases per 1000 live births were early onset, and 0.24 cases per 1000 live births were late-onset infection. Although the estimated incidence of early-onset group B streptococcal infection is 0.5 per 1000 births in the UK overall, incidence varies geographically from 0.21 per 1000 live births in Scotland to 0.73 per 1000 live births in Northern Ireland. Overall, the USA and the UK have relatively similar incidences. One population-based study (427,000 live births) carried out in the USA in 2004 found that the prevalence of early-onset group B streptococcus infections in the USA has decreased from 2.0 per 1000 live births in 1990 to 0.3 per 1000 live births in 2004. This is thought to be a result of the increasing use of maternal intrapartum antibiotic prophylaxis.

AETIOLOGY/RISK FACTORS The main risk factor for group B streptococcal infection in the baby is maternal group B streptococcal infection, which is transmitted *in utero*. Bacteria originating in the maternal genital tract can infect the amniotic fluid via intact or ruptured membranes. Neonatal infection can result from fetal aspiration or ingestion of the infected amniotic fluid. Infection of the neonate can also occur during birth, when the neonate moves through the vagina, with systemic infection occurring via the umbilical cord, respiratory tract, or skin abrasions. Other risk factors for group B streptococcal infection include prematurity, low birthweight, prolonged rupture of membranes, intrapartum fever, chorioamnionitis, maternal ethnicity (black and hispanic mothers are at increased risk compared with white mothers), endometritis, heavy maternal colonisation, and frequent vaginal examinations during labour and delivery. Lower maternal age (less than 20 years) and cigarette smoking have been suggested to be associated with an increased risk of early-onset group B streptococcal infection, but these associations have not been proven. Other factors that may increase the risk of group B streptococcal infection include lower socioeconomic status, and maternal urinary tract infection during the third trimester (quantitative estimates of the increase in risk are not available). The role of group B streptococcal colonisation of fathers, siblings, and close household contacts in the development of late-onset group B streptococcal infection is unclear. Late-onset group B streptococcus sepsis is predominantly associated with serotype 3, with cases evenly distributed, presenting from 8–90 days after birth.

PROGNOSIS Group B streptococcal infection is a frequent cause of neonatal morbidity and mortality. Untreated, mortality from symptomatic early-onset group B streptococcal infection approaches 100%. The combined morbidity and mortality in early-onset group B streptococcal infection exceeds 50%, despite the use of appropriate antibiotics and supportive treatment. In the UK, one study has estimated that early-onset group B streptococcus infection causes more than 40 neonatal deaths and around 25 cases of long-term disability every year, whereas late-onset group B streptococcus infection causes around 16 deaths and 40 cases of long-term disability every year. Even with immediate initiation of antibiotic treatment, mortality with early-onset group B streptococcal infection has been reported to be as high as about 30%. Mortality is particularly high: among babies born prematurely, with low birthweight; after prolonged rupture of membranes; and in babies who develop respiratory distress, sepsis, meningitis, or leukopenia. Even with aggressive interventions, premature infants have a four- to 15-fold higher risk of mortality compared with term infants with early-onset group B streptococcus disease. One population-based study (427,000 live births) carried out in the USA in 2004 found that the mortality rate for preterm infants with early-onset group B streptococcus infection was 23%. The morbidity rate in late-onset group B streptococcal infection has been estimated at 4–6%. Late-onset group B streptococcus infection typically presents as bacteraemia or meningitis. Less frequently, late-onset group B streptococcus infection may cause septic arthritis, cellulitis, or focal infections such as osteomyelitis. Late-onset group B streptococcal infection tends to have a less fulminant onset and is less often fatal than early-onset infection. One observational study reported a mortality rate of 14% with early-onset group B streptococcal infection compared with 4% with late-onset infection. Infants with a blood pH of below 7.25, birthweight below 2500 grams, absolute neutrophil count of below 1500 cells per mm^3, hypotension, apnoea, and pleural effusion may be at higher risk of mortality. Little information is available concerning long-term sequelae for survivors of neonatal group B streptococcal infection.

David Evans

KEY POINTS

- About 50% of term and 80% of preterm babies develop jaundice, which usually appears 2–4 days after birth, and usually resolves spontaneously after 1–2 weeks.

  Jaundice is caused by bilirubin deposition in the skin. Most jaundice in newborn infants is a result of increased red cell breakdown and decreased bilirubin excretion.

  Breastfeeding, haemolysis, and some metabolic and genetic disorders also increase the risk of jaundice.

  Unconjugated bilirubin can be neurotoxic, causing an acute or chronic encephalopathy that may result in cerebral palsy, hearing loss, and seizures.

- Phototherapy provided by conventional or fibreoptic lights in hospital reduces neonatal jaundice compared with no treatment (as assessed by serum bilirubin levels), although we don't know which is the best regimen to use.

  We don't know whether home phototherapy is more or less effective than hospital phototherapy as we found no studies comparing the two treatments.

- There is consensus that exchange transfusion reduces serum bilirubin levels and prevents neurodevelopmental sequelae, although we found no studies to confirm this.

  Exchange transfusion has an estimated mortality of 3–4 per 1000 exchanged infants, and 5–10% permanent sequelae in survivors.

  We don't know whether albumin infusion is beneficial.

- Tin-mesoporphyrin is not currently licensed for routine clinical use in the UK or USA, and further long-term studies are warranted to confirm its place in clinical practice.

  However, tin-mesoporphyrin reduced the need for phototherapy (as assessed by serum bilirubin levels) when given either to preterm infants on the first day, or to jaundiced term or near-term infants within the first few days of life.

(i) **Please visit www.clinicalevidence.bmj.com for full text and references**

What are the effects of treatments for unconjugated hyperbilirubinaemia in term and preterm infants?	
Beneficial	• Hospital phototherapy
Likely To Be Beneficial	• Exchange transfusion*
Unknown Effectiveness	• Albumin infusion • Home versus hospital phototherapy • Tin-mesoporphyrin

Search date November 2006

*Although we found no RCTs, there is general consensus that exchange transfusion is effective in reducing serum bilirubin levels.

DEFINITION Neonatal jaundice refers to the yellow coloration of the skin and sclera of newborn babies that results from hyperbilirubinaemia.

INCIDENCE/PREVALENCE Jaundice is the most common condition requiring medical attention in newborn babies. About 50% of term and 80% of preterm babies develop jaundice in the first week of life. Jaundice is also a common cause of readmission to hospital after early discharge of newborn babies. Jaundice usually appears 2–4 days after birth and disappears 1–2 weeks later, usually without the need for treatment.

AETIOLOGY/RISK FACTORS Jaundice occurs when there is accumulation of bilirubin in the skin and mucous membranes. In most infants with jaundice, there is no underlying disease, and the jaundice is termed physiological. Physiological jaundice typically presents on the second or third day of life, and results from the increased production of bilirubin (owing to increased circulating red cell mass and a shortened red cell lifespan) and the decreased excretion of bilirubin (owing to low concentrations of the hepatocyte binding protein, low activity of glucuronosyl transferase, and increased enterohepatic circulation) that normally occur in newborn babies. Breast-fed infants are more likely to develop jaundice within the first week of life; this is thought to be an exacerbated physiological jaundice caused by a lower calorific intake and increased enterohepatic circulation of bilirubin. Prolonged unconjugated jaundice, persisting beyond the second week, is also seen in breast-fed infants. The mechanism for this later "breast milk jaundice syndrome" is still not completely understood. Non-physiological causes include blood group incompatibility (Rhesus or ABO problems), other causes of haemolysis, sepsis, bruising, and metabolic disorders. Gilbert's and Crigler–Najjar syndromes are rare causes of neonatal jaundice.

PROGNOSIS In the newborn baby, unconjugated bilirubin can penetrate the blood–brain barrier and is potentially neurotoxic. Acute bilirubin encephalopathy consists of initial lethargy and hypotonia, followed by hypertonia (retrocollis and opisthotonus), irritability, apnoea, and seizures. Kernicterus refers to the yellow staining of the deep nuclei of the brain — namely, the basal ganglia (globus pallidus); however, the term is also used to describe the chronic form of bilirubin encephalopathy, which includes symptoms such as athetoid cerebral palsy, hearing loss, failure of upward gaze, and dental enamel dysplasia. The exact level of bilirubin that is neurotoxic is unclear, and kernicterus at autopsy has been reported in infants in the absence of markedly elevated levels of bilirubin. Recent reports suggest a resurgence of kernicterus in countries in which this complication had virtually disappeared. This has been attributed mainly to early discharge of newborns from hospital.

Darcie Kiddoo

KEY POINTS

- Nocturnal enuresis affects 15–20% of 5-year-old children, 5% of 10-year-old children, and 1–2% of people aged 15 years and over. Without treatment, 15% of affected children will become dry each year.

  Nocturnal enuresis is not diagnosed in children younger than 5 years, and treatment may be inappropriate for children younger than 7 years.

- Enuresis alarms increase the number of dry nights compared with no treatment, and may be more effective than TCAs at reducing treatment failure and relapse.

  Combining the use of alarms with dry bed training may increase the number of dry nights, but we don't know whether adding TCAs to alarms is also beneficial.

- We don't know whether using an alarm clock set to wake the child before the time of likely enuresis is more likely to lead to dry nights compared with waking every 3 hours.

- Desmopressin and TCAs reduce the number of wet nights compared with placebo, but do not seem effective once treatment is discontinued, and can cause adverse effects which, in the case of TCAs, include potentially fatal overdose.

  We don't know whether desmopressin is more or less effective at reducing wet nights than TCAs or enuresis alarms.

  An alert has been issued in the UK regarding rare but serious adverse effects including hyponatraemia, water intoxication, and convulsions associated with desmopressin nasal spray, and the primary nocturnal enuresis indication has been withdrawn from the nasal spray in the UK.

- We don't know whether dry bed training, anticholinergic drugs, acupuncture or laser acupuncture, or hypnotherapy are effective at increasing dry nights, or how they compare with other treatments.

(i) **Please visit www.clinicalevidence.bmj.com for full text and references**

What are the effects of interventions for relief of symptoms of nocturnal enuresis?	
Beneficial	• Desmopressin (while treatment continues)
	• Dry bed training plus enuresis alarm
	• Enuresis alarm
Trade-off Between Benefits And Harms	• TCAs (imipramine, desipramine)
Unknown Effectiveness	• Anticholinergic drugs (oxybutynin, tolterodine, hyoscyamine)
	• Desmopressin plus enuresis alarm
	• Dry bed training
	• Hypnotherapy
	• Laser acupuncture

	• Standard home alarm clock
Unlikely To Be Beneficial	• Desmopressin (after treatment discontinuation)

Search date March 2007

DEFINITION Nocturnal enuresis is the involuntary discharge of urine at night in a child aged 5 years or older in the absence of congenital or acquired defects of the central nervous system or urinary tract. Disorders that have bedwetting as a symptom (termed "nocturnal incontinence") can be excluded by a thorough history, examination, and urinalysis. "Monosymptomatic" nocturnal enuresis is characterised by night-time symptoms only and accounts for 85% of cases. Nocturnal enuresis is defined as primary if the child has not been dry for a period of more than 6 months, and secondary if such a period of dryness preceded the onset of wetting. Most management strategies are aimed at children aged 7 years and older.

INCIDENCE/PREVALENCE Between 15–20% of 5-year-olds, 7% of 7-year-olds, 5% of 10-year-olds, 2–3% of 12–14-year-olds, and 1–2% of people aged 15 years and over wet the bed twice a week on average.

AETIOLOGY/RISK FACTORS Nocturnal enuresis is associated with several factors, including small functional bladder capacity, nocturnal polyuria, and, most commonly, arousal dysfunction. Linkage studies have identified associated genetic loci on chromosomes 8q, 12q, 13q, and 22q11.

PROGNOSIS Nocturnal enuresis has widely differing outcomes, from spontaneous resolution to complete resistance to all current treatments. About 1% of children remain enuretic until adulthood. Without treatment, about 15% of children with enuresis become dry each year. We found no RCTs on the best age at which to start treatment in children with nocturnal enuresis. Anecdotal experience suggests that reassurance is sufficient below the age of 7 years. Behavioural treatments, such as moisture or wetting alarms, require motivation and commitment from the child and a parent. Anecdotal experience suggests that children under the age of 7 years may not exhibit the commitment needed.

Gerald McGarry

KEY POINTS

- Up to 9% of children may have recurrent nosebleeds, usually originating from the anterior septum, but many grow out of the problem.

  Nosebleeds may be associated with local inflammation and trauma, including picking the nose.

- Antiseptic cream may reduce nosebleeds compared with no treatment and may be as effective as silver nitrate cautery.

  Antiseptic creams may smell and taste unpleasant.

  Silver nitrate cautery is usually painful even if local anaesthesia is used.

  Simultaneous bilateral cautery is not recommended owing to the possible increased risk of perforation of the septum.

  We don't know whether petroleum jelly speeds up resolution of recurrent bleeding compared with no treatment.

(i) **Please visit www.clinicalevidence.bmj.com for full text and references**

What are the effects of treatments for recurrent idiopathic epistaxis in children?

Likely To Be Beneficial	• Antiseptic cream
Unknown Effectiveness	• Cautery • Petroleum jelly

Search date January 2006

DEFINITION Recurrent idiopathic epistaxis is recurrent, self-limiting, nasal bleeding for which no specific cause is identified. There is no consensus on the frequency or severity of recurrences.

INCIDENCE/PREVALENCE A cross-sectional study of 1218 children (aged 11–14 years) found that 9% had frequent episodes of epistaxis. It is likely that only the most severe episodes are considered for treatment.

AETIOLOGY/RISK FACTORS In children, most epistaxis occurs from the anterior part of the septum in the region of Little's area. Initiating factors include local inflammation, mucosal drying, and local trauma (including nose picking). Epistaxis caused by other specific local (e.g. tumours) or systemic (e.g. clotting disorders) factors is not considered here.

PROGNOSIS Recurrent epistaxis is less common in people over 14 years old, and many children "grow out" of this problem.

David E Arterburn

KEY POINTS

- Obesity is the result of long-term energy imbalances, where daily energy intake exceeds daily energy expenditure.

  Along with long-term health problems, obesity in children is associated with short term psychosocial problems, including social marginalisation, low self-esteem, and impaired quality of life.

  Most obese adolescents stay obese as adults.

- Obesity is increasing among children and adolescents, with 14% of boys and 17% of girls in the UK aged 2–15 years obese in 2004.

- Multifactorial interventions (behavioural, dietary, and physical) may help overweight and obese children to lose weight when the interventions are targeted at the family.

  Interventions involving problem solving may increase the effectiveness of multifactorial interventions.

- We don't know if behavioural, dietary, or physical interventions alone can help overweight and obese children lose weight.

(i) **Please visit www.clinicalevidence.bmj.com for full text and references**

What are the effects of lifestyle interventions for the treatment of childhood obesity?

Likely To Be Beneficial	• Multifactorial interventions
Unknown Effectiveness	• Behavioural interventions alone • Diet alone • Physical activity alone

Search date August 2006

DEFINITION Obesity is a chronic condition characterised by an excess of body fat. It is most often defined by the BMI, which is highly correlated with body fat. BMI is weight in kilograms divided by height in metres squared (kg/m^2). In children and adolescents, BMI varies with age and sex. It typically rises during the first months after birth, falls after the first year and rises again around the sixth year of life. Thus, a given BMI value is usually compared against reference charts to obtain a ranking of BMI percentile for age and sex. The BMI percentile indicates the relative position of the child's BMI as compared with a historical reference population of children of the same age and sex. Worldwide, there is little agreement on the definition of overweight and obesity among children; however, a BMI above the 85th percentile is generally considered to be at least "at risk for overweight" in the USA and UK. A BMI above the 95th percentile is variably defined as overweight or obese but generally indicates a need for intervention.

INCIDENCE/PREVALENCE The prevalence of obesity (generally BMI above the 95th percentile) is steadily increasing among children and adolescents. In the UK in 2004, it was estimated that 14% of boys and 17% of girls aged 2–15 were obese. The prevalence of overweight among children and adolescents in the US increased from 14% in 1999–2000 to 16% in 2003–2004 among girls and from 14% to 18% among boys.

AETIOLOGY/RISK FACTORS Obesity is the result of long-term energy imbalances, where daily energy intake exceeds daily energy expenditure. Energy balance is modulated by a myriad of factors, including metabolic rate, appetite, diet, and physical activity. Although these factors are influenced by genetic traits in a moderate number of children, the

(continued over)

(from previous page)

increase in obesity prevalence in the past few decades cannot be explained by changes in the human gene pool, and is more often attributed to environmental changes that promote excessive food intake and discourage physical activity. The risk of childhood obesity is related to childhood diet and sedentary time. Other risk factors are parental obesity, low parental education, social deprivation, infant feeding patterns, early or more rapid puberty (both a risk factor and an effect of obesity), extreme (both high and low) birthweights, and gestational diabetes. Specifically, physical activity levels have decreased over the years and now only 36% of children and adolescents in the USA are meeting recommended levels of physical activity. Less commonly, obesity may also be induced by drugs (e.g. high-dose glucocorticoids), neuroendocrine disorders (e.g. Cushing's syndrome), or inherited disorders (e.g. Down's syndrome and Prader–Willi syndrome). In this review, we have considered treatment of children for overweight and obesity in a clinical setting (not broader public-health settings — e.g. interventions given to a whole school). We have included interventions given to the children, their parents, or both.

PROGNOSIS Most obese adolescents will become obese adults. For example, a 5-year longitudinal study of obese adolescents age 13–19 years found that 86% remained obese as young adults. Obesity is associated with a higher prevalence of insulin resistance, elevated blood lipids, increased blood pressure, and impaired glucose tolerance, which in turn may increase the risk of several chronic diseases in adulthood, including hypertension, dyslipidaemia, diabetes, CVD, sleep apnoea, osteoarthritis, and some cancers. Perhaps the most significant short term morbidities for overweight/obese children are psychosocial, and include social marginalisation, low self-esteem, and impaired quality of life. Clinicians should emphasise improvements in diet, physical activity, and health independently of changes in body weight.

KEY POINTS

- **OME (glue ear) usually presents with concerns about the child's behaviour, performance at school, or language development.**

  Children usually only have mild hearing impairment and few other symptoms.

  Up to 80% of children have been affected by the age of 4 years, but prevalence declines beyond 6 years of age.

  Non-purulent middle-ear infections can occur in children or adults after upper respiratory tract infection or AOM.

  At least half of cases resolve within 3 months and 95% within a year, but complications such as tympanic membrane perforation, tympanosclerosis, otorrhoea, and cholesteatoma can occur.

- **Risk of OME is increased with passive smoking, bottle feeding, low socioeconomic group, and exposure to many other children.**

  However, there is no evidence to show whether interventions to modify these risk factors reduce the risk of OME.

- **Autoinflation with a nasal balloon may improve effusions, but other devices have not been shown to be effective.**

  Purpose-manufactured nasal balloons may improve effusions over 2 weeks to 3 months, but long-term efficacy is unknown. Children may find autoinflation difficult.

- **Oral antibiotics, antihistamines plus oral decongestants, or mucolytics may be of no benefit in OME, and can cause adverse effects.**

  Antibiotics can cause adverse effects in up to a third of children with OME.

  Antihistamines can cause behavioural changes, seizures, and blood pressure variability.

- **Oral corticosteroids are unlikely to improve symptoms in OME, and can cause growth retardation.**

  We don't know whether intranasal corticosteroids are of benefit.

- **Ventilation tubes may improve short-term outcomes, but the clinical effect size is small. They may also increase the risk of tympanic membrane abnormalities.**

  Ventilation tubes improve hearing for the first 2 years, but have no longer-term benefit, and may not affect cognition or language development.

  Adenoidectomy may improve hearing when performed with tympanostomy, but the clinical significance of the improvements are unclear.

(i) **Please visit www.clinicalevidence.bmj.com for full text and references**

What are the effects of interventions to prevent OME in children?	
Unknown Effectiveness	• Modifying risk factors to prevent OME

What are the effects of pharmacological, mechanical, and surgical interventions to treat OME in children?

Likely To Be Beneficial	• Autoinflation with purpose-manufactured nasal balloon
Trade-off Between Benefits And Harms	• Oral corticosteroids • Ventilation tubes • Ventilation tubes plus adenoidectomy
Unknown Effectiveness	• Adenoidectomy alone • Autoinflation (with devices other than purpose-manufactured nasal balloon) • Intranasal corticosteroids
Unlikely To Be Beneficial	• Antibiotics (oral) • Mucolytics
Likely To Be Ineffective Or Harmful	• Antihistamines plus oral decongestants

Search date March 2007

DEFINITION OME or "glue ear", is serous or mucoid but not mucopurulent fluid in the middle ear. Children usually present with hearing impairment and speech problems. In contrast to those with AOM (see review on p 64), children with OME do not suffer from acute ear pain, fever, or malaise. Hearing impairment is usually mild and often identified when parents express concern regarding their child's behaviour, performance at school, or language development.

INCIDENCE/PREVALENCE OME is commonly seen in paediatric practice, and accounts for 25–35% of all cases of otitis media. One study in the UK found that, at any time, 5% of children aged 5 years had persistent (at least 3 months) bilateral hearing impairment associated with OME. The prevalence declines considerably beyond 6 years of age. Studies in the USA and Europe have estimated that about 50–80% of children aged 4 years have been affected by OME at some time. One study in the USA estimated that, between the ages of 2 months and 2 years, 91.1% of young children will have one episode of middle-ear effusion, and 52.2% will have bilateral involvement. OME is the most common reason for referral for surgery in children in the UK. The number of general practitioner consultations for OME increased from 15.2/1000 (2–10-year-olds) a year to 16.7/1000 a year between 1991 and 2001. Middle-ear effusions also occur infrequently in adults after upper respiratory tract infection or after air travel, and may persist for weeks or months after an episode of AOM.

AETIOLOGY/RISK FACTORS Contributory factors include upper respiratory tract infection and narrow upper respiratory airways. Case-control studies have identified risk factors, including age 6 years or younger, day-care centre attendance, large number of siblings, low socioeconomic group, frequent upper respiratory tract infection, bottle feeding, and household smoking. These factors may be associated with about twice the risk of developing OME.

PROGNOSIS Data from one prospective study of children aged 2–4 years showed that 50% of OME cases resolved within 3 months and 95% within a year. In 5% of preschool children, OME (identified by tympanometric screening) persisted for at least 1 year. One cohort study of 3-year-olds found that 65% of OME cases cleared spontaneously within 3 months. Most children aged 6 years or older will not have further problems. The disease is ultimately self-limiting in most cases. However, one large cohort study (534 children) found that middle-ear disease increased reported hearing difficulty at 5 years of age (OR 1.44, 95% CI 1.18 to 1.76) and was associated with delayed language development in children up to 10 years of age. Hearing impairment is the most common complication of OME. Most children with OME have fluctuating or persistent hearing deficits with mild to moderate degrees of hearing loss, averaging 27 decibels. The type of hearing impairment is usually conductive, but it may be sensorineural, or both. The sensorineural type is usually permanent. Tympanic membrane perforation, tympanosclerosis, otorrhoea, and cholesteatoma occur more frequently among children with OME than among those without OME.

Perinatal asphyxia

William McGuire

KEY POINTS

- Estimates of the incidence of perinatal asphyxia vary. In resource-rich countries, severe perinatal asphyxia (causing death or severe neurological impairment) is 1/1000 live births; in resource-poor countries, studies suggest an incidence of 5–10/1000 live births.

- Limited evidence from three small, weak RCTs suggests that mortality may be lower in infants treated with antioxidants compared with placebo.

- There is limited evidence that hypothermia reduces mortality and neurodevelopmental disability in infants with perinatal asphyxia.

- Limited evidence from one small RCT suggests that a magnesium sulphate/dopamine combination may be more effective than no treatment in reducing a combined outcome of mortality, abnormal scans, and failure to feed.

- Small RCTs with flawed methods suggest that anticonvulsants are of no benefit in reducing mortality or improving neurodevelopmental outcomes in term infants with perinatal asphyxia.

- Resuscitation in air lowered mortality in infants with perinatal asphyxia compared with resuscitation in 100% oxygen. However, current clinical practice is to use 100% oxygen.

- Limited evidence from a systematic review, which reported problems with publication bias in the RCTs it identified, suggests that hyperbaric oxygen treatment lowers rates of mortality and adverse neurological outcomes in infants with perinatal asphyxia and hypoxic–ischaemic encephalopathy. This treatment, although widely used in China, is not standard practice in other countries.

- We don't know whether calcium channel blockers, corticosteroids, fluid restriction, hyperventilation, inotrope support, mannitol, or opiate antagonists are helpful in infants with perinatal asphyxia.

ⓘ **Please visit www.clinicalevidence.bmj.com for full text and references**

What are the effects of interventions in term or near-term newborns with perinatal asphyxia?

Unknown Effectiveness	
	• Antioxidants
	• Calcium channel blockers
	• Corticosteroids
	• Fluid restriction
	• Head and/or whole-body hypothermia
	• Hyperbaric oxygen treatment
	• Hyperventilation
	• Inotrope support
	• Magnesium sulphate
	• Mannitol
	• Opiate antagonists

	• Resuscitation in air (may lower mortality compared with resuscitation using higher concentrations of oxygen but 100% oxygen remains standard practice)
Unlikely To Be Beneficial	• Anticonvulsants (prophylactic)

Search date March 2007

DEFINITION The clinical diagnosis of perinatal asphyxia is based on several criteria, the two main ones being evidence of cardiorespiratory and neurological depression (defined as an Apgar score remaining less than 7 at 5 minutes after birth) and evidence of acute hypoxic compromise with acidaemia (defined as an arterial blood pH of less than 7 or base excess greater than 12 mmol/L). In many settings, especially resource-poor countries, it may be impossible to assess fetal or neonatal acidaemia. In the immediate postpartum period when resuscitation is being undertaken, it may not be possible to determine whether the neurological and cardiorespiratory depression is secondary to hypoxia–ischaemia, or to another condition such as feto-maternal infection, or metabolic disease. Consequently, resuscitation and early management will often be of suspected rather than confirmed perinatal asphyxia. This review deals with perinatal asphyxia in term and near-term newborns.

INCIDENCE/PREVALENCE Estimates of the incidence of perinatal asphyxia vary depending on the definitions used. In resource-rich countries, the incidence of severe perinatal asphyxia (causing death or severe neurological impairment) is about 1/1000 live births. In resource-poor countries, perinatal asphyxia is probably much more common. Data from hospital-based studies in such settings suggest an incidence of 5–10/1000 live births. However, this probably represents an underestimate of the true community incidence of perinatal asphyxia in resource-poor countries.

AETIOLOGY/RISK FACTORS Perinatal asphyxia may occur *in utero*, during labour and delivery, or in the immediate postnatal period. There are numerous causes, including placental abruption, cord compression, transplacental anaesthetic or narcotic administration, intrauterine pneumonia, severe meconium aspiration, congenital cardiac or pulmonary anomalies, and birth trauma. Postnatal asphyxia can be caused by an obstructed airway, maternal opiates — which can cause respiratory depression — or congenital sepsis.

PROGNOSIS Worldwide, perinatal asphyxia is a major cause of death and of acquired brain damage in newborn infants. The prognosis depends on the severity of the asphyxia. Only a minority of infants with severe encephalopathy after perinatal asphyxia survive without handicap. However, there are limited population-based data on long-term outcomes after perinatal asphyxia, such as cerebral palsy, developmental delay, visual and hearing impairment, and learning and behavioural problems. After an asphyxial event, there may be an opportunity to intervene to minimise brain damage. The first phase of brain damage — early cell death — results from primary exhaustion of the cellular energy stores. Early cell death can occur within minutes. Immediate resuscitation to restore oxygen supply and blood circulation aims to limit the extent of this damage. A secondary phase of neuronal injury may occur several hours after the initial insult. The mechanisms believed to be important in this process include oxygen free-radical production, intracellular calcium entry, and apoptosis. Treatments during the postresuscitation phase aim to block these processes, thereby limiting secondary cell damage and minimising the extent of any brain damage.

David Creery and Angelo Mikrogianakis

KEY POINTS

- SIDS is the sudden death of an infant aged under 1 year that remains unexplained after review of the clinical history, examination of the scene of death, and postmortem.

  The incidence varies among countries, with 0.7 cases being reported per 1000 live births in England and Wales in 1996, and 0.8 cases per 1000 in the US.

  Because of the obvious difficulties in performing RCTs to study the effects of interventions in reducing the risk of SIDS, we report only observational evidence in this review.

- Campaigns that have advised avoiding prone sleeping have significantly reduced the incidence of SIDS.

  Observational studies have additionally shown that the incidence of prone positioning is dramatically reduced after national advice campaigns.

- Advice to avoid tobacco smoke exposure seems to reduce the incidence of SIDS.

  National campaigns that advise mothers to avoid tobacco-smoke exposure also seem to lead to a reduction in maternal smoking rates.

- Some campaigns included advice to avoid overheating, overwrapping, and bed sharing and advice to breastfeed, although it is not clear whether this contributed to the observed reduction in SIDS.

- We didn't find any studies looking at the effects of advice to avoid soft sleeping surfaces or to promote soother use.

(i) **Please visit www.clinicalevidence.bmj.com for full text and references**

What are the effects of interventions to reduce the risk of SIDS?

Beneficial	• Advice to avoid prone sleeping*
Likely To Be Beneficial	• Advice to avoid tobacco smoke exposure*
Unknown Effectiveness	• Advice to avoid bed sharing*
	• Advice to avoid overheating or overwrapping*
	• Advice to avoid soft sleeping surfaces*
	• Advice to breastfeed*
	• Advice to promote soother use*

Search date July 2005

*Observational evidence only; RCTs unlikely to be conducted.

DEFINITION SIDS is the sudden death of an infant aged under 1 year that remains unexplained after review of the clinical history, examination of the scene of death, and postmortem.

INCIDENCE/PREVALENCE The incidence of SIDS has varied over time and among nations (incidence per 1000 live births of SIDS in 1996: The Netherlands 0.3, Japan 0.4, Canada 0.5, England and Wales 0.7, USA 0.8, and Australia 0.9).

AETIOLOGY/RISK FACTORS By definition, the cause of SIDS is not known. Observational studies have found an association between SIDS and several risk factors, including prone sleeping position, prenatal or postnatal exposure to tobacco smoke, soft sleeping surfaces, hyperthermia/overwrapping, bed sharing (particularly with mothers who smoke), lack of breastfeeding, and lack of soother use. The risk of SIDS is increased in families in which there has already been a sudden infant death.

PROGNOSIS Prognosis is not applicable.

Sleep disorders in children

Paul Montgomery and Danielle Dunne

KEY POINTS

- Sleep disorders may affect 20–30% of young children, and include excessive daytime sleepiness, problems getting to sleep (dysomnias), or undesirable phenomena during sleep (parasomnias), such as sleep terrors, and sleep-walking.

  Children with physical or learning disabilities are at increased risk of sleep disorders. Other risk factors include being the first-born child, having a difficult temperament or having had colic, and increased maternal respon-siveness.

- There is a paucity of evidence about effective treatments for sleep disorders in children, especially about parasomnias, but behavioural interventions may be the best first-line approach.

- Extinction and graduated extinction interventions improve settling and reduce night wakes compared with placebo in healthy children, and in children with learning disabilities.

  Graduated extinction may be less distressing for parents, and therefore may have better compliance.

  Sleep hygiene interventions may reduce bedtime tantrums in healthy children compared with placebo, with similar effectiveness to graduated extinction.

  Sleep hygiene plus graduated extinction may reduce bedtime tantrums in children with physical or learning disabilities.

  We don't know whether combining behavioural therapy with benzodi-azepines or with chloral improves sleep or parasomnias.

- Melatonin may improve sleep onset and sleep time compared with placebo in healthy children, but we don't know if it is beneficial in children with disabilities, if it improves parasomnias, or what its long-term effects might be.

  We don't know whether antihistamines, exercise, light therapy, or sleep restriction improve dysomnias or parasomnias in children.

  We don't know whether safety or protective interventions, scheduled waking, extinction, or sleep hygiene are effective in children with paras-omnias.

(i) **Please visit www.clinicalevidence.bmj.com for full text and references**

What are the effects of treatments for dysomnias in children?

Likely To Be Beneficial	• Extinction and graduated extinction for dysomnia in both healthy children and those with learning difficulties • Sleep hygiene for dysomnia in otherwise healthy children
Trade-off Between Benefits And Harms	• Melatonin for dysomnia in otherwise healthy children
Unknown Effectiveness	• Antihistamines for dysomnia • Behavioural therapy plus benzodiazepines, or plus chloral and derivatives for dysomnia • Exercise for dysomnia

- Light therapy for dysomnia
- Melatonin for dysomnia in children with physical or learning difficulties
- Sleep hygiene for dysomnia in children with physical or learning difficulties
- Sleep restriction for dysomnia

What are the effects of treatments for parasomnias in children?

Unknown Effectiveness	
	• Antihistamines for parasomnia
	• Behavioural therapy plus benzodiazepines, or plus chloral and derivatives for parasomnia
	• Exercise for parasomnia
	• Extinction and graded extinction approaches for parasomnia
	• Light therapy for parasomnia
	• Melatonin for parasomnia
	• Safety/protective interventions for parasomnia
	• Scheduled waking for parasomnia
	• Sleep hygiene for parasomnia
	• Sleep restriction for parasomnia

Search date September 2006

DEFINITION The International Classification of Sleep Disorders-2 (ICSD-2) defines more than 80 sleep disorders, many of which apply to children — although often in different ways — as much as to adults. Sleep problems can be divided into two broad areas: too much sleep (dysomnias), or too little sleep (parasomnias). **Dysomnias** are disorders that produce either excessive daytime sleepiness, or difficulty initiating or maintaining sleep. They can be intrinsic, extrinsic, or circadian rhythm sleep disorders. Dysomnias include: primary insomnia, primary hypersomnia, narcolepsy, breathing-related sleep disorders, and circadian rhythm sleep disorder. **Parasomnias** are undesirable phenomena that occur predominantly during sleep. They are caused by inappropriately timed activation of physiological systems. Parasomnias include: nightmare disorder, sleep terror disorder, and sleepwalking disorder. **Children with physical or learning disabilities:** Sleep problems tend to be greater in prevalence and severity in this population. For example, pain is related to sleep disturbance, and attention paid to helping the child sleep better is likely to improve recovery. Across a range of physical problems, there are reports in the literature of sleep disturbance associated with them. In most cases, research is limited and the mechanisms are unclear. Children with visual impairment are prone to circadian rhythm problems: their light perception is poor, and the primary cue for sleep onset is lost. Many medications are known to cause sleep problems — such as severe drowsiness with many antiepileptic drugs. Learning disabilities vary considerably in the range of conditions covered by this global term. However, some conditions such as Smith–Magenis, Prader–Willi, and Williams syndrome have sleep disturbance as cardinal features. Others, such as Down's syndrome and mucopolysaccharidoses, are associated with sleep-related breathing problems. Treatment for these groups of children needs to be tailored to their particular problems, and may be problematic for anatomical and neurological reasons. Nevertheless, in large part, these sleep problems should be regarded as treatable, and careful investigation of these problems is required.

(continued over)

(from previous page)

INCIDENCE/PREVALENCE Sleep problems, primarily settling problems and frequent night wakings, are experienced by about 20–30% of children aged 1–5 years, but cultural differences would seem to play at least some role. These sleep disturbances often persist in later childhood: 40–80% of children displaying sleep problems when aged 15–48 months were found to have persistent sleep disorders 2–3 years later. In toddlers, settling and night waking problems are dominant, with rates about 20–25%. A second peak in sleep problems occurs in adolescence, where sleep-timing problems including delayed sleep phase syndrome occur. Such children have difficulty getting off to sleep, and then problems getting up in the morning for school. Across the age range, sleep-related breathing problems occur at rates about 2%. Narcolepsy is thought to occur with a prevalence of 4–6/10,000 in the USA in adults, with the onset of symptoms tending to occur in the second decade. **Children with physical or learning disabilities:** Prevalence of sleep disorders tends to be even greater in children with physical or learning disabilities: about 86% of children aged up to 6 years, 81% of children aged 6–11 years, and 77% of children aged 12–16 years with physical or learning disabilities suffer from severe sleep problems. We found no separate data for dysomnias and parasomnias.

AETIOLOGY/RISK FACTORS Evidence of the aetiology of sleep disorders in children is generally limited; however, the proportion of rapid eye movement (REM, active sleep) is greater in infants than in adults. REM is frequently associated with awakenings, and infants with a sleep disorder often need assistance to resume sleep after such arousals. Factors related to sleep disorders are: having had colic, being the first-born child, and the child having a difficult temperament (e.g. low sensory threshold, negative mood, decreased adaptability). Other factors have been suggested, such as being born prematurely, and low birthweight; however, evidence of such associations is contradictory. These factors may influence the onset of a sleep disorder, but the factors influencing the maintenance of a sleep problem are likely to be different. Increased maternal responsiveness is associated with the maintenance of sleep disorders in children.

PROGNOSIS Children with excessive daytime sleepiness or night waking are likely to suffer from impaired daytime functioning without treatment, and their parents are likely to have increased stress. In addition to these effects, children with parasomnias are at serious risk of accidental injuries. Between 40–80% of children aged 15–48 months displaying sleep problems had persistent sleep problems 2–3 years later. **Children with physical or learning disabilities:** Children with learning disabilities and sleep disorders are more likely to have greater challenging behaviour than those without sleep problems. This naturally affects the quality of life of the parents, frequently resulting in maternal stress, mothers displaying less affection for their children, and marital discord. For children with epilepsy, sleep disorders may exacerbate their condition: a persistent lack of sleep has been associated with an increased frequency of seizures.

KEY POINTS

- Up to 11.3% of girls and 3.6% of boys will have had a UTI by the age of 16, and recurrence of infection is common.

   Vesicoureteric reflux is identified in up to 40% of children being investigated for a first UTI, and is a risk factor for, but weak predictor of, renal scarring.

   Renal scarring occurs in 5–15% of children within 1–2 years of their first presentation with UTI, and is associated with increased risks of progressive renal damage. The risk of scarring probably diminishes over time.

- There is consensus that antibiotics are beneficial in children with UTI compared with no treatment, although few studies have been done to confirm this.

   We don't know whether immediate empirical antibiotic treatment is more effective at resolving symptoms or preventing renal scarring compared with treatment after a delay of 24 hours.

   Immediate treatment may reduce the risk of renal scarring compared with treatment delayed for more than 4 days.

   Longer courses of antibiotics don't seem to be more effective at treating uncomplicated, non-recurrent UTI or pyelonephritis than short (2–4 days) courses, and may be associated with more adverse effects. However, a single dose of oral antibiotics may be less effective than longer courses of the same antibiotic.

   Oral antibiotics may be as effective as intravenous antibiotics at treating UTI (including pyelonephritis) and preventing complications in children without vesicoureteric reflux or renal scarring.

- Prophylactic antibiotics may reduce the risk of recurrent UTI, but can cause adverse effects. We don't know the optimum duration of treatment.

   Immunotherapy, used either in addition to prophylactic antibiotics or on its own, may reduce recurrence of UTI, but studies so far have been small.

- Surgical correction of moderate to severe functional abnormalities may be no more effective than medical management in preventing UTI recurrence or complications, and increases morbidity associated with surgery.

   Children with minor functional anomalies do not seem to develop renal scarring, and so may not benefit from surgery.

ⓘ Please visit www.clinicalevidence.bmj.com for full text and references

What are the effects of treatment of acute UTI in children?	
Likely To Be Beneficial	• Antibiotics (more effective than placebo)*
	• Longer courses (7–10 days) of oral antibiotics (increased cure rates compared with single-dose regimens)

	● Oral antibiotics (as effective as initial intravenous antibiotics in children without severe vesicoureteric reflux or renal scarring)
Unknown Effectiveness	● Immediate empirical antibiotic treatment (unclear benefit compared with delayed treatment, based on microscopy and culture)
Unlikely To Be Beneficial	● Longer (7–14 days) courses of initial intravenous antibiotics (no more effective than shorter [3–4 days] courses of intravenous antibiotics in children with acute pyelonephritis) ● Longer (7–14 days) courses of oral antibiotics (no more effective than shorter [2–4 days] courses for non-recurrent lower UTI in the absence of renal tract abnormality)
Likely To Be Ineffective Or Harmful	● Prolonged delay in antibiotic treatment (more than 4 days)*

What are the effects of interventions to prevent recurrence of UTI in children?

Likely To Be Beneficial	● Immunotherapy ● Prophylactic antibiotics
Unknown Effectiveness	● Surgical correction of minor functional anomalies
Unlikely To Be Beneficial	● Surgical correction of moderate to severe vesicoureteric reflux (grades III–IV, as effective as medical management but with surgical risks)

Search date December 2006

*Based on consensus. RCTs would be considered unethical.

DEFINITION UTI is defined by the presence of a pure growth of more than 10^5 colony-forming units of bacteria per millilitre of urine. Lower counts of bacteria may be clinically important, especially in boys, and in specimens obtained by urinary catheter. Any growth of typical urinary pathogens is considered clinically important if obtained by suprapubic aspiration. In practice, three age ranges are usually considered on the basis of differential risk and different approaches to management: children under 1 year; young children (1–4, 5, or 7 years, depending on the information source); and older children (up to 12–16 years). Recurrent UTI is defined as a further infection by a new organism. Relapsing UTI is defined as a further infection with the same organism.

INCIDENCE/PREVALENCE Boys are more susceptible to UTI than girls before the age of 6 months; thereafter, the incidence is substantially higher in girls than in boys. Estimates of the true incidence of UTI depend on rates of diagnosis and investigation. Observational studies have found that UTIs have been diagnosed in Sweden in at least 2.2% of boys and 2.1% of girls by the age of 2 years, in 7.8% of girls and 1.7% of boys by the age of 7 years, and in the UK in 11.3% of girls and 3.6% of boys by the age of 16 years.

AETIOLOGY/RISK FACTORS The normal urinary tract is sterile. Contamination by bowel flora may result in urinary infection if a virulent organism is involved, or if the child is immunosuppressed. In neonates, infection may originate from other sources. *Escherichia coli* accounts for about 75% of all pathogens. *Proteus* is more common in boys (one study found that proteus caused 33% of UTIs in boys aged 1–16 years, compared with 0% of UTIs in girls aged 1–16). **Obstructive anomalies** are found in 0–4%, and **vesicoureteric reflux** in 8–40% of children being investigated for their first UTI. One meta-analysis of 12 cohort studies (537 children admitted to hospital for UTI, 1062 kidneys) found that 36% of all kidneys had some scarring on DMSA scintigraphy, and that 59% of children with vesicoureteric reflux on micturating cystourethrography had at least one scarred kidney (pooled positive likelihood ratio 1.96, 95% CI 1.51 to 2.54; pooled negative likelihood ratio 0.71, 95% CI 0.58 to 0.85). There was evidence of heterogeneity in likelihood ratios among studies. The authors concluded that vesicoureteric reflux is a weak predictor of renal damage in children admitted to hospital. Thus, although vesicoureteric reflux is a major risk factor for adverse outcome, other factors, some of which have not yet been identified, are also important. **Family history:** Vesicoureteric reflux itself runs in families: in one review article, the incidence of reflux in siblings ranged from 26% (a cohort of asymptomatic siblings) to 86% (siblings with a history of UTI) compared with a rate of less than 1% in the general population. Although some gene variants seem more common in children who suffer renal damage, no clear link has yet been established between specific genes and an adverse outcome. Local or systemic immune problems are also likely to be factors in the development of UTI.

PROGNOSIS **Recurrence:** A study in the UK found that 78% of girls and 71% of boys presenting with UTI within the first year of life experienced recurrence, and that 45% of girls and 39% of boys presenting after their first year of life developed further infections. **Vesicoureteric reflux:** In a longitudinal study, 84% of children (572 children with UTI and vesicoureteric reflux) had spontaneous resolution during medical follow-up at between 5–15 years. **Renal scarring:** A systematic review of imaging in childhood UTI suggested that renal scarring (assessed with intravenous pyelogram [IVP] or dimercaptosuccinic acid [DMSA] scan) occurs in 5–15% of children within 1–2 years of their first diagnosed UTI. Between 32–70% of these scars were noted at the time of initial assessment, suggesting a high level of pre-existing scarring, perhaps caused by previously unrecognised infection. This percentage did not substantially alter, despite an increasing referral rate, during the 3 years studied. One meta-analysis of 12 cohort studies (537 children admitted to hospital for UTI, 1062 kidneys) found that 36% of all kidneys had some scarring on DMSA scintigraphy, and that 59% of children with vesicoureteric reflux on micturating cystourethrography had at least one scarred kidney (pooled positive likelihood ratio 1.96, 95% CI 1.51 to 2.54; pooled negative likelihood ratio 0.71, 95% CI 0.58 to 0.85). However, there was evidence of heterogeneity in likelihood ratios among studies. The authors concluded that vesicoureteric reflux is a weak predictor of renal damage in children admitted to hospital. A retrospective population-based study in the UK suggested that 4.3% of boys and 4.7% of girls develop scarring (assessed using DMSA scans after their first referral for UTI). **New or progressive renal scarring and recurrent UTI:** The systematic review reported on four studies that provided at least 2 years' follow-up: new renal scars developed in 1.6–23% of children, and existing renal scars progressed in 6–34%. It is unclear whether figures for new scars included any children who were previously unscarred. The highest rates of scarring were associated with the highest rates of recurrent UTI. A further study showed that, in children aged 5 years and over, abnormal DMSA scans were noted in 64/118 (55%) children presenting with recurrent UTI, whereas 7/44 (15%) who presented with "first UTI" had scarring (OR for recurrences causing scarring: OR 6.3; 95% CI 2.6 to 15.2). However, recurrent UTI may be less important as a risk factor for scarring in older children: one study showed that, in children with initially normal scans at 3 or 4 years of age, 5/176 (3%) children aged 3 years at presentation, and 0/179 (0%) aged 4 years at presentation had developed scarring between 2 and 11 years later. Of those children who developed scarring, 4/5 (80%) had a definite history of recurrent UTI, in all cases 3 or more episodes (OR for recurrences causing scarring: 11.5; 95% CI 1.3 to 106.1). Another study (287 children with severe vesicoureteric reflux treated either medically or surgically for any UTI) used serial DMSA scintigraphy to evaluate the risk of renal scarring over 5 years. It found that younger children (aged below 2 years) were at greater risk of renal scarring than older children, regardless of treatment for the infection (AR for deterioration in DMSA scan over 5 years: 21/86 (24%) for younger children v 27/201 (13%) for older children; RR 1.82, 95% CI 1.09 to 3.03). It is likely that children who present when older, and who are found to have

(continued over)

(from previous page)

scarring, will have had one or more previous UTI that remained undiagnosed. Many children seem to lose their susceptibility to renal damage with age. **Consequences for longer term:** One long-term follow-up study in the UK found that children with renal scarring and vesicoureteric reflux at presentation, or just one of these followed by documented UTI, were associated with an increased risk of progressive renal damage compared with children presenting without these features (RR of progressive renal damage: 17, 95% CI 2.5 to 118). Renal scarring may be associated with future complications, such as poor renal growth, recurrent adult pyelonephritis, impaired glomerular function, early hypertension, and end-stage renal failure. A combination of recurrent UTI, severe vesicoureteric reflux, and the presence of renal scarring at first presentation is associated with the worst prognosis.

Dereck Hunt

KEY POINTS

- Diabetic foot ulceration is full-thickness penetration of the dermis of the foot in a person with diabetes. Severity is classified using the Wagner system, which grades it from 1 to 5.

  The annual incidence of ulcers among people with diabetes is 2.5–10.7% in resource-rich countries, and the annual incidence of amputation for any reason is 0.25–1.8%.

  For people with healed diabetic foot ulcers, the 5-year cumulative rate of ulcer recurrence is 66% and of amputation is 12%.

- The most effective preventive measure for major amputation appears to be screening and referral to a foot-care clinic if high-risk features are present.

  Other interventions for reducing the risk of foot ulcers include wearing therapeutic footware, and increasing patient education for prevention, but we found no sufficient evidence to ascertain the effectiveness of these treatments.

- Pressure off-loading with total-contact casting or non-removable fibreglass casts successfully improves healing of ulcers.

  Removable-cast walkers rendered irremovable seem equally effective, but have the added benefit of requiring less technical expertise for fitting.

  We don't know whether pressure off-loading with felted foam or pressure-relief half-shoe is effective in treating diabetic foot ulcers.

- Human skin equivalent (applied weekly for a maximum of 5 weeks) seems more effective at promoting ulcer healing than saline moistened gauze.

  Human cultured dermis does not appear effective at promoting healing.

- Topical growth factors appear to increase healing rates, but there has been little long-term follow-up of people treated with these factors.

- Systemic hyperbaric oxygen seems effective in treating people with severely infected ulcers, although it is unclear whether it is useful in people with non-infected, non-ischaemic ulcers.

- We don't know whether debridement or wound dressings are effective in healing ulcers.

  However, debridement with hydrogel and dimethyl sulfoxide wound dressings does appear to help ulcer healing.

  Debridement and wound dressings have been included together because the exact mechanism of the treatment can be unclear (e.g. hydrogel).

ⓘ **Please visit www.clinicalevidence.bmj.com for full text and references**

What are the effects of interventions to prevent foot ulcers and amputations in people with diabetes?

Likely To Be Beneficial	• Screening and referral to foot-care clinics
Unknown Effectiveness	• Education • Therapeutic footwear

What are the effects of treatments in people with diabetes with foot ulceration?

Likely To Be Beneficial	• Human skin equivalent

	• Pressure off-loading with total contact or non-removable cast for plantar ulcers
	• Systemic hyperbaric oxygen (for infected ulcers)
	• Topical growth factors
Unknown Effectiveness	• Debridement or wound dressings
	• Pressure off-loading with felted foam or pressure-relief half-shoe
	• Systemic hyperbaric oxygen (for non-infected non-ischaemic ulcers)
Unlikely To Be Beneficial	• Human cultured dermis

Search date September 2006

DEFINITION Diabetic foot ulceration is full-thickness penetration of the dermis of the foot in a person with diabetes. Ulcer severity is often classified using the Wagner system. **Grade 1** ulcers are superficial ulcers involving the full skin thickness but no underlying tissues. **Grade 2** ulcers are deeper, penetrating down to ligaments and muscle, but not involving bone or abscess formation. **Grade 3** ulcers are deep ulcers with cellulitis or abscess formation, often complicated with osteomyelitis. Ulcers with localised gangrene are classified as **Grade 4**, and those with extensive gangrene involving the entire foot are classified as **Grade 5**.

INCIDENCE/PREVALENCE Studies conducted in Australia, Finland, the UK, and the USA have reported the annual incidence of foot ulcers among people with diabetes as 2.5–10.7%, and the annual incidence of amputation for any reason as 0.25–1.8%.

AETIOLOGY/RISK FACTORS Long-term risk factors for foot ulcers and amputation include duration of diabetes, poor glycaemic control, microvascular complications (retinopathy, nephropathy, and neuropathy), PVD, foot deformities, and previous foot ulceration or amputation. Strong predictors of foot ulceration are altered foot sensation, foot deformities, and previous foot ulcer or amputation of the other foot (altered sensation: RR 2.2, 95% CI 1.5 to 3.1; foot deformity: RR 3.5, 95% CI 1.2 to 9.9); previous foot ulcer: RR 1.6, 95% CI 1.2 to 2.3; previous amputation: RR 2.8, 95% CI 1.8 to 4.3).

PROGNOSIS In people with diabetes, foot ulcers frequently co-exist with vascular insufficiency (although foot ulcers can occur in people with no vascular insufficiency) and may be complicated by infection. Amputation is indicated if disease is severe or does not improve with conservative treatment. As well as affecting quality of life, these complications of diabetes account for a large proportion of the healthcare costs of dealing with diabetes. For people with healed diabetic foot ulcers, the 5-year cumulative rate of ulcer recurrence is 66%, and of amputation is 12%. Severe infected foot ulcers are associated with an increased risk of mortality.

Amaryllis Campbell

KEY POINTS

- Type 1 diabetes occurs when the pancreas produces too little insulin or no insulin at all, because of destruction of the pancreatic islet beta cells, usually attributable to an autoimmune process.

  It is estimated that slightly more than 218,000 people develop type 1 diabetes worldwide annually, of whom about 40% are children.

  Most people with type 1 diabetes require insulin for survival, and are described as insulin dependent. Untreated, they will experience increasing blood glucose levels, progressing to ketoacidosis or non-ketotic hyperosmolar states resulting in coma and death.

- Glycaemic control typically worsens in adolescence, owing to a combination of physical and psychological change and development.

  We don't know whether intensive treatment programmes which incorporate an education component are any more successful than conventional treatment for adolescents with type 1 diabetes.

  There is some evidence that educational and psychosocial interventions may improve quality of life in adolescents with type 1 diabetes.

  We found no good evidence on which to base advice to adolescents about the optimum frequency of blood glucose self-monitoring or of insulin administration.

- Intensive treatment programmes in adults do seem to improve glycaemic control, but require significant investment of time and resources.

  Better glycaemic control is associated with higher rates of hypoglycaemia, which may not be acceptable to some people with type 1 diabetes.

- While regular self-monitoring of blood glucose is recommended to adults with type 1 diabetes, there are no reliable data on which to base advice about optimum frequency of blood glucose self-testing.

- Continuous subcutaneous insulin infusion seems effective at improving glycated haemoglobin levels and quality of life compared with multiple daily subcutaneous injections.

  However, it is associated with increased risks of diabetic ketoacidosis owing to disconnection or malfunction of the pump, and infection.

(i) **Please visit www.clinicalevidence.bmj.com for full text and references**

What are the effects of interventions in adolescents with type 1 diabetes?	
Likely To Be Beneficial	• Educational interventions (compared with controls)
Unknown Effectiveness	• Different frequencies of insulin administration • Different frequencies of blood glucose self-monitoring • Intensive treatment programmes (compared with conventional treatment programmes)

What are the effects of interventions in adults with type 1 diabetes?

Trade-off Between Benefits And Harms	• Continuous subcutaneous insulin infusion (compared with multiple daily subcutaneous insulin injections) • Intensive treatment programmes (compared with conventional treatment programmes)
Unknown Effectiveness	• Different frequencies of blood glucose self-monitoring • Educational interventions (compared with controls)

Search date December 2005

DEFINITION The term diabetes mellitus encompasses a group of disorders characterised by chronic hyperglycaemia with disturbances of carbohydrate, fat, and protein metabolism resulting from defects of insulin secretion, insulin action, or both. The WHO definition recognises diabetes as a progressive disorder of glucose metabolism in which individuals may move between normoglycaemia, impaired glucose tolerance or impaired fasting glycaemia, and frank hyperglycaemia. Type 1 diabetes occurs when the pancreas produces too little insulin or no insulin at all, because of destruction of the pancreatic islet beta cells, usually attributable to an autoimmune process. Markers of autoimmune destruction (autoantibodies to islet cells, autoantibodies to insulin, or autoantibodies to both islet cells and insulin, and to glutamic acid decarboxylase) can be found in 85–90% of individuals with type 1 diabetes when fasting diabetic hyperglycaemia is first detected. The definition of type 1 diabetes also includes individuals with beta cell destruction who are prone to ketoacidosis but for which no specific cause can be found. However, it excludes those forms of beta cell destruction for which a specific cause can be found (e.g. cystic fibrosis, pancreatitis, cancer of the pancreas). Type 2 diabetes results from defects in both insulin secretion and insulin action. The risk of type 2 diabetes increases with age and lack of physical activity, and occurs more frequently in individuals with obesity, hypertension, and dyslipidaemia (the metabolic syndrome). It occurs more frequently in women with previous gestational diabetes. There is also evidence of a familial predisposition. Type 2 diabetes is not covered in this review. **Diagnosis:** In the presence of symptoms (such as thirst, passing increased volumes of urine, blurring of vision, and weight loss), diabetes may be diagnosed on the basis of a single random elevated plasma glucose (at least 11.1 mmol/L). In the absence of symptoms, the diagnosis should be based on at least one additional blood glucose result in the diabetic range, either from a random or fasting (plasma blood glucose at least 7.0 mmol/L) sample, or from the oral glucose tolerance test (plasma blood glucose (at least 11.1 mmol/L 2 hours after a 75 g glucose load). **Population:** For the purpose of this review, we have included adolescents and adults with type 1 diabetes, but excluded pregnant women and people who are acutely unwell: for example, after surgery or MI.

INCIDENCE/PREVALENCE It is estimated that slightly more than 218,000 people develop type 1 diabetes worldwide annually, of whom about 40% are children. The incidence varies considerably between populations, with 60,000 new cases occurring annually in Europe, 45,000 new cases in South East Asia, 36,000 new cases in North America, and the lowest number of new cases, 6900 annually, in Africa. There seems to be a worldwide increase in the incidence of type 1 diabetes in both high- and low-incidence populations. The prevalence of type 1 diabetes is currently estimated at 5.3 million people worldwide, which varies between populations, reflecting both the variation in incidence rates and differing population structures and mortality.

AETIOLOGY/RISK FACTORS Two main aetiological forms of type 1 diabetes are recognised. Autoimmune diabetes mellitus results from autoimmune mediated destruction of the beta cells of the pancreas. The rate of destruction varies, but all individuals with this form of diabetes eventually become dependent on insulin for survival. Peak incidence of autoimmune diabetes is during childhood and adolescence, but it may occur at any age. There is a genetic predisposition, and people with this type of diabetes may have other autoimmune disorders. Certain viruses have also been associated with beta cell destruction, including rubella, Coxsackie B, and cytomegalovirus. Other environmental factors are probably also contributory, but these are poorly defined and understood. Idiopathic diabetes (in which the cause is unidentified) is more common in individuals of African and Asian origin.

PROGNOSIS Untreated, most people with type 1 diabetes, particularly those with autoimmune diabetes mellitus, will experience increasing blood glucose levels, progressing to ketoacidosis or non-ketotic hyperosmolar states resulting in coma and death. The course of idiopathic diabetes may be more varied, with some people experiencing permanent lack of insulin and a tendency to ketoacidosis, although in others the requirement for insulin treatment may fluctuate. However, most people with type 1 diabetes require insulin for survival, and are described as insulin dependent. The long-term effects of diabetes include retinopathy, nephropathy, and neuropathy. Individuals with diabetes mellitus are also at increased risk of cardiovascular, cerebrovascular, and peripheral vascular disease. Good glycaemic control can reduce the risk of developing diabetic complications.

Diabetes: glycaemic control in type 2

Bala Srinivasan, Nick Taub, Kamlesh Khunti, and Melanie Davies.

KEY POINTS

- Diabetes mellitus is now seen as a progressive disorder of glucose metabolism; it affects about 5% of the population worldwide, over 85% of whom have type 2 diabetes.

  Type 2 diabetes is often associated with obesity, hypertension, and dyslipidaemia (the metabolic syndrome), which are powerful predictors of CVD.

  Type 2 diabetes is a disease in which glucose levels rise over time, with or without treatment and irrespective of the type of treatment given. This rise may lead to microvascular and macrovascular complications.

- Most people with type 2 diabetes will eventually need treatment with oral hypoglycaemic agents.

  Metformin reduces glycated haemoglobin by 1–2% and reduces mortality compared with diet alone, without increasing weight, but it can cause hypoglycaemia compared with placebo.

  Sulphonylureas reduce HbA1c by 1–2% compared with diet alone. Older sulphonylureas can cause weight gain and hypoglycaemia, but the risk of these adverse effects may be lower with newer-generation sulphonylureas.

  Meglitinides (nateglinide, repaglinide) may reduce HbA1c by 0.4–0.9% compared with placebo, but may cause hypoglycaemia.

  Combined oral drug treatment may reduce HbA1c levels more than monotherapy, but increases the risk of hypoglycaemia.

  Insulin is no more effective than sulphonylureas in improving glucose control in people with newly diagnosed type 2 diabetes, and is associated with a higher rate of major hypoglycaemic episodes, and with weight gain.

- Individual or group intensive educational programmes may reduce HbA1c compared with usual care, although studies have been of poor quality.

- Insulin improves glycaemic control in people with inadequate control of HbA1c from oral drug treatment, but is associated with weight gain, and an increased risk of hypoglycaemia.

  Adding metformin to insulin improves glucose control compared with insulin alone, but increases gastrointestinal adverse effects. However, the combination may cause less weight gain than insulin alone.

- Monitoring of blood glucose levels has not been shown to improve glycaemic control in people not being treated with insulin.

- Diet may be less effective than metformin or sulphonylureas in improving glucose control, although sulphonylureas were associated with higher rates of hypoglycaemia. However, there is consensus that weight reduction in people with type 2 diabetes can improve glycaemic control, as well as conferring other health benefits.

(i) **Please visit www.clinicalevidence.bmj.com for full text and references**

What are the effects of interventions for glycaemic control in adults with type 2 diabetes?

Beneficial	• Metformin (more effective than placebo or diet alone) • Sulphonylureas (reduce HbA1c compared with placebo or diet alone; newer sulphonylureas reduce hypoglycaemia compared with older sulphonylureas)
Likely To Be Beneficial	• Diet • Education (compared with usual care)

	• Intensive-treatment programmes (compared with usual care) • Meglitinides (nateglinide, repaglinide more effective than placebo, may be as effective as older or newer sulphonylureas)
Trade-off Between Benefits And Harms	• Combined oral drug treatment (compared with monotherapy) • Insulin (better than continuation of oral drug treatment if HbA1c is inadequately controlled) • Insulin plus metformin versus insulin alone (improved HbA1c levels compared with insulin alone, but increased gastrointestinal adverse effects)
Unknown Effectiveness	• Blood glucose self-monitoring • Insulin analogues versus conventional insulin (insufficient evidence to assess how they compare) • Insulin delivered by continuous subcutaneous infusion (probably as effective as multiple daily injections)
Unlikely To Be Beneficial	• Insulin versus sulphonylureas as initial treatment (no added benefit and causes more hypoglycaemic episodes and more weight gain)

Search date October 2006

DEFINITION The term diabetes mellitus encompasses a group of disorders characterised by chronic hyperglycaemia with disturbances of carbohydrate, fat, and protein metabolism resulting from defects of insulin secretion, insulin action, or both. Type 2 diabetes is the most common form of diabetes, and defects of both insulin action and insulin secretion are usually present by the time of diagnosis. The WHO now recognises diabetes as a progressive disorder of glucose metabolism in which individuals may move between normoglycaemia (fasting plasma venous glucose less than 6.1 mmol/L), impaired glucose tolerance (fasting plasma venous glucose less than 7.0 mmol/L and plasma glucose between 7.8 mmol/L and 11.1 mmol/L after 2 hours of 75 g oral glucose load), or impaired fasting glycaemia (fasting venous plasma glucose between 6.1 mmol/L and 7.0 mmol/L), and frank hyperglycaemia (fasting plasma venous glucose 7.0 mmol/L or more or 11.1 mmol/L or more 2 hours after 75 g oral glucose load). As a consequence of the inability of the body to use glucose as an energy source, blood glucose levels rise and symptoms such as thirst, polyuria, blurring of vision, or weight loss may develop. **Diagnosis:** In the presence of symptoms, diabetes may be diagnosed on the basis of a single random elevated plasma glucose (11.1 mmol/L or more). In the absence of symptoms, the diagnosis should be based on blood glucose results in the diabetes range taken at different time points, either from a random sample, or fasting (plasma blood glucose 7.0 mmol/L or more), or from the oral glucose tolerance test (plasma blood glucose 11.1 mmol/L or more 2 hours after 75 g glucose load). **Population:** For the purpose of this review, we have excluded pregnant women and acutely unwell adults (e.g. after surgery or MI).

INCIDENCE/PREVALENCE Type 2 diabetes constitutes about 85–95% of all diabetes in resource-rich countries and accounts for an even higher percentage in resource-poor countries. It is estimated that, in 2006, some 194 million people worldwide, or 5% of the adult population, have diabetes. This is an increase in prevalence from 177 million in

(continued over)

(from previous page)

2000. It is predicted that the prevalence of diabetes will continue to increase and reach 333 million, or 6%, by 2025. By 2025, the region with the greatest number of people with diabetes is expected to be South-East Asia, with about 82 million people with type 2 diabetes. Incidence and prevalence figures for children and adolescents are unreliable, but there is some evidence that type 2 diabetes is becoming more common in adolescents and young adults, especially in resource-poor countries.The overall estimated prevalence of 5% for type 2 diabetes conceals considerable variation in prevalence, which ranges from less than 2% in some African countries to over 14% in some populations.

AETIOLOGY/RISK FACTORS By definition, the specific reasons for the development of the defects of insulin secretion and insulin action that characterise type 2 diabetes are unknown. The risk of type 2 diabetes increases with age and lack of physical activity, and occurs more frequently in people with obesity, hypertension, and dyslipidaemia (the metabolic syndrome). Features of the metabolic syndrome can be present for up to 10 years before disorders of glycaemic control become apparent, and are powerful predictors of CVD and abnormal glucose tolerance (impaired glucose tolerance or diabetes). Type 2 diabetes also occurs more frequently in women with previous gestational diabetes, and certain ethnic groups. There is also evidence of a familial, probably genetic, predisposition.

PROGNOSIS People with type 2 diabetes have blood glucose levels which have been shown to rise progressively from the time of diagnosis, with or without treatment, and irrespective of the type of treatment given. Blood glucose levels above the normal range have been shown to be associated not only with the presence of symptoms, but with an increased risk of long-term microvascular and macrovascular complications.

Jigisha Patel

KEY POINTS

- Dyslipidaemia is characterised by decreased circulating levels of high-density lipoprotein cholesterol (HDL-C) and increased circulating levels of triglycerides and low-density lipoprotein cholesterol (LDL-C).

    Dyslipidaemia is a major contributor to the increased risk of heart disease found in people with diabetes.

    An increase of 1 mmol/L LDL-C is associated with a 1.5-fold increase in the risk of CHD in people with type 2 diabetes.

    A diagnosis of diabetic dyslipidaemia requiring pharmacological treatment is determined by the person's lipid profile and level of cardiovascular risk. The classification of cardiovascular risk and lipid targets for drug treatment differ between the UK, USA, and the rest of Europe. We used the United Kingdom Prospective Diabetes Study (UKPDS) risk calculator to estimate 10-year cardiovascular risk and categorised a greater than 15% risk as "higher" risk and less than 15% "lower risk" according to the UK clinical guidelines. We found no RCTs of a solely lower-risk population, although some studies were excluded because of insufficient data to calculate risk. In clinical practice, most people with diabetes are increasingly considered to be at high cardiovascular risk regardless of the presence or absence of other risk factors.

- Statins are highly effective at improving cardiovascular outcomes in people with diabetes.

    Statins reduce cardiovascular mortality in people with type 2 diabetes with and without known CVD, and regardless of baseline total and LDL-C concentrations.

    Different statins seem to have similar efficacy at reducing LDL-C.

- Combining statins with other treatments (such as ezetimibe or a fibrate) seems to reduce LDL-C more than statin treatments alone.

    Combinations could be useful in people with mixed dyslipidaemia where one drug fails to control all lipid parameters.

- Fibrates seem to have a beneficial effect on cardiovascular mortality and morbidity by reducing triglyceride levels.

    In people with mixed dyslipidaemia, statins may also be required.

- Intensive treatment programmes involving multiple interventions (people seen by a nurse every 4–6 weeks) seem to be better at reducing cholesterol than usual-care programmes.

- Fish oils may reduce triglyceride levels, but also seem to increase LDL-C levels, making them of limited benefit to most diabetic patients.

- Nicotinic acid seems efficacious at increasing HDL-C and may reduce triglycerides, but should probably only be used in combination with a statin in people with mixed dyslipidaemia, or in those unable to tolerate fibrates.

    Nicotinic acid seems to increase the incidence of flushing, particularly in female patients.

    We don't know whether either anion exchange resins or ezetimibe are useful in treating dyslipidaemia in people with diabetes, but they could perhaps be used in combination with a statin if the statin alone fails to achieve lipid targets.

Please visit www.clinicalevidence.bmj.com for full text and references

What are the effects of interventions for dyslipidaemia in people with diabetes?

Beneficial	• Statins
Likely To Be Beneficial	• Combined treatments (for lipid modification) • Fibrates • Intensive multiple-intervention treatment programmes (for lipid modification)
Trade-off Between Benefits And Harms	• Fish oil (for lipid modification) • Nicotinic acid (for lipid modification)
Unknown Effectiveness	• Anion exchange resins • Ezetimibe

Search date January 2006

DEFINITION The term dyslipidaemia is used to describe a group of conditions in which there are abnormal levels of lipids and lipoproteins in the blood. Abnormalities of lipid metabolism are present in people with both type 1 and type 2 diabetes. The nature of these abnormalities is complex, but the core components of diabetic dyslipidaemia are elevated circulating levels of triglycerides and decreased circulating levels of high-density lipoprotein cholesterol (HDL-C). In addition, the number of small dense lipoprotein particles is raised. As a consequence, although the cholesterol content of these particles may be low, small, dense low-density lipoprotein cholesterol (LDL-C) is raised. Total cholesterol and LDL-C may be normal if glycaemic control is adequate. Triglycerides and cholesterol are the main lipids of interest. The main classes of lipoprotein considered in this review are low-density lipoproteins (LDL) and high-density lipoproteins (HDL). **Diagnosis:** A diagnosis of diabetic dyslipidaemia requiring drug treatment is determined by the person's lipid profile and level of cardiovascular risk. The classification of cardiovascular risk and lipid targets for drug treatment differ between the UK and USA, and the rest of Europe. While it is accepted that people with diabetes are at high risk of CVD, in the UK and USA this high-risk group is stratified further in an attempt to target those people most likely to benefit from therapeutic intervention. However, the European guidelines on CVD prevention classify all people with type 2 diabetes, and type 1 diabetes and microalbuminuria as high risk. These targets apply to people with type 2 diabetes. Both in the UK and USA it is acknowledged that there is a case for offering drug treatment at lower lipid levels in people who are at high cardiovascular risk. In the USA, an "optional" goal for LDL-C of 1.81 mmol/L (70 mg/dL) is considered in people with high cardiovascular risk. Although these targets apply to people with type 2 diabetes, in clinical practice they are often extrapolated to people with type 1 diabetes. **Population:** For the purposes of this review we have included studies of adults with type 1 and type 2 diabetes, including those with concurrent hypertension, and have used UK (NICE) guidelines to determine level of risk. The UKPDS [United Kingdom Prospective Diabetes Study] tool, which includes data from people with diabetes, was used to calculate level of cardiovascular risk only. Subpopulations are described in detail in the description of individual studies where appropriate. Studies of children were excluded. Studies of adults with diabetes and microalbuminuria or nephropathy are covered in a separate review (see diabetic nephropathy, p 145).

INCIDENCE/PREVALENCE Type 1 diabetes mellitus: In people with well-controlled type 1 diabetes, the incidence of dyslipidaemia is comparable to that of the general population. However, there are no detailed data on the incidence and prevalence of dyslipidaemia in people with type 1 diabetes mellitus. **Type 2 diabetes mellitus:** Dyslipidaemia is common in people with type 2 diabetes. A survey of 498 adults with type 2 diabetes (representing a projected population size of 13,369,754 in the general US population of adults) estimated that over 70% of people have an LDL-C greater than the US treatment goal of less than

2.6 mmol/L less than 100 mg/dL; some have estimated this figure to be greater than 80%). Over half of men and two thirds of women have an HDL-C level below US recommended goals of greater than 1.0 mmol/L, while over half of men and women have elevated triglyceride levels. Only 28.2% of people with diabetes were on lipid-modifying drugs, and only 3% were controlled to US targets for all lipids.

AETIOLOGY/RISK FACTORS In people with diabetes mellitus, insulin insufficiency or insulin resistance can affect lipid metabolism. **Type 1 diabetes mellitus:** Little is understood about the cause of dyslipidaemia in people with type 1 diabetes. In poorly controlled type 1 diabetes, and in those with nephropathy, the typical cluster of abnormalities seen in diabetic dyslipidaemia does occur, and is associated with a much greater cardiovascular risk than in people without diabetes. **Type 2 diabetes mellitus:** Impaired insulin action may not be the only cause of dyslipidaemia. Central/visceral obesity may increase the amount of free fatty acids released into the portal circulation increasing hepatic triglyceride production, while high-fat meals, typical of a Western diet, may exacerbate postprandial hypertriglyceridaemia. Impaired insulin action in people with type 2 diabetes is thought to result in the loss of suppression of lipolysis (the breakdown of triglycerides into free fatty acids and glycerol) in adipose tissue. This leads to an increased release of free fatty acids into the portal circulation and, consequently, increased delivery of free fatty acids to the liver. The effect of this process is increased production of triglycerides by the liver and a decreased production of HDL-C. In addition, there is impaired clearance of triglycerides from the circulation. This resulting hypertriglyceridaemia alters the activity of other enzymes, which leads to the formation of small dense LDL particles and increased catabolism of HDL.

PROGNOSIS CVD is 2–6 times more frequent in people with diabetes, compared with those without diabetes, and progresses more rapidly when it occurs. Overall, it is the most common cause of death in people with diabetes, with at least 50% of deaths in type 2 diabetes caused by CHD. Dyslipidaemia is one of the major contributors to this increased cardiovascular risk. Lipid abnormalities are important predictors of CHD in people with type 2 diabetes. High LDL-C, high triglycerides, and low HDL-C have all been reported as predictors for cardiovascular risk. A 1.57-fold increase in CHD risk has been reported to be associated with a 1 mmol/L increase in LDL-C and a 15% decrease in risk with a 0.1 mmol/L increase in HDL-C concentration.

140 | Diabetes: prevention of cardiovascular events

Ronald Sigal, Janine Malcolm, and Amel Arnaout

KEY POINTS

- People with diabetes mellitus have 2–4 times the risk of CVD, and are up to 3 times more likely to die after an MI, compared with normoglycaemic people.

- Intensive treatment of multiple risk factors in people with type 2 diabetes and microalbuminuria reduces the risk of CVD compared with conventional treatment.

  Promotion of smoking cessation is likely to reduce cardiovascular events in people with diabetes, although no studies have specifically studied this.

- Tight control of blood pressure and reduction of cholesterol reduces the risk of cardiovascular events in people with hypertension and diabetes.

  ACE inhibitors, angiotensin receptor antagonists, beta-blockers, calcium channel blockers, and diuretics have all been shown to have similar antihypertensive effects.

  Reduction of cholesterol with statins reduces cardiovascular morbidity and mortality in people with diabetes regardless of initial cholesterol levels, and fibrates may also be beneficial.

  Aspirin and clopidogrel have not been consistently shown to reduce cardiovascular events or mortality in people with diabetes and CVD compared with controls, and increase the risk of bleeding.

  Intensive blood glucose control reduces the risk of cardiovascular events in people with type 1 diabetes, but has not been consistently shown to reduce cardiovascular morbidity or mortality in people with type 2 diabetes.

- CABG reduces 4-year mortality compared with PTCA in people with diabetes, although longer-term benefits are unclear.

  PTCA may reduce short-term mortality or MI compared with thrombolysis in people with diabetes and acute MI.

  Adding glycoprotein IIb/IIIa inhibitors reduces cardiovascular morbidity and mortality compared with placebo in people with acute coronary syndrome or undergoing PTCA plus stenting.

(i) **Please visit www.clinicalevidence.bmj.com for full text and references**

What are the effects of promoting smoking cessation in people with diabetes?	
Likely To Be Beneficial	• Smoking cessation*

What are the effects of controlling blood pressure in people with diabetes?	
Beneficial	• Antihypertensive treatment (compared with no antihypertensive treatment) • Lower target blood pressures
Trade-off Between Benefits And Harms	• Different antihypertensive drugs

What are the effects of treating dyslipidaemia in people with diabetes?

Beneficial	• Statins
Likely To Be Beneficial	• Aggressive versus moderate lipid lowering with statins • Fibrates • Low versus standard statin dose in older people

What are the effects of antiplatelet drugs in people with diabetes?

Likely To Be Beneficial	• Adding glycoprotein IIb/IIIa inhibitors to heparin in acute coronary syndromes • Clopidogrel
Trade-off Between Benefits And Harms	• Aspirin
Unlikely To Be Beneficial	• Adding clopidogrel to heparin in acute coronary syndromes

What are the effects of blood glucose control in prevention of CVD in people with diabetes?

Likely To Be Beneficial	• Intensive versus conventional glycaemic control • Metformin versus diet alone as initial treatment in overweight or obese people with type 2 diabetes

What are the effects of treating multiple risk factors in prevention of CVD in people with diabetes?

Beneficial	• Intensive multiple-risk factor treatment

What are the effects of revascularisation procedures in people with diabetes?

Beneficial	• Coronary artery bypass graft compared with PTCA • Stent plus glycoprotein IIb/IIIa inhibitors in people undergoing PTCA
Likely To Be Beneficial	• PTCA compared with thrombolysis
Trade-off Between Benefits And Harms	• CABG compared with PTCA plus stent

Search date November 2004

*No RCT but observational evidence suggests some benefit.

DEFINITION Diabetes mellitus: Diabetes mellitus is a group of disorders characterised by hyperglycaemia, defined as a fasting plasma glucose at least 7.0 mmol/L or at least 11.1 mmol/L 2 hours after a 75 g oral glucose load, on two or more occasions. Intensive treatment is designed to achieve blood glucose values as close to the non-diabetic range as possible. The components of such treatment are education, counselling, monitoring, self-management, and pharmacological treatment with insulin or oral anti-diabetic agents to achieve specific glycaemic goals. **CVD:** Atherosclerotic disease of the heart and/or the coronary, cerebral, or peripheral vessels leading to clinical events such as acute MI, congestive heart failure, sudden cardiac death, stroke, gangrene, and/or need for revascularisation procedures. **Population:** In previous versions of *BMJ Clinical Evidence*, we attempted to differentiate between primary and secondary prevention in this review. However, in middle-aged and older people with type 2 diabetes, this distinction may not be clinically important. We are not aware of any intervention that has been shown to be effective in secondary prevention but ineffective in primary prevention, or vice versa, in people with diabetes. In most cases, a large proportion of people with diabetes entered into CVD prevention trials are middle-aged and older, with additional cardiovascular risk factors, and a large portion of these actually have undiagnosed CVD.

INCIDENCE/PREVALENCE Diabetes mellitus is a major risk factor for CVD. In the USA, a survey of deaths in 1986 suggested that 60–75% of people with diabetes die from cardiovascular causes. The annual incidence of CVD is increased in people with diabetes (men: RR 2–3; women: RR 3–4, adjusted for age and other cardiovascular risk factors). About 45% of middle-aged and older white people with diabetes have evidence of coronary artery disease compared with about 25% of people without diabetes in the same populations. In a Finnish population-based cohort study (1059 people with diabetes and 1373 people without diabetes, aged 45–64 years), the 7-year risk of acute MI was as high in adults with diabetes without previous cardiac disease (20.2/100 person years) as it was in people without diabetes with previous cardiac disease (18.8/100 person years).

AETIOLOGY/RISK FACTORS Diabetes mellitus increases the risk of CVD. Cardiovascular risk factors in people with diabetes include conventional risk factors (age, prior CVD, cigarette smoking, hypertension, dyslipidaemia, sedentary lifestyle, family history of premature CVD) and more diabetes-specific risk factors (elevated urinary protein excretion, poor glycaemic control). Conventional risk factors for CVD contribute to an increase in the relative risk of CVD in people with diabetes to about the same extent as in those without diabetes. One prospective cohort study (164 women and 235 men with diabetes [mean age 65 years] and 437 women and 1099 men without diabetes [mean age 61 years] followed for mortality for a mean of 3.7 years after acute MI) found that significantly more people with diabetes died compared with people without diabetes (116/399 [29%] with diabetes *v* 204/1536 [13%] without diabetes; RR 2.2, 95% CI 1.8 to 2.7). It also found that the mortality risk after MI associated with diabetes was higher for women than for men (adjusted HR 2.7, 95% CI 1.8 to 4.2 for women *v* 1.3, 95% CI 1.0 to 1.8 for men). Physical inactivity is a considerable risk factor for cardiovascular events in both men and women. Another cohort study (5125 women with diabetes) found that participation in little (less than 1 hour a week) or no physical activity compared with physical activity for at least 7 hours a week was associated with a doubling of the risk of a cardiovascular event. A third cohort study (1263 men with diabetes, mean follow-up 12 years) found that low baseline cardiorespiratory fitness increased overall mortality compared with moderate or high fitness (RR 2.9, 95% CI 2.1 to 3.6), and overall mortality was higher in those reporting no recreational exercise in the previous 3 months than in those reporting any recreational physical activity in the same period (RR 1.8, 95% CI 1.3 to 2.5). The absolute risk of CVD is almost the same in women as in men with diabetes. Diabetes-specific cardiovascular risk factors include the duration of diabetes during adulthood (the years of exposure to diabetes before age 20 years add little to the risk of CVD); raised blood glucose concentrations (reflected in fasting blood glucose or HbA1c); and any degree of microalbuminuria (albuminuria 30–299 mg/24 hours). People with diabetes and microalbuminuria have a higher risk of coronary morbidity and mortality compared with people with normal levels of urinary albumin and a similar duration of diabetes (RR 2–3). Clinical proteinuria increases the risk of mortality from cardiac events in people with type 2 diabetes (RR 2.61, 95% CI 1.99 to 3.43) and type 1 diabetes (RR 9) compared with people with the same type of diabetes who have normal albumin excretion. An epidemiological analysis of people with diabetes enrolled in the Heart Outcomes Prevention Evaluation cohort study (3498 people with diabetes and at least 1 other cardiovascular risk factor, age over 55 years, of whom 1140 [32%] had microalbuminuria at baseline; 5 years' follow-up) found a higher risk for major cardiovascular events in those with microalbuminuria (albumin:creatinine ratio [ACR] at least 2.0 mg/mmol) than in those without microalbuminuria (adjusted RR 1.97, 95% CI 1.68 to 2.31), and for all-cause mortality (RR 2.15, 95% CI 1.78 to 2.60). It also found an association between ACR and the risk of major cardiovascular events (ACR 0.22–0.57 mg/mmol: RR 0.63 to 1.14; ACR 0.58–1.62 mg/mmol: RR 1.11, 95% CI 0.86 to 1.43; ACR 1.62–1.99 mg/mmol: RR 1.89, 95% CI 1.52 to 2.36).

PROGNOSIS Diabetes mellitus increases the risk of mortality or serious morbidity after a coronary event (RR 1.5–3.0). This excess risk is partly accounted for by increased prevalence of other cardiovascular risk factors in people with diabetes. A systematic review (search date 1998, 15 prospective cohort studies) found that, in people with diabetes admitted to hospital for acute MI, "stress hyperglycaemia" was associated with significantly higher mortality in hospital compared with lower blood glucose levels (RR 1.7, 95% CI 1.2 to 2.4). One large prospective cohort study (91,285 men aged 40–84 years) found that, compared with men with no diabetes and no CHD, there was higher all-cause and CHD mortality at 5 years' follow-up in men with diabetes with or without CHD, than in men with coronary artery disease alone, with the highest risk in men with both risk factors). Multivariate analysis did not materially alter these associations. Diabetes mellitus alone is associated with a twofold increase in risk for all-cause mortality, with a threefold increase in risk of death from CHD, and, in people with pre-existing CHD, with a 12-fold increase in risk of death from CHD compared with people with neither risk factor.

144 | Diabetes: treating hypertension

Sandeep Vijan

KEY POINTS

- Among people with diabetes, around 40% of those aged 45 years, and more than 60% of those aged 75 years and over, will have a blood pressure greater than 140/90 mm Hg.

  Major cardiac events occur in approximately 5% of people with diabetes and untreated hypertension each year, and the risk is higher in those with other risk factors such as diabetic nephropathy.

- We cannot be sure how different treatments compare in people with diabetes and hypertension. However, evidence suggests that either ACE inhibitors or diuretics are effective first-line treatments.

  ACE inhibitors reduce the risks of cardiovascular and renal disease compared with placebo, but can cause cough and angio-oedema.

  Diuretics such as chlorthalidone reduce cardiovascular events compared with placebo, but may increase glucose, cholesterol, and uric acid levels.

  Diuretics seem as effective as ACE inhibitors at preventing cardiovascular events, and may be more effective than calcium channel blockers at reducing the risk of heart failure.

  Beta-blockers may be as effective as ACE inhibitors at reducing cardiovascular events, microvascular events, or diabetes-related death, but may cause weight gain and increase the need for glucose-lowering treatment.

  Calcium channel blockers seem as effective as diuretics, more effective than beta-blockers, and less effective than ACE inhibitors at reducing cardiovascular events overall, but may be less effective at preventing heart failure compared with chlorthalidone.

  Angiotensin II receptor antagonists may reduce cardiovascular events compared with beta-blockers in people with diabetes, hypertension, and left ventricular hypertrophy.

  We don't know whether alpha-blockers reduce cardiovascular events in people with diabetes and hypertension.

- It seems likely that more-intensive treatment to achieve a greater reduction in blood pressure leads to a greater reduction in cardiovascular events and overall mortality. However, it is difficult to specify a target blood pressure in people with diabetes and hypertension.

Please visit www.clinicalevidence.bmj.com for full text and references

What are the effects of antihypertensives in people with diabetes?	
Beneficial	• ACE inhibitors • Diuretics
Likely To Be Beneficial	• Angiotensin II receptor antagonists (reduce cardiovascular events compared with beta-blockers) • Beta-blockers (similar reduction in cardiovascular and microvascular events to ACE inhibitors, but may cause weight gain and increase the need for glucose-lowering therapy) • Calcium channel blockers (similar reduction in cardiovascular events to diuretics but less effective than ACE inhibitors)
Unknown Effectiveness	• Alpha-blockers

What are the effects of different blood pressure targets in people with diabetes?

Beneficial	• Lower blood pressure targets (more effective than higher targets)

Search date February 2007

DEFINITION Hypertension in diabetes is classically defined as a systolic blood pressure of 140 mm Hg or greater or a diastolic blood pressure of 90 mm Hg or greater. Hypertension is broken into three stages. **Pre-hypertension** is a systolic blood pressure of 120–139 mm Hg or a diastolic blood pressure of 80–89 mm Hg. **Stage 1 hypertension** is a systolic blood pressure of 140–159 mm Hg or diastolic blood pressure of 90–99 mm Hg. **Stage 2 hypertension** is a systolic blood pressure of 160 mm Hg or greater or a diastolic blood pressure of 100 mm Hg or greater. However, guidelines now suggest that pharmacological therapy should be instituted in any person with diabetes and hypertension, regardless of stage. This review focuses on adults with diabetes with stage 1 or 2 hypertension, but with no diagnosis of CHD or diabetic retinopathy. Most studies on the subject do not differentiate between type 1 and type 2 diabetes; but the underlying epidemiology and ages of the populations studied suggest that more than 95% of study participants are likely to have type 2 diabetes. The control of hypertension in people with diabetic retinopathy, p 148, and those with diabetic nephropathy, p 145 is described in separate reviews.

INCIDENCE/PREVALENCE Hypertension is highly prevalent among people with diabetes. It is about 1.5–3.0 times more common in people with type 2 diabetes than in the age-matched general population. Using a diagnostic threshold of 140/90 mm Hg, about 40% of people with diabetes have hypertension at age 45 years, and more than 60% have hypertension by age 75 years. About 30% of people with type 1 diabetes eventually develop hypertension, usually after they develop diabetic nephropathy. The prevalence of hypertension varies depending on the population studied (see aetiology below).

AETIOLOGY/RISK FACTORS The cause of hypertension is multifactorial, complex, and not fully understood. In the general population, there are several major risk factors for hypertension; specific risk factors are not clearly different in the diabetic population. Age is the predominant factor — data suggest that prevalence increases with age. People with at least one parent with hypertension are about twice as likely to develop hypertension. African-Americans have a 7–10% increase in prevalence compared with non-Hispanic white Americans. Obese people also have greater risk: for each unit increase in BMI, the prevalence increases by about 1.0–1.5%. Insulin resistance is associated with development of hypertension.

PROGNOSIS Untreated hypertension in people with diabetes is associated with high rates of CVD (such as MI, heart failure, and stroke) and microvascular disease (such as renal disease [including albuminuria, renal insufficiency, and end-stage renal disease] and diabetic retinopathy). In the placebo groups of major trials of hypertension control in type 2 diabetes, major cardiac events occurred in about 4–6% of people annually, and were substantially higher in populations with additional risk factors such as diabetic nephropathy.

Diabetic nephropathy

Michael Shlipak

KEY POINTS

- Up to a third of people with type 1 or 2 diabetes will develop microalbuminuria or macroalbuminuria after 20 years. Smoking, poor glycaemic control, male sex, older age, and ethnicity are also risk factors.

  Microalbuminuria can also be caused by hypertension, which often complicates type 2 diabetes and makes the diagnosis more difficult.

  Diabetic nephropathy increases the risk of end-stage renal disease and mortality, and is associated with increased cardiovascular risk.

- In people with type 1 diabetes, ACE inhibitors reduce progression of early nephropathy while, in people with late nephropathy, they reduce the risk of end-stage renal failure and death.

  Intensive glycaemic control reduces progression of nephropathy compared with conventional control in people with early renal disease, but we don't know whether glycaemic control is effective in people with late nephropathy.

  We don't know whether angiotensin II receptor antagonists, dietary protein restriction, or tight control of blood pressure reduce the risks of renal or CVD, or improve survival, in people with early or late nephropathy.

- In people with type 2 diabetes, ACE inhibitors reduce progression from early to late nephropathy and may reduce cardiovascular events, but we don't know whether they are beneficial in late nephropathy.

  Angiotensin II receptor antagonists may reduce progression of nephropathy in people with early or late nephropathy.

  Lowering of diastolic blood pressure, even if not raised initially, reduces the risk of progression of early nephropathy, but we don't know whether it is effective in late nephropathy.

  We don't know whether protein restriction or tight glycaemic control are beneficial in early or late nephropathy.

(i) **Please visit www.clinicalevidence.bmj.com for full text and references**

What are the effects of treatments in people with type 1 diabetes and early nephropathy?	
Beneficial	• ACE inhibitors in early-nephropathy, type 1 diabetes (reduce progression to late nephropathy) • Glycaemic control in early-nephropathy, type 1 diabetes (reduced progression to late nephropathy)
Unknown Effectiveness	• Angiotensin II receptor antagonists in early-nephropathy, type 1 diabetes • Protein restriction in early-nephropathy, type 1 diabetes • Tight control of blood pressure in early-nephropathy, type 1 diabetes

What are the effects of treatments in people with type 1 diabetes and late nephropathy?	
Beneficial	• Captopril in late-nephropathy, type 1 diabetes
Unknown Effectiveness	• Angiotensin II receptor antagonists in late-nephropathy, type 1 diabetes

- Glycaemic control in late-nephropathy, type 1 diabetes
- Protein restriction in late-nephropathy, type 1 diabetes
- Tight control of blood pressure in late-nephropathy, type 1 diabetes

What are the effects of treatments in people with type 2 diabetes and early nephropathy?

Beneficial	• ACE inhibitors in early-nephropathy, type 2 diabetes • Angiotensin II receptor antagonists in early-nephropathy, type 2 diabetes • Tight control of blood pressure in early-nephropathy, type 2 diabetes (reduced progression to late nephropathy)
Unknown Effectiveness	• Glycaemic control in early-nephropathy, type 2 diabetes • Protein restriction in early-nephropathy, type 2 diabetes

What are the effects of treatments in people with type 2 diabetes and late nephropathy?

Beneficial	• Angiotensin II receptor antagonists in late nephropathy, type 2 diabetes
Unknown Effectiveness	• ACE inhibitors in late-nephropathy, type 2 diabetes • Glycaemic control in late-nephropathy, type 2 diabetes • Protein restriction in late-nephropathy, type 2 diabetes • Tight control of blood pressure in late-nephropathy, type 2 diabetes

Search date November 2006

DEFINITION Diabetic nephropathy is a clinical syndrome in people with diabetes, characterised by albuminuria on at least two occasions separated by 3–6 months. Diabetic nephropathy is usually accompanied by hypertension, progressive rise in proteinuria, and decline in renal function. In type 1 diabetes, five stages have been proposed. Of these, stages 1 and 2 are equivalent to preclinical nephropathy, and are detected only by imaging or biopsy. Stage 3 is synonymous with early nephropathy — the clinical term used in this review. Stage 4 nephropathy is also known clinically as late nephropathy, and this term will be used for the remainder of this review. Stage 5 represents the progression to end-stage renal disease (ESRD). **Population:** For the purpose of this review, we have included people with diabetes and both early and late nephropathy. Early nephropathy presents as

(continued over)

(from previous page)

microalbuminuria, usually defined by albuminuria level of 30–300 mg a day (or albumin/creatinine ratio of 30–300 mg/g [3.4–34.0 mg/mmol]). Late nephropathy presents as macroalbuminuria, characterised by albuminuria greater than 300 mg a day (or albumin/creatinine ratio greater than 300 mg/g [34 mg/mmol]). The treatment of people with diabetes and ESRD is not covered in this review.

INCIDENCE/PREVALENCE The worldwide prevalence of diabetes in 1997 was 124 million, and this is expected to increase to 221 million by 2010. In the UK, 1.4 million people had been diagnosed with diabetes in 1998, and estimates suggest that a million more have diabetes which has not yet been diagnosed. After 20 years of type 1 or 2 diabetes, the cumulative risk of proteinuria is 27–28%, and the overall prevalence of microalbuminuria and macroalbuminuria is 30–35%. In addition, the incidence of diabetic nephropathy is increasing, partly because of the growing epidemic of type 2 diabetes, and because of increased life expectancies: for example, in the USA, the incidence has increased by 150% in the past decade.

AETIOLOGY/RISK FACTORS Duration of diabetes, older age, male sex, smoking status, and poor glycaemic control have all been found to be risk factors in the development of nephropathy. In addition, certain ethnic groups seem to be at greater risk (see prognosis). Microalbuminuria is less pathognomonic of nephropathy among people with type 2 diabetes because hypertension, which is a common complication, can also cause microalbuminuria. Hypertension can also cause renal insufficiency; so, the time to development of renal insufficiency can be shorter in type 2 diabetes than in type 1. For people who have an atypical course, renal biopsy may be advisable. In addition, there are some differences in the progression of type 1 and type 2 diabetic nephropathy. In people with type 2 diabetes, albuminuria is more often present at diagnosis. Hypertension is also more common in type 2 diabetic nephropathy. Finally, microalbuminuria is less predictive of late nephropathy in people with type 2 diabetes compared with type 1.

PROGNOSIS People with microalbuminuria are at increased risk for progression to macroalbuminuria and ESRD. The natural history of diabetic nephropathy is better defined in type 1 than type 2 diabetes. In type 2 diabetes, the course can be more difficult to predict, primarily because the date of onset of diabetes is less commonly known, and comorbid conditions can contribute to renal disease. Without specific interventions, about 80% of people with type 1 diabetes, and 20–40% of people with type 2 diabetes with microalbuminuria will progress to macroalbuminuria. Diabetic nephropathy is associated with poor outcomes. In the USA, diabetes accounts for 48% of all new cases of ESRD. In the UK it is the most common cause of ESRD, accounting for 20% of cases. People with type 1 diabetes and proteinuria have been found to have a 40-fold greater risk of mortality than people without proteinuria. The prognostic significance of proteinuria is less extreme in type 2 diabetes, although people with proteinuria have a fourfold risk of death compared with people without proteinuria. In addition, increased cardiovascular risk has been associated with albuminuria in people with diabetes. African-Americans, Native Americans, and Mexican Americans have a much higher risk of developing ESRD in the setting of diabetes compared with white people. In the USA, African-American people with diabetes progress to ESRD at a considerably more rapid rate than white people with diabetes. In England, the rates for initiating treatment for ESRD are 4.2 and 3.7 times higher for African-Caribbeans and Indo-Asians respectively than for white people. Native Americans of the Pima tribe, in southwestern USA, have much higher rates of diabetic nephropathy compared with white people, and also progress to ESRD at a faster rate.

Efstratios Mendrinos, Alexandros N Stangos, Constantin J Pournaras

KEY POINTS

- Diabetic retinopathy is the most common cause of blindness in the UK, with older people and those with worse diabetic control, hypertension, and hyperlipidaemia most at risk.

  Diabetic retinopathy can cause microaneurysms, haemorrhages, exudates, changes to blood vessels, and retinal thickening.

- Peripheral retinal laser photocoagulation reduces the risk of severe visual loss compared with no treatment in people with preproliferative (moderate/severe non-proliferative) retinopathy and maculopathy.

  We don't know if any one type of laser treatment is superior.

  We don't know whether peripheral laser photocoagulation is beneficial in people with background or preproliferative (non-proliferative) retinopathy without maculopathy.

- The benefits of laser photocoagulation are more notable in people with proliferate retinopathy than in those with maculopathy.

  Focal macular laser photocoagulation reduces the risk of moderate visual loss in eyes with clinically significant macular oedema plus mild to moderate preproliferative (moderate/severe non-proliferative) diabetic retinopathy, compared with no treatment.

  Grid photocoagulation to zones of retinal thickening may improve visual acuity in eyes with diffuse maculopathy.

  Photocoagulation is unlikely to be beneficial in eyes with maculopathy but without clinically significant macular oedema.

- Intravitreal triamcinolone acetonide improves visual acuity and reduces macular thickness in eyes with macular oedema refractory to previous macular laser photocoagulation, but repeated injections are needed to maintain benefit.

  Secondary ocular hypertension and progression of cataract are common complications with intravitreal triamcinolone; infectious endophthalmitis is rare.

- Vitrectomy can reduce visual loss if performed early in people with vitreous haemorrhage, especially if they have severe proliferative retinopathy.

  We don't know whether vitrectomy is beneficial in people with vitreous haemorrhage plus maculopathy.

(i) **Please visit www.clinicalevidence.bmj.com for full text and references**

What are the effects of laser treatments in people with diabetic retinopathy?	
Beneficial	• Focal macular photocoagulation in people with clinically significant macular oedema
	• Peripheral retinal laser photocoagulation in people with preproliferative (moderate/severe non-proliferative) retinopathy and maculopathy

	• Peripheral retinal laser photocoagulation in people with proliferative retinopathy
Likely To Be Beneficial	• Grid photocoagulation to zones of retinal thickening in people with diffuse maculopathy
Unknown Effectiveness	• Peripheral retinal laser photocoagulation in people with background or preproliferative (non-proliferative) retinopathy without maculopathy
Unlikely To Be Beneficial	• Focal macular photocoagulation in people with maculopathy but without clinically significant macular oedema.

What are the effects of drug treatments for diabetic retinopathy?

Likely To Be Beneficial	• Corticosteroids (intravitreal)

What are the effects of treatments for vitreous haemorrhage?

Beneficial	• Vitrectomy in people with severe vitreous haemorrhage and proliferative retinopathy (if performed early)
Unknown Effectiveness	• Vitrectomy in people with vitreous haemorrhage and maculopathy

Search date March 2007

DEFINITION Diabetic retinopathy is characterised by varying degrees of microaneurysms, haemorrhages, exudates (hard exudates), venous changes, new vessel formation, and retinal thickening. It can involve the peripheral retina, the macula, or both. The range of severity of retinopathy includes background (mild non-proliferative), preproliferative (moderate/severe non-proliferative), proliferative and advanced retinopathy. Involvement of the macula can be focal, diffuse, ischaemic, or mixed.

INCIDENCE/PREVALENCE Diabetic eye disease is the most common cause of blindness in the UK, responsible for 12% of registrable blindness in people aged 16–64 years.

AETIOLOGY/RISK FACTORS Risk factors include age, duration and control of diabetes, raised blood pressure, and hyperlipidaemia.

PROGNOSIS Natural history studies from the 1960s found that at least half of people with proliferative diabetic retinopathy progressed to Snellen visual acuity of less than 6/60 (20/200) within 3–5 years. After 4 years' follow-up, the rate of progression to less than 6/60 (20/200) visual acuity in the better eye was 1.5% in people with type 1 diabetes, 2.7% in people with non-insulin-dependent type 2 diabetes, and 3.2% in people with insulin-dependent type 2 diabetes.

KEY POINTS

- Acute cholecystitis causes unremitting right upper quadrant pain, anorexia, nausea, vomiting and fever, and can lead to perforations, abscess formation, or fistulae if untreated.

   About 95% of people with acute cholecystitis have gallstones.

   It is thought that blockage of the bile duct by a gallstone or local inflammation can lead to acute cholecystitis, but we don't know whether bacterial infection is also necessary.

- Early cholecystectomy within 7 days of onset of symptoms is the treatment of choice for acute cholecystitis.

   Early surgery reduces the duration of hospital admission compared with delayed surgery, but does not reduce mortality or complications.

   Up to a quarter of people scheduled for delayed surgery may require urgent operations because of recurrent or worsening symptoms.

- Laparoscopic cholecystectomy reduces the duration of admission and may improve intraoperative and postoperative outcomes compared with open cholecystectomy, but increases the risk of bile duct injury.

   Up to a quarter of people having laparoscopic cholecystectomy may need conversion to open surgery because of risks of complications or uncontrolled bleeding.

   We don't know whether minilaparoscopic surgery leads to further reductions in duration of admission or improved outcomes compared with laparoscopic surgery.

(i) **Please visit www.clinicalevidence.bmj.com for full text and references**

What are the effects of treatments for acute cholecystitis?	
Beneficial	• Early cholecystectomy (reduces hospital stay and the need for emergency surgery compared with delayed cholecystectomy) • Laparoscopic cholecystectomy (reduced hospital stay and may improve intraoperative and postoperative outcomes compared with open cholecystectomy)
Trade-off Between Benefits And Harms	• Observation alone (resulting in a 30% failure rate and a 36% rate of gallstone-related complications) • Open cholecystectomy (conversion from laparoscopic to open cholecystectomy necessary in 4–27% of people but may increase intraoperative and postoperative complications)
Unknown Effectiveness	• Minilaparoscopic cholecystectomy

Search date December 2005

DEFINITION Acute cholecystitis results from obstruction of the cystic duct, usually by a gallstone, followed by distension and subsequent chemical or bacterial inflammation of the gallbladder. People with acute cholecystitis usually have unremitting right upper quadrant

(continued over)

(from previous page)

pain, anorexia, nausea, vomiting, and fever. About 95% of people with acute cholecystitis have gallstones (calculous cholecystitis) and 5% lack gallstones (acalculous cholecystitis). Severe acute cholecystitis may lead to necrosis of the gallbladder wall, known as gangrenous cholecystitis. This review does not include people with acute cholangitis, which is a severe complication of gallstone disease and generally a result of bacterial infection.

INCIDENCE/PREVALENCE The incidence of acute cholecystitis among people with gallstones is unknown. Of people admitted to hospital for biliary tract disease, 20% have acute cholecystitis. The number of cholecystectomies carried out for acute cholecystitis has increased from the mid-1980s to the early 1990s, especially in elderly people. Acute calculous cholecystitis is three times more common in women than in men up to the age of 50 years, and is about 1.5 times more common in women than in men thereafter.

AETIOLOGY/RISK FACTORS Acute calculous cholecystitis seems to be caused by obstruction of the cystic duct by a gallstone or local mucosal erosion and inflammation caused by a stone, but cystic duct ligation alone does not produce acute cholecystitis in animal studies. The role of bacteria in the pathogenesis of acute cholecystitis is not clear; positive cultures of bile or gallbladder wall are found in 50–75% of cases. The cause of acute acalculous cholecystitis is uncertain and may be multifactorial, including increased susceptibility to bacterial colonisation of static gallbladder bile.

PROGNOSIS Complications of acute cholecystitis include perforation of the gallbladder, pericholecystic abscess, and fistula caused by gallbladder wall ischaemia and infection. In the USA the overall mortality from untreated complications is about 20%.

Rick Nelson

KEY POINTS

- Chronic anal fissures typically occur in the midline, with visible sphincter fibres at the fissure base, anal papillae, sentinel piles, and indurated margins.

    Anal fissures are a common cause of anal pain during, and for 1–2 hours after, defecation. The cause is not fully understood, but low intake of dietary fibre may be a risk factor.

    Chronic fissures typically have a cyclical history of intermittent healing and recurrence, but about 35% will eventually heal, at least temporarily, without intervention.

    Atypical features, such as multiple, large, or irregular fissures, or those not in the midline, may indicate underlying malignancy, STDs, or trauma.

- There is consensus that the nitric oxide donor glyceryl trinitrate is an effective first-line treatment for chronic anal fissure. However, studies have differed widely, and it is less effective than surgical treatment at healing fissures.

    Topical glyceryl trinitrate increases the risk of headaches.

- Internal anal sphincterotomy has been found to improve fissure healing compared with treatment with nitric oxide donors (such as topical glyceryl trinitrate) and botulinum A toxin–haemagglutinin complex.

    Internal anal sphincterotomy increases fissure healing compared with anal stretch/dilation, and anal stretch/dilation is more likely to cause flatus incontinence.

    We don't know whether internal anal sphincterotomy is better or worse than anal advancement flap in improving patient satisfaction or fissure healing.

- We do not know whether calcium channel blockers are more or less effective than placebo or other treatments at healing fissures.

    Oral administration of diltiazem may increase nausea, vomiting, headache, rash, and altered smell, compared with topical application, and may not be more effective.

(i)   Please visit www.clinicalevidence.bmj.com for full text and references

What are the effects of non-surgical treatments for chronic anal fissure?	
Likely To Be Beneficial	• Nitric oxide donors (topical glyceryl trinitrate, isosorbide mononitrate, isosorbide dinitrate; likely to be beneficial as a first-line treatment, but less effective than internal anal sphincterotomy)*
Unknown Effectiveness	• Botulinum A toxin-haemagglutinin complex (botulinum A toxin-hc) • Botulinum A toxin–haemagglutinin complex (botulinum A toxin-hc) plus nitrates • Calcium channel blockers (diltiazem, nifedipine)

What are the effects of surgical treatments for chronic anal fissure?

Beneficial	• Internal anal sphincterotomy
Unknown Effectiveness	• Anal advancement flap (limited evidence as effective as internal anal sphincterotomy based on one small RCT)
Unlikely To Be Beneficial	• Anal stretch/dilation (compared with internal anal sphincterotomy)

Search date January 2007

*Categorisation is based on limited evidence and consensus that nitric oxide donors are beneficial.

DEFINITION An anal fissure is an ulcer or tear in the squamous epithelium of the distal anal canal, usually in the posterior midline. People with an anal fissure usually experience pain during defecation and for 1–2 hours afterwards. Multiple fissures, large, irregular, or large and irregular fissures, or fissures off the midline are considered atypical. Atypical fissures may be caused by malignancy, chemotherapy, STDs, inflammatory bowel disease, or other traumas. Treatments for atypical fissures are not included in this review. It is not clear what the best treatment strategy is in people who present with a painless anal fissure, and in whom an atypical aetiology has been ruled out. **Acute anal fissures** have shraply demarcated, fresh mucosal edges, often with granulation tissue at the base. Acute fissures are believed to often heal spontaneously. **Chronic anal fissures:** Fissures persisting for longer than 4 weeks, or recurrent fissures, are generally defined as chronic. Chronic anal fissures have distinct anatomical features, such as visible sphincter fibres at the fissure base, anal papillae, sentinel piles, and indurated margins. Most published studies only require the presence of one of these signs or symptoms of chronicity to classify a fissure as chronic. This review deals only with chronic anal fissures.

INCIDENCE/PREVALENCE Anal fissures are a common cause of anal pain in all age groups, but we found no reliable evidence about precise incidence.

AETIOLOGY/RISK FACTORS The cause of anal fissure is not fully understood. Low intake of dietary fibre may be a risk factor for the development of acute anal fissure. People with anal fissure often have raised resting anal canal pressures with anal spasm, which may give rise to ischaemia.

PROGNOSIS Chronic fissure typically has a cyclical pain history, with intermittent healing and then recurrence. One systematic review found healing rates of about 35% without intervention, depending on the length of study follow-up.

David Humes, William Speake, and John Simpson

KEY POINTS

- The incidence of acute appendicitis is falling, although the reasons are unclear.

    The lifetime risk is approximately 7–9% in the USA, making appendicectomy the most common abdominal surgical emergency.

    Potential causes of appendicitis include faecoliths, lymphoid hyperplasia, and caecal carcinoma, all of which can lead to obstruction of the appendix lumen.

    Mortality from acute appendicitis is less than 0.3%, but rises to 1.7% after perforation.

- Spontaneous resolution of acute appendicitis has been reported in at least 8% of episodes. Very limited evidence suggests that conservative treatment of acute appendicitis with antibiotics may reduce pain and morphine consumption, but that a third of people are likely to be readmitted with acute appendicitis requiring surgery within 1 year.

- Standard treatment for acute appendicitis is appendicectomy.

    Clinical trials to compare surgery with no surgery would be considered unethical, and have not been done.

    There is some evidence that laparoscopic appendicectomy in adults reduces wound infections, postoperative pain, duration of hospital stay, and time off work compared with open surgery, but may increase the risk of intra-abdominal abscesses.

    Limited evidence suggests that laparoscopic surgery in children may reduce wound infections and duration of hospital stay compared with open surgery, but it has not been shown to reduce other complications.

- The most common complication of appendicectomy is wound infection, with intra-abdominal abscess formation less common.

    Treatment with surgery plus antibiotics reduces wound infections and intra-abdominal abscesses compared with surgery alone in adults with simple or complicated appendicitis.

    However, in children, the benefit of antibiotics may be limited to those with complicated appendicitis.

(i) **Please visit www.clinicalevidence.bmj.com for full text and references**

What are the effects of treatments for acute appendicitis?	
Beneficial	• Surgery plus antibiotics
Likely To Be Beneficial	• Laparoscopic surgery versus open surgery (in children)
Trade-off Between Benefits And Harms	• Antibiotics versus surgery

	• Laparoscopic surgery versus open surgery (in adults)
Unknown Effectiveness	• Antibiotics (versus no treatment/placebo) • Surgery (versus no treatment)
Likely To Be Ineffective Or Harmful	• Stump inversion at open appendicectomy versus simple ligation

Search date November 2006

DEFINITION Acute appendicitis is acute inflammation of the vermiform appendix.

INCIDENCE/PREVALENCE The incidence of acute appendicitis is falling, although the reason is unclear. The reported lifetime risk of appendicitis in the USA is 8.7% in men and 6.7% in women, and about 35,000 cases are reported annually in England. Appendicitis is the most common abdominal surgical emergency requiring operation.

AETIOLOGY/RISK FACTORS The cause of appendicitis is uncertain, although various theories exist. Most relate to luminal obstruction, which prevents escape of secretions, and inevitably leads to a rise in intraluminal pressure within the appendix. This can lead to subsequent mucosal ischaemia, and the stasis provides an ideal environment for bacterial overgrowth. Potential causes of the obstruction are faecoliths (often because of constipation), lymphoid hyperplasia, or caecal carcinoma.

PROGNOSIS The prognosis of untreated appendicitis is unknown, although spontaneous resolution has been reported in at least 1/13 (8%) episodes. The recurrence of appendicitis after conservative management, and recurrent abdominal symptoms in certain people suggest that chronic appendicitis and recurrent acute or subacute appendicitis may also exist. The standard treatment for acute appendicitis is appendicectomy. RCTs comparing treatment versus no treatment would be regarded as unethical. The mortality from acute appendicitis is less than 0.3%, rising to 1.7% after perforation. The most common complication of appendicectomy is wound infection, occurring in 5–33% of cases. Intra-abdominal abscess formation occurs less frequently, in 2% of appendicectomies. A perforated appendix in childhood does not seem to have subsequent negative consequences for female fertility.

Hemant M Kocher

KEY POINTS

- Chronic pancreatitis is characterised by long-standing inflammation of the pancreas owing to a wide variety of causes, including recurrent acute attacks of pancreatitis.

  Chronic pancreatitis affects 3–9 people in 100,000; 70% of cases are alcohol induced.

- Pancreatic enzyme supplements reduce steatorrhoea in people with chronic pancreatitis, but it seems that they have no effect on pain.

  We don't know whether consuming a low-fat diet or avoiding alcohol consumption improves symptoms of chronic pancreatitis. We also don't know if calcium or vitamin/antioxidant supplements are effective.

- There is consensus that tramadol is the most effective oral opioid analgesic for reducing pain in people with chronic pancreatitis, but also that it is associated with gastrointestinal adverse effects.

  We don't know whether nerve blocks are effective.

- There is consensus that endoscopic and surgical pseudocyst decompression or ductal decompression have both benefits and harms; it is unclear which technique is best, and choice often depends on local expertise.

  There is consensus that, despite complications, biliary decompression is essential in people with chronic pancreatitis who have biliary obstruction.

- Resection using pancreaticoduodenectomy may be equivalent to localised excision of the pancreatic head in improving symptoms, but it reduces quality of life and increases intraoperative and postoperative complications. In clinical practice, resection using pancreaticoduodenectomy is usually reserved for when other surgical options, such as pseudocyst or duct decompression, are not feasible because of severity of disease.

  There is consensus that distal pancreatectomy may be a viable option in people with chronic pancreatitis limited to the tail of the pancreas, with most efficacy when multiple pseudocysts are present. It is associated with complications in 15–50% of people.

(i) **Please visit www.clinicalevidence.bmj.com for full text and references**

What are the effects of lifestyle interventions in people with chronic pancreatitis?

Likely To Be Beneficial	• Avoiding alcohol consumption*
Unknown Effectiveness	• Low-fat diet

What are the effects of dietary supplements in people with chronic pancreatitis?

Likely To Be Beneficial	• Pancreatic enzyme supplements (for reducing steatorrhoea)
Unknown Effectiveness	• Calcium supplements
	• Vitamin/antioxidant supplements

What are the effects of drug interventions in people with chronic pancreatitis?

Trade-off Between Benefits And Harms	• Opioid analgesics (consensus that tramadol is more effective than other opioid analgesics but associated with gastrointestinal adverse effects)*

What are the effects of nerve blocks for pain relief in people with chronic pancreatitis?

Unknown Effectiveness	• Nerve blocks

What are the effects of different invasive treatments for specific complications of chronic pancreatitis?

Trade-off Between Benefits And Harms	• Biliary decompression (consensus that, despite complications, essential for biliary obstruction)*
	• Method of ductal decompression (both endoscopic and surgical decompression have benefits and harms)*
	• Method of pseudocyst decompression (both endoscopic and surgical decompression have benefits and harms)*
	• Resection using distal pancreatectomy in people with disease limited to the tail the of pancreas*
	• Resection using pancreaticoduodenectomy (Kausch–Whipple or pylorus-preserving) in people with more severe disease limited to the head of the pancreas

Search date May 2006

*Based on consensus.

DEFINITION Pancreatitis is inflammation of the pancreas. The inflammation may be sudden (acute) or ongoing (chronic). **Acute pancreatitis** usually involves a single "attack", after which the pancreas returns to normal. **Chronic pancreatitis** is characterised by long-standing inflammation of the pancreas owing to a wide variety of causes, including recurrent acute attacks of pancreatitis. Symptoms of chronic pancreatitis include recurring or persistent abdominal pain, and impaired exocrine function. The most reliable test of exocrine function is the demonstration of increased faecal fat — although this test is frequently not performed if imaging is consistent (particularly calcification of the pancreatic gland on computerised tomography scan). **Diagnosis:** There is no consensus on the diagnostic criteria for chronic pancreatitis. Typical symptoms include pain radiating to back, and people may present with malabsorption, malnutrition, and pancreatic endocrine insufficiency. However, these symptoms may be seen in people with more common disorders such reflux disease, peptic ulcers (also more common in heavy drinkers), and also in more serious diseases such as pancreatic or periampullary cancers. Diagnostic tests for chronic pancreatitis include faecal elastase measurement (to prove pancreatic insufficiency) and imaging. Biopsy may be required to resolve diagnostic uncertainty.

INCIDENCE/PREVALENCE The annual incidence of chronic pancreatitis has been estimated in one prospective study and several retrospective studies to be between three and nine cases per 100,000 population. Prevalence is estimated between 0.04% and 5%. Alcoholic chronic pancreatitis is usually diagnosed after a long history of alcohol abuse, and is the most common cause.

AETIOLOGY/RISK FACTORS The TIGAR-O system describes the main predisposing factors for chronic pancreatitis as: **T**oxic-metabolic (which includes alcohol induced [70% of all cases], smoking, hypercalcaemia, hyperlipidaemia, and chronic renal failure); **I**diopathic (which includes tropical pancreatitis and may form up to 20% of all cases); **G**enetic (which includes cationic trypsinogen, CFTR, and SPINK1 mutation); **A**utoimmune (which includes solitary and syndromic); **R**ecurrent and severe acute pancreatitis (which includes post-necrotic and radiation induced); and **O**bstructive (which includes pancreatic divisum and duct obstruction owing to various causes). Although 70% of people with chronic pancreatitis report excessive consumption of alcohol (more than 150 g/day) over a long period (more than 20 years), only 1/10 heavy drinkers develop chronic pancreatitis, suggesting underlying genetic predisposition or polymorphism, although a link has not been established conclusively.

PROGNOSIS Mortality in people with chronic pancreatitis is higher than in the general population, with mortality at 10 years after diagnosis estimated at 70–80%. Diagnosis is usually made at 40–48 years age. Reported causes of mortality in people with chronic pancreatitis are: complications of disease as well as treatment; development of pancreatic cancer or diabetes; and continual exposure to risk factors for mortality, such as smoking and alcohol.

David Humes, John Simpson and Robin Spiller

KEY POINTS

- Diverticula (mucosal outpouching through the wall of the colon) affect over 5% of adults aged 40 years and older, but only 10–25% of affected people will develop symptoms such as lower abdominal pain.

  Recurrent symptoms are common, and 5% of people with diverticula eventually develop complications such as perforation, obstruction, haemorrhage, fistulae, or abscesses.

  Use of NSAIDs, corticosteroids, and opiate analgesics have been associated with an increased risk of perforation of diverticula, while calcium antagonists may protect against these complications.

- Dietary fibre supplementation, and laxatives such as methylcellulose and lactulose are widely used to treat uncomplicated diverticular disease, but we don't know whether they reduce symptoms or prevent complications.

  Antibiotics (rifaximin) plus dietary fibre supplementation may improve symptoms more than fibre alone, but increase the risk of adverse effects.

  We don't know whether mesalazine is also beneficial at improving symptoms in uncomplicated diverticular disease, or at reducing complications after acute diverticulitis, as no good-quality studies have been found.

  We don't know whether elective open or laparoscopic colonic resection improve symptoms in people with uncomplicated diverticular disease.

- Acute diverticulosis is often treated with intravenous fluids, limiting oral intake, and broad-spectrum antibiotic use. However, we don't know whether such medical treatment improves symptoms and cure rates in people with acute diverticulitis.

- Surgery is usually performed for people with peritonitis caused by perforated acute diverticulitis, but we don't know whether it improves outcomes compared with no surgery, or if any one surgical technique is better at preventing complications.

(i) **Please visit www.clinicalevidence.bmj.com for full text and references**

What are the effects of treatments for uncomplicated diverticular disease?	
Likely To Be Beneficial	• Rifaximin (plus dietary fibre supplementation v dietary fibre supplementation alone) for uncomplicated disease
Unknown Effectiveness	• Antispasmodics for uncomplicated disease • Bran and ispaghula husk for uncomplicated disease • Elective surgery for uncomplicated disease • Lactulose for uncomplicated disease • Mesalazine for uncomplicated disease • Methylcellulose for uncomplicated disease

What are the effects of treatments to prevent complications of diverticular disease?	
Unknown Effectiveness	• Advice to increase fibre intake for preventing complications

	• Mesalazine for preventing complications

What are the effects of treatments for acute diverticulitis?

Unknown Effectiveness	• Medical treatment for acute diverticulitis
	• Surgery for acute diverticulitis

Search date March 2007

DEFINITION Colonic diverticula are mucosal outpouchings through the large bowel wall. They are often accompanied by structural changes (elastosis of the taenia coli, muscular thickening, and mucosal folding). They are usually multiple, and occur most frequently in the sigmoid colon. The majority of people with colonic diverticula are asymptomatic, with little to find on clinical examination, while 20% develop symptoms at some point. If diverticula are associated with symptoms, then this is termed diverticular disease. If asymptomatic, then the condition is known as diverticulosis. People who go on to develop complications associated with diverticula (inflammation, perforation, fistulae, abscess formation, obstruction, or haemorrhage) are referred to as having complicated diverticular disease. People with uncomplicated diverticular disease may report abdominal pain (principally colicky left iliac fossa pain), bloating, and altered bowel habit, and may have mild left iliac fossa tenderness on examination. Acute diverticulitis occurs when a diverticulum becomes acutely inflamed. People with acute diverticulitis typically present with severe left iliac fossa pain associated with fever, malaise, and altered bowel habit with left iliac fossa tenderness, associated with general signs of infection, such as fever and tachycardia.

INCIDENCE/PREVALENCE In the UK the incidence of diverticulosis increases with age; about 5% of people are affected in their fifth decade of life, and about 50% by their ninth decade. Diverticulosis is common in resource-rich countries, although there is a lower prevalence of diverticulosis in Western vegetarians consuming a diet high in fibre. Diverticulosis is almost unknown in rural Africa and Asia.

AETIOLOGY/RISK FACTORS There is an association between low-fibre diets and diverticulosis of the colon. Prospective observational studies have found that both physical activity and a high-fibre diet are associated with a lower risk of developing diverticular disease. Case-control studies have found an association between perforated diverticular disease and NSAIDs, corticosteroids, and opiate analgesics, and have found that calcium antagonists have a protective effect. People in Japan, Singapore, and Thailand develop diverticula that affect mainly the right side of the colon.

PROGNOSIS Inflammation will develop in 10–25% of people with diverticula at some point. It is unclear why some people develop symptoms and some do not. Even after successful medical treatment of acute diverticulitis, almost two thirds of people suffer recurrent pain in the lower abdomen. Recurrent diverticulitis is observed in 7–42% of people with diverticular disease, and after recovery from the initial attack the calculated yearly risk of suffering a further episode is 3%. About 50% of recurrences occur within 1 year of the initial episode, and 90% occur within 5 years. Complications of diverticular disease (perforation, obstruction, haemorrhage, and fistula formation) are each seen in about 5% of people with colonic diverticula when followed up for 10–30 years. In the UK, the incidence of perforation is four cases per 100,000 people a year, leading to approximately 2000 cases annually. Intra-abdominal abscess formation is also a recognised complication.

162 | Colorectal cancer

Praveen Roy and Reuben Last

KEY POINTS

- Colorectal cancer is the third most common malignancy in resource-rich countries, and about a quarter of people present with intestinal obstruction or perforation.

  Risk factors for colorectal cancer are mainly dietary and genetic.

  Overall 5-year survival is about 50%, with half of people having surgery experiencing recurrence of the disease.

- Adjuvant chemotherapy reduces mortality compared with surgery alone in people who have Dukes' A, B, or C colorectal cancer.

  Adding levamisole to fluorouracil may not increase survival compared with fluorouracil alone.

  High- or low-dose folinic acid may be as effective at reducing mortality as fluorouracil.

  Severe adverse effects occur in up to 30% of people given adjuvant chemotherapy, and these are life threatening in 5% of people.

- Preoperative radiotherapy may modestly reduce local tumour recurrence and mortality compared with surgery alone in people with rectal cancer.

  Postoperative radiotherapy may be as effective as preoperative radiotherapy.

- Routine intensive follow-up may reduce the time to detection of recurrence, and may increase survival in people with colorectal cancer compared with less intensive follow-up.

- We don't know whether total mesorectal excision reduces recurrence of rectal cancer compared with conventional surgery, but it increases stool frequency and the risk of anastomotic leakage.

 Please visit www.clinicalevidence.bmj.com for full text and references

What are the effects of treatments for colorectal cancer?

Beneficial	• Adjuvant chemotherapy
Likely To Be Beneficial	• Routine intensive follow-up
Trade-off Between Benefits And Harms	• Preoperative radiotherapy
Unknown Effectiveness	• Total mesorectal excision

Search date August 2005

DEFINITION Colorectal cancer is a malignant neoplasm arising from the lining (mucosa) of the large intestine (colon and rectum). Nearly two thirds of colorectal cancers occur in the rectum or sigmoid colon. Colorectal cancer may be categorised as A, B, or C Dukes'.

INCIDENCE/PREVALENCE Colorectal cancer is the third most common malignancy in resource-rich countries. It accounts for about 20,000 deaths each year in the UK and 60,000 deaths each year in the USA. Although the incidence of, and mortality from, colorectal cancer has changed little over the past 40 years, the incidence of the disease has fallen recently in both the UK and the USA. In the UK, about a quarter of people with colorectal cancer present with either intestinal obstruction or perforation.

AETIOLOGY/RISK FACTORS Colon cancer affects almost equal proportions of men and women, most commonly between the ages of 60 and 80 years. Rectal cancer is more common in men. The pathogenesis of colorectal cancer involves genetic and environmental factors. The most important environmental factor is probably diet.

PROGNOSIS Overall 5-year survival is about 50% and has not changed over the past 40 years. Disease-specific mortality in both USA and UK cancer registries is decreasing, but the reasons for this are unclear. Surgery is undertaken with curative intent in over 80% of people, but about half experience cancer recurrence.

Colorectal cancer screening

Carmen Lewis

KEY POINTS

- Colorectal cancer is a malignant neoplasm arising from the lining of the large intestine. Nearly two thirds of colorectal cancers occur in the rectum or sigmoid colon.

  It is the third most common cancer in resource-rich countries, accounting for about 20,000 deaths each year in the UK, and 60,000 each year in the USA.

  Screening is defined (and distinguished from testing on demand) as any organised or systematic testing of asymptomatic people.

- Annual or biennial faecal occult blood testing, followed by further investigation in people with a positive test, decreases colorectal cancer-related mortality compared with no screening.

- We found no evidence that examined combining faecal occult blood test plus flexible sigmoidoscopy for screening of colorectal cancer.

- A single flexible sigmoidoscopy (followed by an immediate colonoscopy and follow-up colonoscopies at 2 and 6 years in people found to have polyps on sigmoidoscopy screening) seems to reduce colorectal cancer rates, but not colorectal cancer mortality, compared with no screening.

- Flexible sigmoidoscopy can produce false positives by detecting polyps which do not have malignant potential, and has been reported by some people to be painful.

- We don't know how effective colonoscopy is in detecting colorectal cancer in healthy people, although the intervention is associated with rare but serious morbidity, including perforation and bleeding.

- Although we found no evidence examining either computed tomography colography or double contrast barium enema in healthy people, evidence in people at a high risk of colorectal cancer suggests that they may be useful diagnostic tools.

(i) **Please visit www.clinicalevidence.bmj.com for full text and references**

What are the effects of screening for colorectal cancer?	
Beneficial	• Faecal occult blood test (annual or biennial testing, followed by further investigation if positive)
Likely To Be Beneficial	• Flexible sigmoidoscopy (single test, followed by colonoscopy if positive)
Unknown Effectiveness	• Colonoscopy • Combination of faecal occult blood test plus flexible sigmoidoscopy • Computed tomography colography • Double contrast barium enema

Search date November 2006

DEFINITION Colorectal cancer is a malignant neoplasm arising from the lining (mucosa) of the large intestine (colon and rectum). Nearly two thirds of colorectal cancers occur in the rectum or sigmoid colon. Colorectal cancer may be classified as A, B, or C Dukes'. More recently, stage D has been proposed to classify people with advanced and widespread regional involvement (metastasis). Screening is defined (and distinguished from testing on demand) as any organised or systematic testing of asymptomatic people. In this review we have included studies of screening in men and women over 45 years of age (with no upper age limit) not known to be at high risk for colorectal cancer. People at high risk of colorectal cancer are defined as those with one or more first-degree relatives with colorectal cancer, or personal history of inflammatory bowel disease, polyps, or colorectal cancer.

INCIDENCE/PREVALENCE Colorectal cancer is the third most common cancer in resource-rich countries. It accounts for about 20,000 deaths each year in the UK, and 60,000 each year in the USA. Over most of the last 40 years the incidence of, and mortality from, colorectal cancer changed little. However, recently, both the incidence and mortality have fallen in the UK and the USA. In the UK, about a quarter of people with colorectal cancer present with either intestinal obstruction or perforation.

AETIOLOGY/RISK FACTORS Colon cancer affects almost equal proportions of men and women, most commonly between the ages of 60 and 80 years. Rectal cancer is more common in men. The pathogenesis of colorectal cancer involves genetic and environmental factors. The most important environmental factor is probably diet. People with a personal or family history of colorectal cancer or polyps, or a personal history of inflammatory bowel disease, are at higher risk of developing colorectal cancer.

PROGNOSIS Overall 5-year survival after colorectal cancer is about 50%. Disease-specific mortality in both UK and US cancer registries is decreasing, but the reasons for this are unclear. Surgery is undertaken with curative intent in over 80% of people, but about half experience cancer recurrence.

Frank Frizelle and Murray Barclay

KEY POINTS

- People with chronic idiopathic constipation can be divided into two main categories: those with difficulty defecating (but with normal bowel-motion frequency) and those with a transit abnormality (which can present as infrequent defecation).

  Although there are defined criteria for the diagnosis of constipation, in practice, diagnostic criteria are less rigid and in part depend on the perception of normal bowel habit.

  Constipation is highly prevalent, with approximately 12 million general practitioner prescriptions for laxatives being written in England in 2001.

- Increasing fibre intake and exercise may improve the symptoms and prevalence of constipation. We haven't found sufficient evidence that examines the effects of other non-drug interventions such as increasing fluid intake or performing biofeedback, although biofeedback may be useful for constipation caused by anismus.

- Despite this lack of firm evidence, a number of poorer-quality studies have implicated these lifestyle interventions as being potentially beneficial.

- Macrogols (polyethylene glycols) improve symptoms of constipation without any serious adverse effects.

- Ispaghula husk (psyllium) seems to improve overall symptoms of constipation more effectively than lactulose.

- The osmotic laxatives lactitol and lactulose seem equally effective in improving the frequency of bowel movements.

- We don't know if other osmotic laxatives such as magnesium salts, or phosphate or sodium citrate enemas are effective.

- We don't know whether other bulk-forming laxatives such as methylcellulose or sterculia are effective for improving symptoms of constipation.

- We don't know the effectiveness of stimulant laxatives such as bisacodyl, cascara, glycerol/glycerine suppositories, or senna.

- Although generally considered beneficial, we found no evidence examining the use of paraffin or seed oils for treating constipation.

(i) **Please visit www.clinicalevidence.bmj.com for full text and references**

What are the effects of non-drug interventions in adults with idiopathic chronic constipation?	
Likely To Be Beneficial	• Exercise or advice to exercise • High-fibre diet or advice to consume a high-fibre diet
Unknown Effectiveness	• Biofeedback • Increasing fluids or advice to increase fluids

What are the effects of other treatments in adults with idiopathic chronic constipation?	
Beneficial	• Macrogols (polyethylene glycols)
Likely To Be Beneficial	• Ispaghula husk (psyllium) • Lactitol

	• Lactulose
Unknown Effectiveness	• Bisacodyl
	• Cascara
	• Docusate
	• Glycerol/glycerin suppositories
	• Magnesium salts
	• Methylcellulose
	• Paraffin
	• Phosphate enemas
	• Seed oils/arachis oil
	• Senna
	• Sodium citrate enemas
	• Sterculia

Search date October 2006

DEFINITION Bowel habits and perception of bowel habits vary widely within and among populations, making constipation difficult to define. People with constipation can be divided into two main categories: those with difficulty defecating (but normal bowel-motion frequency) and those with a transit abnormality (which can present as infrequent defecation). The Rome II criteria is a standardised tool that diagnoses chronic constipation on the basis of two or more of the following symptoms for at least 12 weeks in the preceding year: straining at defecation on at least a quarter of occasions; stools that are lumpy/hard on at least a quarter of occasions; sensation of incomplete evacuation on at least a quarter of occasions; and three or fewer bowel movements a week. In practice, however, diagnostic criteria are less rigid and are in part dependent on perception of normal bowel habit. Typically, chronic constipation is diagnosed when a person has bowel actions twice a week or less, for two consecutive weeks, especially in the presence of features such as straining at stool, abdominal discomfort, and sensation of incomplete evacuation. **Population:** For the purposes of this review we included all RCTs stating that all participants had chronic constipation, whether or not this diagnosis was made according to strict Rome II criteria. Where the definitions of constipation in the RCTs differ markedly from those presented here, we have made this difference explicit. In this review, we deal with chronic constipation not caused by a specific underlying disease (sometimes known as idiopathic constipation) in adults aged over 18 years, although we have included adults with anismus. We excluded studies in pregnant women and in people with constipation associated with underlying specific organic diseases such as dehydration, autonomic neuropathy, spinal cord injury, bowel obstruction, irritable bowel syndrome, or paralytic ileus. We excluded people with Parkinson's disease and dementia, people who were postoperative, or who were terminally ill. Opioid-induced constipation was also excluded. This review does not cover interventions, such as dantron, which are recommended for use only in terminally ill people. **Diagnosis:** The diagnosis of constipation is initially based on history (see above). Specific tests available for further investigation include thyroid function tests, calcium concentration, barium enema or colonoscopy, defecation proctogram, anorectal manometry, and colon transit time studies.

INCIDENCE/PREVALENCE Twelve million general practitioner prescriptions were written for laxatives in England in 2001. Prevalence data are limited by small samples and problems with definition. One UK survey of 731 women found that 8.2% had constipation meeting Rome II criteria, and 8.5% defined themselves as being constipated. A larger survey (1892 adults) found that 39% of men and 52% of women reported straining at stool on more than

(continued over)

(from previous page)

a quarter of occasions. Prevalence rises in the elderly. Several surveys from around the world suggest that, in a community setting, prevalence among the elderly is about 20%.

AETIOLOGY/RISK FACTORS One systematic review suggested that factors associated with an increased risk of constipation included low-fibre diet, low fluid intake, reduced mobility, consumption of drugs such as opioids and anticholinergic antidepressants, and Parkinson's disease.

PROGNOSIS Untreated constipation can lead to faecal impaction (with resulting faecal incontinence), particularly in elderly and confused people. Constipation has been suggested as a risk factor for haemorrhoids and diverticular disease; however, evidence of causality is lacking.

Alexander C von Roon, George E Reese, Timothy R Orchard, and Paris P Tekkis

KEY POINTS

- Crohn's disease is a long-term chronic condition of the gastrointestinal tract.

  It is characterised by transmural, granulomatous inflammation that occurs in a discontinuous pattern, with a tendency to form fistulae.

  The cause is unknown but may depend on interactions between genetic predisposition, environmental triggers, and mucosal immunity.

- First-line treatment to induce remission of acute disease is corticosteroids.

  Budesonide is generally recommended in mild to moderate ileocaecal disease, because it is only slightly less effective in inducing remission than prednisolone, and has a superior adverse-effect profile.

  Prednisolone or methylprednisolone are generally recommended for severe or more extensive disease, because of their superior efficacy.

- Azathioprine and mercaptopurine are effective in inducing remission and healing fistulae in Crohn's disease, provided that at least 17 weeks' treatment are given. Monitoring for myelosuppression is obligatory.

  Aminosalicylates (mesalazine, sulfasalazine) may reduce disease activity, but we don't know which is the best regimen to induce remission.

  Methotrexate 25 mg weekly increases remission rates, and has a corticosteroid-sparing effect. There is consensus that it is also effective for maintenance.

  Cytokine inhibitors (e.g. infliximab) are effective in inducing and maintaining remission in Crohn's disease, but the long-term adverse-effect profile is unclear; they are therefore generally reserved for treatment of disease that is refractory to treatment with corticosteroids or other immunomodulators.

  Antibiotics and ciclosporin are unlikely to be beneficial in inducing remission.

- Bowel-sparing surgery to induce remission may be preferable to extensive resection, in order to avoid short bowel syndrome. Segmental and subtotal colectomy have similar remission rates.

- Laparoscopic resection may reduce postoperative hospital stay, but we don't know whether strictureplasty is effective.

- Azathioprine has been shown to be beneficial in maintaining remission in Crohn's disease, either alone or after surgery, and has a corticosteroid-sparing effect, but is associated with important adverse effects.

  Ciclosporin, oral corticosteroids, or aminosalicylates alone are unlikely to be beneficial in maintaining remission.

  After surgery, aminosalicylates are likely to be beneficial in maintaining remission.

  Methotrexate and infliximab may also maintain remission compared with placebo.

  Smoking cessation reduces the risk of relapse, and enteral nutrition may be effective. Fish oil and probiotics have not been shown to be effective.

(i) **Please visit www.clinicalevidence.bmj.com for full text and references**

What are the effects of medical treatments to induce remission in adults with Crohn's disease?

Beneficial	• Corticosteroids (oral) to induce remission • Infliximab to induce remission
Likely To Be Beneficial	• Aminosalicylates to induce remission (improved Crohn's Disease Activity Index compared with placebo)

	• Methotrexate to induce remission
Trade-off Between Benefits And Harms	• Azathioprine or mercaptopurine to induce remission
Unlikely To Be Beneficial	• Antibiotics to induce remission
Likely To Be Ineffective Or Harmful	• Ciclosporin to induce remission

What are the effects of lifestyle interventions to maintain remission in adults with Crohn's disease?

Beneficial	• Smoking cessation
Likely To Be Beneficial	• Enteral nutrition (compared with unrestricted diet)
Unknown Effectiveness	• Fish oil • Probiotics

What are the effects of surgical interventions to induce remission in adults with small-bowel Crohn's disease?

Likely To Be Beneficial	• Laparoscopic versus open ileocaecal resection (reduced postoperative hospital stay) • Limited versus extended resection
Unknown Effectiveness	• Strictureplasty

What are the effects of surgical interventions to induce remission in adults with colonic Crohn's disease?

Likely To Be Beneficial	• Segmental colectomy

What are the effects of medical interventions to maintain remission in adults with Crohn's disease?

Likely To Be Beneficial	• Infliximab to maintain remission • Methotrexate to maintain remission
Trade-off Between Benefits And Harms	• Azathioprine to maintain remission
Likely To Be Ineffective Or Harmful	• Aminosalicylates to maintain remission • Ciclosporin to maintain remission • Corticosteroids (oral) to maintain remission

What are the effects of medical interventions to maintain remission after surgery in adults with Crohn's disease?

| Likely To Be Beneficial | • Aminosalicylates to maintain remission after surgery |
| | • Azathioprine/mercaptopurine to maintain remission after surgery |

Search date March 2007

DEFINITION Crohn's disease is a chronic inflammatory condition of the gastrointestinal tract, characterised by transmural granulomatous inflammation, a discontinuous pattern of distribution, and fistulae. Although any part of the digestive tract from mouth to anus may be affected, Crohn's disease most frequently occurs in the terminal ileum, ileocaecal region, colon, and perianal region. The disease may be further classified into inflammatory, fistulating, and stricturing disease. The symptoms vary, but commonly include diarrhoea, abdominal pain, weight loss, blood or mucus in the stool, perineal pain, discharge, and irritation resulting from perianal fistulae. Extraintestinal manifestations of the disease include arthritis, uveitis, and skin rash. **Diagnosis:** There is no single gold standard for the diagnosis of Crohn's disease. Diagnosis is made by clinical evaluation and a combination of endoscopic, histological, radiological, and biochemical investigations. Internationally accepted criteria for the diagnosis of Crohn's disease have been defined by Lennard–Jones. After exclusion of infection, ischaemia, irradiation, and malignancy as causes for intestinal inflammation, a combination of three or more of the following findings on clinical examination, radiological investigation, endoscopy, and histological examination of endoscopic biopsies or excised specimens is considered diagnostic: chronic inflammatory lesions of the oral cavity, pylorus or duodenum, small bowel or anus; a discontinuous disease distribution (areas of abnormal mucosa separated by normal mucosa); transmural inflammation (fissuring ulcer, abscess, or fistula); fibrosis (stricture); lymphoid aggregates or aphthoid ulcers; retention of colonic mucin on biopsy in the presence of active inflammation; and granulomata (of the non-caseating type and not caused by foreign bodies). Further macroscopic findings not included in the Lennard–Jones classification that are considered diagnostic for Crohn's disease include fat wrapping, cobblestoning, and thickening of the intestinal wall. Laboratory findings consistent with Crohn's disease include anaemia, thrombocytosis, raised C-reactive protein levels, and a raised erythrocyte sedimentation rate. It may be difficult to distinguish Crohn's disease from ulcerative colitis, particularly when only the colon is affected. In 10–15% of patients originally diagnosed as having Crohn's disease, the diagnosis changes to ulcerative colitis during the first year.

INCIDENCE/PREVALENCE Estimates of the incidence of Crohn's disease worldwide vary considerably. In Europe, incidence rates range from 0.7 (Croatia) to 9.8 (Scotland) new cases per 100,000 people per year, whereas in North America these range from 3.6 (California) to 15.6 (Manitoba, Canada). The incidence of Crohn's disease is increasing, with incidence rates in the UK, Italy, Iceland, Finland, and the USA having doubled between 1955 and 1995. Crohn's disease is most commonly diagnosed in late adolescence and early adulthood, but the mean age at diagnosis in North American studies ranges from 33.4 to 45 years. Crohn's disease appears to affect women more commonly than men. In a systematic review of North American cohort studies of Crohn's disease, the percentage of females affected by the disease varied from 48% to 66%, and was above 50% in nine out of 11 studies.

AETIOLOGY/RISK FACTORS The true aetiology of Crohn's disease remains unknown. Current aetiological theories suggest that the disease results from a genetic predisposition, regulatory defects in the gut mucosal immune system, and environmental triggers. Defects in the gut mucosal immune system are mainly related to disordered activity of T cells (a type of white blood cell). Environmental triggers that have been linked with Crohn's disease include smoking, diet (high sugar intake), and the balance of beneficial and harmful bacteria in the gut. Finally, debate has raged since *Mycobacterium avium paratuberculosis* was

(continued over)

(from previous page)

cultured from intestinal tissue of people with Crohn's disease, with little agreement on whether this bacterium is an infective cause of Crohn's disease.

PROGNOSIS Crohn's disease is a lifelong condition, with periods of active disease alternating with periods of remission. The disease causes significant disability, with only 75% of sufferers being fully capable of work in the year of diagnosis, and 15% of people unable to work after 5–10 years of disease. At least 50% of people with Crohn's disease require surgical treatment during the first 10 years of disease, and approximately 70–80% will require surgery during their lifetime. People with Crohn's disease are at higher risk than those without the disease of developing colorectal and small-bowel cancer. **Mortality:** Mortality rates among people with Crohn's disease are slightly higher than in those without it. A systematic review of seven population-based cohort studies found that estimates of standardised mortality ratios were greater than 1 in six of the seven studies, with estimates ranging from 0.72 (95% CI 0.49 to 1.01) to 2.16 (95% CI 1.54 to 2.94). The review also found that mortality rates in Crohn's disease have not changed during the past 40 years.

Paul Moayyedi, Brendan Delaney, and David Forman

KEY POINTS

- Up to 25% of people have symptoms of GORD, but only 25–40% of these people have oesophagitis visible on endoscopy.

  Although obesity, smoking, alcohol, and certain foods are considered to be risk factors, we don't know that they are actually implicated in GORD.

  About 80% of people with GORD will have recurrent symptoms if treatment is stopped, and severe oesophagitis may result in oesophageal stricture or Barrett's oesophagus.

- Proton pump inhibitors increase healing in GORD compared with placebo and H_2 antagonists, but we don't know if one specific drug is more effective than the others.

  H_2 receptor antagonists reduce the risk of persistent oesophagitis compared with placebo, and may improve symptoms more than antacids.

- We don't know whether antacids/alginates, or lifestyle advice to lose weight or raise the head of the bed are beneficial in improving symptoms of GORD or in preventing recurrence.

- The motility stimulant cisapride may increase endoscopic healing of the oesophagus and reduce the risk of relapse, but has been associated with heart rhythm problems.

- Standard- or low-dose proton pump inhibitors reduce relapse of oesophagitis and reflux symptoms compared with placebo or H_2 antagonists, but we don't know which is the optimum drug regimen.

  H_2 antagonists may reduce the risk of relapse of reflux symptoms, although they have not been shown to prevent recurrence of oesophagitis.

- Laparoscopic or open surgery (Nissen fundoplication) may improve endoscopic oesophagitis compared with medical treatment, although studies have given conflicting results.

  Laparoscopic surgery seems to be as effective as open surgery with lower risks of operative morbidity and shorter duration of admission, but both types of surgery may have serious complications.

ⓘ **Please visit www.clinicalevidence.bmj.com for full text and references**

What are the effects of initial treatment of GORD associated with oesophagitis?	
Beneficial	• H_2 receptor antagonists
	• Proton pump inhibitors
Unknown Effectiveness	• Antacids/alginates
	• Lifestyle advice/modification
Likely To Be Ineffective Or Harmful	• Motility stimulants

What are the effects of maintenance treatment of GORD associated with oesophagitis?

Beneficial	• Proton pump inhibitors
Likely To Be Beneficial	• H₂ receptor antagonists
Trade-off Between Benefits And Harms	• Laparoscopic surgery • Open surgery
Unknown Effectiveness	• Antacids/alginates • Lifestyle advice/modification
Likely To Be Ineffective Or Harmful	• Motility stimulants

Search date July 2005

DEFINITION GORD is defined as reflux of gastroduodenal contents into the oesophagus, causing symptoms sufficient to interfere with quality of life. People with GORD often have symptoms of heartburn and acid regurgitation. GORD can be classified according to the results of upper gastrointestinal endoscopy. Currently, the most validated method is the Los Angeles classification, in which an endoscopy showing mucosal breaks in the distal oesophagus indicate the presence of oesophagitis, which is graded in severity from grade A (mucosal breaks of less than 5 mm in the oesophagus) to grade D (circumferential breaks in the oesophageal mucosa). Alternatively, severity may be graded according to the Savary–Miller classification (grade I: linear, non-confluent erosions, to grade IV: severe ulceration or stricture).

INCIDENCE/PREVALENCE Surveys from Europe and the USA suggest that 20–25% of the population have symptoms of GORD, and 7% have heartburn daily. In primary-care settings, about 25–40% of people with GORD have oesophagitis on endoscopy, but most have endoscopy-negative reflux disease.

AETIOLOGY/RISK FACTORS We found no evidence of clear predictive factors for GORD. Obesity is reported to be a risk factor for GORD, but epidemiological data are conflicting. Smoking and alcohol are also thought to predispose to GORD, but observational data are limited. It has been suggested that some foods — such as coffee, mints, dietary fat, onions, citrus fruits, or tomatoes — may predispose to GORD. However, we found insufficient data on the role of these factors. We found limited evidence that drugs that relax the lower oesophageal sphincter, such as calcium channel blockers, may promote GORD. Twin studies suggest that there may be a genetic predisposition to GORD.

PROGNOSIS GORD is a chronic condition, with about 80% of people relapsing once medication is discontinued. Many people therefore require long-term medical treatment or surgery. Endoscopy-negative reflux disease remains stable, with a minority of people developing oesophagitis over time. However, people with severe oesophagitis may develop complications such as oesophageal stricture or Barrett's oesophagus.

Haemorrhoids 175

R Justin Davies

KEY POINTS

- Haemorrhoids are cushions of submucosal vascular tissue located in the anal canal starting just distal to the dentate line. Haemorrhoidal disease occurs when there are symptoms such as bleeding, prolapse, pain, thrombosis, mucus discharge, and pruritus.

  Incidence is difficult to ascertain as many people with the condition will never consult with a medical practitioner, although one study found 10 million people in the US complaining of the disease.

- First- and second-degree haemorrhoids are classically treated with some form of non-surgical ablative/fixative intervention, third degree treated with rubber band ligation or haemorrhoidectomy, and fourth degree with haemorrhoidectomy.

- Rubber band ligation is known to be highly effective in treating first, second, and some third-degree haemorrhoids.

  Rubber band ligation can produce some immediate adverse effects, and the clinician should therefore always gain informed consent.

- Closed haemorrhoidectomy appears to be an effective treatment for relieving symptoms in people with first- to fourth-degree haemorrhoids.

  Although effective, closed haemorrhoidectomy seems to be associated with greater postoperative complications compared with haemorrhoidal artery ligation or stapled haemorrhoidectomy.

- Open excisional haemorrhoidectomy may also be effective in treating all grades of haemorrhoids, although it produces similar levels of adverse effects compared with closed haemorrhoidectomy.

- Infrared coagulation may be as effective as rubber band ligation and injection sclerotherapy in the treatment of first- and second-degree haemorrhoids.

- We found insufficient evidence to judge the effectiveness of injection sclerotherapy or haemorrhoidal artery ligation.

- While stapled haemorrhoidectomy seems effective in treating people with more severe haemorrhoids, some of the adverse effects are potentially life threatening, and so the procedure should only ever be carried out by a fully trained colorectal surgeon.

Please visit www.clinicalevidence.bmj.com for full text and references

What are the effects of treatments for haemorrhoidal disease?	
Beneficial	• Rubber band ligation
Likely To Be Beneficial	• Closed haemorrhoidectomy • Infrared coagulation/photocoagulation • Open excisional (Milligan–Morgan/diathermy) haemorrhoidectomy
Trade-off Between Benefits And Harms	• Stapled haemorrhoidectomy
Unknown Effectiveness	• Haemorrhoidal artery ligation

• Injection sclerotherapy

Search date March 2005

DEFINITION Haemorrhoids are cushions of submucosal vascular tissue located in the anal canal starting just distal to the dentate line. These vascular cushions are a normal anatomical structure of the anal canal, and their existence does not necessarily indicate actual haemorrhoidal disease. Haemorrhoidal disease occurs when there are symptoms such as bleeding, prolapse, pain, thrombosis, mucus discharge, and pruritus. Rectal bleeding is the most common manifestation of haemorrhoidal disease. The bleeding tends to be bright red in nature and occurs on the toilet tissue or drips into the toilet bowl. Haemorrhoids can occur internally, externally, or can be mixed (internal and external components). If prolapse occurs, a perianal mass may be evident with defecation. Haemorrhoids are traditionally graded into four degrees. **First degree (or grade):** The haemorrhoids bleed with defecation but do not prolapse. First-degree haemorrhoids associated with mild symptoms are usually secondary to leakage of blood from mildly inflamed, thin walled veins or arterioles. Conservative management with dietary manipulation (addition of fibre) and attention to anal hygiene is often adequate. Recurrent rectal bleeding may require ablation of the vessels with non-surgical ablative techniques, such as injection sclerotherapy, infrared coagulation, or rubber band ligation. Infrared coagulation is used infrequently in clinical practice in the UK today, whereas rubber band ligation and injection sclerotherapy are very commonly used. **Second degree:** The haemorrhoids prolapse with defecation and reduce spontaneously. Second-degree haemorrhoids can be treated with rubber band ligation or other non-surgical ablative techniques. **Third degree:** The haemorrhoids prolapse and require manual reduction. In third-degree haemorrhoids, where there is significant destruction of the suspensory ligaments, relocation and fixation of the mucosa to the underlying muscular wall is generally necessary. Prolapse can be treated with rubber band ligation initially, but haemorrhoidectomy may be required, especially if prolapse is seen in more than one position. **Fourth degree:** The haemorrhoids prolapse and cannot be reduced. If treatment is necessary, fourth-degree haemorrhoids require haemorrhoidectomy. Haemorrhoids are thought to be associated with chronic constipation, straining to defecate, pregnancy, and low dietary fibre. Frequency, duration, and severity of haemorrhoidal symptoms, such as bleeding, prolapse, or both, determine the type of treatment. Often, absent or episodic symptoms do not require treatment, and the presence of symptoms does not mandate invasive treatment. Some people decline treatment if they can be appropriately reassured that there is no other more serious cause for their symptoms.

INCIDENCE/PREVALENCE Haemorrhoids are thought to be common in the general population, but we found no reliable data regarding incidence. Data from the National Center for Health Statistics found that 10 million people in the USA complained of haemorrhoids, leading to a prevalence rate of 4.4%. However, a true figure for prevalence of haemorrhoids is unknown, as there will be many people with the condition who never consult a medical practitioner.

AETIOLOGY/RISK FACTORS The cause of haemorrhoids remains unknown, but it is thought that the downward slide of the anal vascular cushions is the most likely explanation. Other possible causes include straining to defecate, erect posture, and obstruction of venous return from raised intra-abdominal pressure: for example, in pregnancy. It is thought that there may be a hereditary predisposition in some individuals, thought possibly to be due to a congenital weakness of the venous wall.

PROGNOSIS The prognosis is generally excellent, as many symptomatic episodes will often settle with conservative measures only. If further intervention is required, the prognosis remains very good, although recurrent symptoms may occur. Early in the clinical course of haemorrhoids, prolapse reduces spontaneously. Later, the prolapse may require manual reduction and might result in mucus discharge which can cause pruritus ani. Pain is usually not a symptom of internal haemorrhoids unless the haemorrhoids are prolapsed. Pain may be associated with thrombosed external haemorrhoids. Death from bleeding haemorrhoids is an incredibly rare event.

Alex Ford, Cliodna McNulty, Brendan Delaney, and Paul Moayyedi

KEY POINTS

- The principal effect of *Helicobacter pylori* infection is lifelong chronic gastritis, affecting 50–80% of adults born before 1950 in resource-rich countries, and up to 20% of younger adults.

  H pylori infection can be identified indirectly by the C13 urea breath test, and stool antigen tests, which are more accurate than serology.

  Transmission and prevalence rates are higher where there is childhood poverty. Adult reinfection rates are less than 1% a year.

  About 15% of people with *H pylori* infection will develop a peptic ulcer, and 1% will develop gastric cancer during their lifetime.

- Eradication of *H pylori* makes healing of duodenal ulcers more likely, and reduces the risk of bleeding with gastric and duodenal ulcers, either alone or when added to antisecretory drug treatment. Eradication also greatly reduces the risk of recurrence of a duodenal ulcer.

  However, we don't know whether eradication increases healing of gastric ulcers, or reduces recurrence after healing of a gastric ulcer.

  Eradication of *H pylori* may reduce the risk of NSAID-related ulcers in people without previous ulcers. However, we don't know whether it reduces NSAID-related ulcers or bleeding in people with previous ulcers.

- In areas of low prevalence of *H pylori*, few ulcers are caused by *H pylori* infection. Eradication may be less effective in preventing ulcers in these areas compared with higher-prevalence areas.

- Eradication of *H pylori* reduces symptoms of dyspepsia, but not of GORD.

  Eradicating *H pylori* has been shown to reduce dyspeptic symptoms in people with non-ulcer dyspepsia or uninvestigated dyspepsia compared with placebo.

- Despite the association between *H pylori* infection and gastric cancer, no studies have shown a reduced risk after eradication treatment.

  Gastric B cell lymphoma lesions may regress after *H pylori* eradication, but we don't know this for sure.

- Triple regimens seem to be more effective than dual regimens, with 2 weeks of triple treatment more effective than 1 week of triple treatment.

  A 3-day quadruple regimen is as effective as a 1-week triple regimen, but has fewer adverse effects.

  Antibiotics can cause adverse effects such as nausea and diarrhoea. Bismuth may turn the stools black.

Please visit www.clinicalevidence.bmj.com for full text and references

What are the effects of *Helicobacter pylori* eradication treatment in people with a proven duodenal ulcer?	
Beneficial	• *Helicobacter pylori* eradication for healing and preventing recurrence of duodenal ulcer

What are the effects of *Helicobacter pylori* eradication treatment for people with a proven gastric ulcer?	
Beneficial	• *Helicobacter pylori* eradication for healing and preventing recurrence of gastric ulcer

What are the effects of *Helicobacter pylori* eradication treatment in people with NSAID-related peptic ulcers?

Unknown Effectiveness	• *Helicobacter pylori* eradication for healing of NSAID-related peptic ulcers

What are the effects of *Helicobacter pylori* eradication treatment for preventing NSAID-related peptic ulcers in people with previous ulcers or dyspepsia?

Unknown Effectiveness	• *Helicobacter pylori* eradication for prevention of NSAID-related peptic ulcers in people with previous ulcers or dyspepsia

What are the effects of *Helicobacter pylori* eradication treatment for preventing NSAID-related peptic ulcers in people without previous ulcers?

Likely To Be Beneficial	• *Helicobacter pylori* eradication for the prevention of NSAID-related peptic ulcers in people without previous ulcers (more effective than placebo and as effective as antisecretory treatment)

What are the effects of *Helicobacter pylori* eradication treatment in people with proven GORD?

Unlikely To Be Beneficial	• *Helicobacter pylori* eradication in *Helicobacter pylori*-positive people with GORD

What are the effects of *Helicobacter pylori* eradication treatment in people with localised B cell lymphoma of the stomach?

Unknown Effectiveness	• *Helicobacter pylori* eradication for localised gastric B cell lymphoma

What are the effects of *Helicobacter pylori* eradication treatment on the risk of developing gastric cancer?

Unknown Effectiveness	• *Helicobacter pylori* eradication for prevention of gastric cancer

What are the effects of *Helicobacter pylori* eradication treatment in people with proven non-ulcer dyspepsia?

Beneficial	• *Helicobacter pylori* eradication for non-ulcer dyspepsia

What are the effects of *Helicobacter pylori* eradication treatment in people with uninvestigated dyspepsia?

Beneficial	• *Helicobacter pylori* eradication in people with uninvestigated dyspepsia (more effective than placebo)*

Do *Helicobacter pylori* eradication treatments differ in their effects?

Likely To Be Beneficial	• Quadruple regimen (as effective as triple regimen) • Three-day quadruple regimen (as effective as 1-week triple regimen but with fewer adverse effects) • Triple regimen (more effective than dual regimen) • Two-week triple regimen (more effective than 1-week triple regimen)
Unknown Effectiveness	• Different triple regimens (relative effects of different drug combinations on clinical outcomes unclear)

Search date September 2006

*Endoscopy should not be delayed in people at risk of malignancy.

DEFINITION *Helicobacter pylori* is a Gram-negative flagellated spiral bacterium found in the stomach. Infection with *H pylori* is predominantly acquired in childhood. *H pylori* infection is not associated with a specific type of dyspeptic symptom. The organism is associated with lifelong chronic gastritis, and may cause other gastroduodenal disorders. **Diagnosis:** *H pylori* can be identified indirectly by serology or by the C13 urea breath test. The urea breath test is more accurate than serology, with a sensitivity and specificity greater than 95%, and indicates active infection, whereas serology may lack specificity, and cannot be used reliably as a test of active infection. Thus, the urea breath test is the test of choice where prevalence, and hence predictive value of serology, may be low, or where a "test of cure" is required. In some areas, stool antigen tests that have a similar performance to the urea breath test are now available. **Population:** This review focuses on *H pylori*-positive people throughout.

INCIDENCE/PREVALENCE In resource-rich countries, *H pylori* prevalence rates vary with year of birth and social class. Prevalence in many resource-rich countries tends to be much higher (50–80%) in individuals born before 1950 compared with prevalence (less than 20%) in individuals born more recently. In many resource-poor countries, the infection has a high prevalence (80–95%) irrespective of the period of birth. Adult prevalence is believed to represent the persistence of a historically higher rate of infection acquired in childhood, rather than increasing acquisition of infection during life.

AETIOLOGY/RISK FACTORS Overcrowded conditions associated with childhood poverty lead to increased transmission and higher prevalence rates. Adult reinfection rates are low — less than 1% a year.

PROGNOSIS *H pylori* infection is believed to be causally related to the development of duodenal and gastric ulceration, B cell gastric lymphoma, and distal gastric cancer. About 15% of people infected with *H pylori* will develop a peptic ulcer, and 1% of people will develop gastric cancer during their lifetimes. One systematic review of observational studies (search date 2000, 16 studies, 1625 people) found that the frequency of peptic ulcer disease in people taking NSAIDs was greater in those who were *H pylori*-positive than in those who were *H pylori*-negative (peptic ulcer: 341/817 [42%] in *H pylori*-positive NSAID users v 209/808 [26%] in *H pylori*-negative NSAID users; OR 2.12, 95% CI 1.68 to 2.67).

Andre Chow, Sanjay Purkayastha, Thanos Athanasiou, Paris Tekkis, and Ara Darzi

KEY POINTS

- The main risk factors for inguinal hernia are male sex and increasing age.

  Complications of inguinal hernia include strangulation, intestinal obstruction, and infarction. Recurrence can occur after surgery.

- The consensus is that surgery is the treatment of choice for inguinal hernia, although few good-quality studies have compared surgery with expectant management.

- Open suture repair is a well established surgical treatment for people with unilateral inguinal hernia, but it seems to be less effective at preventing recurrence, and prolongs recovery compared with other techniques.

  Open mesh repair reduces the risk of recurrence compared with open suture repair, without increasing the rate of surgical complications.

  Totally extraperitoneal (TEP) laparoscopic repair may lead to less pain, faster recovery, and similar recurrence rates compared with open mesh repair, but studies have given inconclusive results.

  Transabdominal preperitoneal (TAPP) laparoscopic repair reduces pain and speeds up recovery compared with open mesh repair, but the two procedures have similar recurrence rates.

- Open suture repair may be associated with longer recovery times compared with open mesh repair or TAPP laparoscopic repair in people with bilateral inguinal hernia.

  Open mesh repair seems as effective as TEP, but may prolong recovery and increase complication rates compared with TAPP laparoscopic repair.

- Open suture repair may be associated with an increased recovery time compared with open mesh repair in people with recurrent inguinal hernia.

  We do not know how open suture repair compares with TEP or TAPP laparoscopic repair in people with recurrent inguinal hernia.

  TAPP and TEP laparoscopic repair may both reduce recovery time compared with open mesh repair, but complication rates seem to be similar.

(i) **Please visit www.clinicalevidence.bmj.com for full text and references**

What are the effects of elective treatments for primary unilateral inguinal hernia in adults?

Beneficial	• Open mesh repair (reduced recurrence compared with open suture repair, with no increase in surgical complications) • Totally extraperitoneal (TEP) laparoscopic repair (reduced pain and time to return to usual activities compared with open repair) • Transabdominal preperitoneal (TAPP) laparoscopic repair (reduced pain and time to return to usual activities compared with open repair)
Likely To Be Beneficial	• Open suture repair (conventional, well-established surgical technique, but less effective for improving clinically important outcomes than open mesh repair, laparoscopic repair)*
Unknown Effectiveness	• Expectant management

What are the effects of elective treatments for primary bilateral inguinal hernia in adults?

Likely To Be Beneficial	• Open mesh repair (may reduce length of hospital stay compared with open suture repair) • Open suture repair (conventional, well-established surgical technique, but may be less effective in improving clinically important outcomes than open mesh repair or transabdominal preperitoneal (TAPP) laparoscopic repair)* • Totally extraperitoneal (TEP) laparoscopic repair (similar outcomes to open mesh repair) • Transabdominal preperitoneal (TAPP) laparoscopic repair (may reduce time to return to normal activities compared with open repair)
Unknown Effectiveness	• Expectant management

What are the effects of elective treatments for recurrent inguinal hernia in adults?

Likely To Be Beneficial	• Open mesh repair (slightly reduced length of hospital stay compared with open suture repair; other effects uncertain) • Open suture repair (conventional, well established surgical technique but may be less effective than open mesh repair or transabdominal preperitoneal (TAPP) laparoscopic repair) in improving clinically important outcomes* • Totally extraperitoneal (TEP) laparoscopic repair (may reduce time to return to normal activities compared with open mesh repair) • Transabdominal preperitoneal (TAPP) laparoscopic repair (may reduce time to return to normal activities compared with open repair; other effects uncertain)
Unknown Effectiveness	• Expectant management

Search date September 2006

*Based on clinical experience and consensus.

DEFINITION Inguinal hernia is an out-pouching of the peritoneum, with or without its contents, which occurs through the muscles of the anterior abdominal wall at the level of the inguinal canal in the groin. It almost always occurs in men because of the inherent weakness of the abdominal wall where the spermatic cord passes through the inguinal canal. A portion of bowel may become caught in the peritoneal pouch, and present as a lump in the groin. The hernia may extend into the scrotum, and can cause discomfort or ache. Primary hernias relate to the first presentation of a hernia and are distinct from

(continued over)

(from previous page)

recurrent hernias. A hernia is described as reducible if it occurs intermittently (e.g. on straining or standing) and can be pushed back into the abdominal cavity, and is described as irreducible if it remains permanently outside the abdominal cavity. Inguinal hernia is usually a long-standing condition, and diagnosis is made clinically, on the basis of these typical symptoms and signs. The condition may occur in one groin (unilateral hernia) or both groins simultaneously (bilateral hernia), and may recur after treatment (recurrent hernia). Occasionally, hernia may present acutely because of complications (see prognosis below). Clinical experience and consensus suggest that surgical intervention is an effective treatment for inguinal hernia. However, surgery is associated with complications (see outcomes below); therefore, much of this review examines the relative effectiveness and safety of different surgical techniques. Inguinal hernias are frequently classified as direct or indirect, depending on whether the hernia sac bulges directly through the posterior wall of the inguinal canal (direct hernia), or rather passes through the internal inguinal ring alongside the spermatic cord, and follows the course of the inguinal canal (indirect hernia). However, none of the studies that we identified distinguished between these two types of inguinal hernia. Identified studies gave little detail about the severity of hernia among included participants. In general, studies explicitly excluded people with irreducible or complicated hernia, large hernia (extending into the scrotum), or serious comorbidity, and those at high surgical risk (e.g. because of coagulation disorders). In this review, we deal only with non-acute, uncomplicated inguinal hernias in adults.

INCIDENCE/PREVALENCE In resource-rich countries inguinal hernia is usually repaired surgically. Surgical audit data therefore provide reasonable estimates of incidence. We found one nationally mandated guideline, which reported that in 2001–2002 there were about 70,000 inguinal hernia surgeries performed in England, involving 0.14% of the population and requiring over 100,000 NHS hospital bed-days. Of these procedures, 62,969 were for the repair of primary hernias and 4939 for the repair of recurrent hernias. A similar number of inguinal hernia repairs were undertaken in public healthcare settings in England in 2002–2003. In the USA, estimates based on cross-sectional data suggest that about 700,000 inguinal hernia repairs were undertaken in 1993. A national survey of general practices, covering about 1% of the population of England and Wales in 1991–1992, found that about 95% of people presenting to primary-care settings with inguinal hernia were male. It found that the incidence rose from about 11/10,000 person years in men aged 16–24 years to about 200/10,000 person years in men aged 75 years or above.

AETIOLOGY/RISK FACTORS Age and male sex are risk factors (see incidence/prevalence above). Chronic cough and manual labour involving heavy lifting are conventionally regarded as risk factors because they lead to high intra-abdominal pressure. Obesity has also been suggested as a risk factor. However, we found no reliable data to quantify these risks.

PROGNOSIS We found few reliable data on untreated prognosis. Strangulation, intestinal obstruction, and infarction are the most important acute complications of untreated hernia, and are potentially life threatening. National statistics from England found that 5% of primary inguinal hernia repairs were undertaken as emergencies (presumably because of acute complications) in 1998–1999. Older age, longer duration of hernia, and longer duration of irreducibility are thought to be risk factors for acute complications, although we found no reliable data to quantify these effects.

Niek de Wit, Gregory Rubin, and Roger H Jones

KEY POINTS

- **Irritable bowel syndrome (IBS) causes abdominal pain and bloating, and diarrhoea or constipation, in the absence of identifiable structural or biochemical disorders.**

  The prevalence of IBS varies depending on the criteria used to diagnose it, but ranges from about 5% to over 15%.

  IBS is associated with abnormal gastrointestinal motor function and enhanced visceral perception, as well as psychosocial and genetic factors.

  People with IBS have an increased likelihood of having a cholecystectomy or hysterectomy compared with people without IBS.

- **Antidepressants may reduce the symptoms of IBS compared with placebo, although studies have been of poor quality and have given inconclusive results.**

- **Antispasmodics may improve symptoms of IBS compared with placebo, but studies have given conflicting results.**

- **The $5HT_3$ receptor antagonist alosetron may be more effective than mebeverine at reducing symptoms in women with diarrhoea-predominant IBS, but we don't know whether it is effective in men.**

  We don't know whether other $5HT_3$ receptor antagonists are beneficial in IBS as we found no studies.

- **Loperamide may reduce stool frequency in diarrhoea-predominant IBS, but may not improve other symptoms compared with placebo.**

- **$5HT_4$ receptor antagonists such as tegaserod may improve symptoms in women with constipation-predominant IBS compared with placebo, but we don't know whether they are beneficial in men.**

  CAUTION: Tegaserod may be associated with serious diarrhoea, and alosetron may be associated with ischaemic colitis.

- **Soluble fibre supplementation may improve overall symptoms in people with IBS, and both soluble and insoluble fibre supplementation may improve constipation, although studies have been of poor quality.**

- **CBT may reduce symptoms in the short term, but studies have been of poor quality and have given conflicting results. We don't know whether it is beneficial in the longer term. We don't know if hypnotherapy can reduce symptoms.**

(i) **Please visit www.clinicalevidence.bmj.com for full text and references**

What are the effects of treatments in people with irritable bowel syndrome?	
Likely To Be Beneficial	• Antidepressants (amitriptyline, clomipramine, desipramine, doxepin, mianserin, trimipramine, fluoxetine) • Antispasmodics • Soluble-fibre supplementation (reduces global symptoms)
Trade-off Between Benefits And Harms	• $5HT_4$ receptor agonists (tegaserod) • Alosetron
Unknown Effectiveness	• $5HT_3$ receptor antagonists other than alosetron • CBT

- Hypnotherapy
- Insoluble-fibre supplementation
- Loperamide

Search date June 2006

DEFINITION Irritable bowel syndrome (IBS) is a chronic non-inflammatory condition characterised by abdominal pain, altered bowel habit (diarrhoea or constipation), and abdominal bloating, but with no identifiable structural or biochemical disorder. Symptom based criteria, such as the Manning criteria, the Rome I criteria, and the Rome II criteria, aid diagnosis but their main use is in defining populations in clinical trials. The Rome criteria also subcategorise IBS according to predominant symptoms (diarrhoea, constipation, or alternating between diarrhoea and constipation). In practice, the division between constipation-predominant and diarrhoea-predominant IBS may not be clear-cut in all people. Restriction of trial entry to a subcategory of IBS limits the generalisability of study results.

INCIDENCE/PREVALENCE Estimates of incidence and prevalence vary depending on the diagnostic criteria used to define IBS. One cross-sectional postal survey (4476 people aged 20–69 years) in Teeside, UK, defined IBS as recurrent abdominal pain on more than six occasions during the previous year plus two or more of the Manning criteria. It estimated prevalence in the UK to be 16.7% (95% CI 15.4% to 18.0%) overall, with a prevalence of 22.8% (95% CI 20.8% to 24.8%) among women and 10.5% (95% CI 8.9% to 12.1%) among men. A cross-sectional postal survey (4500 people aged above 17 years) in Australia found prevalences of IBS of 13.6% (95% CI 12.3% to 14.8%) using the Manning criteria, 6.9% (95% CI 6.0% to 7.8%) using the Rome I criteria, and 4.4% (95% CI 3.5% to 5.1%) using the Rome II criteria.

AETIOLOGY/RISK FACTORS The pathophysiology of IBS is not certain, but abnormal gastrointestinal motor function and enhanced visceral perception appear important. Other determinants include psychosocial factors such as a history of childhood abuse, genetic predisposition, and a history of enteric mucosal inflammation. We found no reliable prospective data to measure these associations.

PROGNOSIS A retrospective study reviewed the medical records of people with IBS (112 people aged 20–64 years when diagnosed with IBS at the Mayo Clinic, USA, in 1961–1963). IBS was defined as the presence of abdominal pain associated with either disturbed defecation or abdominal distension, and the absence of organic bowel disease. Over a 32-year period, death rates were similar among people with IBS compared with age- and gender-matched controls. One postal survey (4432 adults aged 20–69 years) found that people with IBS are significantly more likely than controls to have had a cholecystectomy (OR 1.9, 95% CI 1.2 to 3.2). A paper reporting on the same survey population (2238 women aged 20–69 years) found that women with IBS were significantly more likely than controls to have had a hysterectomy (OR 1.6, 95% CI 1.1 to 2.2). We found no reliable estimates of the duration of IBS if left untreated.

Adrian O'Sullivan and Hemant M Kocher

KEY POINTS

- **Pancreatic cancer is the fourth most common cause of cancer death in higher-income countries, with 5-year survival only 10% (range 7% to 25%), even in people presenting with early-stage cancer.**

  Risk factors include age, smoking, chronic pancreatitis, a family history, and dietary factors. Diabetes mellitus may also increase the risk.

- **In people with pancreatic cancer considered suitable for complete tumour resection, pancreaticoduodenectomy (Kausch–Whipple procedure) or pylorus-preserving pancreaticoduodenectomy (Traverso–Longmire procedure) may prolong survival compared with non-surgical treatment, although no large RCTs have been found.**

  Pylorus-preserving pancreaticoduodenectomy may lead to similar quality of life and survival compared with Kausch–Whipple pancreaticoduodenectomy.

  Extended lymphadenectomy is associated with increases in adverse effects compared with standard lymphadenectomy, without conferring any survival benefit.

- **Somatostatin and its analogues, particularly octreotide, prevent complications (pancreatic leak and intra-abdominal collections) of pancreatic surgery, but do not reduce mortality.**

  We don't know which anastomosis (pancreaticogastrostomy or pancreaticojejunostomy) is more effective for preventing pancreatic leak, although there are observational data suggesting that pancreaticogastrostomy may be preferable.

  Pancreatic duct occlusion does not assist in preventing complications associated with pancreatic leak when added to anastomosis. When used alone, duct occlusion increases pancreatic fistula, and pancreatic endocrine and exocrine insufficiency, and cannot therefore be recommended.

  We don't know if fibrin glue is effective for preventing pancreatic leak.

- **Adjuvant fluorouracil-based chemotherapy increases median and 5-year survival in people with completely resected pancreatic cancer compared with no chemotherapy.**

  Adjuvant chemoradiotherapy does not seem to improve survival in people with resected pancreatic cancer.

  We don't know whether adjuvant gemcitabine-based chemotherapy increases survival compared with no chemotherapy in people with resected pancreatic cancer. Trials are underway and we await their results.

- **In people with non-resectable pancreatic cancer, gemcitabine or fluorouracil monotherapy seem preferable to combination chemotherapy based on either drug.**

  We found insufficient evidence to recommend chemoradiation over chemotherapy alone in people with non-resectable pancreatic cancer.

(i) **Please visit www.clinicalevidence.bmj.com for full text and references**

What are the effects of surgical treatments in people with pancreatic cancer considered suitable for complete tumour resection?

Unknown Effectiveness	• Pancreaticoduodenectomy versus non-surgical treatment

	• Pylorus-preserving pancreaticoduodenectomy (compared with Kausch–Whipple procedure)
Unlikely To Be Beneficial	• Extended (radical) versus standard lymphadenectomy in people receiving pancreaticoduodenectomy

What are the effects of interventions to prevent pancreatic leak after pancreaticoduodenectomy in people with pancreatic cancer considered suitable for complete tumour resection?

Likely To Be Beneficial	• Somatostatin and somatostatin analogues
Unknown Effectiveness	• Fibrin glue • Pancreaticojejunostomy versus pancreaticogastrostomy reconstruction (unclear from RCT evidence which is better, but observational evidence supports pancreaticogastrostomy)
Likely To Be Ineffective Or Harmful	• Pancreatic duct occlusion

What are the effects of adjuvant treatments in people with completely resected pancreatic cancer?

Beneficial	• Fluorouracil-based chemotherapy (adjuvant) for resected pancreatic cancer (increases survival compared with surgery alone)
Unknown Effectiveness	• Chemoradiotherapy for resected pancreatic cancer • Gemcitabine-based chemotherapy (adjuvant) for resected pancreatic cancer

What are the effects of interventions in people with non-resectable (locally advanced or advanced) pancreatic cancer?

Beneficial	• Fluorouracil-based chemotherapy for non-resectable pancreatic cancer (increases survival compared with supportive care)
Likely To Be Beneficial	• Fluorouracil-based monotherapy for non-resectable pancreatic cancer (may be less effective than gemcitabine monotherapy; as effective as fluorouracil-based combination chemotherapy with fewer adverse effects) • Gemcitabine-based monotherapy for non-resectable pancreatic cancer (may be more

	effective than fluorouracil monotherapy and as effective as gemcitabine-based combination chemotherapy with fewer adverse effects)
Unknown Effectiveness	● Chemoradiotherapy

Search date November 2006

*RCTs comparing surgery versus no surgery may be considered unethical in people with pancreatic cancer considered suitable for complete tumour resection.

DEFINITION In this review, the term "pancreatic cancer" refers to primary ductal adenocarcinoma of the pancreas. Other pancreatic malignancies such as neuroendocrine and serous cystic tumours of the pancreas are not considered. Symptoms of pancreatic cancer include pain, jaundice, nausea, weight loss, anorexia, and symptoms associated with gastrointestinal obstruction and diabetes. Pancreatic cancer is staged using the tumour, node, metastasis (TNM) and American Joint Committee on Cancer (AJCC) classification systems. A pancreatic tumour is considered resectable if the tumour appears to be localised to the pancreas without invasion into major blood vessels, or distant spread to liver, lungs, or bone. Earlier detection of tumours increases the possibility of resection. Other factors that influence resectability include perceived perioperative risk based on other co-morbidities.

INCIDENCE/PREVALENCE Pancreatic cancer is the eighth most common cancer in the UK, with an annual incidence in England and Wales of about 12/100,000. It is the fourth most common cause of cancer death in higher-income countries, responsible for about 30,000 deaths each year in the USA. Prevalence is similar in men and women, with 5–10% presenting with resectable disease.

AETIOLOGY/RISK FACTORS Pancreatic cancer is more likely to develop in people who smoke and have high alcohol intake. Dietary factors, such as lack of fruit and vegetables, are also reported risk factors. One population-based cohort study of more than 2000 people suggested that there was a 1% chance of developing pancreatic cancer within 3 years of diagnosis in people diagnosed with new-onset diabetes mellitus. However, estimates of the magnitude of increased risk of pancreatic cancer in people with diabetes vary. Additional risk factors include chronic sporadic pancreatitis — which carries a fivefold increased risk of developing pancreatic cancer — and, in some cases, a family history of pancreatic cancer.

PROGNOSIS Prognosis in people with pancreatic cancer is poor. The overall median survival worldwide is less than 6 months, with an overall 5-year survival rate of 0.4–5.0%. The surgical resection rate worldwide is between 2.6% and 9.0%, with a median survival of 11–20 months, and a 5-year survival rate of 7–25%, with few long-term survivors. Tumour resection is graded from R0 to R2, with R0 meaning no tumour remains after surgery (confirmed by histology); R1 meaning surgeon believes no tumour remains but histology demonstrates positive margins; and R2 meaning that the surgeon was unable to remove all macroscopic tumour completely.

Charles Bailey

KEY POINTS

- Stomach cancer is usually an adenocarcinoma arising in the stomach, and includes tumours arising at or just below the gastro-oesophageal junction (type II and III junctional tumours). Only non-metastatic stomach cancers are considered here.

  The incidence varies among countries and by gender, with about 80 cases per 100,000 people in Japanese men, 30/100,000 in Japanese women, 18/100,000 in British men, and 10/100,000 in British women.

- With regard to surgical resection, subtotal gastrectomy seems to be as effective as total gastrectomy.

  In practice, surgeons sometimes recommend total gastrectomy "de principe" in people with poorly differentiated "diffuse" cancer to prevent infiltration of microscopic tumour deposits into the proximal resection margin.

- Removal of adjacent organs (spleen and distal pancreas) is associated with increased morbidity and mortality compared with gastrectomy alone.

  Current consensus is that adjacent organs should only be removed to ensure complete tumour removal, or when required because of trauma during surgery.

- We found no sufficient evidence to judge the effectiveness of radical lymphadenectomy compared with conservative lymphadenectomy.

- Adjuvant chemoradiotherapy seems to improve survival compared with surgery alone in people with resectable stomach adenocarcinoma.

- Adjuvant chemotherapy might also be effective compared with surgery alone, although the evidence is somewhat varied.

(i) **Please visit www.clinicalevidence.bmj.com for full text and references**

What are the effects of radical versus conservative surgical resection?	
Likely To Be Beneficial	• Subtotal gastrectomy for resectable distal tumours (as effective as total gastrectomy)
Unknown Effectiveness	• Radical versus conservative lymphadenectomy
Likely To Be Ineffective Or Harmful	• Removal of adjacent organs

What are the effects of adjuvant chemotherapy?	
Likely To Be Beneficial	• Adjuvant chemoradiotherapy
	• Adjuvant chemotherapy

Search date August 2006

DEFINITION Stomach cancer is usually an adenocarcinoma arising in the stomach and includes tumours arising at or just below the gastro-oesophageal junction (type II and III junctional tumours). Tumours are staged according to degree of invasion and spread. Only non-metastatic stomach cancers are considered in this review.

INCIDENCE/PREVALENCE The incidence of stomach cancer varies among countries and by sex (incidence per 100,000 population a year in Japanese men is about 80, Japanese women 30, British men 18, British women 10, white American men 11, and white American women 7). Incidence has declined dramatically in North America, Australia, and New Zealand since 1930, but the decline in Europe has been slower. In the USA, stomach cancer remains relatively common among particular ethnic groups, especially Japanese-Americans and some Hispanic groups. The incidence of cancer of the proximal stomach and gastro-oesophageal junction is rising rapidly in many European populations and in North America. The reasons for this are poorly understood.

AETIOLOGY/RISK FACTORS Distal stomach cancer is strongly associated with lifelong infection with *Helicobacter pylori* and poor dietary intake of antioxidant vitamins (A, C, and E). In Western Europe and North America, distal stomach cancer is associated with relative socioeconomic deprivation. Proximal stomach cancer is strongly associated with smoking (OR about 4), and is probably associated with GORD, obesity, high fat intake, and medium to high socioeconomic status.

PROGNOSIS Invasive stomach cancer (stages T2–T4) is fatal without surgery. Mean survival without treatment is less than 6 months from diagnosis. Intramucosal or submucosal cancer (stage T1) may progress slowly to invasive cancer over several years. In the USA, over 50% of people recently diagnosed with stomach cancer have regional lymph node metastasis or involvement of adjacent organs. The prognosis after macroscopically and microscopically complete resection (R0) is related strongly to disease stage, particularly penetration of the serosa (stage T3) and lymph node involvement. Five-year survival rates range from over 90% in intramucosal cancer to about 20% in people with stage T3N2 disease. In Japan, the 5-year survival rate for people with advanced disease is reported to be about 50%, but the explanation for the difference remains unclear. Comparisons between Japanese and Western practice are confounded by factors such as age, fitness, and disease stage, as well as by tumour location, because many Western series include gastro-oesophageal junction adenocarcinoma, which is associated with a much lower survival rate after surgery.

Jose Acuin

KEY POINTS

- Chronic suppurative otitis media (CSOM) causes recurrent or persistent discharge (otorrhoea) through a perforation in the tympanic membrane, and can lead to thickening of the middle-ear mucosa, mucosal polyps, and cholesteatoma.

  CSOM is a common cause of hearing impairment, disability, and poor scholastic performance, and can occasionally lead to fatal intracranial infections and acute mastoiditis, especially in resource-poor countries.

- Topical antibiotics either alone or in combination with topical corticosteroids may improve symptoms compared with placebo or either treatment alone in adults, although few adequate studies have been found. There is consensus that topical antibiotics should be combined with ear cleansing.

  We don't know whether topical antiseptics, topical corticosteroids, or systemic antibiotics are beneficial in reducing symptoms.

  It is possible that antibiotics against gram-negative bacteria may reduce ear discharge more than other classes of antibiotics or placebo.

- We don't know whether tympanoplasty with or without mastoidectomy improves symptoms compared with no surgery or other treatments in adults or children with CSOM.

- In children with CSOM, the benefits of ear cleansing are unknown, although this treatment is usually recommended for children with ear discharge.

  We don't know whether topical antiseptics, topical or systemic antibiotics, or topical corticosteroids, alone or in combination with antibiotics, improve symptoms in children with CSOM compared with placebo or other treatments.

  It is possible that topical antibiotics improve resolution of ear discharge compared with topical antiseptics, but they may increase the risk of ototoxicity.

(i) **Please visit www.clinicalevidence.bmj.com for full text and references**

What are the effects of treatments for chronic suppurative otitis media in adults?	
Likely To Be Beneficial	• Antibiotics (topical) in adults • Antibiotics (topical) plus corticosteroids (topical) in adults
Unknown Effectiveness	• Antibiotics (systemic) in adults (unclear if as effective as topical) • Antibiotics (topical plus systemic) in adults (unclear if more effective than topical alone) • Antiseptics (topical) in adults • Corticosteroids (topical) in adults • Ear cleansing in adults • Tympanoplasty (with or without mastoidectomy) in adults

What are the effects of treatments for chronic suppurative otitis media in children?

Unknown Effectiveness	• Antibiotics (systemic) in children
	• Antibiotics (topical) in children
	• Antibiotics (topical) plus corticosteroids (topical) in children
	• Antiseptics (topical) in children
	• Corticosteroids (topical) in children
	• Ear cleansing in children
	• Tympanoplasty (with or without mastoidectomy) in children

Search date January 2007

DEFINITION Chronic suppurative otitis media (CSOM) is persistent inflammation of the middle ear or mastoid cavity. Synonyms include "chronic otitis media (without effusion)", chronic mastoiditis, and chronic tympanomastoiditis. CSOM is characterised by recurrent or persistent ear discharge (otorrhoea) over 2–6 weeks through a perforation of the tympanic membrane. Typical findings may also include thickened granular middle-ear mucosa, mucosal polyps, and cholesteatoma within the middle ear. CSOM is differentiated from chronic OME, in which there is an intact tympanic membrane with fluid in the middle ear but no active infection. CSOM does not include chronic perforations of the eardrum that are dry, or only occasionally discharge, and have no signs of active infection. CSOM with cholesteatoma is not dealt with in this review.

INCIDENCE/PREVALENCE The worldwide prevalence of CSOM is 65–330 million people, and 39–200 million (60%) suffer from clinically significant hearing impairment.

AETIOLOGY/RISK FACTORS CSOM is assumed to be a complication of AOM, but the risk factors for CSOM are not clear. Frequent upper respiratory tract infections and poor socioeconomic conditions (overcrowded housing, and poor hygiene and nutrition) may be related to the development of CSOM. Improvement in housing, hygiene, and nutrition in Maori children was associated with a halving of the prevalence of CSOM between 1978 and 1987. See also AOM, p 64. The most commonly isolated microorganisms are *Pseudomonas aeruginosa* and *Staphylococcus aureus*; *P aeruginosa* has been particularly implicated in the causation of bony necrosis and mucosal disease. However, a systematic review found no clear evidence that antibiotics are effective in preventing the progression of acute to CSOM even among children who are at high risk for the disease.

PROGNOSIS The natural history of CSOM is poorly understood. The perforation may close spontaneously in an unknown portion of cases, but persists in others leading to mild to moderate hearing impairment (about 26–60 dB increase in hearing thresholds), based on surveys among children in Africa, Brazil, India, and Sierra Leone, and among the general population in Thailand. In many resource-poor countries, CSOM represents the most frequent cause of moderate hearing loss (40–60 dB). Persistent hearing loss during the first 2 years of life may increase learning disabilities and poor scholastic performance. Progressive hearing loss may occur among those in whom infection persists and discharge recurs. Less frequently, spread of infection may lead to life-threatening complications such as intracranial infections and acute mastoiditis. The frequency of serious complications fell from 20% in 1938 to 2.5% in 1948 worldwide and is currently estimated to be about 0.7% to 3.2% worldwide. This is believed to be associated with increased use of antibiotic treatment, tympanoplasty, and mastoidectomy. Otitis media was estimated to have caused 3599 deaths and a loss of almost 1.5 DALYs in 2002, 90% of which were in resource-poor countries. Most of these deaths were probably as a result of CSOM, because AOM is a self-limiting infection (see review on AOM, p 64).

Ear wax

George Browning

KEY POINTS

- Ear wax only becomes a problem if it causes a hearing impairment, or other ear-related symptoms.

   Ear wax is more likely to accumulate and cause a hearing impairment when normal extrusion is prevented: for example, by hearing aids, or by the use of cotton buds to clean the ears.

   Ear wax can visually obscure the ear drum, and may need to be removed for diagnostic purposes.

- For such a commonly occurring condition, there is little high-quality evidence available to guide practice.

- Ear syringing is generally considered effective, but evidence is limited.

   Syringing can clear wax from the ear canal in up to 100% of ears when performed alone, or after the use of wax softeners.

   Ear syringing may be associated with vertigo and tympanic membrane perforation in some people. Pain, damage to the skin of the ear canal, and otitis externa are other possible adverse effects.

- Other mechanical methods of removing ear wax by trained staff using instruments — such as microsuction — are probably effective, although the evidence is limited.

   Mechanical removal of wax with suction, probes, or forceps is considered effective, but can cause trauma to the ear canal, depending on the experience and training of the operator, and the adequacy of visualisation.

- Benefits of wax softeners are unknown when used prior to syringing or alone.

   The use of wax softeners prior to syringing may increase clearance rate, but the evidence is limited.

   Evidence is too limited to show whether wax softeners alone are effective in clearing wax, or whether one type of softener is more effective than another.

(i) **Please visit www.clinicalevidence.bmj.com for full text and references**

What are the effects of methods to remove ear wax?	
Trade-off Between Benefits And Harms	• Ear syringing*
Unknown Effectiveness	• Manual removal (other than ear syringing)* • Wax softeners alone • Wax softeners prior to syringing

Search date June 2007

*Although many practitioners consider these to be standard treatments, we found no RCTs of these interventions.

DEFINITION Ear wax is normal and becomes a problem only if it produces hearing impairment, pain, or other ear-related symptoms. Ear wax may also need to be removed if it prevents inspection of the ear drum. The term "impacted wax" is used in different ways, and can merely imply the coexistence of wax obscuring the ear drum with symptoms in that ear.

INCIDENCE/PREVALENCE We found four surveys of the prevalence of impacted wax. The studies were carried out in a variety of populations, and used a variety of definitions of impacted wax. Prevalence ranged from 7–35%. It is unclear how these figures relate to prevalence in the general population.

AETIOLOGY/RISK FACTORS Factors that prevent the normal extrusion of wax from the ear canal (e.g. wearing a hearing aid, using cotton buds to clean ears) increase the chance of ear wax accumulating.

PROGNOSIS Most ear wax emerges from the external canal spontaneously; one small RCT that included a no-treatment group found that 32% of ears with impacted wax showed some degree of spontaneous resolution after 5 days (26.3% described as moderately clear; 5.3% described as completely clear). Without impaction or adherence to the drum, there is likely to be minimal, if any, hearing loss.

194 | Menière's disease

Adrian James and Marc Thorp

KEY POINTS

- Menière's disease causes recurrent vertigo, hearing loss, tinnitus, and fullness or pressure in the ear, and mainly affects adults aged 40–60 years.

  Menière's disease is progressive at first but fluctuating, and episodes can occur in clusters.

  Vertigo usually resolves but hearing deteriorates, and symptoms other than hearing loss and tinnitus usually improve regardless of treatment.

- We do not know whether anticholinergic drugs, benzodiazepines, phenothiazines, cinnarizine, or betahistine improve symptoms in an acute attack of Menière's disease, as no good-quality studies have been found.

- Betahistine seems no more effective than placebo at preventing hearing loss in people with Menière's disease.

  We do not know whether betahistine reduces the frequency or severity of vertigo, tinnitus or aural fullness.

  We do not know whether diuretics, trimetazidine, dietary modification, psychological support, or vestibular rehabilitation improve tinnitus or hearing, or reduce the frequency of attacks of Menière's disease.

(i) **Please visit www.clinicalevidence.bmj.com for full text and references**

What are the effects of treatments for acute attacks of Menière's disease?	
Unknown Effectiveness	• Anticholinergics
	• Benzodiazepines
	• Betahistine
	• Cinnarizine
	• Phenothiazines

What are the effects of interventions to prevent attacks and delay disease progression of Menière's disease?	
Unknown Effectiveness	• Betahistine (for vertigo or tinnitus or aural fullness)
	• Dietary modification
	• Diuretics
	• Psychological support
	• Trimetazidine
	• Vestibular rehabilitation
Unlikely To Be Beneficial	• Betahistine (for hearing loss)

Search date January 2006

DEFINITION Menière's disease is characterised by recurrent episodes of spontaneous rotational vertigo, sensorineural hearing loss, tinnitus, and a feeling of fullness or pressure in the ear. It may be unilateral or bilateral. Acute episodes can occur in clusters of about 6–11 a year, although remission may last several months. The diagnosis is made clinically.

It is important to distinguish Menière's disease from other types of vertigo that might occur independently with hearing loss and tinnitus, and respond differently to treatment (e.g. benign positional vertigo, acute labyrinthitis). Strict diagnostic criteria help to identify the condition. In this review, we have applied the classification of the American Academy of Otolaryngology — Head and Neck Surgery to assess the diagnostic rigour used in RCTs.

INCIDENCE/PREVALENCE Menière's disease is most common between 40–60 years of age, although younger people may be affected. In Europe, the incidence is about 50–200/100,000 a year. A survey of general practitioner records of 27,365 people in the UK in the 1950s found an incidence of 43 affected people in a 1-year period (157/100,000). Diagnostic criteria were not defined in this survey. A survey of over 8 million people in 1973 in Sweden found an incidence of 46/100,000 a year with diagnosis strictly based on the triad of vertigo, hearing loss, and tinnitus. From smaller studies, the incidence appears to be lower in Japan (17/100,000, based on national surveys of hospital attendances in 1977, 1982, and 1990) and in Uganda.

AETIOLOGY/RISK FACTORS Menière's disease is associated with endolymphatic hydrops (raised endolymph pressure in the membranous labyrinth of the inner ear), but a causal relationship remains unproved. Specific disorders associated with hydrops (such as temporal bone fracture, syphilis, hypothyroidism, Cogan's syndrome, and Mondini dysplasia) can produce symptoms similar to those of Menière's disease.

PROGNOSIS Menière's disease is progressive at first but fluctuates unpredictably. It is difficult to distinguish natural resolution from the effects of treatment. Significant improvement in vertigo is usually seen in the placebo arms of RCTs. Acute attacks of vertigo often increase in frequency during the first few years after presentation and then decrease in frequency in association with sustained deterioration in hearing. In most people, vertiginous episodes eventually cease completely. In one 20-year cohort study in 34 people, 28 (82%) people had at least moderate hearing loss (mean pure-tone hearing loss greater than 50 dB) and 16 (47%) developed bilateral disease. Symptoms other than hearing loss improve in 60–80% of people irrespective of treatment.

Middle-ear pain and trauma during air travel

Arin Basu

KEY POINTS

- Changes in air pressure during air travel can cause ear-drum pain and perforation, vertigo, and hearing loss. Barotitis is inflammation of the ear drum caused by air-pressure changes.

  It has been estimated that 10% of adults and 22% of children might have damage to the ear drum after a flight, although perforation is rare.

  Symptoms usually resolve spontaneously.

- Nasal balloon inflation may reduce symptoms of barotitis in people during air travel.

- Oral pseudoephedrine may reduce symptoms in adults with previous ear pain during flights.

  We don't know whether oral pseudoephedrine is also beneficial in children, but it can cause drowsiness.

- We don't know whether topical nasal decongestants can prevent symptoms of barotrauma.

(i) **Please visit www.clinicalevidence.bmj.com for full text and references**

Preventing middle-ear pain during air travel	
Likely To Be Beneficial	• Nasal balloon inflation • Pseudoephedrine (oral) in adults
Unknown Effectiveness	• Nasal decongestants (topical) • Pseudoephedrine (oral) in children

Search date April 2007

DEFINITION The effects of air travel on the middle ear, as a result of changes in air pressure, can include ear-drum pain, vertigo, hearing loss, and ear-drum perforation.

INCIDENCE/PREVALENCE The prevalence of symptoms depends on the altitude, type of aircraft, and characteristics of the passengers. One point prevalence study found that, in commercial passengers, 20% of adult and 40% of child passengers had negative pressure in the middle ear after flight, and that 10% of adults and 22% of children had otoscopic evidence of damage to the ear drum. We found no data on the incidence of perforation, which seems to be extremely rare in commercial passengers.

AETIOLOGY/RISK FACTORS During aircraft descent, the pressure in the middle ear drops relative to that in the ear canal. A narrow, inflamed, or poorly functioning Eustachian tube impedes the necessary influx of air. As the pressure difference between the middle and outer ear increases, the ear drum is pulled inward.

PROGNOSIS In most people, symptoms resolve spontaneously. Experience in military aviation shows that most ear-drum perforations will heal spontaneously.

Daniel Hajioff

KEY POINTS

- Otitis externa is thought to affect 10% of people at some stage of life and can present as acute, chronic, or necrotising forms.

    Otitis externa may be associated with eczema of the ear canal and is more common in swimmers, humid environments, people with absence of ear wax or narrow ear canals, hearing-aid users, and after mechanical trauma.

    The most common pathogens are *Pseudomonas aeruginosa* and *Staphylococcus aureus.*.

    Fungal overgrowth can occur, especially after prolonged antibiotic use.

- Topical anti-infective agents may improve symptoms and signs of otitis externa.

    Methylprednisolone–neomycin drops are probably more effective than placebo in reducing signs and symptoms of otitis externa over 28 days.

    We do not know whether any one regimen should be used in preference to other possible treatments.

    We don't know whether antifungal agents improve symptoms of otitis externa.

- Topical corticosteroids may reduce signs and symptoms of otitis externa, but few good-quality studies have been found.

    Topical budesonide is probably more effective than placebo in reducing signs and symptoms of otitis externa.

    Low-potency corticosteroids maybe as effective as higher-potency corticosteroids after 1 week.

    There is no evidence to compare topical corticosteroids with topical anti-infective agents.

- Oral antibiotics have not been shown to be beneficial.

    Adding oral co-trimoxazole to topical anti-infective agents does not improve symptoms compared with topical agents alone.

- Topical acetic acid may increase cure when used with topical anti-infective agents and corticosteroids, but is less effective than this combination when used alone.

- Prophylactic treatments to prevent otitis externa (topical acetic acid, topical corticosteroids, or water exclusion), and specialist aural toilet, have not been evaluated in clinical trials.

Please visit www.clinicalevidence.bmj.com for full text and references

What are the effects of empirical treatment for otitis externa?	
Likely To Be Beneficial	• Topical aluminium acetate drops (as effective as topical antibiotics)
	• Topical antibacterials (with or without corticosteroids)
	• Topical corticosteroids
Unknown Effectiveness	• Oral antibiotics
	• Specialist aural toilet

	• Topical acetic acid (insufficient evidence to demonstrate effectiveness compared with placebo)
	• Topical antifungals (with or without corticosteroids)
Unlikely To Be Beneficial	• Oral antibiotics plus topical anti-infective agents (no better than topical anti-infective agents alone)

What are the effects of prophylactic treatments for otitis externa?

Unknown Effectiveness	• Topical acetic acid spray or drops
	• Topical corticosteroids
	• Water exclusion

Search date March 2006

DEFINITION Otitis externa is inflammation, often with infection, of the external ear canal. This inflammation is usually generalised throughout the ear canal, and is therefore often referred to as "diffuse otitis externa". This review excludes localised inflammations such as furuncles. Otitis externa has acute (less than 6 weeks), chronic (more than 3 months), and necrotising (malignant) forms. Acute otitis externa may present as a single episode, or recur. It causes pain with aural discharge and associated hearing loss. If the ear canal is visible, it appears red and inflamed. *Pseudomonas aeruginosa* and *Staphylococcus aureus* are the most frequent bacterial pathogens in otitis externa. Fungal overgrowth (e.g. with *Aspergillus niger*) is also quite common, especially after prolonged antibiotic treatment. Chronic otitis externa may result in canal stenosis with associated hearing loss, for which it may be difficult to fit hearing aids. Necrotising otitis externa is defined by destruction of the temporal bone, usually in people with diabetes or in people who are immunocompromised, and can be life threatening. In this review, we look at the empirical treatment of acute and chronic otitis externa only.

INCIDENCE/PREVALENCE Otitis externa is common in all parts of the world. The incidence is not known precisely, but 10% of people are thought to have been affected at some time. The condition affects children, but is more common in adults. It accounts for a large proportion of the workload of otolaryngology departments, but milder cases are often managed in primary care.

AETIOLOGY/RISK FACTORS Otitis externa may be associated with local or generalised eczema of the ear canal. It is more common in swimmers, in humid environments, in people with an absence of ear wax or narrow external ear canals, in hearing aid users, and after mechanical trauma.

PROGNOSIS We found few reliable data. Many cases of otitis externa resolve spontaneously over several weeks or months. Acute episodes have a tendency to recur, although the risk of recurrence is unknown. Experience suggests that chronic inflammation affects a small proportion of people after a single episode of acute otitis externa, and may rarely lead to canal stenosis.

Christos C Georgalas, Neil S Tolley, and Antony Narula

KEY POINTS

- Diagnosis of acute tonsillitis is clinical, and it can be difficult to distinguish viral from bacterial infections.

  Rapid antigen testing has a very low sensitivity in the diagnosis of bacterial tonsillitis, but more accurate tests take longer to deliver results.

  Bacteria are cultured from few people with tonsillitis. Other causes include infectious mononucleosis from Epstein–Barr virus infection, cytomegalovirus, toxoplasmosis, HIV, hepatitis A, and rubella.

- Acute tonsillitis with group A beta haemolytic streptococci can occasionally cause rheumatic fever and acute glomerulonephritis, which can be prevented by treatment with penicillin.

  In resource-rich countries these complications are so rare that routine aggressive antibiotic use cannot be justified.

- Tonsillectomy, with or without adenoidectomy, is one of the most frequently performed surgical procedures in the UK.

- We don't know if tonsillectomy is beneficial in adults with recurrent acute tonsillitis, as we found no studies.

- In children, the effectiveness of tonsillectomy has to be judged against the potential harms. Tonsillectomy is more beneficial in people with severe symptoms while, in populations with a low incidence of tonsillitis, the modest benefit may be outweighed by the morbidity associated with the surgery.

- The use of diathermy in tonsillectomy is associated with reduced rates of primary bleeding, but increased rates of secondary and overall bleeding. Adequate training in the appropriate use of diathermy during tonsillectomy is important.

- Adequate training in the appropriate use of diathermy during tonsillectomy is important. In deciding which method to apply, the surgeon should consider the underlying characteristics of patients, as well as the relative importance of secondary compared with primary bleeding, and intraoperative blood loss compared with postoperative pain. Overall, cold steel dissection tonsillectomy seems to have the lowest rates of postoperative haemorrhage and postoperative pain, although it is associated with slightly increased intraoperative bleeding. The use of diathermy in tonsillectomy must be weighted against its potential harms.

Please visit www.clinicalevidence.bmj.com for full text and references

What are the effects of tonsillectomy in children and adults with acute recurrent or chronic throat infections?	
Beneficial	• Cold steel tonsillectomy compared with diathermy tonsillectomy in children and adults
Trade-off Between Benefits And Harms	• Tonsillectomy versus antibiotics in children
Unknown Effectiveness	• Tonsillectomy versus antibiotics in adults

Search date November 2006

DEFINITION The definition of severe recurrent throat infections is arbitrary, but recent criteria have defined severe tonsillitis as five or more episodes of true tonsillitis a year, symptoms for at least a year, and episodes that are disabling and prevent normal functioning. However, in most cases, the severity of recurrent throat infections depends on many factors, and cannot be judged solely on the basis of its incidence. This definition does not include tonsillitis caused by infectious mononucleosis, which usually occurs as a single episode. However, acute tonsillitis in this situation may be followed by recurrent tonsillitis in some people. Tonsillitis may occur in isolation or as part of a generalised pharyngitis. The clinical distinction between tonsillitis and pharyngitis is unclear in the literature, and the condition is often referred to simply as "acute sore throat". A sore throat lasting for 24–48 hours as part of the prodrome of minor upper respiratory tract infection is excluded from this definition. Diagnosis of acute tonsillitis is primarily clinical, with the main interest being in whether the illness is viral or bacterial — this being of relevance if antibiotics are being considered. Studies have attempted to distinguish viral from bacterial sore throat on clinical grounds, but the results are conflicting, suggesting a lack of reliable diagnostic criteria. Investigations to assist with this distinction include throat swabs and serological tests, including the rapid antigen test and the antistreptolysin O titre. Rapid antigen testing is convenient and popular in North America, but has doubtful sensitivity (61–95%), at least when measured against throat swab results, although specificity is higher (88–100%). However, the inevitable delay in reporting of both swabs and the antistreptolysin O titre reduce their value in the routine clinical situation.

INCIDENCE/PREVALENCE Recurrent sore throat has an incidence in general practice in the UK of 100 per 1000 population a year. Acute tonsillitis is more common in childhood.

AETIOLOGY/RISK FACTORS Common bacterial pathogens include beta haemolytic and other streptococci. Bacteria are cultured only from a minority of people with tonsillitis. The role of viruses is uncertain. In tonsillitis associated with infectious mononucleosis, the most common infective agent is the Epstein–Barr virus (present in 50% of children and 90% of adults with the condition). Cytomegalovirus infection may also result in the clinical picture of infectious mononucleosis, and the differential diagnosis also includes toxoplasmosis, HIV, hepatitis A, and rubella.

PROGNOSIS We found no good data on the natural history of tonsillitis or recurrent sore throat in children or adults. People in RCTs randomised to medical treatment (courses of antibiotics as required) have shown a tendency towards improvement over time. Recurrent severe tonsillitis results in considerable morbidity, including time lost from school or work. The most common complication of acute tonsillitis is peritonsillar abscess, but we found no good evidence on its incidence. Rheumatic fever and acute glomerulonephritis are recognised complications of acute tonsillitis associated with group A beta haemolytic streptococci. These diseases are rare in resource-rich countries, but do occasionally occur. They are still a common problem in certain populations, notably Australian aboriginals, and may be effectively prevented in closed communities by the use of penicillin. A recently updated systematic review found that antibiotics reduced the incidence of these diseases. However, in resource-rich countries, these diseases are so rare that routine aggressive antibiotic use is not justified. The review also found that antibiotics shorten the duration of illness by about 16 hours overall.

Aziz Sheikh, Sukhmeet Singh Panesar, Sangeeta Dhami, and Sarah Salvilla

KEY POINTS

- Seasonal allergic rhinitis causes sneezing, with an itchy, blocked, or running nose, and affects up to 25% of people in resouce-rich countries.

  Symptoms are caused by an IgE-mediated type 1 hypersensitivity reaction to air borne allergens such as pollen or fungal spores, and may also cause eye, respiratory, and systemic problems.

- Oral antihistamines reduce symptoms and improve quality of life compared with placebo, but can cause drowsiness.

  Intranasal antihistamines may improve symptoms compared with placebo, although studies have given conflicting results, but we don't know whether they are as effective as oral antihistamines.

  We don't know whether oral decongestants reduce symptoms compared with placebo, but combined treatment with pseudoephedrine plus oral antihistamines may be more effective compared with either treatment alone.

- CAUTION: astemizole and terfenadine may be associated with cardiac adverse effects.

- The oral leukotriene receptor antagonist montelukast improves symptoms and quality of life compared with placebo, but combination treatment with montelukast plus loratadine may be no more effective than either treatment alone.

  We don't know whether intranasal ipratropium bromide reduces symptoms as no studies were found.

- Intranasal corticosteroids improve symptoms compared with placebo.

  Systematic corticosteroids may improve symptoms compared with placebo, but are associated with well-documented adverse effects.

(i) **Please visit www.clinicalevidence.bmj.com for full text and references**

What are the effects of treatments for seasonal allergic rhinitis in adolescents and adults?	
Beneficial	• Antihistamines (oral acrivastine, brompheniramine, cetirizine, levocetirizine, ebastine, fexofenadine, loratadine, desloratidine, rupatadine, and mizolastine) • Corticosteroids (intranasal) • Pseudoephedrine plus antihistamines (oral)
Likely To Be Beneficial	• Corticosteroids (systemic) • Leukotriene receptor antagonists (oral) • Leukotriene receptor antagonists plus antihistamines (oral) • Levocabastine (intranasal)
Unknown Effectiveness	• Azelastine (intranasal) • Decongestants (oral) alone

	• Ipratropium bromide (intranasal)
Likely To Be Ineffective Or Harmful	• Astemizole (oral) • Terfenadine (oral)

Search date September 2005

DEFINITION Seasonal allergic rhinitis is a symptom complex that may affect several organ systems. Symptoms will typically consist of seasonal sneezing, nasal itching, nasal blockage, and watery nasal discharge. Eye symptoms (red eyes, itchy eyes, and tearing) are also common. Other symptoms may include peak seasonal coughing, wheezing and shortness of breath, oral allergy syndrome (manifesting as an itchy, swollen oropharynx on eating stoned fruits), and systemic symptoms such as tiredness, fever, a pressure sensation in the head, and itchiness. Confirming the presence of pollen hypersensitivity using objective allergy tests such as skin prick tests, detection of serum specific IgE, and nasal provocation challenge testing may improve diagnostic accuracy. This review focuses on people aged 12 years and over.

INCIDENCE/PREVALENCE Seasonal allergic rhinitis is found throughout the world. Epidemiological evidence suggests that there is considerable geographical variation in its prevalence. Prevalence is highest in socioeconomically developed countries, where the condition may affect as much as 25% of the population. Prevalence and severity are increasing. It is thought that improved living standards and reduced risk of childhood infections may lead to immune deviation of T helper cells in early life, which may, in turn, increase susceptibility to seasonal allergic rhinitis (the so called "hygiene hypothesis"). Although people of all ages may be affected, the peak age of onset is adolescence.

AETIOLOGY/RISK FACTORS The symptoms of seasonal allergic rhinitis are caused by an IgE-mediated type 1 hypersensitivity reaction to grass, tree, or weed pollen. Allergy to other seasonal aeroallergens such as fungal spores may also provoke symptoms. Typically, symptoms become worse during the relevant pollen season, and outdoors when pollen exposure is increased. Risk factors include a personal or family history of atopy or other allergic disorders, male sex, birth order (increased risk being seen in first born), and small family size.

PROGNOSIS Seasonal allergic rhinitis may impair quality of life — interfering with work, sleep, and recreational activities. Other allergic problems such as asthma and eczema frequently coexist, adding to the impact of rhinitis.

Kim Ah-See

KEY POINTS

- Acute sinusitis is defined pathologically, by transient inflammation of the mucosal lining of the paranasal sinuses lasting less than 4 weeks.

  Clinically, it is characterised by nasal congestion, rhinorrhoea, facial pain, hyposmia, sneezing, and, if more severe, additional malaise and fever.

  It affects 1–5% of the adult population each year in Europe.

- In clinically, and in radiologically/bacteriologically diagnosed, acute sinusitis, corticosteroids (intra-nasal spray) may reduce symptoms compared with placebo.

- In clinically diagnosed acute sinusitis, there is currently little evidence from RCTs to support the use of amoxicillin, co-amoxiclav (amoxicillin–clavulanate), or doxycycline over placebo in terms of clinical cure rate.

  We found no RCTs on the effects of cephalosporins or macrolides compared with placebo in clinically diagnosed acute sinusitis.

- In people with acute sinusitis radiologically or bacteriologically confirmed as caused by a bacterial infection, antibiotics seem to be effective.

  Amoxicillin and co-amoxiclav improve early clinical cure rates, but are associated with adverse gastrointestinal effects.

  Cephalosporins and macrolides also seem as effective as amoxicillin, and with fewer adverse effects.

  We found insufficient evidence to judge the efficacy of doxycycline.

  Long-term antibiotic regimens (6–10-day courses) do not seem any more effective than short-term treatments (3–5-day courses), but do seem to produce more adverse effects.

  We found insufficient evidence to draw conclusions on which is the most effective dosage regimen for antibiotics.

  CAUTION: Since the last update of this review, the acute sinusitis indication for telithromycin has been withdrawn by the FDA as the risks benefits ratio is no longer favourable (12 February 2007).

- We found no studies examining the effectiveness of antihistamines, decongestants, steam inhalation, or saline nasal washes in sinusitis diagnosed either clinically or based on radiological or bacteriological results.

(i) **Please visit www.clinicalevidence.bmj.com for full text and references**

What are the effects of treatments in people with clinically diagnosed acute sinusitis?	
Likely To Be Beneficial	• Corticosteroids (intra-nasal)
Unknown Effectiveness	• Antihistamines
	• Decongestants (xylometazoline, phenylephrine, pseudoephedrine)
	• Saline nasal washes
	• Steam inhalation
Unlikely To Be Beneficial	• Antibiotics (amoxicillin, co-amoxiclav, doxycycline, cephalosporins, macrolides)

What are the effects of treatments in people with radiologically or bacteriologically confirmed acute sinusitis?

Likely To Be Beneficial	• Cephalosporins or macrolides (fewer adverse effects than amoxicillin or co-amoxiclav) • Corticosteroids (intra-nasal)
Trade-off Between Benefits And Harms	• Amoxicillin or co-amoxiclav (more adverse effects than cephalosporins or macrolides)
Unknown Effectiveness	• Antihistamines • Decongestants (xylometazoline, phenylephrine, pseudoephedrine) • Different dosages of antibiotics (amoxicillin, co-amoxiclav, doxycycline, cephalosporins, macrolides) • Doxycycline • Long-course antibiotic regimens: amoxicillin, co-amoxiclav, doxycycline, cephalosporins, macrolides (no more effective than short-course regimens, and more adverse effects) • Saline nasal washes • Steam inhalation

Search date August 2007

DEFINITION Acute sinusitis is defined pathologically, by transient inflammation of the mucosal lining of the paranasal sinuses lasting less than 4 weeks. Clinically, it is characterised by nasal congestion, rhinorrhoea, facial pain, hyposmia, sneezing, and, if more severe, by additional malaise and fever. The diagnosis is usually made clinically (on the basis of history and examination, but without radiological or bacteriological investigation). Clinically diagnosed acute sinusitis is less likely to be caused by bacterial infection compared with acute sinusitis confirmed by radiological or bacteriological investigation. In this review, we have excluded studies in children, in people with symptoms for more than 4 weeks (chronic sinusitis), and in people with symptoms after facial trauma. We have made it clear in each section whether we are dealing with clinically diagnosed acute sinusitis or acute sinusitis with clinical symptoms that have also been confirmed by bacteriological or radiological investigation, because the effects of treatment may be different in these groups.

INCIDENCE/PREVALENCE Each year in Europe 1–5% of adults are diagnosed with acute sinusitis by their general practitioners. Extrapolated to the British population, this is estimated to cause 6 million restricted working days a year. Most people with acute sinusitis are assessed and treated in a primary-care setting. The prevalence varies according to whether diagnosis is made on clinical grounds, or on the basis of radiological or bacteriological investigation.

AETIOLOGY/RISK FACTORS One systematic review (search date 1998) reported that about 50% of people with a clinical diagnosis of acute sinusitis have bacterial sinus infection. The usual pathogens in acute bacterial sinusitis are *Streptococcus pneumoniae* and *Haemophilus influenzae*, with occasional infection with *Moraxella catarrhalis*. Preceding viral upper respiratory-tract infection is often the trigger for acute bacterial sinusitis, with about 0.5% of common colds becoming complicated by the development of acute sinusitis.

PROGNOSIS One meta-analysis of RCTs found that up to two thirds of people with acute sinusitis had spontaneous resolution of symptoms without active treatment. One non-systematic review reported that people with acute sinusitis are at risk of chronic sinusitis and irreversible damage to the normal mucociliary mucosal surface. One further non-systematic review reported rare life-threatening complications, such as orbital cellulitis and meningitis, after acute sinusitis. However, we found no reliable data to measure these risks.

Julian Savage, Stephanie Cook, and Angus Waddell

KEY POINTS

- Up to 18% of people in industrialised societies have mild tinnitus, which severely affects daily life in 0.5% of people.

  Tinnitus can be associated with hearing loss, acoustic neuromas, drug toxicity, ear diseases, and depression.

  Tinnitus can last for many years, and can interfere with sleep and concentration.

- There is insufficient evidence to show that antidepressant drugs improve tinnitus symptoms.

  Antidepressant drugs can improve depression in people with tinnitus.

  TCAs are associated with adverse effects such as dry mouth, blurred vision, and constipation.

- CBT is ineffective in reducing tinnitus loudness, but does improve quality of life in people with tinnitus.

  We do not know whether acupuncture, hypnosis, psychotherapy, electro-magnetic stimulation, hearing aids, tinnitus-masking devices, tinnitus retraining therapy, baclofen, cinnarizine, gingko biloba, hyperbaric oxygen, lamotrigine, nicotinamide, acamprosate, or zinc are effective in people with tinnitus, because very few studies have been carried out.

  We do not know whether benzodiazepines or carbamazepine improve symptoms of tinnitus, and they have adverse effects that can outweigh any possible benefits.

(i) **Please visit www.clinicalevidence.bmj.com for full text and references**

What are the effects of treatments for chronic tinnitus?

Trade-off Between Benefits And Harms	• Antidepressant drugs
Unknown Effectiveness	• Acamprosate
	• Acupuncture
	• Baclofen
	• Benzodiazepines (alprazolam)
	• Cinnarizine
	• Electromagnetic stimulation/ear-canal magnets
	• Ginkgo biloba
	• Hearing aids
	• Hyperbaric oxygen
	• Hypnosis
	• Lamotrigine
	• Nicotinamide
	• Psychotherapy
	• Tinnitus masking devices
	• Tinnitus retraining therapy

	• Zinc
Likely To Be Ineffective Or Harmful	• Carbamazepine

Search date December 2006

DEFINITION Tinnitus is the perception of sound in the ear or head which does not arise from the external environment, from within the body (e.g. vascular sounds), or from auditory hallucinations related to mental illness. This review is concerned with tinnitus for which tinnitus is the only, or the predominant, symptom in an affected person.

INCIDENCE/PREVALENCE Up to 18% of the general population in industrialised countries are mildly affected by chronic tinnitus, and 0.5% report tinnitus having a severe effect on their ability to lead a normal life.

AETIOLOGY/RISK FACTORS Tinnitus can occur as an isolated idiopathic symptom, or in association with any type of hearing loss. Tinnitus can be a particular feature of presbycusis (age-related hearing loss), noise-induced hearing loss, Menière's disease (see review on Menière's disease, p 194), or the presence of an acoustic neuroma. In people with toxicity from aspirin or quinine, tinnitus can occur with hearing thresholds remaining normal. Tinnitus is also associated with depression, although it can be unclear whether the tinnitus is a manifestation of the depressive illness or a factor contributing to its development. Studies involving people with tinnitus caused by Menière's disease, acoustic neuroma, chronic otitis media, head injury, barotraumas, or other clear pathology, have been excluded from this review. This review is principally concerned with idiopathic tinnitus with or without degenerative sensorineural hearing loss.

PROGNOSIS Tinnitus can have an insidious onset, with a long delay before clinical presentation. It can persist for many years or for decades, particularly when associated with a sensorineural hearing loss. Tinnitus can cause disruption of sleep patterns, inability to concentrate, and depression.

Hyperthyroidism (primary)

Birte Nygaard

KEY POINTS

- Hyperthyroidism is characterised by high levels of serum thyroxine and triiodothyronine, and low levels of thyroid-stimulating hormone.

  Thyrotoxicosis is the clinical effect of high levels of thyroid hormones, whether or not the thyroid gland is the primary source.

  The main causes of hyperthyroidism are Graves' disease, toxic multinodular goitre, and toxic adenoma.

  About 20 times more women than men have hyperthyroidism.

- There is consensus that antithyroid drugs (carbimazole, propylthiouracil, and thiamazole) are effective in treating hyperthyroidism, although we found no evidence comparing them with placebo or with each other.

  We found no evidence that antithyroid drugs plus thyroxine (block-replace regimens) improved relapse rates compared with titration regimens.

  Higher-dose antithyroid drugs work better when taken for longer (more than 18 months) than for a shorter time (6 months).

  The doses of antithyroid drugs reported in the studies we found are higher than are generally used in practice.

- There is also consensus that radioactive iodine (radioiodine) is effective for hyperthyroidism.

  We don't know whether radioactive iodine increases risk of thyroid and extrathyroid cancer.

  Radioactive iodine can worsen ophthalmopathy in people with Graves' disease.

  Giving antithyroid drugs to people having radioiodine may increase the proportion of people with persistent or recurrent hyperthyroidism or who need further treatment.

- There is consensus that thyroidectomy is effective for hyperthyroidism.

  Total thyroidectomy is more effective than subtotal thyroidectomy for hyperthyroidism.

  Replacement thyroxine will need to be given to people who become hypothyroid after thyroidectomy.

- There may be some improvement in bone mineral density and thyroid-stimulating hormone levels after treatment with antithyroid treatment in women who have subclinical hyperthyroidism.

(i) **Please visit www.clinicalevidence.bmj.com for full text and references**

What are the effects of drug treatments for primary hyperthyroidism?	
Likely To Be Beneficial	• Antithyroid drugs (carbimazole, propylthiouracil, and thiamazole)*
	• Radioactive iodine (effective in people without ophthalmopathy; may increase ophthalmopathy in people with Graves' disease)*
Unlikely To Be Beneficial	• Adding thyroxine to antithyroid drugs (carbimazole, propylthiouracil, and thiamazole) for primary hyperthyroidism

	• Antithyroid drugs (carbimazole, propylthiouracil, and thiamazole) plus radioactive iodine compared with radioiodine alone

What are the effects of surgical treatments for primary hyperthyroidism?

Likely To Be Beneficial	• Thyroidectomy*

What are the effects of treatments for subclinical hyperthyroidism?

Likely To Be Beneficial	• Radioactive iodine treatment for subclinical hyperthyroidism

Search date June 2007

*Based on consensus, as RCTs would be considered unethical.

DEFINITION Hyperthyroidism is characterised by high levels of serum thyroxine (T4), high levels of serum triiodothyronine (T3), or both, and low levels of thyroid-stimulating hormone (TSH, also known as thyrotropin). Subclinical hyperthyroidism is characterised by decreased levels of TSH (less than 0.1 mU/L) but with levels of T4 and T3 within the normal range (total T4: 60–140 nmol/L; total T3: 1.0–2.5 nmol/L, depending on assay type). The terms hyperthyroidism and thyrotoxicosis are often used synonymously; however, they refer to slightly different conditions. Hyperthyroidism refers to overactivity of the thyroid gland leading to excessive production of thyroid hormones. Thyrotoxicosis refers to the clinical effects of unbound thyroid hormones, whether or not the thyroid gland is the primary source. Secondary hyperthyroidism due to pituitary adenomas, thyroiditis, iodine-induced hyperthyroiditis, and treatment of children and pregnant or lactating women are not covered in this review. Hyperthyroidism can be caused by Graves' disease (diffusely enlarged thyroid gland on palpation, ophthalmopathy, and dermopathy), toxic multinodular goitre (thyrotoxicosis and increased radioiodine uptake with multinodular goitre on palpation), or toxic adenoma (benign hyperfunctioning thyroid neoplasm presenting as a solitary thyroid nodule). We have not included treatment of Graves' ophthalmopathy in this review, although we do report on worsening of Graves' ophthalmopathy with radioiodine. We have also not included euthyroid sick syndrome (a condition seen in people with, for example, pneumonia, MI, cancer, and depression — it is characterised by low levels of TSH and T3). **Diagnosis:** The diagnosis of hyperthyroidism is established by a raised serum total or free T4 or T3 hormone levels, reduced TSH level, and high radioiodine uptake in the thyroid gland along with features of thyrotoxicosis. The usual symptoms are irritability, heat intolerance and excessive sweating, palpitations, weight loss with increased appetite, increased bowel frequency, and oligomenorrhoea. People with hyperthyroidism also often have tachycardia, fine tremors, warm and moist skin, muscle weakness, and eyelid retraction or lag.

INCIDENCE/PREVALENCE Hyperthyroidism is more common in women than in men. One study (2779 people in the UK, median age 58 years, 20 years' follow-up) found an incidence of clinical hyperthyroidism of 0.8/1000 women a year (95% CI 0.5/1000 women/year to 1.4/1000 women/year). The study reported that the incidence was negligible in men. The incidence of hyperthyroidism is higher in areas of low iodine intake than in areas with high iodine intake, because suboptimal iodine intake induces nodular goitre, and by time the nodules become autonomic, hyperthyroidism develops. In Denmark, an area characterised by moderate iodine insufficiency, the overall incidence of hyperthyroidism (defined as low levels of TSH) is 9.7%, compared with 1.0% in Iceland, an area of high iodine intake. The prevalence in this Danish study was 38.7/100,000 a year in women and 2/100,000 a year in men.

(continued over)

(from previous page)

AETIOLOGY/RISK FACTORS Smoking is a risk factor, with an increased risk of both Graves' disease (OR 2.5, 95% CI 1.8 to 3.5) and toxic nodular goitre (OR 1.7, 95% CI 1.1 to 2.5). In areas with high iodine intake, Graves' disease is the major cause, whereas, in areas of low iodine intake, the major cause is nodular goitre. A correlation between diabetes mellitus and thyroid dysfunction has been described. In a Scottish population with diabetes, the overall prevalence of thyroid disease was found to be 13%, highest in women with type 1 diabetes (31%). As a result of screening, new thyroid disease was diagnosed in 7% of people with diabetes (hyperthyroidism in 1%).

PROGNOSIS Clinical hyperthyroidism can be complicated by severe cardiovascular or neuropsychiatry manifestations requiring admission to hospital or urgent treatment. **Mortality:** One population-based 10-year cohort study of 1191 people aged 60 years and over found a higher mortality among people who had a low initial TSH level. The excess in mortality was attributable to CVD. However, the people in this study who had low TSH level may have had a higher prevalence of other illnesses, and adjustment was done only for age and sex, not for co-morbidity. We found another population-based study evaluating 3888 people with hyperthyroidism. No increase was found in all-cause mortality or serious vascular events in people whose hyperthyroidism was treated and stabilised, but an increased risk of dysrhythmias was found in people treated for hyperthyroidism compared with standard population (standardised incidence ratio 2.71, 95% CI 1.63 to 4.24). **Atrial fibrillation in people with overt hyperthyroidism:** We found one cohort study evaluating the incidence of atrial fibrillation in people aged over 60 years with low serum TSH concentrations (up to 0.1 mU/L). It found that low serum TSH concentrations were associated with an increased risk of atrial fibrillation (diagnosed by ECG) at 10 years (61 people with low TSH, 1576 people with normal TSH; incidence of atrial fibrillation: 28/1000 person-years with low TSH values v 11/1000 person-years with normal TSH values; 13/61 [21%] with low TSH values v 133/1576 [8%] with normal TSH values; RR 2.53, 95% CI 1.52 to 4.20; RR calculated by *BMJ Clinical Evidence*). A population-based study including 40,628 people diagnosed with hyperthyroidism in Denmark from 1977 to 1999 found that 8.3% were diagnosed with atrial fibrillation or flutter within ± 30 days from the date of diagnosis of hyperthyroidism. **Quality of life:** Left untreated, thyroid problems can adversely effect quality of life in many ways, which can continue in the long term. In a long-term follow-up (179 people, treated for 14–21 years before investigation), people with Graves' disease, compared with a large Swedish reference population, had diminished vital and mental quality-of-life aspects even after years of treatment. **Fracture rate and bone mineral density:** Hip and spine bone mineral density levels can decrease if hyperthyroidism is untreated. However, when treated, bone mineral density can increase to normal levels. The risk of hip fracture is also higher in people with hyperthyroidism. Progression from subclinical to overt hyperthyroidism is seen in people with nodular goitre, but not in people found by screening to be without other signs of thyroid disease. A meta-analysis (search date 1996) based on data from screening studies estimated that each year 1.5% of women and 1.0% of men who had a low TSH level and normal free T4 and T3 levels developed an elevated free T4 or free T3 level. Ophthalmopathy is a complication of Graves' hyperthyroidism. Treatment can be problematic and usually involves topical corticosteroids and external radiation of the eye muscles. **Thyroid volume and the nodularity of the gland influence the cure rate of hyperthyroidism:** In a controlled study (124 people with newly diagnosed hyperthyroidism), remission rates were calculated after treatment with a combined antithyroid drug plus T4 for about 2 years. People with Graves' disease with no goitre or a small goitre had a significantly better outcome compared with people with Graves' disease with a medium-sized or large goitre. Most people with multinodular goitre had a relapse within the first year after stopping medication.

Birte Nygaard

KEY POINTS

- Primary hypothyroidism is defined as low levels of blood thyroid hormone due to destruction of the thyroid gland. This destruction is usually caused by autoimmunity, or an intervention such as surgery, radioiodine, or radiation.

  It can be classified as clinical (overt), when diagnosed by characteristic features, raised levels of thyroid-stimulating hormone (TSH), and reduced levels of T4, or subclinical, when serum TSH is raised, but serum T4 is normal and there are no symptoms of thyroid dysfunction.

  Hypothyroidism is six times more common in women, affecting up to 40/10,000 each year (compared with 6/10,000 men).

- There is consensus that levothyroxine is effective in treating clinical (overt) hypothyroidism, but evidence is sparse.

  Treatment can lead to hyperthyroidism, reduction of bone mass in postmenopausal women, and increased risk of atrial fibrillation.

  We found no evidence that levothyroxine plus liothyronine improves symptoms more than levothyroxine alone.

- We don't know how effective levothyroxine is in treating people with subclinical hypothyroidism, as studies have been too small to detect any clinically relevant differences.

Please visit www.clinicalevidence.bmj.com for full text and references

What are the effects of treatments for clinical (overt) hypothyroidism?	
Beneficial	• Levothyroxine (L-thyroxine)*
Unlikely To Be Beneficial	• Levothyroxine (L-thyroxine) plus liothyronine compared with levothyroxine (L-thyroxine) alone (no evidence of improved outcomes with levothyroxine plus liothyronone compared with levothyroxine alone)

What are the effects of treatments for subclinical hypothyroidism?	
Unknown Effectiveness	• Levothyroxine (L-thyroxine)

Search date January 2007

*No RCT evidence, but there is clinical consensus that levothyroxine is beneficial in clinical (overt) hypothyroidism. A placebo-controlled trial would be considered unethical.

DEFINITION Hypothyroidism is characterised by low levels of blood thyroid hormone. **Clinical (overt) hypothyroidism** is diagnosed on the basis of characteristic clinical features, consisting of mental slowing, depression, dementia, weight gain, constipation, dry skin, hair loss, cold intolerance, hoarse voice, irregular menstruation, infertility, muscle stiffness and pain, bradycardia, hypercholesterolaemia, combined with a raised blood level of thyroid stimulating hormone (TSH) (serum TSH levels over 12 mU/L), and a low-serum thyroxine (T4) level (serum T4 under 60 nmol/L). **Subclinical hypothyroidism** is diagnosed when serum TSH is raised (serum TSH levels over 4 mU/L) but serum T4 is normal, with minor or no symptoms or signs of thyroid dysfunction. **Primary hypothyroidism** occurs after

(continued over)

(from previous page)

destruction of the thyroid gland due to autoimmunity (the most common cause), or medical intervention such as surgery, radioiodine, and radiation. **Secondary hypothyroidism** occurs after pituitary or hypothalamic damage, and results in insufficient production of TSH. Secondary hypothyroidism is not covered in this review. **Euthyroid sick syndrome** is diagnosed when tri-iodothyronine (T3) levels are low, serum T4 is low, and TSH levels are normal or low. Euthyroid sick syndrome is not covered in this review.

INCIDENCE/PREVALENCE Hypothyroidism is more common in women than in men (in the UK, female:male ratio of 6:1). One study (2779 people in the UK with a median age of 58 years) found that the incidence of clinical (overt) hypothyroidism was 40/10,000 women a year and 6/10,000 men a year. The prevalence was 9.3% in women and 1.3% in men. In areas with high iodine intake, the incidence of hypothyroidism can be higher than in areas with normal or low iodine intake. In Denmark, where there is moderate iodine insufficiency, the overall incidence of hypothyroidism is 1.4/10,000 a year, increasing to 8/10,000 a year in people over 70 years. The incidence of subclinical hypothyroidism increases with age. Up to 10% of women over the age of 60 have subclinical hypothyroidism (evaluated from data from the Netherlands and USA).

AETIOLOGY/RISK FACTORS Primary thyroid gland failure can occur as a result of chronic autoimmune thyroiditis, radioactive iodine treatment, or thyroidectomy. Other causes include drug adverse effects (e.g. amiodarone and lithium), transient hypothyroidism due to silent thyroiditis, subacute thyroiditis, or postpartum thyroiditis.

PROGNOSIS In people with subclinical hypothyroidism, the risk of developing clinical (overt) hypothyroidism is described in the UK Whickham Survey (25 years' follow-up; for women: OR 8, 95% CI 3 to 20; for men: OR 44, 95% CI 19 to 104; if both a raised TSH and positive antithyroid antibodies were present; for women: OR 38, 95% CI 22 to 65; for men: OR 173, 95% CI 81 to 370). For women, the survey found an annual risk of 4.3% a year (if both raised serum TSH and antithyroid antibodies were present) and 2.6% a year (if raised serum TSH was present alone); the minimum number of people with raised TSH and antithyroid antibodies who would need treating to prevent this progression to clinical (overt) hypothyroidism in one person over 5 years is 5–8. **CVD:** A large cross-sectional study (25,862 people with serum TSH between 5.1 mU/L and 10.0 mU/L) found significantly higher mean-total cholesterol concentrations in people who were hypothyroid compared with people who were euthyroid (5.8 mmol/L v 5.6 mmol/L). Another study (124 elderly women with subclinical hypothyroidism, 931 women who were euthyroid) found a significantly increased risk of MI in women with subclinical hypothyroidism (OR 2.3, 95% CI 1.3 to 4.0) and of aortic atherosclerosis (OR 1.7, 95% CI 1.1 to 2.6). **Mental health:** Subclinical hypothyroidism is associated with depression. People with subclinical hypothyroidism may have depression that is refractory to both antidepressant drugs and thyroid hormone alone. Memory impairment, hysteria, anxiety, somatic complaints, and depressive features without depression have been described in people with subclinical hypothyroidism.

David E Arterburn, David E DeLaet, and Daniel P Schauer

KEY POINTS

- About a third of the US population and a quarter of the UK population are obese, with increased risks of hypertension, dyslipidaemia, diabetes, CVD, osteoarthritis, and some cancers.

  Less than 10% of overweight or obese adults aged 40–49 years revert to a normal body weight after 4 years.

  Nearly 5 million US adults used prescription weight-loss medication between 1996 and 1998, but a quarter of all users were not overweight.

- Diethylpropion, mazindol, orlistat, phentermine, rimonabant, and sibutramine may promote modest weight loss (an additional 1–7 kg lost) in obese adults having lifestyle interventions compared with placebo, but they can all cause adverse effects.

  Diethylpropion, phentermine, and mazindol have been associated with heart and lung problems in case reports and series.

  Sibutramine has been associated with cardiac arrhythmias and cardiac arrest in case reports.

  Orlistat may be less effective at promoting weight loss compared with sibutramine, although studies have shown contradictory results.

  We don't know whether combining orlistat and sibutramine treatment leads to greater weight loss than either treatment alone.

- Bariatric surgery (vertical banded gastroplasty, gastric bypass or gastric banding) may increase weight loss compared with no surgery in morbidly obese people.

  Bariatric surgery may result in loss of over 20% of body weight, which may be largely maintained for 10 years.

  Operative and postoperative complications are common, and up to 2% of people die within 30 days of surgery. However, surgery may reduce long-term mortality compared with no surgery.

  We don't know which surgical technique is the most effective or least harmful.

  We don't know how biliopancreatic diversion or sleeve gastrectomy compare with other treatments.

(i) **Please visit www.clinicalevidence.bmj.com for full text and references**

What are the effects of drug treatments in adults with obesity?	
Trade-off Between Benefits And Harms	• Diethylpropion
	• Mazindol
	• Orlistat
	• Phentermine
	• Rimonabant
	• Sibutramine
Unknown Effectiveness	• Sibutramine plus orlistat

What are the effects of bariatric surgery in adults with morbid obesity?

Likely To Be Beneficial	• Bariatric surgery (more effective than non-surgical treatment for clinically important weight loss in morbidly obese adults; but operative complications common) • Gastric banding • Gastric bypass • Vertical banded gastroplasty
Unknown Effectiveness	• Biliopancreatic diversion (no studies comparing biliopancreatic diversion versus other bariatric techniques) • Sleeve gastrectomy (no studies comparing sleeve gastrectomy versus other bariatric techniques)

Search date July 2005

DEFINITION Obesity is a chronic condition characterised by an excess of body fat. It is most often defined by the BMI, a mathematical formula that is highly correlated with body fat. BMI is weight in kilograms divided by height in metres squared (kg/m²). Worldwide, adults with BMIs between 25–30 kg/m² are categorised as overweight, and those with BMIs above 30 kg/m² are categorised as obese. Nearly 5 million US adults used prescription weight-loss medication between 1996 and 1998. A quarter of users were not overweight. Inappropriate use of prescription medication is more common among women, white people, and Hispanic people. The National Institutes of Health in the USA has issued guidelines for obesity treatment, which indicate that all obese adults (BMI above 3 kg/m²) and all adults with a BMI of 27 kg/m² or more and obesity-associated chronic diseases are candidates for drug treatment. Morbidly obese adults (BMI above 4 kg/m²) and all adults with a BMI of 35 kg/m² or more and obesity-associated chronic diseases are candidates for bariatric surgery.

INCIDENCE/PREVALENCE Obesity has increased steadily in many countries since 1900. In the UK in 2002, it was estimated that 23% of men and 25% of women were obese. In the past decade alone, the prevalence of obesity in the USA has increased from 22.9% between 1988 and 1994, to 32.2% in 2004.

AETIOLOGY/RISK FACTORS Obesity is the result of long-term mismatches in energy balance, where daily energy intake exceeds daily energy expenditure. Energy balance is modulated by a myriad of factors, including metabolic rate, appetite, diet, and physical activity. Although these factors are influenced by genetic traits, the increase in obesity prevalence in the past few decades cannot be explained by changes in the human gene pool, and is more often attributed to environmental changes that promote excessive food intake and discourage physical activity. Less commonly, obesity may also be induced by drugs (e.g. high-dose glucocorticoids), or be secondary to a variety of neuroendocrine disorders such as Cushing's syndrome and polycystic ovary syndrome.

PROGNOSIS Obesity is a risk factor for several chronic diseases, including hypertension, dyslipidaemia, diabetes, CVD, sleep apnoea, osteoarthritis, and some cancers. The relationship between increasing body weight and mortality is curvilinear, where mortality is highest among adults with very low body weight (BMI below 18.5 kg/m²) and among adults with the highest body weight (BMI below 35 kg/m²). Obese adults have more annual admissions to hospitals, more outpatient visits, higher prescription-drug costs, and worse health-related quality of life compared with normal-weight adults. Less than 10% of overweight or obese adults aged 40–49 years revert to a normal body weight after 4 years.

Cathy Williams

KEY POINTS

- Amblyopia is reduced visual acuity not immediately correctable by glasses, in the absence of ocular pathology.

    It is commonly associated with squint (strabismus), or with refractive errors that result in different visual inputs to each eye during the sensitive period of visual development (less than 7–8 years of age).

    The cumulative incidence is estimated at 2–4% in children aged up to 15 years.

- Early vision screening before school entry can help detect amblyopia early, and may improve treatment outcomes compared with surveillance or school-entry screening.

    We do not know whether children with a higher risk of eye problems should be targeted for vision screening.

- Most evidence is available for children less than 7 years of age, in whom wearing glasses for up to 30 weeks can improve amblyopia and may cure it. Occlusion treatment (covering the fellow eye using a patch) plus glasses, plus, on occasion, adjuvant treatment, is more effective than glasses alone in children not fully treated with glasses.

    Some older children might improve with treatment, although there are few data available to support this.

- Prescribing patching for the fellow eye for longer periods every day is not more effective at improving amblyopia than prescribing shorter periods of daily patching, but success rates increase in proportion to objectively measured compliance.

    Penalisation, which involves blurring of the fellow eye (usually with a cycloplegic agent, such as atropine) can be as effective as patching for improving amblyopia in children aged less than 7 years.

    We don't know whether active vision therapy or devices to stimulate vision are effective as adjuvant treatment for the treatment of amblyopia.

Please visit www.clinicalevidence.bmj.com for full text and references

What are the effects of interventions to detect amblyopia early?	
Likely To Be Beneficial	• Screening versus usual care
Unknown Effectiveness	• Targeted vision screening versus mass screening

What are the effects of medical treatments for amblyopia?	
Beneficial	• Glasses*
	• Occlusion (patching) plus glasses
Likely To Be Beneficial	• Penalisation
Unknown Effectiveness	• Active vision therapy (visual tasks)

• Devices to stimulate vision

Search date July 2006

*Categorisation based on consensus. Limited RCT evidence available.

DEFINITION Amblyopia is reduced visual acuity not immediately correctable by glasses, in the absence of ocular pathology. It is usually unilateral but can be bilateral. It is associated with complete or partial lack of clear visual input to one eye (deprivation amblyopia or anisometropic amblyopia) or, less often, to both eyes (bilateral deprivation or refractive amblyopia), or to different visual inputs to the two eyes (strabismic amblyopia) during the sensitive period of visual development, which is usually considered to be up to 7 years of age. The severity of amblyopia is often classified according to the visual acuity in the affected eye, using visual acuity testing. "Mild" amblyopia is often classified as being visual acuity of 6/9–6/12, "moderate" amblyopia as being worse than 6/12–6/36, and "severe" amblyopia as being worse than 6/36. Different studies use different definitions of severity, but most assume normal vision (6/6 or better) in the fellow eye. One line of letters or symbols (usually 4 or 5) in a visual-acuity chart constitutes 0.1 LogMAR units. A change in 0.2 LogMAR units is often quoted as being the smallest clinically important change in visual acuity, although some studies use a change of 0.1 LogMAR units or greater, which might be considered clinically marginal. **Diagnosis:** Amblyopia is diagnosed by testing visual acuity in each eye separately, with the person wearing an adequate refractive correction, and after exclusion of ocular pathology. Amblyopia is defined in terms of visual acuity, but other visual functions are affected as well.

INCIDENCE/PREVALENCE It is estimated that the cumulative incidence is 2–4% in children up to 15 years of age. The population prevalence is affected by whether there have been any interventions to prevent or treat the condition.

AETIOLOGY/RISK FACTORS Amblyopia is associated with degraded visual input, either caused by high refractive error (refractive amblyopia, also known as ametropic amblyopia), by different refractive errors in each eye (anisometropic amblyopia), or by conflicting visual inputs between the eyes because of strabismus (strabismic amblyopia). Amblyopia can also be associated with an obstruction to the visual axis — for example, by ptosis or cataract (known as deprivation amblyopia). In a multicentre RCT of 409 children aged from 3 years to under 7 years treated for amblyopia, 38% were strabismic, 37% were anisometropic, and 24% were both strabismic and anisometropic. Whereas strabismus and anisometropia are common causes of amblyopia, less-common causes include ptosis, congenital cataract, and corneal injury or dystrophy, accounting for only up to 3% of cases.

PROGNOSIS Amblyopia is commonly regarded as untreatable after 7–8 years of age, although there is some evidence that treatment can be effective in children aged 7–12 years. Recovery of normal vision becomes progressively less likely in older children. Successfully treated amblyopia might regress in about a quarter of children. The lifetime risk of blindness because of loss of the better-seeing eye is 1.2% (95% CI 1.1% to 1.4%). If the better-seeing eye is lost, the visual acuity of 10% of amblyopic eyes can improve.

Jennifer Arnold and Wilson Heriot

KEY POINTS

- Sight-threatening (late) AMD occurs in 2% of people aged over 50 years in industrialised countries, with prevalence increasing with age.

  Early-stage disease is marked by normal vision, but retinal changes (drusen and pigment changes). Disease progression leads to worsening central vision, but peripheral vision is preserved.

  85% of cases are atrophic (dry) AMD, but exudative (wet) AMD, marked by choroidal neovascularisation, leads to a more rapid loss of sight.

  The main risk factor is age. Hypertension, smoking, and a family history of AMD are also risk factors.

- High-dose antioxidant vitamin and zinc supplementation may reduce progression of moderate AMD, but there is no evidence of benefit in people with no, or mild AMD, or in those with established late AMD in both eyes.

- CAUTION: Beta-carotene, an antioxidant vitamin used in AMD, has been linked to an increased risk of lung cancer in people at high risk of this disease.

- Photodynamic treatment with verteporfin reduces the risk of developing moderate or severe loss of visual acuity and legal blindness in people with vision initially better than 20/100 or 20/200, compared with placebo.

  Photodynamic treatment is associated with an initial loss of vision and photosensitive reactions in a small proportion of people.

- Thermal laser photocoagulation can reduce severe visual loss in people with exudative AMD. It is frequently associated with an immediate and permanent reduction in visual acuity if the lesion involves the central macula, but it remains a proven effective treatment for extrafoveal choroidal neovascularisation.

  About half of people treated with thermal lasers show recurrent choroidal neovascularisation within 3 years.

  We don't know whether laser treatment of drusen prevents progression of disease, and it may increase short-term rates of choroidal neovascularisation.

- Antiangiogenesis treatment using vascular endothelial growth factor (VEGF) inhibitors such as ranibizumab or pegaptanib reduces the risk of moderate vision loss, and may improve vision at 12 and 24 months.

  Antiangiogenesis treatment using anecortave acetate may be as effective as photodynamic therapy in reducing vision loss.

- Studies investigating external beam radiotherapy have given contradictory results, and have failed to show an overall benefit in AMD.

- Subcutaneous interferon alfa-2a and submacular surgery have not been shown to improve vision, and are associated with potentially severe adverse effects.

- We found no RCT evidence on the effects of transpupillary thermotherapy.

(i) **Please visit www.clinicalevidence.bmj.com for full text and references**

What are the effects of interventions to prevent progression of early- or late-stage AMD?

Likely To Be Beneficial	• Antioxidant vitamin plus zinc supplementation
Unknown Effectiveness	• Laser to drusen

What are the effects of treatments for exudative AMD?	
Beneficial	• Antiangiogenesis treatment using pegaptanib (reduces moderate vision loss compared with placebo) • Antiangiogenesis treatment using ranibizumab (reduces moderate vision loss and increases vision gain and visual acuity compared with placebo or photodynamic therapy) • Photodynamic treatment with verteporfin
Likely To Be Beneficial	• Antiangiogenesis treatment using anecortave acetate
Trade-off Between Benefits And Harms	• Thermal laser photocoagulation
Unknown Effectiveness	• External beam radiation • Transpupillary thermotherapy
Likely To Be Ineffective Or Harmful	• Antiangiogenesis treatment using interferon alfa-2a (subcutaneous) • Submacular surgery

Search date March 2006

DEFINITION AMD typically affects those aged 50 years and older. It has two clinical stages: **early AMD**, marked by drusen and pigmentary change, and usually associated with normal vision; and **late or sight-threatening AMD**, associated with a decrease in central vision. Late-stage AMD has two forms: **atrophic (or dry) AMD**, characterised by geographic atrophy; and **exudative (or wet) AMD**, characterised by choroidal neovascularisation (CNV), which eventually causes a disciform scar.

INCIDENCE/PREVALENCE AMD is a common cause of blindness registration in industrialised countries. Atrophic AMD is more common than the more sight-threatening exudative AMD, affecting about 85% of people with AMD. Late (sight-threatening) AMD is found in about 2% of all people aged over 50 years, and prevalence rises with age (0.7–1.4% of people aged 65–75 years; 11–19% of people above 85 years).

AETIOLOGY/RISK FACTORS Proposed hypotheses for the cause of atrophic and exudative AMD involve vascular factors and oxidative damage, coupled with genetic predisposition. Age is the strongest risk factor. Systemic risk factors include smoking, and a family history of AMD. Complement factor H (HF1), a major inhibitor of the alternative complement pathway, seems to play a major role in the pathogenesis of AMD blindness. Haplotype analysis reveals that multiple HF1 variants confer elevated or reduced risk of AMD (proportion of people with 1 at-risk haplotype: 50% of AMD cases v 29% of controls; OR 2.46, 95% CI 1.95 to 3.11; proportion of people with homozygotes for this halotype: 24% of AMD cases v 8% of controls; OR 3.51, 95% CI 2.13 to 5.78). These results are supported by other laboratories, and suggest that retinal and pigment epithelial destruction may be related to defective protection from immunological activity, rather than senescence or oxidative injury alone. However, the trigger for complement activation is unknown. A link between a genetic trait (Y402H variant of CFH) and a modifiable lifestyle risk — smoking — has been established by logistic regression modelling of gene–gene and gene–environment interactions in a case-controlled data set. The study authors estimated that CFH, LOC387715, and cigarette smoking together explain 61% of the patient-attributable risk of

AMD, with adjusted percentage estimates of 20% for smoking, 36% for LOC387715, and 43% for CFH. Ocular risk factors for the development of exudative AMD include the presence of soft drusen, macular pigmentary change, CNV in the other eye, and previous cataract surgery. Hypertension, diet (especially intake of antioxidant micronutrients), and oestrogen are suspected as causal agents for atrophic and exudative AMD, but the effects of these factors remain unproved.

PROGNOSIS AMD impairs central vision, which is required for reading, driving, face recognition, and all fine visual tasks. **Atrophic AMD** progresses slowly over many years, and time to legal blindness is highly variable (usually about 5–10 years). **Exudative AMD** is more often threatening to vision; 90% of people with serious visual loss caused by AMD have the exudative type. This condition usually manifests with a sudden worsening and distortion of central vision. One study estimated (based on data derived primarily from cohort studies) that the risk of developing exudative AMD in people with bilateral soft drusen was 1–5% at 1 year and 13–18% at 3 years. The observed 5-year rate in a population survey was 7%. Most eyes (estimates vary from 60% to 90%) with exudative AMD progress to legal blindness and develop a central defect (scotoma) in the visual field. Peripheral vision is preserved, allowing the person to be mobile and independent. The ability to read with visual aids depends on the size and density of the central scotoma, and the degree to which the person retains sensitivity to contrast. Once exudative AMD has developed in one eye, the other eye is at high risk (cumulative estimated incidence: 10% at 1 year, 28% at 3 years, and 42% at 5 years).

John Epling

KEY POINTS

- Conjunctivitis causes irritation, itching, foreign-body sensation, and watering or discharge from the eye.

  Most cases in adults are probably due to viral infection, but children are more likely to develop bacterial conjunctivitis than they are viral forms. The main bacterial pathogens are *Staphylococcus* species in adults, and *Haemophilus influenzae*, *Streptoccoccus pneumoniae* and *Moraxella catarrhalis* in children.

  A bacterial cause is more likely if there is glueing of the eyelids, and no itch.

  Contact lens wearers may be more likely to develop gram-negative infections. Bacterial keratitis occurs in up to 30/100,000 contact lens wearers.

  Gonococcal ophthalmia neonatorum can occur in up to 10% of infants exposed to gonorrhoeal exudate during delivery despite prophylaxis, and can be associated with bacteraemia and meningitis.

  Otitis media can occur in 25% of children with *H influenzae* conjunctivitis, and meningitis can develop in 18% of people with meningococcal conjunctivitis.

- Conjunctivitis resolves spontaneously within 2–5 days in more than half of people without treatment, but infectious complications can occur rarely.

- Topical antibiotics may speed up clinical and microbiological cure of bacterial conjunctivitis, but the benefit is small.

  In people with suspected, but not proven, bacterial conjunctivitis, empirical treatment with topical antibiotics may be beneficial. However, this benefit is marginal, so it is advisable to suggest to patients to only take antibiotics if symptoms do not resolve after 1–2 days.

  Clinical and microbiological cure rates are increased in the first week or so in people with culture-positive bacterial conjunctivitis, but there is no good evidence of a longer-term benefit from topical antibiotics.

  Adverse effects of topical antibiotics are mild, but their effect on bacterial resistance is unknown.

- Parenteral antibiotics may cure gonoccocal ophthalmia neonatorum, although we do not know whether they are beneficial in children in Western countries, as we only found studies from Africa. Neonates will usually require investigation for concomitant infections and complications.

  We don't know whether ocular decongestants, saline, or warm compresses are beneficial in people with suspected or proven bacterial conjunctivitis or gonococcal conjunctivitis.

(i) **Please visit www.clinicalevidence.bmj.com for full text and references**

What are the effects of empirical treatment in adults and children with suspected bacterial conjunctivitis?	
Likely To Be Beneficial	• Empirical treatment with topical antibiotics in people with suspected bacterial conjunctivitis if given to patient with advice to use after 1–2 days if symptoms do not resolve
Unknown Effectiveness	• Empirical treatment with ocular decongestants in people with suspected bacterial conjunctivitis

- Empirical treatment with oral antibiotics in people with suspected bacterial conjunctivitis
- Empirical treatment with saline in people with suspected bacterial conjunctivitis
- Empirical treatment with warm compresses in people with suspected bacterial conjunctivitis

What are the effects of treatment in adults and children with bacteriologically proven bacterial conjunctivitis?

Beneficial	• Antibiotics (topical) in people with proven bacterial conjunctivitis
Unknown Effectiveness	• Ocular decongestants in people with proven bacterial conjunctivitis • Saline in people with proven bacterial conjunctivitis • Warm compresses in people with proven bacterial conjunctivitis

What are the effects of treatment in adults and children with clinically proven gonococcal conjunctivitis?

Likely To Be Beneficial	• Antibiotics (parenteral alone or combined with topical) in people with suspected or proven gonococcal conjunctivitis *
Unknown Effectiveness	• Antibiotics (oral) in people with suspected or proven gonococcal conjunctivitis • Ocular decongestants in people with suspected or proven gonococcal conjunctivitis • Saline in people with suspected or proven gonococcal conjunctivitis • Warm compresses in people with clinically suspected or proven gonococcal conjunctivitis

Search date January 2007

DEFINITION Conjunctivitis is any inflammation of the conjunctiva, generally characterised by irritation, itching, foreign-body sensation, and watering or discharge. Treatment is often based on clinical suspicion that the conjunctivitis is bacterial, without waiting for the results of microbiological tests. In this review, therefore, we have distinguished the effects of empirical treatment from effects of treatment in people with culture-positive bacterial conjunctivitis. Bacterial conjunctivitis in contact lens wearers is of particular concern because of the risk of bacterial keratitis — an infection of the cornea accompanying acute or subacute corneal trauma, which is more difficult to treat than conjunctivitis and can threaten vision. Conjunctivitis caused by *N gonorrhoeae* — referred to as ophthalmia neonatorum — is primarily a disease of neonates, caused by exposure of the neonatal conjunctivae to the cervico-vaginal exudate of infected women during parturition. **Diagnosis** The traditional criteria differentiating bacterial from other types of conjunctivitis have been: a yellow–white mucopurulent discharge; a papillary reaction (small bumps with fibrovascular

(continued over)

(from previous page)

cores on the palpebral conjunctiva, appearing grossly as a fine velvety surface); and bilateral infection. A recent systematic review was unable to find any quality research basis for these criteria, but a follow-up study performed by the authors of the review found that glued eyes and the absence of itching were predictive of a bacterial cause. A history of recent conjunctivitis argued against a bacterial cause. If eye pain is moderate or severe and visual acuity is reduced, more serious causes need to be considered. Gonococcal ophthalmia neonatorum is diagnosed by a persistent and increasingly purulent conjunctivitis in exposed infants beginning from 3–21 days after delivery.

INCIDENCE/PREVALENCE We found no good evidence on the incidence or prevalence of bacterial conjunctivitis. Bacterial keratitis is estimated to occur in 10–30/100,000 contact lens wearers. Gonococcal ophthalmia neonatorum occurs at rates of 0–10% in infants who received antibiotic prophylaxis after delivery to mothers with gonorrhoea infection, and in 2–48% of exposed infants without prophylaxis.

AETIOLOGY/RISK FACTORS Conjunctivitis may be infectious (causes include bacteria and viruses) or allergic. In adults, bacterial conjunctivitis is less common than viral conjunctivitis, although estimates vary widely (viral conjunctivitis has been reported to account for 8–75% of acute conjunctivitis). *Staphylococcus* species are the most common pathogens for bacterial conjunctivitis in adults, followed by *Streptococcus pneumoniae* and *Haemophilus influenzae*. In children, bacterial conjunctivitis is more common than the viral form, and is mainly caused by *H influenzae*, *S pneumoniae*, and *Moraxella catarrhalis*. One prospective study (428 children from southern Israel with a clinical diagnosis of conjunctivitis) found that, in 55% of the children, conjunctivitis was caused by *S pneumoniae*, *H influenzae*, or *M catarrhalis*. Narrative reviews suggest that the causative agents of bacterial conjunctivitis and keratitis in contact lens wearers are more frequently gram-negative bacteria (such as *Pseudomonas aeruginosa*), but may include all of the above agents. *Acanthamoeba spp.* infections can be particularly difficult to diagnose and treat, and are most common in contact lens wearers.

PROGNOSIS Most bacterial conjunctivitis is self-limiting. One systematic review (search date 2004) found clinical cure or significant improvement with placebo within 2–5 days in 65% of people. Some organisms cause corneal or systemic complications, or both. Otitis media may develop in 25% of children with *H influenzae* conjunctivitis, and systemic meningitis may complicate primary meningococcal conjunctivitis in 18% of people. Untreated gonococcal ophthalmia neonatorum can cause corneal ulceration, perforation of the globe, and panophthalmitis. Investigations to detect concomitant infections, as well as gonococcal bacteremia and meningitis, and hospitalisation for parenteral treatment of the eye infection, are frequently required.

Cataract 223

David Allen

KEY POINTS

- Cataracts are cloudy or opaque areas in the lens of the eye which can impair vision. Age-related cataracts are defined as occurring in people of 50 years of age, in the absence of known mechanical, chemical, or radiation trauma.

  Cataract accounts for over 47% of blindness worldwide, causing blindness in about 17.3 million people in 1990.

  Surgery for cataract in people with glaucoma may affect glaucoma control.

- Phaco extracapsular extraction successfully improves visual acuity for at least 1 year compared with waiting list controls in people with cataract without ocular co-morbidities.

  When combined with foldable posterior chamber intraocular lens implant, the surgery is more effective at improving vision than manual extracapsular extraction, and with fewer complications.

  This procedure has largely superseded manual extracapsular cataract extraction in resource-rich countries.

- Manual extracapsular extraction has also been shown to be successful in treating cataracts.

  Combined with intraocular lens implant, manual extracapsular extraction is significantly better at improving vision compared with intracapsular extraction plus aphakic glasses.

  This finding may be particularly relevant to treatment in resource-poor countries.

- Intracapsular extraction is likely to be better at improving vision compared with no extraction, although it is not as beneficial as manual extracapsular extraction.

  The rate of complications is also higher with this technique compared with extracapsular extraction.

- In people with glaucoma, concomitant cataract surgery (phaco or manual extracapsular extraction) and glaucoma surgery appears to be more beneficial than cataract surgery alone, in that they both improve vision to a similar extent, but the glaucoma surgery additionally improves intraocular pressure.

  We found no studies comparing different types of cataract surgery in people with glaucoma.

- In people with diabetic retinopathy, phaco extracapsular extraction may improve visual acuity and reduce postoperative inflammation compared with manual extraction.

  We do not know whether adding diabetic retinopathy treatment to cataract surgery is more beneficial than cataract surgery alone.

ⓘ Please visit www.clinicalevidence.bmj.com for full text and references

What are the effects of surgery for age-related cataract without other ocular comorbidity?

Beneficial	• Manual extracapsular extraction (more effective than intracapsular extraction but less effective than phaco extracapsular extraction)

	• Phaco extracapsular extraction (improved visual acuity with fewer complications than manual extracapsular extraction)
Likely To Be Beneficial	• Intracapsular extraction (more effective than no extraction;* less effective than manual extracapsular extraction and has more complications)

What are the effects of treatment for age-related cataract in people with glaucoma?

Likely To Be Beneficial	• Concomitant cataract and glaucoma surgery (reduced intraocular pressure compared with cataract surgery alone)
Unknown Effectiveness	• Cataract surgery (manual or phaco extracapsular extraction) alone • Cataract surgery plus non-concomitant glaucoma surgery

What are the effects of surgical treatments for age-related cataract in people with diabetic retinopathy?

Likely To Be Beneficial	• Cataract surgery (phaco or manual extracapsular extraction) in people with diabetic retinopathy
Unknown Effectiveness	• Adding diabetic retinopathy treatment to cataract surgery (phaco or manual extracapsular extraction)

Search date October 2006

*Based on consensus.

DEFINITION Cataracts are cloudy or opaque areas in the lens of the eye (which should usually be completely clear). This results in changes that can impair vision. **Age-related (or senile) cataract** is defined as cataract occurring in people over 50 years of age in the absence of known mechanical, chemical, or radiation trauma. This review covers treatment for age-related cataract. It does not cover cataract in people with diabetes mellitus or recurrent uveitis: these conditions can affect the surgical outcome. This review also addresses the treatment of age-related cataract in people with glaucoma. Surgery for cataracts in people with glaucoma may affect glaucoma control, and the optimal strategy for treating these conditions when they co-exist is not clear. See also review on glaucoma, p 225.

INCIDENCE/PREVALENCE Cataract accounts for over 47% of blindness worldwide, causing blindness in about 17.3 million people in 1990. A cross-sectional study in a representative sample of an urban population in New South Wales, Australia in 1997 (3654 people aged 49–96 years) found that the prevalence of late cataract (of all types) in people aged 65–74 years was 21.6%, and in people aged 85 years and over it was 67.3%. This rate excluded those people who had already had cataract surgery. The incidence of non-age-related cataract within this population is so small that this can be taken as the effective incidence of age-related cataract. Glaucoma has an overall prevalence of about 2.0% rising to about 4.5% in people aged 70 years or over (the peak age for cataract surgery). The 5-year incidence of nuclear cataract in people aged over 50 years old and with open-angle glaucoma was estimated to be 25% in 2006.

AETIOLOGY/RISK FACTORS Diet, smoking, and exposure to ultraviolet light are thought to be risk factors in the development of age-related cataract. In addition, some people may have a genetic predisposition to development of age-related cataract.

PROGNOSIS Age-related cataract progresses with age, but at an unpredictable rate. Cataract surgery is indicated when the chances of significant visual improvement outweigh the risks of a poor surgical outcome. It is not dependent on reaching a specific visual acuity standard. Cataract surgery may also be indicated where the presence of cataract makes it hard to treat or monitor concurrent retinal disease, such as diabetic retinopathy.

Glaucoma

Rajiv Shah and Richard Wormald

KEY POINTS

- Glaucoma is characterised by progressive optic neuropathy and peripheral visual-field loss. It affects 1–2% of white people aged over 40 years and accounts for 8% of new blind registrations in the UK.

  The main risk factor for glaucoma is raised intraocular pressure, but 40% of people with glaucoma have normal intraocular pressure, and only 10% of people with raised intraocular pressure are at risk of optic nerve damage.

  In black people, glaucoma is more prevalent than in white populations, presents earlier, and is more difficult to control.

  Blindness from glaucoma results from gross loss of visual field or loss of central vision, and can progress quickly without treatment.

- Laser trabeculoplasty plus topical medical treatment is more effective at reducing progression of optic nerve damage in people with primary open-angle or pseudoexfoliation glaucoma, compared with no treatment.

  Topical medical treatment may reduce the risk of developing glaucoma in people with ocular hypertension compared with placebo, and may reduce loss of visual field in people with primary open-angle glaucoma compared with surgery, although studies have shown conflicting results.

- Surgical trabeculectomy may be as effective as topical medical treatment at preventing visual-field loss in primary open-angle glaucoma, but increases the risk of developing cataracts.

  Surgical trabeculectomy may be more effective than laser trabeculoplasty at reducing intraocular pressure, but we don't know which is more effective at maintaining visual fields and acuity.

- Medical treatment may reduce progression of glaucoma compared with placebo in people with primary open-angle glaucoma, although we don't know whether it is also beneficial in normal-tension glaucoma.

  Surgical treatment, with or without medical treatment, may reduce progression of visual-field loss in people with normal-tension glaucoma.

- There is a consensus that medical and surgical treatments are beneficial in people with acute angle-closure glaucoma, although we don't know this for sure.

(i) **Please visit www.clinicalevidence.bmj.com for full text and references**

What are the effects of treatments for established primary open-angle glaucoma, ocular hypertension, or both?	
Likely To Be Beneficial	• Laser trabeculoplasty plus topical medical treatment (compared with no initial treatment or topical medical treatment alone) • Topical medical treatment (in people with primary open-angle glaucoma or ocular hypertension)
Trade-off Between Benefits And Harms	• Surgical trabeculectomy
Unknown Effectiveness	• Laser trabeculoplasty (compared with surgical trabeculectomy)

What are the effects of lowering intraocular pressure in people with normal-tension glaucoma?

Likely To Be Beneficial	• Medical treatment
Trade-off Between Benefits And Harms	• Surgical treatment

What are the effects of treatment for acute angle-closure glaucoma?

Likely To Be Beneficial	• Medical treatment*
	• Surgical treatment*

Search date January 2006

*No placebo controlled RCTs but strong consensus that treatments are effective.

DEFINITION Glaucoma is a group of diseases characterised by progressive optic neuropathy. It is usually bilateral, but asymmetric, and may occur at any intraocular pressure. All forms of glaucoma show optic-nerve damage (cupping, pallor, or both) associated with peripheral visual-field loss. **Primary open-angle glaucoma** occurs in people with an open anterior chamber drainage angle and no secondary identifiable cause. Knowledge of the natural history of these conditions is incomplete, but it is thought that the problem starts with an intraocular pressure that is too high for the optic nerve. However, in a large proportion of people with glaucoma (about 40%) intraocular pressure is within the statistically defined normal range. The term ocular hypertension generally applies to eyes with an intraocular pressure greater than the statistical upper limit of normal (about 21 mm Hg). However, only a relatively small proportion of eyes with raised intraocular pressure have an optic nerve that is vulnerable to its effects (about 10%). However, because intraocular pressure is the main and only modifiable risk factor for the disease, studies on the effectiveness of reducing intraocular pressure often include people who have both ocular hypertension and primary open angle glaucoma. Previously, trialists were anxious about withholding active treatment in overt primary open-angle glaucoma, and so many placebo or no-treatment trials selected people just with ocular hypertension. Trials comparing treatments often include both people with primary open-angle glaucoma and people with ocular hypertension, but in these the outcome is usually intraocular pressure alone. **Normal-tension glaucoma** occurs in people with intraocular pressures that are consistently below the statistical upper limit of normal (21 mm Hg; 2 standard deviations above the population mean). **Acute-angle closure glaucoma** is glaucoma resulting from a rapid and severe rise in intraocular pressure caused by physical obstruction of the anterior chamber drainage angle.

INCIDENCE/PREVALENCE Glaucoma occurs in 1–2% of white people aged over 40 years, rising to 5% at 70 years. Primary open-angle glaucoma accounts for two thirds of those affected, and normal-tension glaucoma for about a quarter. In black people, glaucoma is more prevalent, presents at a younger age with higher intraocular pressures, is more difficult to control, and is the main irreversible cause of blindness in black populations of African origin. Glaucoma-related blindness is responsible for 8% of new blind registrations in the UK.

AETIOLOGY/RISK FACTORS The major risk factor for developing primary open-angle glaucoma is raised intraocular pressure. In one RCT (90 people with intraocular pressure above 22 mm Hg, 1 other glaucoma risk factor, and normal visual fields, mean age 55–56 years), three baseline risk factors were identified to be independently associated with glaucomatous field loss. These were higher intraocular pressure (P = 0.047, intraocular pressure per mm Hg), suspect discs (P = 0.007), and older age (P = 0.034, age per year).

(continued over)

(from previous page)

Lesser risk factors include family history and ethnic origin. The relationship between systemic blood pressure and intraocular pressure may be an important determinant of blood flow to the optic-nerve head and, as a consequence, may represent a risk factor for glaucoma. Systemic hypotension, vasospasm (including Raynaud's disease and migraine), and a history of major blood loss have been reported as risk factors for normal-tension glaucoma in hospital-based studies. Risk factors for acute angle closure glaucoma include family history, female sex, being long-sighted, and cataract. One systematic review (search date 1999, 6 observational studies, 594,662 people with mydriasis) did not find any evidence supporting the theory that routine pupillary dilatation with short-acting mydriatics was a risk factor for acute angle-closure glaucoma.

PROGNOSIS Advanced visual-field loss is found in about 20% of people with primary open-angle glaucoma at diagnosis, and is an important prognostic factor for glaucoma-related blindness. Blindness due to glaucoma results from gross loss of visual field or loss of central vision. Once early field defects have appeared, and where the intraocular pressure is greater than 30 mm Hg, untreated people may lose the remainder of the visual field in 3 years or less. As the disease progresses, people with glaucoma have difficulty moving from a bright room to a darker room, and judging steps and kerbs. Progression of visual-field loss is often slower in normal-tension glaucoma. Acute angle glaucoma leads to rapid loss of vision, initially from corneal oedema and subsequently from ischaemic optic neuropathy.

Nigel H Barker

KEY POINTS

- Ocular infection with herpes simplex virus can cause inflammation of the eyelids, conjunctivae, iris, retina, and cornea, which may lead to scarring, glaucoma, and blindness.

  Infection is common and usually acquired early in life, with 50% of people from higher and 80% from lower socioeconomic groups in the USA having antibodies by the age of 30 years.

  Attacks usually resolve within 1–2 weeks, but 50% of people will experience a recurrence within 10 years.

- Topical antiviral agents and topical interferons increase healing of epithelial keratitis compared with placebo.

  Physicochemical debridement or interferon may speed up healing if added to antiviral agents, but we don't know whether debridement is effective when used alone.

- Topical corticosteroids reduce progression and shorten the duration of stromal keratitis compared with placebo, when added to topical antiviral agents.

  Adding oral aciclovir to topical corticosteroids plus topical antiviral treatment may not increase healing compared with topical treatment alone.

- Long-term oral aciclovir treatment in people with previous ocular epithelial or stromal keratitis reduces recurrence after 1 year compared with placebo.

  Short-term prophylaxis (for 3 weeks) with aciclovir does not seem to reduce the risk of recurrence.

- We don't know whether oral aciclovir reduces recurrence of ocular herpes simplex infection after corneal grafts.

(i) **Please visit www.clinicalevidence.bmj.com for full text and references**

What are the effects of treatments in people with epithelial keratitis?

Beneficial	• Antiviral agents (topical)
	• Interferons (topical)
Unknown Effectiveness	• Debridement

What are the effects of treatments in people with stromal keratitis?

Beneficial	• Adding topical corticosteroids to topical antiviral treatment
Unlikely To Be Beneficial	• Adding oral aciclovir to topical corticosteroids plus topical antiviral treatment

What are the effects of interventions to prevent recurrence of ocular herpes simplex?	
Beneficial	• Long-term (1 year) oral aciclovir
Unlikely To Be Beneficial	• Short-term (3 weeks) oral aciclovir

What are the effects of interventions to prevent recurrence of ocular herpes simplex in people with corneal grafts?	
Unknown Effectiveness	• Oral aciclovir

Search date June 2006

DEFINITION Ocular herpes simplex is usually caused by herpes simplex virus type 1 (HSV-1) but also occasionally by the type 2 virus (HSV-2). Ocular manifestations of HSV are varied and include blepharitis (inflammation of the eyelids), canalicular obstruction, conjunctivitis, corneal complications, iritis, and retinitis. Corneal complications are of two main types: **epithelial keratitis** is inflammation of the cells that form the surface layer of the cornea and **stromal keratitis** is inflammation of the middle layer (stroma) of the cornea. HSV infections are classified as neonatal, primary (HSV in a person with no previous viral exposure), and recurrent (previous viral exposure with humoral and cellular immunity present).

INCIDENCE/PREVALENCE Infections with HSV are usually acquired in early life. A US study found antibodies against HSV-1 in about 50% of people with high socioeconomic status and 80% of people with low socioeconomic status by the age of 30 years. It quoted a report suggesting that overcrowding may be a causal factor. However, only about 20–25% of people with HSV antibodies had any history of clinical manifestations of ocular or cutaneous herpetic disease. Ocular HSV is the most common cause of corneal blindness in high-income countries, and is the most common cause of unilateral corneal blindness in the world. A 33-year study of the population of Rochester, Minnesota, found the annual incidence of new cases of ocular herpes simplex was 8.4/100 000 (95% CI 6.9/100,000 to 9.9/100,000) and the annual incidence of all episodes (new and recurrent) was 20.7/100,000 (95% CI 18.3/100,000 to 23.1/100,000). The prevalence of ocular herpes was 149/100,000 population (95% CI 115/100,000 to 183/100,000). Twelve per cent of people had bilateral disease.

AETIOLOGY/RISK FACTORS Epithelial keratitis results from productive, lytic viral infection of the corneal epithelial cells. Stromal keratitis and iritis are thought to result from a combination of viral infection and compromised immune mechanisms. Observational evidence (346 people with ocular HSV in the placebo arm of an RCT) showed that a previous history of stromal keratitis was a risk factor for the recurrence of stromal keratitis (6/174 [4%] without previous stromal keratitis v 53/172 [32%] with previous stromal keratitis; RR 10.0, 95% CI 4.3 to 23.0; P less than 0.001). Age, sex, ethnicity, and previous history of non-ocular HSV disease were not associated with an increased risk of recurrence.

PROGNOSIS HSV epithelial keratitis tends to resolve spontaneously within 1–2 weeks while stromal keratitis is more likely to result in corneal scarring and loss of vision. In a trial of 271 people treated with topical trifluorothymidine and randomly assigned to receive either oral aciclovir or placebo, the epithelial lesion had resolved completely or was at least less than 1 mm after 1 week of treatment with placebo in 89% of people, and after 2 weeks in 99% of people. Stromal keratitis or iritis occurs in about 25% of people after epithelial keratitis. The effects of HSV stromal keratitis include scarring, tissue destruction, neovascularisation, glaucoma, and persistent epithelial defects. The rate of recurrence of ocular herpes for people with one episode is 10% at 1 year, 23% at 2 years, and 50% at 10 years. The risk of recurrent ocular HSV infection (epithelial or stromal) also increases with the number of previous episodes reported (2 or 3 previous episodes: RR 1.41, 95% CI 0.82 to 2.42; 4 or more previous episodes: RR 2.09, 95% CI 1.24 to 3.50). Of corneal grafts performed in Australia over a 10-year period, 5% were in people with visual disability or with actual or impending corneal perforation after stromal ocular herpes simplex. The recurrence of HSV in a corneal graft has a major effect on graft survival. The Australian Corneal Graft Registry found that, in corneal grafts performed for HSV keratitis, there was at least one HSV recurrence in 58% of corneal grafts that failed over a follow-up period of 9 years.

232 Retinal detachment

David Steel and Scott Fraser

KEY POINTS

- Rhegmatogenous retinal detachment (RRD) is the most common form of retinal detachment, where a retinal "break" allows the ingress of fluid from the vitreous cavity to the subretinal space, resulting in retinal separation. It occurs in about 1 in 10,000 people a year.

  This review considers acute progressive RRD only.

- Cryotherapy and photocoagulation are widely used for preventing progression from retinal breaks or lattice degeneration to RRD, and there is consensus that they are effective, particularly in people with symptomatic flap tears and retinal dialysis.

- There is consensus that scleral buckling, pneumatic retinopexy, and vitrectomy are all effective for treating RRD, but it is unclear how they compare with one another.

  In people receiving vitrectomy for RRD with severe proliferative vitreoretinopathy (occurring as a complication of retinal detachment or previous treatment for retinal detachment), silicone oil and long-acting gas are equally effective for increasing reattachment rates and improving visual acuity; silicone oil is better than short-acting gas.

  We don't know if fluorouracil plus heparin added to infusion solution during vitrectomy surgery for proliferative vitreoretinopathy is effective for increasing reattachment rates and improving visual acuity.

(i) **Please visit www.clinicalevidence.bmj.com for full text and references**

What are the effects of interventions to prevent progression from retinal breaks or lattice degeneration to retinal detachment?	
Likely To Be Beneficial	• Cryotherapy* • Laser photocoagulation*

What are the effects of different surgical interventions in people with rhegmatogenous retinal detachment?	
Likely To Be Beneficial	• Scleral buckling versus other surgical techniques* (consensus that scleral buckling, pneumatic retinopexy, or vitrectomy all effective, but unclear how they compare with one another)

What are the effects of interventions to treat proliferative vitreoretinopathy occurring as a complication of retinal detachment or previous treatment for retinal detachment?	
Likely To Be Beneficial	• Silicone oil or long-acting gas tamponade (silicone oil and long-acting gas equally effective in people receiving vitrectomy for rhegmatogenous

	retinal detachment with severe proliferative vitreoretinopathy, silicone oil better than short-acting gas)
Unknown Effectiveness	• Fluorouracil plus low-molecular-weight heparin added to infusion solution during vitrectomy surgery for proliferative vitreoretinopathy

Search date September 2006

*Based on consensus; no RCT evidence available.

DEFINITION Retinal detachment can be defined as the separation of the neurosensory retina from the underlying retinal pigment epithelium (RPE). Direct apposition of the retina to the RPE is essential for normal retinal function, and retinal detachment involving the foveal centre leads to profound loss of vision in the affected eye. **Rhegmatogenous retinal detachment (RRD)** is the most common form of retinal detachment, where a retinal "break" allows the ingress of fluid from the vitreous cavity to the subretinal space, resulting in retinal separation. Retinal "break" refers to a full-thickness defect in the neurosensory retina. A "break" can include a tear in the retina at the time of posterior vitreous detachment (PVD), an atrophic hole in the retina (associated with lattice degeneration), or retinal dialysis (generally secondary to blunt trauma), and tears associated with retinal necrosis from trauma or inflammation. Rarer causes of retinal detachment include: tractional retinal detachment secondary to fibrous tissue on the surface of the retina, and exudative retinal detachment as a result of choroidal tumours that produce increased fluid flow through the subretinal space, or ocular inflammatory conditions. Retinal detachments can also be a mixture of two or more of the above types. Asymptomatic and non-progressive chronic retinal detachment can also occur. This review considers acute progressive RRD only. **Diagnosis:** RRD is often, but not universally, associated with symptoms of flashes of light (retinal photopsia), visual floaters, and peripheral and usually progressive visual-field loss. It is diagnosed by ophthalmoscopy. Acute RRD is seen as an oedematous folded retina with loss of the normal retinal transparency. The detachment can assume a bullous configuration that moves when the eye moves. There can be associated signs of PVD, as well as vitreous haemorrhage or RPE cells circulating in the vitreous cavity after retinal-break formation. The presence of pigment cells in the anterior vitreous, visible on slit-lamp biomicroscopy (termed "Shafer's sign"), is a sensitive indicator of the presence of a retinal break in a person presenting with an acute PVD. Chronic retinal detachments can be associated with retinal cyst formation and "tidemarks" demarcating the extent of the detachment, as well as subretinal fibrosis.

INCIDENCE/PREVALENCE RRD can occur at any age, but reaches peak prevalence in people aged 60–70 years. It affects men more than women, and white people more than black people. Observational studies from the USA, Europe, and New Zealand found that non-traumatic, phakic (lens intact) RRD occurred in about 6–18/100,000 people a year (i.e. about 1 in 10,000).

AETIOLOGY/RISK FACTORS The occurrence of retinal detachment is related to the interplay between predisposing retinal lesions and vitreoretinal traction, and occurs when fluid moves from the vitreous cavity through a retinal break into the subretinal space. Most (80–90%) retinal detachments are associated with retinal-break formation at the time of PVD. PVD is a naturally occurring phenomenon, occurring with a rapidly increasing prevalence in the 60–70-year-old age group. Most (70%) retinal breaks formed at the time of PVD are seen as tears in the retina, or as holes with a free-floating retinal operculum. Retinal breaks can occur in areas of previously abnormal retina — for example, lattice degeneration. Symptoms and signs of acute PVD are known to be associated with a higher risk of immediate progression to RRD in people with predisposing retinal lesions. However, people with established (chronic) PVD and predisposing retinal lesions who have not immediately progressed to RRD are at lower risk than those without a PVD. Symptomatic retinal tears with persistent vitreoretinal traction (not a complete PVD) have a very high rate of progression to retinal detachment — greater than 50% if left untreated. The risk of retinal

(continued over)

(from previous page)

detachment is increased to a variable extent in people with asymptomatic pre-existing retinal disease or lesions, especially retinal-flap tears, operculated retinal holes after separation of a retinal flap, atrophic retinal holes, lattice degeneration (areas of retinal thinning with abnormal vitreoretinal adhesion), and retinal dialyses. Autopsy studies have shown that about 6–11% of people aged over 20 years have retinal breaks in one form or another. However the chances of an RRD occurring in these asymptomatic eyes with no history of fellow-eye RRD is 0.5% over a follow-up period of 11 years. Similarly, 7–8% of adults have areas of lattice degeneration, but only a small proportion of these lesions progress to RRD. Asymptomatic retinal dialysis is thought to have a high risk of progression to retinal detachment, especially after trauma. Several general factors increase the risk of RRD. RRD has a higher prevalence in short-sighted (myopic) people, with around a 10-fold increased incidence in people with greater than 3 dioptres of myopia. The fellow eye in people with an RRD is at a higher risk, with 2–10% of RRDs being bilateral. Some of these will have pre-existing retinal lesions, but most subsequent RRD (at least 50%, and possibly as high as 80–90%) in the fellow eye will occur from ophthalmoscopically normal areas of retina. Hence prophylaxis to visible abnormal areas may not completely reduce the incidence of fellow-eye RRD. There is also a higher incidence of RDD in people with a family history of retinal detachment, especially in conditions such as Stickler syndrome. People who have had previous cataract surgery also have a higher incidence of RRD. About 0.5–0.6% of people experience RRD after phacoemulsification surgery for cataracts, with the risk being increased by 15–20 times if posterior capsule rupture occurs. About 10% of RRDs are associated with trauma. There are other conditions which, more rarely, increase the risk of RRD, including uveitis — especially CMV retinitis — and other degenerative retinal conditions such as retinoschisis.

PROGNOSIS On presentation, retinal detachment is usually divided into "macula on", when the fovea is still attached and "macula off", where the retina is detached centrally. People with macula-on retinal detachments have good initial visual acuity, and a better prognosis with successful surgery. Rapidly progressive cases are therefore treated as a matter of some urgency. Macula-off retinal detachments have worse visual acuity initially, and have a worse prognosis even with successful detachment surgery. Overall, about 95% of people have anatomically successful repair of RRD, with 70–90% achieving this in one operation. In 90% of successfully repaired macula-on retinal detachments, vision is 6/12 or better, while only 50% of macula-off retinal detachments achieve 6/15, with this level of vision being rare when the macula has been detached for 1 week or more. Reasons for anatomical failure of surgery include new or missed retinal breaks, and proliferative vitreoretinopathy (PVR). Causes of poor visual acuity after successful repair include macular epiretinal membranes (fibrosis), cystoid macular oedema, and foveal photoreceptor degeneration in macula-off retinal detachments.

Anthony W Solomon and David CW Mabey

KEY POINTS

- Active trachoma is caused by chronic infection of the conjunctiva by *Chlamydia trachomatis*, and is the world's leading infectious cause of blindness.

  Infection can lead to scarring of the tarsal conjunctiva, shortening and inversion of the upper eyelid (entropion), and scarring of the eye by eyelashes (trichiasis), leading to blindness.

  Trachoma is a disease of poverty, overcrowding, and poor sanitation. Active disease mainly affects children, but adults are at increased risk of scarring.

- Public health interventions to improve hygiene may reduce the risks of developing trachoma, but studies have given conflicting results.

  Face-washing plus topical antibiotics may be beneficial, but we don't know whether face-washing alone is effective.

  Fly control using insecticide alone, insecticide plus mass antibiotics, or by providing pit latrines, may reduce the risks of trachoma, but is unlikely to be a feasible large-scale approach.

- We don't know whether oral or topical antibiotics reduce the risk of active trachoma compared with placebo or with each other, as few comparable studies have been found.

- Lid-rotation surgery with bilamellar tarsal rotation or tarsal advance and rotation may be effective at correcting entropion and trichiasis compared with other types of surgery.

- We don't know whether posterior lamellar tarsal rotation plus azithromycin is more effective than posterior lamellar tarsal rotation alone at correcting entropion and trichiasis.

(i) **Please visit www.clinicalevidence.bmj.com for full text and references**

What are the effects of interventions to prevent scarring trachoma by reducing the prevalence of active trachoma?

Likely To Be Beneficial	• Face-washing plus topical tetracycline • Fly control using insecticide alone
Unknown Effectiveness	• Antibiotics • Face-washing alone • Fly control through the provision of pit latrines • Fly control using insecticide plus antibiotics • Health education

What are the effects of eyelid surgery for treating entropion and trichiasis?

Likely To Be Beneficial	• Bilamellar tarsal rotation or tarsal advance and rotation (compared with other types of eyelid surgery)
Unlikely To Be Beneficial	• Posterior lamellar tarsal rotation plus azithromycin (compared with surgery alone)

Search date January 2007

DEFINITION Active trachoma is chronic inflammation of the conjunctiva caused by infection with *Chlamydia trachomatis*. The WHO simplified trachoma grading scheme defines active trachoma as TF and/or TI, where TF (trachomatous inflammation — follicular) is the presence of five or more follicles in the central part of the upper tarsal conjunctiva, each at least 0.5 mm in diameter, and TI (trachomatous inflammation — intense) is pronounced inflammatory thickening of the upper tarsal conjunctiva that obscures more than half of the normal deep vessels. **Cicatricial trachoma** is caused by repeated infection with *C trachomatis*; it includes the presence of visible scars on the tarsal conjunctiva (trachomatous scarring), shortening and inversion of the upper eyelid (entropion), and malposition of the lashes so that they abrade the eye (trichiasis). Trachomatous scarring can be present without entropion/trichiasis, but if entropion/trichiasis is present because of trachoma, there will be scarring. Trachoma blindness results from corneal opacification, which occurs because of the mechanical trauma wrought by entropion/trichiasis. **Diagnosis** of trachoma is by clinical examination, using the criteria set out in either the modified WHO grading system or the WHO simplified grading system. The simplified grading system is now the most commonly employed.

INCIDENCE/PREVALENCE Trachoma is the world's leading cause of infectious blindness. Globally, active trachoma affects an estimated 84 million people, most of them children. About 7.6 million people are blind or at risk of blindness as a consequence. Trachoma is a disease of poverty, regardless of geographical region. Cicatricial trachoma is prevalent in large regions of Africa, the Middle East, Asia, and Aboriginal communities in Australia, and there are also small foci in Central and South America. In areas where trachoma is constantly present at high prevalence, active disease is found in more than 50% of preschool children, and may have a prevalence as high as 60–90%, and as many as 75% of women and 50% of men aged over 45 years may show signs of scarring disease. The prevalence of active trachoma decreases with increasing age. Although similar prevalences of active disease are observed in boys and girls, the later sequelae of trichiasis, entropion, and corneal opacification are usually more common in women than men.

AETIOLOGY/RISK FACTORS Active trachoma is associated with youth, poor access to water and sanitation, and close contact between people. Discharge from the eyes and nose may facilitate transmission of ocular *C trachomatis* infection. Sharing a bedroom with someone who has active trachoma is a risk factor for infection. The density of eye-seeking flies in a community is associated with active trachoma. Flies important to trachoma transmission lay their eggs on human faeces lying exposed on the soil, suggesting that access to improved sanitation might help control trachoma.

PROGNOSIS Corneal damage from trachoma is caused by multiple processes. Scarring trachoma damages glandular structures and may cause an inadequate tear film; a dry eye may be more susceptible to damage from inturned lashes and superadded infection by other bacteria and fungi, leading to corneal opacification.

Niaz Islam and Carlos Pavesio

KEY POINTS

- Anterior uveitis is inflammation of the uveal tract, and includes iritis (inflammation of the iris) and iridocyclitis (inflammation of both iris and ciliary body).

  It is usually rare, with an annual incidence of 12/100,000 population, although it is more common in Finland (annual incidence of 23/100,000), probably because of genetic factors, such as high frequency of HLA–B27 in the population.

  It is often self-limiting, but can in some cases lead to complications such as posterior synechiae, cataract, glaucoma, and chronic uveitis.

- Corticosteroid eye drops have been the standard treatment for uveitis since the early 1950s, although the evidence supporting their effectiveness is somewhat sparse.

  Widely known adverse effects of topical corticosteroid eye drops include local irritation, hyperaemia, oedema, and blurred vision.

- The studies examining the effects of NSAID eye drops or mydriatics were either too small or of insufficient quality to judge their effectiveness in treating uveitis.

(i) **Please visit www.clinicalevidence.bmj.com for full text and references**

What are the effects of anti-inflammatory eye drops on acute anterior uveitis?	
Likely To Be Beneficial	• Corticosteroids*
Unknown Effectiveness	• Mydriatics (different drugs or potencies) • NSAID eye drops

Search date February 2007

*Based on consensus; RCTs unlikely to be conducted.

DEFINITION Anterior uveitis is inflammation of the uveal tract, and includes iritis and iridocyclitis. It can be classified according to its clinical course into acute or chronic anterior uveitis, or according to its clinical appearance into granulomatous or non-granulomatous anterior uveitis. **Acute anterior uveitis** is characterised by an extremely painful red eye, often associated with photophobia, and occasionally with decreased visual acuity. **Chronic anterior uveitis** is defined as inflammation lasting over 6 weeks. It is usually asymptomatic, but many people have mild symptoms during exacerbations.

INCIDENCE/PREVALENCE Acute anterior uveitis is rare, with an annual incidence of 12/100,000 population. It is particularly common in Finland (annual incidence 22.6/100,000 population, prevalence 68.7/100,000 population), probably because of genetic factors such as the high frequency of HLA–B27 in the Finnish population. It is equally common in men and women, and more than 90% of cases occur in people older than 20 years of age.

AETIOLOGY/RISK FACTORS No cause is identified in 60–80% of people with acute anterior uveitis. Systemic disorders that may be associated with acute anterior uveitis include ankylosing spondylitis, Reiter's syndrome, Kawasaki's disease, infectious uveitis, Behçet's syndrome, inflammatory bowel disease, interstitial nephritis, sarcoidosis, Vogt–Koyanagi–Harada syndrome, and masquerade syndromes. Acute anterior uveitis also occurs

(continued over)

(from previous page)

in association with HLA–B27 expression not linked to any systemic disease. Acute anterior uveitis may occur after surgery, or as an adverse drug or hypersensitivity reaction.

PROGNOSIS Acute anterior uveitis is often self-limiting, but we found no evidence about how often it resolves spontaneously, in which people, or over what length of time. Complications include posterior synechiae, cataract, glaucoma, and chronic uveitis. In a study of 154 people (232 eyes) with acute anterior uveitis (119 people HLA–B27 positive), visual acuity was better than 20/60 in 209/232 eyes (90%), and 20/60 or worse in 23/232 eyes (10%), including worse than 20/200 (classified as legally blind) in 11/232 eyes (5%).

HIV infection

Martin David Talbot

KEY POINTS

- Infection with HIV usually leads to 8–10 years of asymptomatic infection before immune function deteriorates and AIDS develops.

  Without treatment, about 50% of infected people will die of AIDS over 10 years. With treatment, prognosis depends on age, CD4 cell count, and initial viral load.

- Concurrent STDs increase the risk of transmission of HIV infection. Treating STDs may reduce the risk of an individual acquiring HIV, but we don't know whether it is effective on a population level.

- Antiretroviral treatment (especially combinations including zidovudine) may reduce the risk of HIV infection among healthcare workers who have been exposed to the infection.

- Triple antiretroviral treatments are now standard for people with HIV infection.

  Boosted protease inhibitor-based regimens may be more effective than standard protease-based triple regimens at reducing viral load and preventing HIV progression and death.

  Non-nucleoside reverse transcriptase inhibitor- (NNRTI: efavirenz or nevirapine) based triple regimens increase viral suppression compared with protease inhibitor-based triple regimens, although HIV progression rates may not be reduced.

  Protease inhibitor-based triple regimens are less effective than NNRTI-based triple regimens at reducing viral load. Protease-based regimens may increase cholesterol and triglyceride levels.

  NRTI triple regimens offer similar viral suppression to protease-inhibitor based triple regimens. Some NRTIs (stavudine) may be associated with lipodystrophy.

- We do not know whether early initiation of antiretroviral treatment using triple regimens improves long-term survival compared with delayed treatment. The decision about when to start treatment currently depends on severity of symptoms and CD4 lymphocyte count, so that likely benefits can be balanced against risks of adverse effects of treatment.

ⓘ **Please visit www.clinicalevidence.bmj.com for full text and references**

What are the effects of preventive interventions?	
Likely To Be Beneficial	• Early diagnosis and treatment of STDs (in regions with emerging HIV epidemics) • Postexposure prophylaxis in healthcare workers*
Unknown Effectiveness	• Presumptive mass treatment of STDs

What are the effects of different antiretroviral drug treatment regimens in HIV infection?	
Beneficial	• Boosted protease inhibitor-based triple regimens (may be more effective as standard protease-based triple regimens at reducing viral load)

	• Non-nucleoside reverse transcriptase inhibitor-(NNRTI) based triple regimens (increase viral suppression compared with protease inhibitor-based triple regimens but may not affect progression)
Likely To Be Beneficial	• Nucleoside reverse transcriptase inhibitor- (NRTI) based triple regimens (similar viral suppression to protease inhibitor-based triple regimens) • Protease inhibitor-based triple regimens (similar viral suppression to nucleoside reverse transcriptase inhibitor (NRTI) triple regimens but less effective than non-nucleoside reverse transcriptase inhibitor- (NNRTI) based triple regimens; may also be less effective than boosted protease inhibitor-based regimens)
Unknown Effectiveness	• Early versus delayed antiretroviral treatment using triple antiretroviral regimens

Search date June 2006

*No RCTs: based on consensus and known effectiveness of antiretroviral drugs in the treatment setting.

DEFINITION HIV infection refers to infection with the human immunodeficiency virus (HIV) type 1 or type 2. Clinically, this is characterised by a variable period (about 8–10 years on average) of asymptomatic infection, followed by repeated episodes of illness of varying and increasing severity as immune function deteriorates, resulting in AIDS. The type of illness varies by country, availability of specific treatments for HIV, and prophylaxis for opportunistic infections. Current treatments interrupt the life cycle of the virus without effecting a cure: mutations in the viral genome result in gradual resistance drift and increasing ineffectiveness of drug treatments.

INCIDENCE/PREVALENCE Worldwide estimates suggest that by December 2005 about 38.6 million people were living with HIV. In 2005, there were estimated to be 4.1 million new cases of HIV and 3.3 million deaths from AIDS. About 95% of HIV infections occur in resource-poor countries. By 1999, occupationally acquired HIV infection in healthcare workers had been documented in at least 102 definite and 217 possible cases, although this is likely to be an underestimate.

AETIOLOGY/RISK FACTORS The major risk factor for transmission of HIV is unprotected heterosexual or homosexual intercourse. Other risk factors include needlestick injury, sharing drug-injecting equipment, and blood transfusion. An HIV-infected woman may also transmit the virus to her baby transplacentally, during birth, or through breast milk. This has been reported in 15–30% of pregnant women with HIV infection. Mother-to-child transmission of HIV is dealt with in a separate review (HIV: mother-to-child transmission, p 240). Not everyone exposed to HIV will become infected, although risk increases if exposure is repeated, at high dose, or through blood. There is at least a two- to fivefold greater risk of HIV-infection among people with STDs.

PROGNOSIS Without treatment, about 50% of people infected with HIV will become ill and die from AIDS over about 10 years. A meta-analysis of 13 cohort studies from Europe and the USA looked at 12,574 treatment-naive people starting highly active antiretroviral therapy (HAART) with a combination of at least three drugs. A lower baseline CD4 cell count and higher baseline HIV-1 viral load were associated with an increased probability of progression to AIDS or death. Other independent predictors of poorer outcome were advanced age, infection through injection drug use, and a previous diagnosis of AIDS. The CD4 cell count at initiation was the dominant prognostic factor in people starting HAART.

People with the most favourable prognostic factors (aged under 50 years old, not infected through injection drug use, viral load below 100,000 copies/mL, and CD4 cell count above 350 cells/mL on initiation of HAART) were estimated to have a 3.5% chance of progression to AIDS or death within 3 years. People with the most unfavourable prognostic factors (aged at least 50 years old, infected through intravenous drug use, viral load at least 100,000 copies/mL, and CD4 cell count below 50 cells/mL on initiation of HAART) had an estimated 50% chance of progression to AIDS or death within 3 years. Genetic factors have been shown to affect response to antiretroviral treatment, but were not considered in the meta-analysis. We found one non-systematic review assessing prognosis in people in Africa. It identified one study conducted in rural Uganda, which found similar survival rates (a median 9.8 years from the time of HIV-1 seroconversion), but found that progression to symptomatic disease was faster in Uganda than in resource-rich countries, owing largely to the high background level of morbidity. The review reported that most people in hospital in Africa with HIV have the clinical features of AIDS just before they die, and many are severely immunosuppressed. The review also suggested that morbidity was similar to that in resource-rich countries before the introduction of HAART.

HIV: mother-to-child transmission

Jimmy Volmink and Ben Marais

KEY POINTS

- Without active intervention, the risk of mother-to-child transmission (MTCT) of HIV-1 is high, especially in populations where prolonged breastfeeding is the norm.

    Without antiviral treatment, the risk of transmission of HIV from infected mothers to their children is approximately 15–30% during pregnancy and labour, with an additional 10–20% transmission risk attributed to prolonged breastfeeding.

    HIV-2 is rarely transmitted from mother to child.

    Transmission is more likely in mothers with high viral loads and/or advanced HIV disease.

    Without antiretroviral treatment (ART), 15–30% of vertically infected infants die within the first year of life.

    The long-term treatment of children with ART is complicated by multiple concerns regarding the development of resistance, and by adverse effects.

    From a paediatric perspective, successful prevention of MTCT remains the most important focus.

- Antiretroviral drugs given to the mother during pregnancy or labour, and/or to the baby immediately after birth, reduce the risk of MTCT of HIV-1.

- Reductions in MTCT are possible using simple ART regimens.

    Longer courses of ART are more effective, but the greatest benefit is derived from treatment during late pregnancy, labour, and early infancy.

    Suppression of the maternal viral load to undetectable levels (below 50 copies/mL) using highly active antiretroviral therapy (HAART) offers the greatest risk reduction, and is currently the standard of care offered in most resource-rich countries, where MTCT rates have been reduced to 1–2%.

    Alternative short-course regimens have been tested in resource-limited settings where HAART is not yet widely available. RCTs demonstrate that short courses of antiretroviral drugs have proven efficacy for reducing MTCT. Identifying optimal short-course regimens (drug combination, timing, and cost effectiveness) for various settings remains a focus for ongoing research.

- Avoidance of breastfeeding prevents postpartum transmission of HIV, but formula feeding requires access to clean water and health education.

    The risk of breastfeeding-related HIV transmission needs to be balanced against the multiple benefits that breastfeeding offers. In resource-poor countries, breastfeeding is strongly associated with reduced infant morbidity and improved child survival.

    Modified breastfeeding practices may reduce the risk of HIV transmission while retaining some of its associated benefits.

    In settings where formula feeding is not feasible (no clean water, insufficient health education, significant cultural barriers) modified breastfeeding practices may offer the best compromise.

    Early breastfeeding with weaning around age 4–6 months may offer an HIV-free survival benefit compared with either formula, mixed feeding, or prolonged breastfeeding.

    Heat- or microbicidal-treated expressed breast milk may offer value in particular settings.

- Elective caesarean section at 38 weeks may reduce vertical transmission rates (apart from breast-milk transmission).

The potential benefits of this intervention need to be balanced against the increased risk of surgery-associated complications, high cost, and feasibility issues. These reservations are particularly relevant in resource-limited settings.

- Immunotherapy with HIV hyperimmune globulin or immunoglobulin without HIV antibody does not reduce HIV-1 MTCT risk.
- Vaginal microbicides have not been demonstrated to reduce HIV-1 MTCT risk.
- There is no evidence that vitamin A or multivitamin supplementation reduces the risk of HIV-1 MTCT or infant mortality.

(i) Please visit www.clinicalevidence.bmj.com for full text and references

What are the effects of measures to reduce mother-to-child transmission of HIV?

Beneficial	• Antiretroviral drugs
Likely To Be Beneficial	• Avoiding breastfeeding (formula feeding better, provided there is access to clean water and health education, even in infants receiving antiretroviral treatment) • Elective caesarean section
Unknown Effectiveness	• Immunotherapy • Vaginal microbicides
Likely To Be Ineffective Or Harmful	• Vitamin supplements

Search date January 2007

DEFINITION Mother-to-child transmission (MTCT) of HIV infection is defined as transmission of HIV from an infected mother to her child during gestation, labour, or postpartum through breastfeeding. HIV-1 infection is frequently transmitted from mother to child, although HIV-2 is rarely transmitted in this way. Infected children rarely have symptoms or signs of HIV at birth, but usually develop them over subsequent months.

INCIDENCE/PREVALENCE A review of 13 cohort studies estimated the risk of MTCT of HIV in the absence of antiretroviral treatment (ART), to be 15–20% in Europe, 15–30% in the USA, and 25–35% in Africa. The risk of transmission is estimated to be 15–30% during pregnancy, with an additional transmission risk of 10–20% associated with prolonged breastfeeding. The Joint United Nation's Programme on HIV/AIDS (UNAIDS) estimates that more than 2 million children are infected with HIV-1 worldwide, and that more than 1800 new HIV infections are transmitted daily from mothers to infants. Of these, more than 80% are in sub-Saharan Africa, where more than 500,000 children were newly infected with HIV in 2004 alone.

AETIOLOGY/RISK FACTORS Transmission of HIV to infants is more likely if the mother has a high viral load. A Tanzanian study reported that a viral load of 50,000 copies/mL or more at delivery was associated with a fourfold increase in the risk of early transmission, using polymerase chain reaction (PCR) results at 6 weeks of age (OR 4.21, 95% CI 1.59 to 11.13; P = 0.00 4).Other maternal risk factors include STDs, chorioamnionitis, prolonged rupture of membranes, vaginal mode of delivery, low CD4+ count, advanced maternal HIV disease, obstetric events with bleeding (episiotomy, perineal laceration, and intrapartum

(continued over)

(from previous page)

haemorrhage), young maternal age, and history of stillbirth. A recent multi-centre RCT, conducted in Africa to investigate the ability of a simple anti- and peripartum antibiotic regimen to reduce the incidence of chorioamnionitis and the associated risk of MTCT of HIV-1, failed to demonstrate any protective effect (proportions of HIV-infected children at birth; antibiotics 7%, placebo 8%; P = 0.4 1). Estimations of the timing of MTCT of HIV-1 during pregnancy indicate that the vast majority of transmission (80%) occurs during late pregnancy (3% at less than 14 weeks, 3% at 14–28 weeks, 14% at 28–36 weeks, 50% at 36 weeks to labour, and 30% during labour). Prolonged breastfeeding poses a significant additional risk for MTCT, with about 60% of total transmissions occurring during pregnancy, and 40% via breast milk, in breastfeeding populations. With the use of effective drug regimens to reduce peri-partum MTCT of HIV, prolonged breast or mixed feeding becomes the predominant route of transmission. Late postnatal transmission (beyond 3–6 months) contributes substantially to overall MTCT; this may occur throughout the total period of breastfeeding.

PROGNOSIS The natural history of HIV infection in infancy is variable. It has been estimated that 25% of infants infected with HIV progress rapidly to AIDS or death within the first year of life, although some survive beyond 12 years of age even in the absence of ART. A collaborative European study that documented the natural history of disease in the absence of ART reported 15% mortality during infancy, and 28% mortality by the age of 5 years. However, the prognosis of African children with vertically acquired HIV infection may be worse. In a prospective study conducted in Kigali, Rwanda, the cumulative probability of death in 54 HIV-infected children was 0.26 (95% CI 0.16 to 0.41) at 1 year, 0.45 (95% CI 0.32 to 0.60) at 2 years, and 0.62 (95% CI 0.47 to 0.78) at 5 years. In comparison, the cumulative probability of death in HIV-uninfected children at 5 years of age was 15 times less (0.04, 95%CI: 0.02 to 0.07). Among the HIV-infected children, the cumulative probabilities of developing AIDS were 0.17, 95% CI 0.09 to 0.32 at 1 year, 0.28, 95% CI 0.17 to 0.45 at 2 years, and 0.35, 95% CI 0.22 to 0.53 at 5 years of age. Of the 28 HIV-infected children that died, 9 met the case definition of AIDS. On a population level, HIV accounted for 2% of deaths in 1990, and almost 8% in 1999, in children under 5 years of age living in sub-Saharan Africa. Five countries (Botswana, Namibia, Swaziland, Zambia, and Zimbabwe) reported HIV-attributable mortality rates in excess of 30/1000 in children under the age of 5 years.

John Ioannidis and Taryn Young

KEY POINTS

- Opportunistic infections can occur in up to 40% of people with HIV infection and a CD4 count below 250/mm^3, although the risks are much lower with use of highly active antiretroviral treatment.

- Trimethoprim–sulfamethoxazole or azithromycin may reduce the risk of PCP, but have not been shown to reduce toxoplasmosis infection.

    Atovaquone may prevent PCP and toxoplasmosis in people who cannot take trimethoprim–sulfamethoxazole, although we don't know this for sure.

- Tuberculosis can be prevented by standard prophylaxis in people who are tuberculin skin test positive, but not in those who are tuberculin skin test negative.

    Short-term combination treatment has similar efficacy to long-term isoniazid monotherapy, but has greater risk of adverse effects.

- Azithromycin or clarithromycin may reduce the risk of disseminated *M avium* complex (MAC) disease in people without prior MAC disease.

    Adding rifabutin may reduce the risk of MAC disease compared with other antibiotic regimen, while adding ethambutol decreases the risk of relapse.

    Combination treatment with clarithromycin plus clofazimine may increase mortality and is usually avoided.

- Aciclovir reduces the risk of HSV and VZV infection and overall mortality, but has not been shown to reduce CMV infection.

    Valaciclovir and ganciclovir may reduce the risk of CMV infection, but may be associated with serious adverse effects.

- Fluconazole and itraconazole may reduce the risk of invasive fungal infections or their relapse, but can cause serious adverse effects.

- In people with a CD4 cell count above 100–200/mm^3, discontinuation of prophylactic treatment may not increase the risk of PCP, toxoplasmosis, or MAC infection.

(i) **Please visit www.clinicalevidence.bmj.com for full text and references**

What are the effects of prophylaxis for PCP and toxoplasmosis?

Likely To Be Beneficial	• Atovaquone • Azithromycin (alone or plus rifabutin, compared with rifabutin alone, for PCP prevention) • Trimethoprim–sulfamethoxazole for PCP
Unknown Effectiveness	• Trimethoprim–sulfamethoxazole for toxoplasmosis

What are the effects of antituberculosis prophylaxis in people with HIV infection?

Beneficial	• Antituberculosis prophylaxis versus placebo
Trade-off Between Benefits And Harms	• Isoniazid for 6–12 months (versus combination treatment for 2–3 months — longer treatment regimen, but similar benefits and fewer harms)

What are the effects of prophylaxis for disseminated *M avium* complex (MAC) disease for people without previous MAC disease?

Likely To Be Beneficial	• Azithromycin
	• Clarithromycin
Trade-off Between Benefits And Harms	• Rifabutin plus macrolides

What are the effects of prophylaxis for disseminated *M avium* complex (MAC) disease for people with previous MAC disease?

Likely To Be Beneficial	• Clarithromycin, rifabutin, and ethambutol (more effective than clarithromycin plus clofazimine)
	• Ethambutol added to clarithromycin plus clofazimine
Unknown Effectiveness	• Rifabutin added to clarithromycin plus ethambutol
Likely To Be Ineffective Or Harmful	• Clofazimine added to clarithromycin and ethambutol (higher mortality than clofazimine plus ethambutol)

What are the effects of prophylaxis for CMV, HSV, and VZV?

Beneficial	• Aciclovir
Trade-off Between Benefits And Harms	• Oral ganciclovir (in people with severe CD4 depletion)
	• Valaciclovir
Unknown Effectiveness	• Famciclovir (for recurrent HSV)

What are the effects of prophylaxis for invasive fungal disease in people without previous fungal disease?

| Trade-off Between Benefits And Harms | • Fluconazole or itraconazole |

What are the effects of prophylaxis for invasive fungal disease in people with previous invasive fungal disease?

| Likely To Be Beneficial | • Itraconazole (more effective than placebo for preventing *Penicillium marneffei* relapse) |
| Likely To Be Ineffective Or Harmful | • Itraconazole (less effective than fluconazole for preventing relapse of cryptococcal meningitis) |

What are the effects of discontinuing prophylaxis against opportunistic pathogens in people on highly active antiretroviral treatment (HAART)?	
Likely To Be Beneficial	• Discontinuing prophylaxis for MAC in people with CD4 above 100/mm^3 • Discontinuing prophylaxis for PCP and toxoplasmosis in people with CD4 above 200/mm^3
Unknown Effectiveness	• Discontinuing prophylaxis for CMV in people with CD4 above 100/mm^3

Search date December 2004

DEFINITION Opportunistic infections are intercurrent infections that occur in people infected with HIV. Prophylaxis aims to avoid either the first occurrence of these infections (primary prophylaxis) or their recurrence (secondary prophylaxis, maintenance treatment). This review includes PCP, *Toxoplasma gondii* encephalitis, *Mycobacterium tuberculosis*, *Mycobacterium avium* complex (MAC) disease, CMV disease (most often retinitis), infections from other herpes viruses (HSV and VZV), and invasive fungal disease (*Cryptococcus neoformans*, *Histoplasma capsulatum*, and *Penicillium marneffei*).

INCIDENCE/PREVALENCE The incidence of opportunistic infections is high in people with immune impairment. Data available before the introduction of highly active antiretroviral treatment (HAART) suggest that, with a CD4 below 250/mm^3, the 2-year probability of developing an opportunistic infection is 40% for PCP, 22% for CMV, 18% for MAC, 6% for toxoplasmosis, and 5% for cryptococcal meningitis. The introduction of HAART has reduced the rate of opportunistic infections. One cohort study found that the introduction of HAART decreased the incidence of PCP by 94%, CMV by 82%, and MAC by 64%, as presenting AIDS events. HAART decreased the incidence of events subsequent to the diagnosis of AIDS by 84% for PCP, 82% for CMV, and 97% for MAC.

AETIOLOGY/RISK FACTORS Opportunistic infections are caused by a wide array of pathogens and result from immune-system defects induced by HIV. The risk of developing opportunistic infections increases dramatically with progressive impairment of the immune system. Each opportunistic infection has a different threshold of immune impairment, beyond which the risk increases substantially. Opportunistic pathogens may infect the immunocompromised host *de novo*, but usually they are simply reactivations of latent pathogens in such hosts.

PROGNOSIS Prognosis depends on the type of opportunistic infection. Even with treatment they may cause serious morbidity and mortality. Most deaths due to HIV infection are caused by opportunistic infections.

HIV: treating *pneumocystis* pneumonia (PCP)

Richard Bellamy

KEY POINTS

- *Pneumocystis* pneumonia (PCP) is a common AIDS-defining opportunistic illness in people with HIV infection, but its incidence has fallen with use of prophylactic treatment.

- Without treatment, PCP is likely to be fatal in people with AIDS, so placebo-controlled studies would be considered unethical.

- Most clinicians consider trimethoprim–sulfamethoxazole (co-trimoxazole) standard first-line treatment for PCP.

   Trimethoprim–sulfamethoxazole may be more effective than atovaquone, but is more likely to cause adverse effects. Clindamycin–primaquine, trimethoprim–dapsone, and intravenous pentamidine may be as effective as co-trimoxazole, with similar adverse effect rates.

   Systemic absorption of aerosolised pentamidine is low, so adverse effects are few, but it may be less effective than other treatments in people with severely impaired respiratory function, and is perceived as having a high rate of treatment failure.

- Adjuvant corticosteroids reduce mortality when used early in the treatment of moderate to severe PCP, but we don't know whether they are beneficial in mild PCP.

- Clindamycin–primaquine may be more effective than other treatment options in people who have failed to respond to first-line antipneumocystis treatment, but no high quality studies have been found.

(i) Please visit www.clinicalevidence.bmj.com for full text and references

What are the effects of first-line antipneumocystis treatments for PCP in people infected with HIV?	
Beneficial	• Trimethoprim–sulfamethoxazole (TMP–SMX; co-trimoxazole)
Likely To Be Beneficial	• Atovaquone (but less effective than TMP–SMX)*
	• Clindamycin–primaquine (may be as effective as TMP–SMX)
	• Pentamidine (aerosolised) (but less effective than TMP–SMX)
	• Pentamidine (intravenous) (may be as effective as TMP–SMX)
	• Trimethoprim–dapsone (may be as effective as TMP–SMX)

What are the effects of adjuvant corticosteroids in people receiving first-line antipneumocystis treatments for PCP in people infected with HIV?	
Beneficial	• Adjuvant corticosteroids (in people with moderate to severe PCP)

What are the effects of treatments for PCP in people infected with HIV who have not responded to first-line antipneumocystis treatment?

Unknown Effectiveness	• Treatment after failure of first-line treatment

Search date November 2006

DEFINITION *Pneumocystis* pneumonia (PCP) is caused by the opportunistic fungus *Pneumocystis jiroveci*. The infection occurs in people with impaired immune function. Most cases occur in people infected with HIV, in whom PCP is an AIDS-defining illness. The pneumonia is generally classified as **mild** if arterial oxygen tension (PaO_2) is greater than 70 mm Hg on room air, or if the alveolar–arterial oxygen gradient is less than 35 mm Hg, or both. It is generally classified as **moderate/severe** if PaO_2 is less than 70 mm Hg, or if the alveolar–arterial oxygen gradient is greater than 35 mm Hg, or both. This review focuses on the treatment of PCP in adults infected with HIV. Prevention of PCP is covered under HIV: prevention of opportunistic infections, p 245.

INCIDENCE/PREVALENCE PCP was the most common AIDS-defining illness in resource-rich nations before PCP prophylaxis became widespread, and is still one of the most common AIDS-defining conditions. It is probably also common throughout resource-poor countries, although the prevalence is harder to assess here because of difficulties in making the diagnosis. Before the widespread use of prophylaxis it was estimated that up to 80% of people with AIDS would eventually develop PCP. Widespread use of prophylaxis against PCP, and of highly active antiretroviral treatment have dramatically reduced the incidence of this infection (see HIV: prevention of opportunistic infections, p 245).

AETIOLOGY/RISK FACTORS Risk factors for PCP include HIV infection, primary immune deficiencies, prematurity, cancer, use of immune suppressants after organ transplantation, and prolonged use of high-dose corticosteroids. HIV infection is now responsible for the vast majority of cases of PCP. Among adults with HIV infection, those with a CD4 cell count below 200 cells/mm³ are at highest risk, and the median CD4 cell count at diagnosis of PCP is about 50 cells/mm³.

PROGNOSIS It is generally believed that without treatment PCP would almost certainly be fatal in a person with AIDS. For ethical reasons, no studies have examined short-term prognosis without treatment. People with AIDS and PCP frequently have other serious opportunistic infections, which can adversely affect their prognosis.

Brendan Payne and Richard Bellamy

KEY POINTS

- Tuberculosis is a major opportunistic infection and cause of death in people with HIV, and often presents as non-pulmonary disease.

  In people infected with both HIV and *Mycobacterium tuberculosis*, the annual risk of developing active tuberculosis is 5–10%, more than 10 times the rate for people with *Mycobacterium tuberculosis* infection but without HIV.

  Untreated, mortality from tuberculosis in people with HIV is likely to be very high, and over 5% of people relapse after successful treatment.

- Conventional antituberculous treatment (2 months of rifampicin plus isoniazid plus pyrazinamide, with or without ethambutol, followed by 4–7 months of rifampicin plus isoniazid) is considered beneficial in people with HIV and is standard treatment. Placebo-controlled RCTs of active tuberculosis would therefore be considered unethical and are unlikely to be performed.

  We don't know whether antituberculous treatment regimens containing rifabutin or quinolones are more effective compared with conventional regimens.

  Regimens containing thiacetazone may be less effective at producing negative sputum cultures compared with conventional regimens and may have more adverse effects, including fatal mucocutaneous reactions.

  We don't know whether regimens lasting longer than 6 months are more effective than shorter regimens, but regimens that use rifampicin for at least 5 months are less likely to lead to recurrence compared with regimens that use 3 months or less of rifampicin.

- Adjuvant immunotherapy with *Mycobacterium vaccae* does not increase cure rates or survival compared with placebo vaccination.

- Adjuvant immunotherapy with corticosteroids does not increase survival or decrease tuberculosis recurrence in HIV-positive people with pulmonary or pleural tuberculosis compared with placebo. RCTs found that corticosteroids caused an increased risk of high blood glucose and high blood pressure.

  We don't know whether adjuvant immunotherapy with corticosteroids increases survival in HIV-positive people with tuberculous meningitis or tuberculous pericarditis compared with placebo.

  We don't know whether early initiation of highly active antiretroviral treatment (HAART) improves tuberculosis cure rates compared with delayed initiation of HAART, and there is a risk of interaction with antituberculous drugs.

  We don't know whether directly observed therapy improves cure rates compared with unsupervised treatment in people with HIV.

- We don't know which antimycobacterial treatment combinations are most effective in people with HIV who have failed first-line treatment.

- Secondary prophylaxis with antituberculous drugs after successful completion of conventional antituberculous treatment reduces the risk of tuberculosis recurrence in people with HIV who are not receiving HAART, compared with placebo.

  We don't know whether secondary prophylaxis with antituberculous drugs reduces mortality.

(i) **Please visit www.clinicalevidence.bmj.com for full text and references**

What are the effects of first-line treatments for tuberculosis in people infected with HIV?

Beneficial	• Conventional antituberculous treatment*
Unknown Effectiveness	• Adjuvant immunotherapy with corticosteroids • Antituberculous treatment containing quinolones (compared with alternative regimens) • Antituberculous treatment containing rifabutin (compared with alternative regimens) • Directly observed therapy, short course (compared with unsupervised treatment) • Early initiation of highly active antiretroviral treatment (compared with delayed initiation of highly active antiretroviral treatment) • Longer courses of antituberculous treatment (compared with conventional short course treatment)
Unlikely To Be Beneficial	• Adjuvant immunotherapy with *Mycobacterium vaccae*
Likely To Be Ineffective Or Harmful	• Antituberculous treatment containing 3 months or less of rifampicin (compared with rifampicin for at least 5 months) • Antituberculous treatment containing thiacetazone

What are the effects of second-line treatments for tuberculosis in people infected with HIV?

Unknown Effectiveness	• Antimycobacterial treatment combinations (comparative benefits of different regimens unclear) • Secondary prophylaxis with antituberculous drugs versus placebo after successful completion of conventional antituberculous treatment

Search date January 2007

*Categorisation based on consensus.

DEFINITION HIV infection kills more people than any other infectious disease. Infection with *Mycobacterium tuberculosis* is among the most important HIV-related opportunistic infections, in both resource-rich and resource-poor countries. HIV infection compromises the host's immune defences and can lead to failure to control latent *Mycobacterium tuberculosis* infection, with the subsequent development of active (i.e. symptomatic) tuberculosis. The HIV pandemic has been a major contributing factor in the spread of tuberculosis in many countries. Tuberculosis most commonly affects the lungs, but can also affect many other organs such as lymph nodes, kidneys, liver, gastrointestinal tract, and the central nervous system. In a study of 132 HIV-positive people with tuberculosis in San Francisco, 50 (38%) had solely pulmonary disease, 40 (30%) had solely extrapulmonary disease, and

(continued over)

(from previous page)

42 (32%) had both pulmonary and extrapulmonary disease. In Africa and South America, 40–80% of HIV-positive people presenting with tuberculosis have pulmonary disease. The specific symptoms of tuberculosis depend on the site of infection. Pulmonary disease characteristically presents with cough, haemoptysis, chest pain, and systemic symptoms such as weight loss and night sweats. This review deals with the treatment of active tuberculosis (both pulmonary and extrapulmonary) in people with HIV. Prevention of tuberculosis in people with HIV is covered in a separate review (see review on HIV: prevention of opportunistic infections, p 245).

INCIDENCE/PREVALENCE About a third of the world's population has latent *Mycobacterium tuberculosis* infection. Each year about 740,000 cases of active tuberculosis occur in people who are HIV positive, resulting in 248,000 deaths. HIV infection has been a major factor in the increase in the number of cases of tuberculosis occurring worldwide. Most people infected with HIV live in sub-Saharan Africa. In several countries of this region, over 40% of people who develop tuberculosis are infected with HIV. Tuberculosis is the most frequent cause of death in people infected with HIV in the Democratic Republic of Congo. Reliable data on cause of death in people in other sub-Saharan African countries are rare, but tuberculosis is probably a frequent cause of death among people with HIV.

AETIOLOGY/RISK FACTORS Risk factors for tuberculosis include social factors such as poverty, overcrowding, and homelessness, and medical factors such as steroid treatment. In people co-infected with HIV and *Mycobacterium tuberculosis*, the annual risk of developing active tuberculosis is about 5–10% — more than 10 times greater than for people infected with *Mycobacterium tuberculosis* who do not have HIV. The annual risk of tuberculosis in co-infected people may be higher in resource-poor countries than in established market economies because of additional risk factors such as poor nutrition and poverty. Without preventive treatment about 30% of HIV-positive people with latent tuberculosis will develop active tuberculosis. Preventive treatment aims to reduce this risk.

PROGNOSIS Without treatment, active tuberculosis would probably be fatal in a person infected with HIV. For ethical reasons, no studies have examined the prognosis of active tuberculosis without treatment in people infected with HIV. In one study in the era before highly active antiretroviral treatment in the USA, the median survival of HIV-infected people treated for tuberculosis was 16 months. However, only 13/99 (13%) of the deaths were attributed to tuberculosis. The other common causes of death were PCP (24%), bacterial pneumonia (14%), wasting syndrome (9%), and Kaposi's sarcoma (9%). In Malawi, 47% of HIV-positive people with tuberculosis died during 32 months of follow-up. The most common causes of death among people with HIV in sub-Saharan Africa are wasting syndrome, chronic diarrhoea, cryptococcal meningitis, and chest infection. The differences in cause of death between sub-Saharan Africa and the USA may be attributable to the availability of diagnostic tests as much as to genuine differences in the underlying causes. Recurrence of tuberculosis after completion of treatment is more common among people with HIV than among HIV-uninfected people. In one study in New York, 83/1530 (5.4%) people with HIV who completed tuberculosis treatment had a recurrence of disease compared with 21/1413 (1.5%) HIV-uninfected people who completed tuberculosis treatment. One cohort study in 326 South African mineworkers successfully treated for tuberculosis found a higher recurrence rate of tuberculosis in HIV-positive people, with 16.0 cases per 100 person-years of follow-up compared with 6.4 cases per 100 person-years of follow-up among HIV-negative people. In a randomised trial in Haiti, the tuberculosis recurrence rate among HIV-positive people not receiving post-treatment isoniazid was 7.8 cases per 100 person-years of follow-up compared with 0.4 per 100 person-years of follow-up in HIV-negative people.

Leonila Dans and Elizabeth Martínez

KEY POINTS

- Invasive infection with the parasite *Entamoeba histolytica* can be asymptomatic, or can cause diarrhoea with blood and mucus, abdominal pains, and fever.

  Amoebic dysentery is transmitted in areas where poor sanitation allows contamination of drinking water and food with faeces. In these areas, up to 40% of people with diarrhoea may have amoebic dysentery.

  Fulminant amoebic dysentery is often fatal. Other complications include perforation of the colon, colonic ulcers, amoeboma, and chronic carriage.

- Ornidazole may be effective at curing amoebic dysentery compared with placebo, but can cause nausea and vomiting.

  We don't know whether tinidazole is better than placebo, but it seems to be more effective than metronidazole at reducing symptoms and clearing the infection, with fewer adverse effects.

  Secnidazole and tinidazole may be as effective as ornidazole at curing amoebic dysentery in children.

- We don't know whether emetine or paromomycin are beneficial in treating amoebic dysentery.

🛈 **Please visit www.clinicalevidence.bmj.com for full text and references**

What are the effects of drug treatments for amoebic dysentery in endemic areas?	
Likely To Be Beneficial	• Ornidazole • Secnidazole* • Tinidazole*
Unknown Effectiveness	• Emetine • Paromomycin
Unlikely To Be Beneficial	• Metronidazole*

Search date July 2006

*No placebo-controlled RCTs. Categorisation based on consensus and evidence of similar effectiveness among these drugs.

DEFINITION Amoebic dysentery is caused by the protozoan parasite *Entamoeba histolytica*. Invasive intestinal parasitic infection can result in symptoms of fulminant dysentery, such as fever, chills, bloody or mucous diarrhoea, and abdominal discomfort. The dysentery can alternate, with periods of constipation or remission. This review focuses on amoebic dysentery only, and includes populations with both suspected and documented disease in endemic areas where levels of infection do not exhibit wide fluctuations through time. The term amoebic dysentery encompasses people described as having symptomatic intestinal amoebiasis, amoebic colitis, amoebic diarrhoea, or invasive intestinal amoebiasis. Extraintestinal amoebiasis (e.g. amoebic liver abscess) and asymptomatic amoebiasis are not covered.

INCIDENCE/PREVALENCE We found no accurate global prevalence data for *E histolytica* infection and amoebic dysentery. Estimates on the prevalence of *Entamoeba* infection

(continued over)

(from previous page)

range from 1–40% of the population in Central and South America, Africa, and Asia, and from 0.2–10.8% in endemic areas of resource-rich countries such as the USA. However, these estimates are difficult to interpret, mainly because infection can remain asymptomatic or go unreported, and because many older reports do not distinguish *E histolytica* from the non-pathogenic, morphologically identical species *Entamoeba dispar*. Development and availability of more sophisticated methods (such as the enzyme-linked immunosorbent assay- [ELISA] based test) to differentiate the two species might give a more accurate estimate of its global prevalence. Infection with *E histolytica* is a common cause of acute diarrhoea in resource-poor countries. One survey conducted in Egypt found that 38% of people with acute diarrhoea in an outpatient clinic had amoebic dysentery.

AETIOLOGY/RISK FACTORS Ingestion of cysts from food or water contaminated with faeces is the main route of *E histolytica* transmission. Low standards of hygiene and sanitation, particularly those related to crowding, tropical climate, contamination of food and water with faeces, and inadequate disposal of faeces, all account for the high rates of infection seen in resource-poor countries. It has been suggested that some animals, such as dogs, pigs, and monkeys, may act as reservoir hosts to the protozoa, but this has not been proven. In resource-rich countries, risk factors include communal living, oral and anal sex, compromised immune system, and migration or travel from endemic areas.

PROGNOSIS Amoebic dysentery may progress to amoeboma, fulminant colitis, toxic megacolon and colonic ulcers, and may lead to perforation. Amoeboma may be mistaken for colonic carcinoma or pyogenic abscess. Amoebic dysentery may also result in chronic carriage and the chronic passing of amoebic cysts. Fulminant amoebic dysentery is reported to have 55–88% mortality. It is estimated that more than 500 million people are infected with *E histolytica* worldwide. Between 40,000 and 100,000 will die each year, placing this infection second to malaria in mortality caused by protozoan parasites.

George Swingler

KEY POINTS

- Chickenpox is caused by primary infection with VZV. In healthy people, it is usually a mild, self-limiting illness, characterised by low-grade fever, malaise, and a generalised, itchy, vesicular rash.

    Chickenpox is very contagious — in the UK, USA and Japan, over 80% of people have been infected by the age of 10 years.

    The most common complications are bacterial skin sepsis in children under 5, acute cerebellar ataxia in older children, and varicella pneumonia in adults (which causes 20–30 hospital admissions per 10,000 adults).

- Live attenuated varicella vaccine is effective at preventing chickenpox in healthy children.

    The vaccine does not seem to reduce the incidence of chickenpox in postexposed children, although it does reduce severity of symptoms.

- We found no evidence that looks at the effect of the vaccine in healthy adults.

- Newborns whose mothers' rashes appear in the last 5 days of pregnancy or within 2 days of birth have been reported, in small case series, to have a very high risk of severe chickenpox.

    In these cases, the general consensus is to administer zoster immunoglobulin.

    We haven't found any evidence assessing aciclovir, famciclovir, or valaciclovir for preventing chickenpox in prenatally exposed children.

- Overall, there is sparse evidence examining the effects of vaccines in immunocompromised adults and children.

    We don't know how effective famciclovir, valaciclovir, live attenuated varicella virus, or zoster immunoglobulin are in preventing chickenpox in immunocompromised adults or children.

    Aciclovir (high dose) has been shown to be beneficial in reducing clinical chickenpox in people with HIV infection. We don't know how effective it is in other immunocompromised people to prevent chickenpox.

- Oral aciclovir also seems to effectively treat chickenpox if administered within 24 hours of onset of rash.

    When given later than 24 hours after onset of rash, aciclovir doesn't seem as effective, although the evidence is sparse.

    We haven't found any evidence assessing famciclovir or valaciclovir for treating chickenpox in healthy people.

- In children with malignancy, intravenous aciclovir appears to reduce clinical deterioration from chickenpox.

    We found no evidence assessing how effective aciclovir, famciclovir, or valaciclovir are in treating immunocompromised adults with chickenpox.

(i) **Please visit www.clinicalevidence.bmj.com for full text and references**

What are the effects of interventions to prevent chickenpox in healthy adults and children?	
Beneficial	• Live attenuated vaccine in healthy children
Unknown Effectiveness	• Live attenuated vaccine in healthy adults

What are the effects of interventions to prevent chickenpox in children exposed prenatally?

Unknown Effectiveness	• Aciclovir in children exposed prenatally
	• Famciclovir in children exposed prenatally
	• Valaciclovir in children exposed prenatally
	• Varicella zoster immunoglobulin in children exposed prenatally
	• Zoster immunoglobulin in children exposed prenatally

What are the effects of interventions to prevent chickenpox in immunocompromised adults and children?

Beneficial	• Aciclovir, high dose (more than 320 mg/day) prevention in people with HIV infection
Unknown Effectiveness	• Aciclovir prevention in people with immunocompromise other than HIV
	• Famciclovir (prevention in immunocompromised people)
	• Live attenuated vaccine in immunocompromised people
	• Valaciclovir (prevention in immunocompromised people)
	• Varicella zoster immunoglobulin(prevention in immunocompromised people)
	• Zoster immunoglobulin(prevention in immunocompromised people)

What are the effects of treatments for chickenpox in healthy adults and children?

Likely To Be Beneficial	• Aciclovir (oral) in healthy people (given less than 24 hours after onset of rash)
Unknown Effectiveness	• Aciclovir (oral) treatment in healthy people (given more than 24 hours after onset of rash)
	• Famciclovir (treatment in healthy people)
	• Valaciclovir (treatment in healthy people)

What are the effects of treatments for chickenpox in immunocompromised adults and children?

Likely To Be Beneficial	• Aciclovir (intravenous) for treatment of chickenpox in children with malignancy
Unknown Effectiveness	• Famciclovir (treatment in immunocompromised people)

> • Valaciclovir (treatment in immunocompromised people)

Search date March 2007

DEFINITION Chickenpox is caused by primary infection with VZV. In healthy people, it is usually a mild, self-limiting illness, characterised by low-grade fever, malaise, and a generalised, itchy, vesicular rash.

INCIDENCE/PREVALENCE Chickenpox is extremely contagious. Over 90% of unvaccinated people become infected, but infection occurs at different ages in different parts of the world — over 80% of people have been infected by the age of 10 years in the USA, the UK, and Japan, and by the age of 20–30 years in India, South East Asia, and the West Indies.

AETIOLOGY/RISK FACTORS Chickenpox is caused by exposure to VZV.

PROGNOSIS Infants and children: In healthy children the illness is usually mild and self-limiting. In the USA, mortality in infants and children (aged 1–14 years) with chickenpox is about 7/100,000 in infants, and 1.4/100,000 in children. In Australia, mortality from chickenpox is about 0.5–0.6/100,000 in children aged 1–11 years, and about 1.2/100,000 in infants. Bacterial skin sepsis is the most common complication in children under 5 years of age, and acute cerebellar ataxia is the most common complication in older children; both cause hospital admission in 2–3/10,000 children. **Adults:** Mortality in adults is higher, at about 31/100,000. Varicella pneumonia is the most common complication, causing 20–30 hospital admissions/10,000 adults. Activation of latent VZV infection can cause herpes zoster, also known as shingles (see review on postherpetic neuralgia, p 292). **Cancer chemotherapy:** One case series (77 children with both cancer and chickenpox; 1 child received zoster immune globulin within 72 hours of exposure) found that more children receiving chemotherapy developed progressive chickenpox with multiple organ involvement compared with those in remission (19/60 [32%] of children receiving chemotherapy v 0/17 [0%] of children in remission), and more children died (4/60 [7%] of children receiving chemotherapy v 0/17 [0%] of children in remission). **HIV infection:** One retrospective case series (45 children with AIDS; no treatment reported) found that 25% children with AIDS who acquired chickenpox in hospital developed pneumonia, and 5% died. In a retrospective cohort study (73 children with HIV and chickenpox; 83% with symptomatic HIV; 14 children received varicella zoster immune globulin, 9 within 48 hours of exposure), infection beyond 2 months occurred in 10 children (14%), and recurrent VZV infections occurred in 38 (55%). There was a strong association between an increasing number of recurrences and low CD4 cell counts. Half of recurrent infections involved generalised rashes, and the other half had zoster. **Newborns:** We found no cohort studies of untreated children with perinatal exposure to chickenpox. One cohort study (281 neonates receiving varicella zoster immune globulin because their mothers had developed a chickenpox rash during the month before or after delivery) found that 134 (48%) developed a chickenpox rash and 19 (14%) developed severe chickenpox. Sixteen (84%) of the 19 cases of severe chickenpox occurred in neonates of mothers whose rash had started between 4 days before and 2 days after delivery.

Piero Olliaro

KEY POINTS

- Infection with *Toxoplasma gondii* is asymptomatic or mild in immunocompetent people and leads to lifelong immunity, however, it can have serious consequences in pregnancy.

  About 5 per 1000 non-immune pregnant women may acquire toxoplasma infection, with a 10–100% risk of transmission to the baby.

  Infection is usually acquired from undercooked meat, or fruit and vegetables contaminated with cat faeces.

  Fetal infection can cause eye and brain damage, growth retardation, and intrauterine death.

  Risks of transmission to the baby are higher later in pregnancy, but risks of infection causing harm to the baby are greater earlier in pregnancy.

  Children with subclinical infection at birth may have cognitive, motor, or visual defects that may be difficult to diagnose in early childhood.

- We don't know whether treating infected pregnant women with spiramycin and/or pyrimethamine–sulphonamides reduces the risk of fetal infection, as the few studies that have been done have had conflicting results.

  It is possible that treatment of infection in pregnancy may save the pregnancy without preventing infection, which could increase the prevalence of congenital disease.

Please visit www.clinicalevidence.bmj.com for full text and references

What are the effects on mother and baby of treating toxoplasmosis during pregnancy?

Unknown Effectiveness	• Antiparasitic drugs

Search date March 2004

DEFINITION Toxoplasmosis is caused by the parasite *Toxoplasma gondii*. Infection is asymptomatic or unremarkable in immunocompetent individuals, but leads to a lifelong antibody response. During pregnancy, toxoplasmosis can be transmitted across the placenta and may cause intrauterine death, neonatal growth retardation, mental retardation, ocular defects, and blindness in later life. Congenital toxoplasmosis (confirmed infection of the fetus or newborn) can also present at birth — either as subclinical disease, which may evolve with neurological or ophthalmological disease later in life, or as a disease of varying severity, ranging from mild ocular damage to severe mental retardation.

INCIDENCE/PREVALENCE Reported rates of toxoplasma seroprevalence vary among and within countries, as well as over time. The risk of primary infection is highest in young people, including young women during pregnancy. We found no cohort studies describing annual seroconversion rates in women of childbearing age, or incidence of primary infection. One systematic review (search date 1996) identified 15 studies that reported rates of seroconversion in non-immune pregnant women ranging from 2.4–16/1000 in Europe and from 2–6/1000 in the USA. France began screening for congenital toxoplasmosis in 1978, and during the period 1980–1995 the seroconversion rate during pregnancy in non-immune women was 4–5/1000.

AETIOLOGY/RISK FACTORS Toxoplasma infection is usually acquired by ingesting either sporocysts (from unwashed fruit or vegetables contaminated by cat faeces) or tissue cysts (from raw or undercooked meat). The risk of contracting toxoplasma infection varies with eating habits, contact with cats and other pets, and occupational exposure.

PROGNOSIS One systematic review of studies conducted from 1983–1996 found no population-based prospective studies of the natural history of toxoplasma infection during pregnancy. One systematic review (search date 1997; 9 controlled, non-randomised studies) found that untreated toxoplasmosis acquired during pregnancy was associated with infection rates in children of between 10–100%. We found two European studies that correlated gestation at time of maternal seroconversion with risk of transmission and severity of disease at birth. Risk of transmission increased with gestational age at maternal seroconversion, reaching 70–90% when seroconversion occurred after 30 weeks' gestation. In contrast, the risk of the infant developing clinical disease was highest when maternal seroconversion occurred early in pregnancy. The highest risk of developing early signs of disease (including chorioretinitis and hydrocephaly) was about 10%, recorded when seroconversion occurred between 24 and 30 weeks' gestation. Infants with congenital toxoplasmosis and generalised neurological abnormalities at birth develop mental retardation, growth retardation, blindness or visual defects, seizures, and spasticity. Children with subclinical infection at birth may have cognitive, motor, and visual deficits, which may go undiagnosed for many years. One case-control study (845 school children in Brazil) found mental retardation and retinochoroiditis to be significantly associated with positive toxoplasma serology (population-attributable risk 6–9%).

Marissa Alejandria

KEY POINTS

- Infection with the dengue virus, transmitted by mosquito, ranges from asymptomatic or undifferentiated febrile illness to fatal haemorrhagic fever, and affects up to 100 million people a year worldwide.

  Dengue haemorrhagic fever is characterised by: a sudden onset of high fever; haemorrhages in the skin; gastrointestinal tract, and mucosa; and low platelet counts. Plasma leakage results in fluid in the abdomen and lungs. It typically occurs in children under 15 years.

  Severe dengue haemorrhagic fever is called dengue shock syndrome.

  Dengue haemorrhagic fever and dengue shock syndrome are major causes of hospital admission and mortality in children. Up to 5% of people with dengue haemorrhagic fever die of the infection, depending on availability of appropriate supportive care.

- Intravenous fluids are the standard treatment to expand plasma volume and are likely to be beneficial, but studies to demonstrate their effectiveness would be unethical.

  Crystalloids seem as effective as colloids in children with moderately severe dengue shock syndrome, although we don't know whether they are beneficial in severe dengue shock syndrome.

  There is consensus that blood component transfusion (fresh frozen plasma, packed red blood cells, or platelets) should be added to intravenous fluids in children with coagulopathy or bleeding. The optimal time for beginning transfusion is unclear.

- We don't know whether adding carbazochrome sodium sulfonate (AC-17), corticosteroids, intravenous immunoglobulin, or recombinant activated factor VII to standard intravenous fluids reduces the risks of shock, pleural effusion, or mortality. We also don't know whether adding recombinant activated factor VII to blood component transfusion reduces the risk of bleeding episodes, shock, or mortality. We also don't know whether adding recombitant activated factor VII to blood component transfusion reduces the risk of bleeding episodes, shock, or mortality.

(i) **Please visit www.clinicalevidence.bmj.com for full text and references**

What are the effects of supportive treatments for dengue haemorrhagic fever or dengue shock syndrome in children?

Likely To Be Beneficial	• Adding blood component transfusion to standard intravenous fluids*
	• Crystalloids compared with colloids (evidence crystalloids as effective as colloids in moderately severe dengue shock syndrome; evidence insufficient in severe dengue shock syndrome)
	• Intravenous fluids versus placebo*
Unknown Effectiveness	• Adding carbazochrome sodium sulfonate (AC-17) to standard intravenous fluids
	• Adding corticosteroids to standard intravenous fluids
	• Adding intravenous immunoglobulin to standard intravenous fluids

> - Adding recombinant-activated factor VII to blood component transfusion

Search date November 2006

*Categorisation based on consensus.

DEFINITION Dengue infection is a mosquito-borne arboviral infection. The spectrum of dengue virus infection ranges from asymptomatic or undifferentiated febrile illness to dengue fever and dengue haemorrhagic fever or dengue shock syndrome. An important criterion to consider in the diagnosis of dengue infection is history of travel or residence in a dengue-endemic area within 2 weeks of the onset of fever. **Dengue fever** is an acute febrile illness whose clinical presentation varies with age. Infants and young children may have an undifferentiated febrile disease with a maculopapular rash. Children aged 15 years or older and adults may have either a mild febrile illness, or the classic incapacitating disease (also called "breakbone fever"), presenting with high fever of sudden onset, and non-specific signs and symptoms of: severe headache; pain behind the eyes; muscle, bone, or joint pains; nausea; vomiting; and rash. **Dengue haemorrhagic fever** is characterised by four criteria: acute onset of high fever; haemorrhagic manifestations evidenced by a positive tourniquet test, skin haemorrhages, mucosal and gastrointestinal tract bleeding; thrombocytopenia; and evidence of plasma leakage manifested by a rise or drop in haematocrit, fluid in the lungs or abdomen, or hypoproteinaemia. Dengue haemorrhagic fever is classified into four grades of severity. Presence of thrombocytopenia and haemoconcentration differentiates dengue haemorrhagic fever grades I and II from dengue fever. Grades III and IV dengue haemorrhagic fever are considered **dengue shock syndrome**. This review deals with interventions for dengue haemorrhagic fever and dengue shock syndrome in children.

INCIDENCE/PREVALENCE Dengue fever and dengue haemorrhagic fever are public health problems worldwide, particularly in low-lying areas where *Aedes aegypti*, a domestic mosquito, is present. Cities near to the equator but high in the Andes are free of dengue because *Aedes* mosquitoes do not survive at high altitudes. Worldwide, an estimated 50–100 million cases of dengue fever, and hundreds of thousands of dengue haemorrhagic fever occur yearly. Endemic regions are the Americas, South East Asia, the western Pacific, Africa, and the eastern Mediterranean. Major global demographic changes and their consequences (particularly increases in the density and geographic distribution of the vector with declining vector control; unreliable water supply systems; increasing non-biodegradable container and poor solid waste disposal; increased geographic range of virus transmission owing to increased air travel; and increased population density in urban areas) are responsible for the resurgence of dengue in the past century. The WHO estimates that global temperature rises of 1.0–3.5 °C may increase transmission of dengue fever by shortening the extrinsic incubation period of viruses within the mosquito, adding 20,000–30,000 more fatal cases annually.

AETIOLOGY/RISK FACTORS Dengue virus serotypes 1–4 (DEN 1, 2, 3, 4) belonging to the flavivirus genus are the aetiologic agents. These serotypes are closely related, but antigenically distinct. *Ae aegypti*, the principal vector, transmits the virus to and between humans. Dengue haemorrhagic fever and dengue shock syndrome typically occur in children under the age of 15 years, although dengue fever primarily occurs in adults and older children. Important risk factors influencing who will develop dengue haemorrhagic fever or severe disease during epidemics include the virus strain and serotype, immune status of the host, age, and genetic predisposition. There is evidence that sequential infection or pre-existing antidengue antibodies increases the risk of dengue haemorrhagic fever through antibody dependent enhancement.

PROGNOSIS Dengue fever is an incapacitating disease, but prognosis is favourable in previously healthy adults — although dengue haemorrhagic fever and dengue shock syndrome are major causes of hospital admission and mortality in children. Dengue fever is generally self-limiting, with less than 1% case fatality. The acute phase of the illness lasts for 2–7 days, but the convalescent phase may be prolonged for weeks associated with fatigue and depression, especially in adults. Prognosis in dengue haemorrhagic fever and

(continued over)

(from previous page)

dengue shock syndrome depends on prevention, or early recognition and treatment of shock. Case fatality ranges from 2.5% to 5.0%. Once shock sets in, fatality may be as high as 12–44%. However, in centres with appropriate intensive supportive treatment, fatality can be less than 1%. There is no specific antiviral treatment. The standard treatment is to give intravenous fluids to expand plasma volume. People usually recover after prompt and adequate fluid and electrolyte supportive treatment. The optimal fluid regimen, however, remains the subject of debate. This is particularly important in dengue, where one of the management difficulties is to correct hypovolaemia rapidly without precipitating fluid overload.

Guy de Bruyn

KEY POINTS

- Diarrhoea is watery or liquid stools, usually with an increase in stool weight above 200 g daily and an increase in daily stool frequency.

  An estimated 4000 million cases of diarrhoea occurred worldwide in 1996, resulting in 2.5 million deaths.

- In people from resource-poor countries, antisecretory agents, such as racecadotril, seem to be as effective at improving symptoms of diarrhoea as antimotility agents, such as loperamide, but with fewer adverse effects.

  Empirical treatment with antibiotics also seems to reduce the duration of diarrhoea and improve symptoms in this population, although it can produce adverse effects such as rash, myalgia, and nausea.

  Instructing people to refrain from taking any solid food for 24 hours does not seem a useful treatment, although the evidence for this is sparse.

  We don't know how effective oral rehydration solutions or antibiotics plus antimotility agents are in this population, as we found no RCTs.

- Antisecretory agents, antibiotics, and antimotility agents also seem effective in treating people from resource-rich countries travelling to resource-poor countries.

  We don't know whether antibiotics plus antimotility agents are more effective than either treatment alone or placebo.

  Bismuth subsalicylate is effective in treating travellers' diarrhoea, but less so than loperamide, and with more adverse effects (primarily black tongue and black stools).

  We don't know the effectiveness of oral rehydration solutions or restricting diet in reducing symptoms of diarrhoea in people travelling to resource-poor countires.

- For people from resource-poor countires with mild or moderate diarrhoea, antisecretory agents seem as beneficial as antimotility agents, and cause fewer adverse effects (particularly rebound constipation).

  We found insufficient evidence to allow us to judge the efficacy of antibiotics, antibiotics plus antimotility agents, or oral rehydration solutions in this population.

- Oral rehydration solutions are considered to be beneficial in people from resource-poor countries who have severe diarrhoea.

  Studies have shown that amino acid-based and rice-based oral rehydration solutions are beneficial, but the evidence is less clear about the efficacy of bicarbonate or reduced osmolarity solutions.

- We don't know whether intravenous rehydration is more beneficial than oral rehydration, or enteral rehydration through a nasogastric tube.

  We don't know whether antimotility agents, antisecretory agents, antibiotics, or antiobiotics plus antimotility agents are effective for treating people with severe diarrhoea in resource-poor countries.

Please visit www.clinicalevidence.bmj.com for full text and references

What are the effects of treatments for acute diarrhoea in adults living in resource-rich countries?

Likely To Be Beneficial	• Antimotility agents in resource-rich countries • Antisecretory agents in resource-rich countries
Trade-off Between Benefits And Harms	• Antibiotics (empirical use for mild to moderate diarrhoea) in resource-rich countries
Unknown Effectiveness	• Antibiotics plus antimotility agents in resource-rich countries • Diet in resource-rich countries • Oral rehydration solutions in resource-rich countries

What are the effects of treatments for mild to moderate diarrhoea in adults from resource-rich countries travelling to resource-poor countries?

Likely To Be Beneficial	• Antibiotics (empirical use for mild to moderate diarrhoea) for travellers' diarrhoea • Antimotility agents for travellers' diarrhoea • Bismuth subsalicylate for travellers' diarrhoea (reduced duration of diarrhoea compared with placebo, but less effective than loperamide)
Trade-off Between Benefits And Harms	• Antisecretory agents for travellers' diarrhoea
Unknown Effectiveness	• Antibiotics plus antimotility agents for travellers' diarrhoea • Diet for travellers' diarrhoea • Oral rehydration solutions for travellers' diarrhoea

What are the effects of treatments for mild to moderate diarrhoea in adults living in resource-poor countries?

Likely To Be Beneficial	• Antimotility agents in resource-poor countries • Antisecretory agents for mild to moderate diarrhoea in resource-poor countries
Unknown Effectiveness	• Antibiotics (empirical use) for mild to moderate diarrhoea in resource-poor countries • Antibiotics plus antimotility agents for mild to moderate diarrhoea in resource-poor countries • Oral rehydration solutions for mild to moderate diarrhoea in resource-poor countries

What are the effects of treatments for severe diarrhoea in adults living in resource-poor countries?

Beneficial	• Amino acid rehydration solutions for severe diarrhoea in resource-poor countries
	• Rice-based oral rehydration solution for severe diarrhoea in resource-poor countries
	• Standard oral rehydration solution for severe diarrhoea in resource-poor countries*
Unknown Effectiveness	• Antibiotics (empirical use) for severe diarrhoea in resource-poor countries
	• Antibiotics plus antimotility agents for severe diarrhoea in resource-poor countries
	• Antimotility agents for severe diarrhoea in resource-poor countries
	• Antisecretory agents for severe diarrhoea in resource-poor countries
	• Bicarbonate oral rehydration solution for severe diarrhoea in resource-poor countries
	• Intravenous rehydration (compared with nasogastric tube rehydration or oral rehydration solution alone) for severe diarrhoea in resource-poor countries
	• Reduced osmolarity oral rehydration solution for severe diarrhoea in resource-poor countries

Search date January 2007

*Categorisation based on consensus. RCTs are unlikely to be conducted.

DEFINITION Diarrhoea is watery or liquid stools, usually with an increase in stool weight above 200 g daily and an increase in daily stool frequency. This review covers empirical treatment of suspected infectious diarrhoea in adults.

INCIDENCE/PREVALENCE An estimated 4000 million cases of diarrhoea occurred worldwide in 1996, resulting in 2.5 million deaths. In the USA, the estimated incidence for infectious intestinal disease is 0.44 episodes per person per year (1 episode per person every 2.3 years), resulting in about one consultation with a doctor per person every 28 years. A recent community study in the UK reported an incidence of 19 cases per 100 person-years, of which 3.3 cases per 100 person-years resulted in consultation with a general practitioner. Both estimates derive from population-based studies, including both adults and children. The epidemiology of travellers' diarrhoea is not well understood. Incidence is higher in travellers visiting resource-poor countries, but it varies widely by location and season of travel. The incidence of diarrhoea in adults in resource-poor countries is largely unknown owing to the lack of large-scale surveillance studies in these countries.

AETIOLOGY/RISK FACTORS The cause of diarrhoea depends on geographical location, standards of food hygiene, sanitation, water supply, and season. Commonly identified causes of sporadic diarrhoea in adults in resource-poor countries include *Campylobacter*, *Salmonella*, *Shigella*, *Escherichia coli*, *Yersinia*, protozoa, and viruses. No pathogens are identified in more than half of people with diarrhoea. In returning travellers, about 50% of

(continued over)

(from previous page)

episodes are caused by bacteria such as enterotoxigenic *E coli*, *Salmonella*, *Shigella*, *Campylobacter*, *Vibrio*, enteroadherent *E coli*, *Yersinia*, and *Aeromonas* .

PROGNOSIS In resource-rich countries, death from infectious diarrhoea is rare, although serious complications, including severe dehydration and renal failure, can occur and may necessitate admission to hospital. Elderly people and those in long-term care have an increased risk of death. In resource-poor countries, diarrhoea is reported to cause more deaths in children under 5 years of age than any other condition. Few studies have examined which factors predict poor outcome in adults.

Suzanne Norris and Abdul Hadi Mohsen

KEY POINTS

- Nearly a third of the world's population has been infected by hepatitis B at some point, and at least 350 million people have become chronic carriers. Progressive liver damage occurs in up to 25% of carriers.

    In areas of high endemicity, transmission occurs largely in childhood, from an infected mother to her baby, or between members of a household.

    In areas of low endemicity, transmission usually occurs as a result of sexual activity, intravenous drug use, or occupational exposure.

    The risk of developing hepatitis B depends largely on the vaccination policy of the country of residence, and routine vaccination of all infants is recommended by the WHO.

- Selective vaccination of infants with recombinant or plasma-derived vaccines in countries with high endemicity of hepatitis B reduces occurrence and chronic carrier state.

    Combining vaccine with hepatitis B immunoglobulin is more effective than vaccine alone.

- Universal vaccination of infants with recombinant or plasma-derived vaccines, in countries with high endemicity of hepatitis B, reduces the risk of acute hepatitis, chronic carrier state, and complications of chronic infection, and may be more effective than selective vaccination of high-risk individuals.

    Vaccination of children born to hepatitis B surface antigen- (HBsAg) positive mothers prevents development of a chronic carrier state compared with placebo.

- Universal vaccination of infants or adolescents in low endemic areas may reduce the risk of infection, or of developing a chronic carrier state, but we don't know how different vaccination strategies compare, as no studies have been done.

- Selective vaccination of high-risk individuals in countries with low hepatitis B endemicity may prevent acute infection and development of a chronic carrier state.

    Uptake of vaccination may be low, even in high-risk groups.

- Vaccination is associated generally with mild adverse effects, although more serious autoimmune adverse effects can occur rarely.

- We don't know whether selective vaccination of people with known chronic liver disease not caused by hepatitis B reduces subsequent infection rates, as few studies have been done.

Please visit www.clinicalevidence.bmj.com for full text and references

What are the effects of vaccination against hepatitis B infection in countries with high endemicity?

Beneficial	• Selective vaccination of high-risk individuals (evidence only for children born to hepatitis B surface antigen- (HBsAg) positive mothers; plasma-derived vaccine and recombinant vaccine equally effective, more so when combined with hepatitis B immunoglobulin)
	• Universal vaccination of infants (more effective than placebo or no treatment; limited evidence that it may be better than selective vaccination of high-risk individuals)

What are the effects of vaccination against hepatitis B infection in countries with low endemicity?

Likely To Be Beneficial	• Selective vaccination of high-risk individuals • Universal vaccination of adolescents • Universal vaccination of infants
Unknown Effectiveness	• Selective vaccination of people with known chronic liver disease not caused by hepatitis B

Search date November 2006

DEFINITION Hepatitis B is a viral infectious disease with an incubation period of 40–160 days. Acute hepatitis B infection is characterised by anorexia, vague abdominal discomfort, nausea and vomiting, jaundice, and occasional fever. Illness is associated with deranged liver function tests (especially raised alanine transaminases) and presence of serological markers of acute hepatitis B infection (e.g. hepatitis B surface antigen [HBsAg], anti-HBc IgM).

INCIDENCE/PREVALENCE The incidence of acute hepatitis B, and prevalence of its chronic carrier state, vary widely across the globe. In areas with high endemicity (HBsAg prevalence at least 8%: e.g. South East Asia and Africa), more than half of the population becomes infected at some point. In countries with low endemicity (HBsAg prevalence below 2%: e.g. North America, western Europe, and Australia), most of the population does not become infected. Nearly a third of the world's population has been infected by hepatitis B at some point, and at least 350 million people (5–6% of the world's population) are currently chronic carriers of hepatitis B infection.

AETIOLOGY/RISK FACTORS In countries with high endemicity, most transmissions occur during childhood from an infected mother to her baby (vertical transmission) or from one family member to another (horizontal transmission). Horizontal transmission is thought to be an important route of hepatitis B infection during early childhood, and probably occurs mainly through unnoticed contact with blood from infected family members. In countries with high endemicity, the proportion of chronic HBsAg carriage attributable to vertical transmission has been estimated at 5–50%. The proportion of chronic HBsAg carriage attributable to horizontal transmission is not known, although one survey in China found that 27.2% of families had one or more HBsAg-positive members. In countries with low endemicity, most hepatitis B infections occur later — from sexual activity, intravenous drug use, or occupational exposure. Less frequent causes of infection include household contact, regular haemodialysis, transmission from a healthcare professional, and receipt of infected organs or blood products. The vaccination policy of a country is a large determinant of the risk of developing hepatitis B. Since the development of plasma-derived hepatitis B vaccine in the early 1980s, subsequently replaced by recombinant vaccine, many countries have adopted a policy of universal vaccination of infants. On the basis of disease burden, the WHO recommended that hepatitis B vaccine be incorporated into routine infant and childhood vaccination programmes in countries with high endemicity by 1995 and in all countries by 1997. However, in many countries with low endemicity, universal vaccination policy remains controversial and has still not been adopted. Some of these countries have adopted a policy of selective vaccination of high-risk individuals. Others have adopted a universal adolescent-vaccination policy.

PROGNOSIS Hepatitis B infection resolves after the acute infection in 90–95% of cases. In the remainder (5–10%) it may result in several serious sequelae. Massive hepatic necrosis occurs in 1% of people with acute viral hepatitis, leading to a serious and often fatal condition called acute fulminant hepatitis. Between 2% and 10% of those infected as adults become chronic carriers, indicated by HBsAg persistence for more than 6 months. Chronic carriage is more frequent in those infected as children, and reaches up to 90% in those infected during the perinatal period. Between 20% and 25% of chronic carriers develop a progressive chronic liver disease. In about a quarter to a third of cases, this progresses to cirrhosis and hepatocellular carcinoma. These complications usually arise in older adults, and are major causes of mortality in populations with high hepatitis B endemicity. Observational studies suggest that, in these countries, almost 80% of chronic liver disease and cirrhosis are attributed to hepatitis B, and these complications lead to at least 1 million deaths every year worldwide.

270 | Hepatitis C (chronic)

Abdul Mohsen and Suzanne Norris

KEY POINTS

- Chronic hepatitis C virus infection is defined as persistent, detectable serum hepatitis C virus RNA for a period greater than 6 months, with or without derangement in liver function tests.

  60–85% of people infected with hepatitis C virus will go on to develop chronic hepatitis C, which is now believed to affect 3% of the world's population.

  Complications of chronic hepatitis C virus infection include cirrhosis, compensated and decompensated liver disease, and hepatocellular carcinoma.

  Many people chronically infected with hepatitis C virus remain asymptomatic, including a significant number of those who progress to cirrhosis, so routine screening of people in high-risk groups is advisable.

- Interferon monotherapy produces a sustained virological response in both treatment-naïve people, and people with cirrhosis or advanced fibrosis.

  Interferon also improves liver histology, although it may not be effective in preventing hepatocellular carcinoma in people with cirrhosis.

  Efficacy is dependent upon duration of treatment, with 12-month treatments appearing to be more effective — but also more likely to produce adverse effects — than 6-month treatments.

  6 MU of interferon three times weekly seems no more effective at achieving sustained virological response than 3 MU three times weekly, but is more likely to produce adverse effects.

  Adding ribavirin to interferon regimens further increases the likelihood of achieving sustained virological response, but also increases the risk of anaemia. Efficacy of combination therapy depends on genotype, with genotype 1-infected people requiring 12 months' treatment, and genotype 2- and genotype 3-infected people requiring only 6 months' treatment.

- Peginterferon monotherapy increases the proportion of treatment-naïve people who achieve sustained virological response compared with standard interferon monotherapy.

  180 µg once-weekly doses seem more effective than 135 µg weekly doses.

  Adding ribavirin to peginterferon increases the likelihood of achieving sustained virological response compared with either peginterferon alone or standard interferon plus ribavirin.

- In people previously non-responsive to interferon monotherapy, treatment with interferon alpha plus ribavirin increases the likelihood of achieving sustained virological response.

  This effect appears greater when the interferon dose is higher than 3 MU three times weekly, or the duration of the treatment is 12 months or longer.

  We found no studies examining the effectiveness of peginterferon monotherapy in this population, although, because interferon plus ribavirin is effective, there is consensus that peginterferon plus ribavirin is also likely to be beneficial.

- In people who relapse after interferon monotherapy, treatment with interferon plus ribavirin is more likely than interferon treatment alone to achieve sustained virological response.

  Again, although we found no studies, there is general consensus that peginterferon plus ribavirin is likely to improve the probability of achieving sustained virological response.

- In people coinfected with hepatitis C virus and HIV, peginterferon plus ribavirin is more likely than standard interferon plus ribavirin treatment to achieve sustained virological response.

  We do not know how effective interferon alone or peginterferon alone are in people coinfected with hepatitis C virus and HIV.

(i) **Please visit www.clinicalevidence.bmj.com for full text and references**

What are the effects of interventions in treatment-naïve people with chronic infection but without liver decompensation?

Beneficial	• Interferon in treatment-naïve people
	• Interferon plus ribavirin in treatment-naïve people
	• Peginterferon in treatment-naïve people
	• Peginterferon plus ribavirin in treatment-naïve people

What are the effects of interventions to treat people with chronic infection, but without liver decompensation, who have not responded to interferon treatment?

Beneficial	• Interferon alfa plus ribavirin in non-responders to interferon
Unknown Effectiveness	• Interferon retreatment in non-responders to interferon
	• Peginterferon in non-responders to interferon
	• Peginterferon plus ribavirin in non-responders to interferon

What are the effects of interventions in people with chronic infection, but without liver decompensation, who relapse after interferon treatment?

Beneficial	• Interferon alfa plus ribavirin in people who have relapsed
	• Interferon in people who have relapsed (less effective than interferon alfa plus ribavirin at sustaining virological response)
Likely To Be Beneficial	• Peginterferon plus ribavirin in people who have relapsed*
Unknown Effectiveness	• Peginterferon in people who have relapsed

What are the effects of interventions in people with chronic hepatitis C infection, who also have HIV?

Likely To Be Beneficial	• Interferon alfa plus ribavirin in people coinfected with hepatitis C virus and HIV (increased rates of sustained viral response from baseline but less effective than peginterferon plus ribavirin)
	• Peginterferon plus ribavirin in people co infected with hepatitis C virus and HIV
Unknown Effectiveness	• Interferon in people coinfected with hepatitis C virus and HIV

> • Peginterferon in people coinfected with hepatitis C virus and HIV

Search date May 2006

*We found no RCTs. Categorisation based on consensus.

DEFINITION Hepatitis C virus (HCV), identified in 1989, is a member of the flaviviridae family of spherical, enveloped, positive-strand RNA viruses. There are six different HCV genotypes. Genotype 1 is the most common, and the most resistant to treatment. Chronic HCV infection is defined as persistent, detectable serum HCV RNA for a period greater than 6 months, with or without derangement in liver function tests. This is in contrast to acute HCV infection, in which serum HCV RNA clears within 6 months. Prospective studies have shown that 60–85% of HCV-infected people will develop chronic infection. This review will only deal with interventions used to treat chronic HCV infection without liver decompensation. The effect of treatment is measured by the presence or absence of detectable serum HCV RNA. The loss of detectable HCV RNA at the end of the treatment period is defined as the end of treatment-virological response. The loss of detectable HCV RNA 24 weeks or more after the completion of treatment is termed the sustained virological response (SVR). Response to treatment is defined as the loss of detectable serum HCV RNA. **Non-response** is defined as a failure to clear serum HCV RNA during the treatment period. A **relapse** from treatment is defined as loss of serum HCV RNA during treatment, which reappears during the follow-up period, typically within 24 weeks of treatment episode.

INCIDENCE/PREVALENCE HCV has emerged as a major viral pandemic over the past two decades, with about 3% of the world's population chronically infected. HCV prevalence varies throughout the world, with the highest number of infections reported in Egypt (6–28%). In the USA, an estimated four million people are positive for HCV antibodies, reflecting a prevalence rate of 2%, and about 35,000 new HCV infections are estimated to occur each year. In Europe, the prevalence of HCV infection ranges from about 0.5% to 2%. Diagnosis of HCV infection is often the result of active screening, because many people chronically infected with HCV remain asymptomatic, including a significant number of those who progress to cirrhosis. The true incidence of HCV is therefore difficult to calculate accurately, because this relates to the prevalence of risk factors for HCV transmission, in particular injection drug use.

AETIOLOGY/RISK FACTORS HCV is mainly blood borne, and transmission occurs primarily through exposure to infected blood. This exposure may occur because of the use of infected needles used for injection drug use, blood transfusion or solid organ transplantation from infected donors in the absence of universal screening procedures, maternal (vertical) transmission, unsafe medical practices, and occupational exposure to infected blood. As a result of HCV screening, the absolute risk of acquiring infection through blood components or products is now small — less than 1/400,000 units of blood transfused. HCV vertical transmission is uncommon, with a transmission rate of less than 6%. Poverty, high-risk sexual behaviour, and having less than 12 years of education are linked to an increased risk of infection. However, in some cases, no risk factors can be identified.

PROGNOSIS The spectrum of liver disease and the rate of disease progression vary in people with chronic HCV infection. Complications of chronic HCV infection include cirrhosis, compensated and decompensated liver disease, and hepatocellular carcinoma. Studies suggest that a third of people with chronic HCV infection are "rapid progressors" (time from infection to cirrhosis less than 20 years); a third are "intermediate progressors" (time to cirrhosis 20–50 years); and a third are "slow or non-progressors" (time to cirrhosis more than 50 years). Factors associated with disease progression include: older age at acquisition; male sex; coinfection with HIV, hepatitis B virus, or both; coexisting liver disease; and excessive alcohol consumption. In people who develop cirrhosis, the 5-year risk of decompensation is 15–20%, the 5-year risk of hepatocellular carcinoma is 10%, and in those who develop cirrhosis, the annual risk of hepatocellular carcinoma is 1–5% a year.

Tom Jefferson

KEY POINTS

- Influenza viruses are constantly altering their antigenic structure, and every year the WHO recommends which strains of influenza should be included in vaccines.

  During the autumn–winter months (influenza seasons), influenza circulates more frequently, causing a greater proportion of influenza-like illness, and sometimes serious seasonal epidemics.

  The incidence of infection depends on the underlying immunity of the population.

- When a significantly different form of influenza occurs by mutation, it can greatly increase infection rates, as well as morbidity and mortality (a pandemic).

- Influenza and influenza-like illness (caused by a range of other viruses) are clinically indistinguishable.

  Trials of vaccines assess how to prevent the symptoms and consequences of both, as well as infection rates.

- Vaccines are effective in reducing infection and school absence in children over 2 years old, but there is no evidence that they reduce transmission, hospitalisation, pneumonia, or death.

- Live or inactivated vaccines are effective in reducing infection and in slightly reducing absence from work in adults, but there is no evidence that they reduce transmission, hospitalisation, pneumonia, or death.

- There is poor-quality evidence from cohort studies that vaccines are effective in the institutionalised elderly, but there is little good-quality evidence for the elderly population in general.

- Zanamivir and oseltamivir provide symptomatic relief, or prevent symptoms if administered early in the disease, but do not prevent infection.

  Zanamivir and oseltamivir interrupt household transmission of seasonal influenza, prevent hospitalisations, and reduce, but do not suppress, viral excretion from the nose.

  These agents cause fewer adverse effects than amantadine and rimantadine, and there is less evidence of resistance.

- Although amantadine and rimantadine provide symptomatic relief or prevent symptoms if administered early in influenza A, they engender viral resistance.

  Amantadine and rimantadine do not prevent infection and transmission, and cause harms, especially in a prophylactic role.

- Amantadine was ineffective in the 1968–69 pandemic, and zanamivir, oseltamivir, and newer vaccines are untested in a pandemic.

- Symptomatic relief with echinacea, vitamin C, and decongestants in influenza-like illness is covered in the review common cold, p 491.

- Single studies reporting data for one or two seasons are difficult to interpret, and not easy to generalise from, because of the marked variability of viral circulation.

Please visit www.clinicalevidence.bmj.com for full text and references

What are the effects of vaccines to prevent influenza?

Likely To Be Beneficial	• Vaccines in adults (prevention of cases)

	• Vaccines in children (prevention of symptoms and/or infection)
Unknown Effectiveness	• Vaccines in the elderly (prevention of cases and complications)

What are the effects of antiviral chemoprophylaxis of influenza?

Likely To Be Beneficial	• Orally inhaled zanamivir (prevention of symptoms in influenza A and B)
	• Oseltamivir (oral) (prevention of symptoms in influenza A and B)
Likely To Be Ineffective Or Harmful	• Oral amantadine to prevent influenza*
	• Oral rimantadine to prevent influenza

What are the effects of antiviral medications to treat influenza?

Likely To Be Beneficial	• Orally inhaled zanamivir for early treatment of influenza A or B (reduced duration of symptoms and incidence of complications)
	• Oral oseltamivir for early treatment of influenza A and B (reduced duration of symptoms and incidence of complications)
Likely To Be Ineffective Or Harmful	• Oral amantadine for early treatment of influenza A*
	• Oral rimantadine for early treatment of influenza A*

Search date April 2007

*Categorisation based on consensus.

DEFINITION Influenza is an acute respiratory illness caused by infection with influenza A and B viruses. The illness can affect both the upper and lower respiratory tract and is often accompanied by systemic signs and symptoms, such as abrupt onset of fever, chills, non-productive cough, myalgias, headache, nasal congestion, sore throat, and fatigue. **Diagnosis:** Not all people infected with influenza viruses become symptomatic, and not everybody with the above symptoms will have influenza. This is because different viral and bacterial circulating agents cause an influenza-like illness with a clinical picture each year, which is indistinguishable from influenza. Between 40% and 85% of infections with influenza result in clinical illness, depending on age and pre-existing immunity to the virus. One systematic review (search date 2004, 6 RCTs in Europe, North America, and the southern hemisphere, 7164 people) of symptoms of influenza found that, in all age groups, the likelihood of influenza was decreased by the absence of fever (OR 0.40, 95% CI 0.25 to 0.66), cough (OR 0.42, 95% CI 0.31 to 0.57), or nasal congestion (OR 0.49, 95% CI 0.42 to 0.59). It found that, in people aged 60 or older, the probability of influenza was increased by the combination of fever, cough, and acute onset (OR 5.4, 95% CI 3.8 to 7.7), fever and cough (OR 5.0, 95% CI 3.5 to 6.9), fever alone (OR 3.8, 95% CI 2.8 to 5.0), malaise (OR 2.6, 95% CI, 2.2 to 3.1), or chills (OR, 2.6, 95% CI, 2.0 to 3.2), and also found that influenza was less likely if sneezing was present (OR, 0.47, 95% CI, 0.24 to 0.92). Although influenza is usually diagnosed clinically, genuine influenza infection can only be diagnosed with laboratory confirmation, either by culture, serological responses, or by bedside testing. The rapid bedside diagnostic tests available on the market are mainly antigen-detection immunoassays and (unlike laboratory tests, such as culture or reverse transcription–polymerase chain reaction) can be carried out within 30 minutes. However, the results must be interpreted with caution. During times of low influenza viral circulation, the positive predictive value is low, leading to an increased proportion of false positive results. In times of high viral circulation, the negative predictive value is low, leading to an increased proportion of false negatives. It is also impractical to test all potential influenza cases. If a good surveillance system is in place, with quick feedback, the positive predictive value of clinical diagnosis alone (based on high fever and a cough) will be similar to the bedside test (79–87%). **Population:** For the purpose of this review, we have included trials that assessed both influenza-like illness and influenza, which are clinically indistinguishable. Where appropriate, the applicability of data to influenza pandemic has been discussed.

INCIDENCE/PREVALENCE Seasonal influenza: Circulation of seasonal influenza viruses can vary between years, seasons, and even settings. In temperate areas, seasonal influenza activity typically peaks between late December and early March in the northern hemisphere, and between May and September in the southern hemisphere. In tropical areas, there is no temporal peak in influenza activity through the year. The annual incidence of influenza varies, and depends partly on the underlying level of population immunity to circulating influenza viruses. One localised study in the USA found that serological conversion, with or without symptoms, occurred in 10–20% of people a year, with the highest infection rates in people aged under 20 years. A systematic review in people aged up to 19 years found that the average incidence of influenza was between 5% and 10%. The proportion of people affected by circulating influenza is higher in institutions and in areas of overcrowding. **Pandemic influenza:** The incidence of symptomatic influenza depends on, among other factors, the susceptibility of the host. Occasionally, a new type of influenza virus appears, generated either by direct mutation or by reassortment of the viral genome. Because immunity to this new virus is low, it is able to behave in an aggressive way, causing morbidity and mortality on a global scale, mainly because of the body's inability to prevent the creation of a high viral load, the cytopathic effect of the new virus, and the complications in target organs, such as lungs and airways. Widespread epidemics are known as pandemics. In the 20th century, three pandemics were caused by different influenza A viral subtypes (see aetiology): in 1918–9 (H1N1), 1957 (H2N2), and 1968 (H3N2). **Avian influenza:** Influenza infection may also appear as a zoonotic infection, with direct spread of the avian virus to humans. In April 2003, 87 people in the Netherlands were infected with avian virus H7N7. In most cases, the only symptom was conjunctivitis. However, a 57-year-old vet dealing with veterinary public-health interventions died of acute respiratory distress. An avian virus (H5N1) has been transmitted from bird to human (and occasionally from human to human) sporadically since 1997. Such transmission has frequently taken place in situations of poor hygiene and close proximity between birds and humans.

AETIOLOGY/RISK FACTORS Viral classification: The influenza virus is composed of a protein envelope around an RNA core. On the surface of the envelope are two antigens: neuraminidase (N antigen) and haemagglutinin (H antigen). The influenza virus has a marked propensity to mutate its external antigenic composition to escape the host's immune defences. Given this extreme mutability, a classification of viral subtype A based on H and N typing has been introduced. **Transmission:** Influenza viruses are transmitted primarily from person to person through respiratory droplets disseminated during sneezing, coughing, and talking, and through contact with contaminated surfaces. The incubation period of influenza is 1–4 days, and infected adults are usually contagious from the day before symptom onset until 5 days after symptom onset. **Pandemic influenza:** Pandemics are thought to originate mostly in southern China, where ducks (the animal reservoir and breeding ground for new strains), pigs (which are thought to be the biological intermediate host, or "mixing vessel", and humans live in close proximity. Pigs are considered to be plausible intermediate hosts because their respiratory epithelial cells have receptors for both avian (i.e. duck) and human viral haemagglutinins. Minor changes in viral antigenic configurations, known as "drift", cause local or more circumscribed epidemics.

(continued over)

(from previous page)

PROGNOSIS The symptoms of uncomplicated influenza usually resolve within 1 week, although cough and fatigue may persist. Complications include otitis media, bacterial sinusitis, secondary bacterial pneumonia, and, less commonly, viral pneumonia, respiratory failure, and exacerbations of underlying disease. In the UK, 1.3% of people with influenza-like illness are hospitalised each year (95% CI 0.6% to 2.6%). It is estimated that 300–400 deaths each year are attributable to influenza, rising to in excess of 29,000 during an epidemic. The risk of hospitalisation is highest in people 65 years or older, in young children, and in people with chronic medical conditions. Over 90% of influenza-related deaths during recent seasonal epidemics in the USA have been in people 65 years or older. During influenza pandemics, morbidity and mortality may be high in younger age groups. Severe illness is more common with influenza A infections than with influenza B infections. For pandemic influenza, see incidence.

Diana Lockwood

KEY POINTS

- Leprosy is a chronic granulomatous disease caused by *Mycobacterium leprae*, primarily affecting the peripheral nerves and skin.

    The WHO field leprosy classification is based on the number of skin lesions: single-lesion leprosy (1 lesion), paucibacillary leprosy (2–5 skin lesions), and multibacillary leprosy (more than 5 skin lesions).

    Worldwide, about 720,000 new cases of leprosy are reported each year, and about 2 million people have leprosy-related disabilities.

- Vaccination is the most efficient method of preventing the contraction of leprosy.

    BCG vaccination reduces the incidence of leprosy, although we don't know for sure if BCG vaccination plus killed *M leprae* improves its effectiveness.

    ICRC vaccine prevents leprosy and produces few adverse effects, although its formulation is unclear and we only found evidence in one geographical area.

    Mycobacterium w vaccine reduces the incidence of leprosy compared with placebo, but is less effective than ICRC or BCG (alone or with killed *M leprae*).

- Leprosy is generally treated with multidrug programmes.

    Despite sparse good RCT or cohort study evidence, there is consensus that multidrug treatment (rifampicin plus clofazimine plus dapsone) is highly effective for treating multibacillary leprosy.

    Multidrug treatment with rifampicin plus dapsone is believed to improve skin lesions, nerve impairment, and relapse rates in people with paucibacillary leprosy, despite a lack of good evidence.

    Multiple-dose treatments with rifampicin monthly plus dapsone daily for 6 months are more effective than single-dose treatments with rifampicin plus minocycline plus ofloxacin for treating people with single skin lesions (although both achieve high cure rates).

(i) **Please visit www.clinicalevidence.bmj.com for full text and references**

What are the effects of interventions to prevent leprosy?	
Beneficial	• BCG plus killed *Mycobacterium leprae* vaccine
	• BCG vaccine
Likely To Be Beneficial	• ICRC vaccine
Unlikely To Be Beneficial	• *Mycobacterium w* vaccine (reduced incidence of leprosy, but may be less effective than BCG vaccine alone, BCG plus killed *Mycobacterium leprae* vaccine, or ICRC vaccine)

What are the effects of treatments for leprosy?	
Beneficial	• Multidrug treatment for multibacillary leprosy*
	• Multidrug treatment for paucibacillary leprosy*

- Multiple-dose compared with single-dose treatment for single-skin-lesion leprosy (both achieve high cure rates but multiple dose is likely to achieve a higher rate)

Search date March 2006

*Categorisation based on observational evidence and consensus; RCTs unlikely to be conducted.

DEFINITION Leprosy is a chronic granulomatous disease caused by *Mycobacterium leprae*, primarily affecting the peripheral nerves and skin. The clinical picture depends on the individual's immune response to *M leprae*. At the tuberculoid end of the Ridley–Jopling scale, individuals have good cell-mediated immunity and few skin lesions. At the lepromatous end of the scale, individuals have low reactivity for *M leprae*, causing uncontrolled bacterial spread and skin and mucosal infiltration. Peripheral nerve damage occurs across the spectrum. Nerve damage may occur before, during, or after treatment. Some people have no nerve damage, while others develop anaesthesia of the hands and feet, which puts them at risk of developing neuropathic injury. Weakness and paralysis of the small muscles of the hands, feet, and eyes puts people at risk of developing deformity and contractures. Loss of the fingers and toes is caused by by repeated injury in a weak, anaesthetic limb. These visible deformities cause stigmatisation. Classification is based on clinical appearance and bacterial index of lesions. The WHO field leprosy classification is based on the number of skin lesions: single-lesion leprosy (1 lesion), paucibacillary leprosy (2–5 skin lesions), and multibacillary leprosy (more than 5 skin lesions).

INCIDENCE/PREVALENCE Worldwide, about 720,000 new cases of leprosy are reported each year, and about 2 million people have leprosy-related disabilities. Six major endemic countries (India, Brazil, Myanmar, Madagascar, Nepal, and Mozambique) account for 88% of all new cases. Cohort studies show a peak of disease presentation between 10 and 20 years of age. After puberty, there are twice as many cases in males as in females.

AETIOLOGY/RISK FACTORS *M leprae* is discharged from the nasal mucosa of people with untreated lepromatous leprosy, and spreads, via the recipient's nasal mucosa, to infect their skin and nerves. It is a hardy organism and has been shown to survive outside human hosts in India for many months. Risk factors for infection, when known, include household contact with a person with leprosy. We found no good evidence of an association with HIV infection, nutrition, or socioeconomic status.

PROGNOSIS Complications of leprosy include nerve damage, immunological reactions, and bacillary infiltration. Without treatment, tuberculoid infection eventually resolves spontaneously. Most people with borderline tuberculoid and borderline lepromatous leprosy gradually develop lepromatous infection. Many people have peripheral nerve damage at the time of diagnosis, ranging from 15% in Bangladesh to 55% in Ethiopia. Immunological reactions can occur with or without antibiotic treatment. Further nerve damage occurs through immune-mediated reactions (type 1 reactions) and neuritis. Erythema nodosum leprosum (type 2 reactions) is an immune complex-mediated reaction causing fever, malaise, and neuritis, which occurs in 20% of people with lepromatous leprosy, and 5% with borderline lepromatous leprosy. Secondary impairments (wounds, contractures, and digit resorption) occur in 33–56% of people with established nerve damage. We found no recent information on mortality.

Ashley M Croft

KEY POINTS

- Malaria transmission occurs most frequently in environments with a humidity over 60% and ambient temperature of 25–30 °C. Risks increase with longer visits, and depend on activity.

  Infection can follow a single mosquito bite. Incubation is usually 10–14 days, but can be up to 18 months depending on the strain of parasite.

  Complications are usually due to delayed or inappropriate treatment, but up to 88% of previously healthy travellers recover fully with prompt treatment. Older people have a worse prognosis.

- Many of the studies on prevention of malaria have been performed on people other than travellers, such as residents of endemic malaria areas.

- Various non-drug preventive measures may be effective, but some may have adverse effects.

  There is consensus that skin-applied chemical repellents containing DEET (diethyltoluamide) reduce the risk of insect bites. Picaridin is a newer and possibly more effective repellent than DEET, but it has not yet been evaluated against clinical outcomes.

  Using treated bednets or clothing may be beneficial.

  We don't know whether insecticide sprays or lifestyle changes, such as wearing full-length clothing, dietary supplementation, use of air conditioning or electric fans, mosquito coils or vaporising mats, bath or chemical base oils, skin-applied plant-based repellents, electronic buzzers, outdoor smoke, vaccines, or biological control measures can reduce the risk of malaria infection. Mosquito coils and vaporising mats should not be used indoors.

- Various drug treatments may be effective in preventing malaria, but we cannot be sure which is the most effective drug regimen, and most have adverse effects which can sometimes be serious.

  Atovaquone–proguanil and doxycycline may be beneficial.

  Chloroquine is considered to reduce the risk of malaria in travellers to areas where chloroquine resistance is low, although few studies have been done.

  Mefloquine and chloroquine–proguanil may be beneficial, but their adverse effects must also be considered.

  We don't know whether pyrimethamine–dapsone or pyrimethamine–sulfadoxine are effective.

  Children may be at risk of encephalopathic adverse effects from topical insect repellents containing DEET. There is consensus that chloroquine is effective and safe in preventing malaria in children, but we don't know whether this is the case for any other treatments.

- Insecticide-treated bed nets may be effective in preventing malaria in pregnant women.

  We found no RCT evidence about insecticide-treated clothing in pregnant women, but evidence in non-pregnant adults that it is effective is likely to be generalisable to pregnant women. However, there are attendant risks.

  There is consensus that chloroquine may be beneficial in pregnant women.

- Atovaquone–proguanil may have no more adverse effects than placebo in airline pilots, but we have no direct evidence assessing whether treatments are safe or effective in this occupational group. There is no reason to suggest that evidence of benefit of atovaquone–proguanil, chloroquine, or doxycycline in other adults would not be generalisable to airline pilots.

- CAUTION: Adverse effects of primaquine and amodiaquine limit their use in preventing malaria.

(i) **Please visit www.clinicalevidence.bmj.com for full text and references**

What are the effects of non-drug interventions to prevent malaria in non-pregnant adult travellers?

Likely To Be Beneficial	• Insecticide-treated bed nets in non-pregnant adult travellers • Insecticide-treated clothing in non-pregnant adults • Skin-applied chemical repellents containing DEET or picaridin in non-pregnant adult travellers*
Unknown Effectiveness	• Aerosol insecticides in non-pregnant adult travellers • Air conditioning and electric fans in non-pregnant adult travellers • Bath or chemical base oils in non-pregnant adult travellers • Biological control measures in non-pregnant adults • Dietary supplementation in non-pregnant adult travellers • Electronic buzzers in non-pregnant adult travellers • Lifestyle changes (including full-length clothing, light clothing, behaviour modification) in non-pregnant adult travellers • Mosquito coils and vaporising mats in non-pregnant adult travellers • Outdoor smoke in non-pregnant adult travellers • Skin-applied plant-based repellents in non-pregnant adult travellers

What are the effects of antimalaria drug prophylaxis in non-pregnant adult travellers?

Likely To Be Beneficial	• Atovaquone–proguanil in non-pregnant adult travellers • Chloroquine in non-pregnant adults (in areas of chloroquine sensitivity)* • Doxycycline in non-pregnant adults
Trade-off Between Benefits And Harms	• Chloroquine–proguanil in non-pregnant adults • Mefloquine in non-pregnant adult travellers
Unknown Effectiveness	• Pyrimethamine–dapsone in non-pregnant adult travellers

	• Pyrimethamine–sulfadoxine in non-pregnant adult travellers
Likely To Be Ineffective Or Harmful	• Amodiaquine in non-pregnant adult travellers • Primaquine in non-pregnant adults

What are the effects of antimalaria vaccines in adult and child travellers?

Unknown Effectiveness	• Vaccines in adult and child travellers

What are the effects of antimalaria interventions in child travellers?

Likely To Be Beneficial	• Chloroquine in child travellers (in areas of chloroquine sensitivity)*
Trade-off Between Benefits And Harms	• Topical (skin-applied) insect repellents containing DEET (diethyl-3-methyl-benzamide) in child travellers*

What are the effects of antimalaria interventions in pregnant travellers?

Likely To Be Beneficial	• Chloroquine in pregnant travellers (in areas of chloroquine sensitivity) * • Insecticide-treated bed nets in pregnant travellers • Insecticide-treated clothing in pregnant travellers
Trade-off Between Benefits And Harms	• Skin-applied insect repellents in pregnant travellers

What are the effects of antimalaria interventions in airline pilots?

Likely To Be Beneficial	• Antimalaria drugs (atovaquone–proguanil, chloroquine, doxycycline) in airline pilots

Search date February 2007

*Categorisation based on consensus.

DEFINITION Malaria is an acute parasitic disease of the tropics and subtropics, caused by the invasion and destruction of red blood cells by one or more of four species of the genus *Plasmodium: P falciparum, P vivax, P ovale,* and *P malariae.* The clinical presentation of malaria varies according to the infecting species, and according to the genetics, immune status, and age of the infected person. The most severe form of human malaria is caused by *P falciparum,* in which variable clinical features include spiking fevers, chills, headache, muscular aching and weakness, vomiting, cough, diarrhoea, and abdominal pain; other

(continued over)

(from previous page)

symptoms related to organ failure may supervene, such as acute renal failure, generalised convulsions, and circulatory collapse, followed by coma and death. *P falciparum* accounts for more than 50% of malaria infections in most East Asian countries, over 90% in sub-Saharan Africa, and almost 100% in Hispaniola. Travellers are defined here as visitors from a malaria-free area to a malaria-endemic area, who stay in the endemic area for less than 1 year.

INCIDENCE/PREVALENCE Malaria is the most dangerous parasitic disease of humans, infecting about 5% of the world's population, and causing about one million deaths each year. The disease is strongly resurgent, owing to the effects of war, climate change, large-scale population movements, increased breeding opportunities for vector mosquitoes, rapidly spreading drug and insecticide resistance, and neglect of public health infrastructure. Malaria is currently endemic in more than 100 countries, which are visited by more than 125 million international travellers each year. Cases of malaria acquired by international travellers from industrialised countries probably number 25,000 annually. Of these, about 10,000 are reported and 150 are fatal.

AETIOLOGY/RISK FACTORS Humans acquire malaria from sporozoites transmitted by the bite of infected female anopheline mosquitoes. Of about 3200 mosquito species so far described, some 430 belong to the genus *Anopheles*. Of these, about 70 anopheline species are known to transmit malaria, with about 40 species considered important vectors. When foraging, blood-thirsty female mosquitoes fly upwind searching for the scent trail of an attractive host. Female anophelines are attracted to their human hosts over a range of 7–20 m, through a variety of stimuli, including exhaled carbon dioxide, lactic acid, other host odours, warmth, and moisture. Larger people tend to be bitten by mosquitoes more than smaller individuals. Women receive significantly more mosquito bites in trials than men. Children secrete lower levels of chemical attractants than adults, and therefore usually receive fewer mosquito bites than adults. Malaria transmission does not usually occur at temperatures below 16 °C or above 35 °C, or at altitudes greater than 3000 m above sea level at the equator (lower elevations in cooler climates), because sporozoite development in the mosquito cannot take place. The optimal conditions for transmission are a humidity of over 60%, and an ambient temperature of 25–30 °C. Most of the important vectors of malaria breed in small temporary collections of fresh surface water exposed to sunlight and with little predation, and in sites such as residual pools in drying river beds. Although rainfall provides breeding sites for mosquitoes, excessive rainfall may wash away mosquito larvae and pupae. Conversely, prolonged droughts may be associated with increased malaria transmission if they reduce the size and flow rates of large rivers sufficiently to produce suitable *Anopheles* breeding sites. Anopheline mosquitoes vary in their preferred feeding and resting locations, although most bite in the evening and at night. The *Anopheles* mosquito will feed by day only if unusually hungry. *Anopheles* adults usually fly not more than 2–3 km from their breeding sites, although a flight range of up to 7 km has been observed. One cross sectional study of about 7000 children under the age of 10 years found that, during months of peak transmission, living within 3 km of an *Anopheles* breeding site significantly increased the risk of malaria compared with living 8–10 km away (RR 21.00, 95% CI 2.87 to 153.00). Exceptionally, strong winds may carry *Anopheles* up to 30 km or more. In travellers, malaria risk is related to destination, activity, and duration of travel. A retrospective cohort study (5898 confirmed cases) conducted in Italian travellers between 1989 and 1997 found that the malaria incidence was 1.5/1000 for travel to Africa, 0.11/1000 for travel to Asia, and 0.04/1000 for travel to Central and South America. A survey of approximately 170,000 Swedish travellers found that the prevalence of malaria was lowest among travellers to Central America and the Caribbean (0.01/1000), and higher among travellers to East, Central, and West Africa (prevalence among travellers to East Africa 2.4/1000, Central Africa 3.6/1000, and West Africa 30/1000). A survey of 2131 German travellers to sub-Saharan Africa found that solo travellers were at almost a ninefold greater risk of infection than those on package tours. A case-control study (46 cases, 557 controls) reported that a visit to the tropics for longer than 21 days doubled the malaria risk compared with visits lasting 21 days or less.

PROGNOSIS Malaria can develop after just one anopheline mosquito bite. Human malaria has a usual incubation period of 10–14 days (*P falciparum*, *P vivax*, and *P ovale*) to about 28 days (*P malariae*). Certain strains of *P vivax* and *P ovale* can have a much longer incubation period of 6–18 months. About 90% of malaria attacks in travellers occur at home. About 36% of cases that develop after returning home do so more than 2 months after the traveller's return. People returning from an endemic area with any fever pattern should be considered to have malaria until proved otherwise. Once malaria infection occurs, older travellers are at greater risk of poor clinical outcomes and death. In US travellers between 1966 and 1987, the case fatality rate was 0.4% for people aged 0–19 years, 2.2% for ages 20–39 years, 5.8% for ages 40–69 years, and 30.3% for those aged 70–79 years. Complications and death from malaria are mainly due to inappropriate treatment, or to delayed initiation of treatment. If malaria is diagnosed and treated promptly, about 88% of previously healthy travellers will recover completely.

Aika Omari and Paul Garner

KEY POINTS

- Severe malaria mainly affects children under 5 years old, non-immune travellers, migrants to malarial areas, and people living in areas with unstable or seasonal malaria.

  Cerebral malaria, causing encephalopathy and coma, is fatal in around 20% of children and adults, and neurological sequelae may occur in some survivors.

  Severe malarial anaemia may have a mortality rate of over 13%.

- International consensus has historically regarded quinine as standard treatment for severe falciparum malaria. Controlled trials will generally compare new treatments against this standard.

  We found no clear evidence on the best quinine treatment regimen or route of administration to use, although high-initial-dose quinine clears parasites more rapidly compared with lower-dose quinine, but increases the risk of adverse effects.

  Intravenous artesunate is probably more effective than quinine in reducing mortality from severe malaria.

  Intramuscular artemether and rectal artemisinin, artemether, artesunate, and dihydroartemisinin may be as effective as quinine in reducing mortality from severe malaria.

  We don't know how intramuscular arteether compares with quinine.

  Routine use of phenobarbitone in cerebral malaria may reduce convulsions compared with placebo, but can increase mortality.

  Dexamethasone has not been shown to reduce mortality from severe malaria, and it increases the risk of gastrointestinal bleeding and seizures.

- We don't know whether initial blood transfusion or exchange blood transfusion reduce mortality from severe malaria as no adequate-quality studies have been found. Blood transfusion is associated with adverse effects, but is clinically essential in some circumstances.

Please visit www.clinicalevidence.bmj.com for full text and references

What are the effects of antimalarial treatments for complicated falciparum malaria in non-pregnant people?	
Likely To Be Beneficial	• High-initial-dose quinine (reduced parasite- and fever-clearance times, but no significant difference in mortality compared with standard regimes) • Intramuscular artemether (as effective as quinine) • Intravenous artesunate versus quinine • Quinine* • Rectal artemisinin and its derivatives
Unknown Effectiveness	• Intramuscular arteether versus quinine • Intramuscular versus intravenous quinine

What are the effects of adjunctive treatment for complicated falciparum malaria in non-pregnant people?	
Unknown Effectiveness	• Exchange blood transfusion • Initial blood transfusion
Likely To Be Ineffective Or Harmful	• Dexamethasone • Phenobarbitone

Search date December 2006

*Based on consensus. RCTs would be considered unethical.

DEFINITION Falciparum malaria is caused by protozoan infection of red blood cells with *Plasmodium falciparum* and comprises a variety of syndromes. This review deals with clinically complicated malaria (i.e. malaria that presents with life-threatening conditions, including coma, severe anaemia, renal failure, respiratory distress syndrome, hypoglycaemia, shock, spontaneous haemorrhage, and convulsions). The diagnosis of cerebral malaria should be considered where there is encephalopathy in the presence of malaria parasites. A strict definition of cerebral malaria requires the presence of unrousable coma and no other cause of encephalopathy (e.g. hypoglycaemia, sedative drugs), in the presence of *P falciparum* infection. This review does not currently cover the treatment of malaria in pregnancy.

INCIDENCE/PREVALENCE Malaria is a major health problem in the tropics, with 300–500 million clinical cases occurring annually and an estimated 1.1–2.7 million deaths each year as a result of severe malaria. Over 90% of deaths occur in children under 5 years old, mainly from cerebral malaria and anaemia. In areas where the rate of malaria transmission is stable (endemic), those most at risk of acquiring severe malaria are children under 5 years old, because adults and older children have partial immunity, which offers some protection. In areas where the rate of malaria transmission is unstable (non-endemic), severe malaria affects both adults and children. Non-immune travellers and migrants are also at risk of developing severe malaria.

AETIOLOGY/RISK FACTORS Malaria is transmitted by the bite of infected female anopheline mosquitoes. Certain haemoglobins such as haemoglobin S and haemoglobin C are protective against severe malaria (see aetiology in review on malaria: prevention in travellers, p 279).

PROGNOSIS In children under 5 years of age with cerebral malaria, the estimated case fatality of treated malaria is 19%, although reported hospital-case fatality may be as high as 40%. Neurological sequelae persisting for more than 6 months may occur in some survivors, and include ataxia, hemiplegia, speech disorders, behavioural disorders, epilepsy, and blindness. Severe malarial anaemia may have a case-fatality rate higher than 13%. In adults, the mortality of cerebral malaria is 20%; this rises to 50% in pregnancy.

Malaria: uncomplicated, caused by *Plasmodium falciparum*

David Taylor-Robinson, Katharine Jones, and Paul Garner

KEY POINTS

- Uncomplicated malaria is when the person has symptomatic infection with malaria parasites but no signs of vital organ disturbance.

   Uncomplicated malaria can progress to severe malaria, become chronic, or resolve, depending on host immunity and access to appropriate treatment.

   Severe malaria is more likely to develop in people with no prior immunity, and accounts for over one million deaths worldwide each year.

   The choice between treatment regimens depends partly on background drug-resistance patterns in the relevant country or region.

- Evidence suggests that artemether–lumefantrine is more effective than amodiaquine plus sulfadoxine–pyrimethamine.

- Artesunate plus amodiaquine is more effective at curing a current infection than amodiaquine plus sulfadoxine–pyrimethamine, but, in terms of people being parasite free at day 28, there is little to choose between them, since the risk of new infections appears greater with artesunate plus amodiaquine.

- Amodiaquine plus sulfadoxine–pyrimethamine achieves higher cure rates than artesunate plus sulfadoxine–pyrimethamine. Gametocyte clearance is better with artesunate plus sulfadoxine–pyrimethamine.

   Public health specialists believe that amodiaquine resistance will progress rapidly and limit the usefulness of the non-artemisinin combination if it is used regularly. On the other hand, amodiaquine and sulfadoxine–pyrimethamine are currently available in many countries, whereas artemisinin supplies are limited.

- Evidence suggests that a six-dose regimen of artemether–lumefantrine is more effective than a four-dose regimen.

- Both artemether–lumefantrine (6 doses) and artesunate plus amodiaquine were effective, but artemether–lumefantrine (6 doses) was superior in some trials.

- Artesunate plus mefloquine performs better than artemether–lumefantrine in terms of cure in areas where this has been studied.

- The choice between artesunate plus amodiaquine and artesunate plus sulfadoxine–pyrimethamine depends on background drug-resistance patterns in the relevant country or region.

(i) **Please visit www.clinicalevidence.bmj.com for full text and references**

Are artemisinin combination treatments more effective than non-artemisinin combinations treatments in people living in endemic areas (excluding South-East Asia)?	
Likely To Be Beneficial	• Artemether–lumefantrine (6 doses) (more effective than amodiaquine plus sulfadoxine–pyrimethamine)
Trade-off Between Benefits And Harms	• Artesunate (3 days) plus amodiaquine (possibly more effective than amodiaquine plus sulfadoxine–pyrimethamine)
Unlikely To Be Beneficial	• Artesunate (3 days) plus sulfadoxine–pyrimethamine (possibly less effective than amodiaquine plus sulfadoxine–pyrimethamine)

Which artemisinin combination treatment is most effective in people living in endemic areas?

Likely To Be Beneficial	• Artemether–lumefantrine (6 doses) (more effective than a 4-dose regimen)
	• Artemether–lumefantrine (6 doses) (possibly more effective than artesunate plus amodiaquine)
Unknown Effectiveness	• Artemether–lumefantrine (6 doses) versus artesunate plus sulfadoxine–pyrimethamine
	• Artesunate plus amodiaquine versus artesunate plus sulfadoxine–pyrimethamine (relative benefits unclear)
Unlikely To Be Beneficial	• Artemether–lumefantrine (6 doses) (possibly less effective than artesunate [3 days] plus mefloquine)

Search date November 2006

DEFINITION Malaria is a parasite transmitted by *Anopheles* mosquitoes. There are four types of human malaria: *falciparum*, *vivax*, *ovale*, and *malariae*. The *falciparum* type is the most important cause of illness and death, and *Plasmodium falciparum*, the responsible organism, is known to develop resistance to antimalarial drugs. This review covers treatments for *falciparum* malaria only, in a population of adults and children living in endemic malarial areas, exposed (seasonally or all year round) to malaria. It does not cover treatment of malaria in non-immune travellers, pregnant women, and people infected with HIV. Repeated episodes of *falciparum* malaria result in temporary and incomplete immunity. Therefore, adults living in areas where malaria is common are often found to be "semi-immune" — presenting with asymptomatic or chronic forms of malaria, with clinical episodes attenuated by their immunity. '**Severe malaria**' is defined as a form of symptomatic malaria with signs of vital organ disturbance WHO 2000). Any person with symptomatic malaria who does not develop any such signs is defined as having '**uncomplicated malaria**'. This review assesses the effectiveness of antimalarial drugs only in people with uncomplicated malaria.

INCIDENCE/PREVALENCE Malaria is a major health problem in the tropics, with 300–500 million new clinical cases annually, most of them cases of uncomplicated malaria. An estimated 1.1–2.7 million deaths occur annually as a result of severe *falciparum* malaria.

AETIOLOGY/RISK FACTORS The malaria parasite is transmitted by infected *Anopheles* mosquitoes. Risk factors for developing the disease include exposure to infected mosquitoes (living in an endemic area; housing that allows mosquitoes to enter, and absence of mosquito nets; and living in an area where *Anopheles* mosquitoes can thrive). Risk factors in relation to severity of the illness relate to host immunity, determined mainly by exposure to the parasite, and therefore varying with level of transmission in the area, and the age of the host. Malaria is uncommon in the first 6 months of life (fetal haemoglobin is protective); it is, however, common in children over 6 months of age. In areas of intense transmission, infection is attenuated by host immunity in older age groups; however, morbidity and mortality can also be high in adults in areas of less-intense transmission.

PROGNOSIS Uncomplicated malaria may progress to severe malaria, become chronic, or resolve with effective treatment or the development of improved immunity. The outcome is therefore dependent on host immunity and access to effective treatment. In the absence of effective treatment, people with no or low immunity are at increased risk of developing severe malaria (see review on malaria: severe, life threatening, p 284) resulting in high morbidity and mortality.

Jailson B Correia and C A Hart

KEY POINTS

- *Neisseria meningitides* (the meningococcus) causes sporadic cases of conjunctivitis, septic arthritis, meningitis and septicaemia in temperate countries, but regular epidemics occur in sub-Saharan Africa.

    Transmission is via close contact, with young children and students most at risk of infection and of death in the UK.

    About 10–15% of people carry the meningococcus in the throat, but invasive disease is associated with recent acquisition of a virulent strain.

    In resource-rich countries, mortality is up to 25% for people with septicaemia, but less than 1% for meningitis alone.

- Antibiotics can reduce carriage of meningococci in the throat compared with placebo, but we don't know whether this leads to a reduced risk of meningococcal disease, as no studies have been found.

- Prophylactic antibiotics may reduce the risks of infection in contacts, although no good-quality studies have been found that confirm this.

- We don't know whether pre-admission parenteral penicillin is beneficial, as we found no studies, but the potential benefits of early treatment are likely to outweigh any harm from its use.

- Adding corticosteroids to treatment reduces mortality in adults with bacterial meningitis of any cause, but we don't know whether it is beneficial in the subgroup of people with meningococcal meningitis.

    Corticosteroids may not prevent neurological sequelae in adults.

    Adding corticosteroids to treatment reduces severe hearing loss in children, but has not been shown to reduce mortality, and we don't know whether it is beneficial in the subgroup with meningococcal disease.

- We don't know whether adding corticosteroids is beneficial in children or adults with meningococcal septicaemia, as no studies have been found.

    Corticosteroids have not been shown to reduce mortality in adults or children with severe sepsis.

(i) **Please visit www.clinicalevidence.bmj.com for full text and references**

What are the effects of interventions to prevent meningococcal disease in contacts and carriers?	
Likely To Be Beneficial	• Antibiotics for throat carriage (reduce carriage, but unknown effect on risk of disease)
	• Prophylactic antibiotics (sulfadiazine) in contacts*

What are the effects of interventions to treat suspected cases of meningococcal disease before admission to hospital?	
Unknown Effectiveness	• Pre-admission parenteral penicillin in suspected cases*

What are the effects of treatments for meningococcal meningitis on admission in children?	
Likely To Be Beneficial	• Adding corticosteroids (reduced severe hearing loss in bacterial meningitis of any cause, but no

	difference in mortality and unknown effectiveness in meningococcal meningitis)

What are the effects of treatments for meningococcal meningitis on admission in adults?

Likely To Be Beneficial	• Adding corticosteroids (reduced mortality in bacterial meningitis of any cause, but unknown effectiveness in meningococcal meningitis)

What are the effects of treatments for meningococcal septicaemia in children?

Unknown Effectiveness	• Adding corticosteroids

What are the effects of treatments for meningococcal septicaemia in adults?

Unknown Effectiveness	• Adding corticosteroids

Search date May 2004

*Based on consensus or observational evidence. RCTs unlikely to be conducted.

DEFINITION Meningococcal disease is any clinical condition caused by *Neisseria meningitidis* (the meningococcus) groups A, B, C, W135, or other serogroups. These conditions include purulent conjunctivitis, septic arthritis, meningitis, and septicaemia with or without meningitis. In this review we cover meningococcal meningitis and meningococcal septicaemia with or without meningitis.

INCIDENCE/PREVALENCE Meningococcal disease is sporadic in temperate countries, and is most commonly caused by group B or C meningococci. The annual incidence in Europe varies from less than 1 case/100,000 people in France, up to 4–5 cases/100,000 people in the UK and Spain, and in the USA it is 0.6–1.5 cases/100,000 people. Occasional outbreaks occur among close family contacts, secondary-school pupils, military recruits, and students living in halls of residence. Sub-Saharan Africa has regular epidemics in countries lying in the expanded "meningitis belt", reaching 500 cases/100,000 people during epidemics, which are usually due to serogroup A, although recent outbreaks of serogroup W135 cause concern. In sub-Saharan Africa, over 90% of cases present with meningitis alone.

AETIOLOGY/RISK FACTORS The meningococcus colonises and infects healthy people, and is transmitted by close contact, probably by exchange of upper respiratory tract secretions. The risk of transmission is greatest during the first week of contact. Risk factors include crowding and exposure to cigarette smoke. In the UK, children younger than 2 years have the highest incidence of meningococcal disease, with a second peak between ages 15–24 years. There is currently an increased incidence of meningococcal disease among university students, especially among those in their first term and living in catered accommodation, although we found no accurate numerical estimate of risk from close contact in, for example, halls of residence. Close contacts of an index case have a much higher risk of infection than do people in the general population. The risk of epidemic spread is higher with groups A and C meningococci than with group B meningococci. It is not known what makes a meningococcus virulent. Certain clones tend to predominate at different times and in different groups. Carriage of meningococcus in the throat has been reported in 10–15% of people; recent acquisition of a virulent meningococcus is more likely to be associated with invasive disease.

(continued over)

(from previous page)

PROGNOSIS Mortality is highest in infants and adolescents, and is related to disease presentation and availability of therapeutic resources. In resource-rich countries, case fatality rates have been around 19–25% for septicaemia, 10–12% for meningitis plus septicaemia, and less than 1% in meningitis alone, but an overall reduction in mortality was observed in recent years in people admitted to paediatric intensive-care units.

Tim Weller

KEY POINTS

- Methicillin–resistant *Staphylococcus aureus* (MRSA) has a gene that makes it resistant to methicillin as well as other beta lactam antibiotics including flucloxacillin, cephalosporins and carbapenems.

  MRSA can be part of the normal body flora (colonisation), especially in the nose, but can cause infection, especially in people with prolonged hospital admissions, with underlying disease, or after antibiotic use.

  About 40% of *S aureus* in blood cultures in the UK is resistant to methicillin.

- Glycopeptides (teicoplanin, vancomycin) and linezolid seem to have similar efficacy at curing MRSA infection.

  Trimethoprim–sulfamethoxazole may be as effective as vancomycin at curing MRSA infection in injecting drug users, with similar toxicity.

- We don't know whether macrolides (azithromycin, clarithromycin, erythromycin), quinolones (ciprofloxacin, levofloxacin, moxifloxacin), tetracyclines (doxycycline, minocycline, oxytetracycline), clindamycin, daptomycin, fusidic acid, quinupristin–dalfopristin, or rifampicin are effective at curing MRSA infection, as we found no adequate studies.

  Ciprofloxacin has been used in combination with rifampicin or fusidic acid for MRSA bone and joint infections. Fusidic acid or rifampicin should not be used as monotherapy as resistance rapidly develops.

  Clindamycin may be used in preference to macrolides in susceptible MRSA infections, as bioavailability may be better and resistance less likely.

  Oral tetracyclines are recommended for minor MRSA infections.

- Mupirocin nasal ointment may improve eradication of colonised MRSA compared with placebo, and may be as effective as topical fusidic acid plus oral trimethoprim–sulfamethoxazole and more effective than tea tree oil, although studies have given conflicting results.

  We don't know whether antiseptic body washes, chlorhexidine–neomycin nasal cream, or systemic antimicrobials are effective at clearing MRSA colonisation.

ⓘ **Please visit www.clinicalevidence.bmj.com for full text and references**

What are the effects of treatment for MRSA infections at any body site?

Trade-off Between Benefits And Harms	• Linezolid (compared with glycopeptides) • Teicoplanin, vancomycin (glycopeptides) (compared with linezolid, quinupristin–dalfopristin, or trimethoprim–sulfamethoxazole)
Unknown Effectiveness	• Azithromycin, clarithromycin, erythromycin (macrolides) • Ciprofloxacin, levofloxacin, moxifloxacin (quinolones) • Clindamycin • Daptomycin • Doxycycline, minocycline, oxytetracycline (tetracyclines) • Fusidic acid

- Quinupristin–dalfopristin

- Rifampicin

- Trimethoprim

- Trimethoprim–sulfamethoxazole (compared with vancomycin)

What are the effects of treatment for MRSA nasal or extra-nasal colonisation?

Likely To Be Beneficial	• Mupirocin nasal ointment
Unknown Effectiveness	• Antiseptic body washes • Chlorhexidine–neomycin nasal cream • Mupirocin nasal ointment for 5 days (compared with more than 5 days) • Systemic antimicrobials
Unlikely To Be Beneficial	• Tea tree preparations

Search date July 2005

DEFINITION Methicillin-resistant *Staphylococcus aureus* (MRSA) is an organism resistant to methicillin by means of the *mecA* gene. This confers resistance to all beta lactam antibiotics, including flucloxacillin, oxacillin, cephalosporins, and carbapenems. Antimicrobial resistance is defined as the failure of the antimicrobial to reach a concentration in the infected tissue high enough to inhibit the growth of the infecting organism. MRSA presents in the same way as susceptible *S aureus*. It can be part of the normal flora (colonisation) or it can cause infection. The phenomena of colonisation and infection should be treated as separate entities. **MRSA colonisation:** Growth of MRSA from a body fluid or swab from any body site. The most common site of colonisation is the anterior nares but MRSA can also be found in other areas such as the axillae, abnormal skin (e.g. eczema), urine, and throat. There should be no signs or symptoms of infection. The colonised site may act as a reservoir of MRSA, which then causes infection at another site or can be passed on to others. Although the colonised patient (or staff member) does not need treatment, a course of decolonisation treatment may be given in order to eradicate carriage and prevent future infections or transmission. **MRSA infection:** Growth of MRSA from a sterile body site (e.g. blood culture or cerebrospinal fluid) or growth of MRSA from a non-sterile body site (e.g. wound, urine, or sputum) in the presence of symptoms or signs of infection. MRSA infections are also accompanied by fever and signs of inflammation, including skin/soft tissue, wound, bone and joint, nosocomial pneumonia, endocarditis, and prosthetic material. MRSA is becoming an increasingly important issue as a community-acquired infection in people who have not been recently admitted to hospital or had medical problems. However, the investigation of treatment strategies for community compared with nosocomial MRSA is ongoing, and will not be covered here.

INCIDENCE/PREVALENCE The incidence of MRSA varies from country to country. The UK, Ireland, and southern Europe (e.g. Spain, Italy, and Greece) have a high incidence when compared with northern Europe and Scandinavia. The most objective measure of incidence is the percentage of *S aureus* found in blood cultures that are resistant to methicillin. This currently stands at about 40% in the UK.

AETIOLOGY/RISK FACTORS Risk factors for MRSA colonisation include: prolonged stay in hospital, severe underlying disease, prior antibiotics, exposure to colonised people, and admission to a high-risk unit (critical care, renal unit, etc).

PROGNOSIS The virulence of MRSA has been found to be equal to that of methicillin-susceptible *S aureus* in animal models and case-control studies. However, as MRSA tends to affect more elderly and debilitated people, the overall morbidity and mortality of people with MRSA is found to be higher if this is not taken into account. A meta-analysis of 31 cohort studies found that mortality associated with MRSA bacteraemia was significantly higher than that of methicillin-susceptible *S aureus* bacteraemia (mean mortality not reported; OR 1.93, 95% CI 1.54 to 2.42).

294 | Postherpetic neuralgia

David Wareham

KEY POINTS

- Pain that occurs after resolution of acute herpes zoster infection can be severe. It may be accompanied by itching and follows the distribution of the original infection.

  The main risk factor for postherpetic neuralgia is increasing age; it is uncommon in people under 50 years, but develops in 20% of people aged 60–65 years who have had acute herpes zoster, and in more than 30% of those people aged over 80 years.

  Up to 2% of people with acute herpes zoster may continue to have postherpetic pain for 5 years or more.

- Oral antiviral agents (aciclovir, famciclovir, valaciclovir, and netivudine), taken during acute herpes zoster infection, may reduce the duration of postherpetic neuralgia compared with placebo.

  We don't know whether topical antiviral drugs, TCAs, or corticosteroids taken during an acute attack reduce the risks of postherpetic neuralgia, as few good-quality studies have been found.

  Corticosteroids may cause dissemination of herpes zoster infection.

  We don't know whether the use of dressings during an acute attack reduces the risk of postherpetic neuralgia, as we found no studies.

- Gabapentin and TCAs may reduce pain at up to 8 weeks compared with placebo in people with established postherpetic neuralgia.

  Adverse effects of TCAs are dose related and may be less frequent in postherpetic neuralgia compared with depression, as lower doses are generally used.

  Opioid analgesic drugs are likely to be effective in reducing pain associated with postherpetic neuralgia, but they can cause sedation and other well known adverse effects.

  We don't know whether dextromethorphan is effective at reducing postherpetic neuralgia.

  We don't know whether topical anaesthesia or topical counterirritants such as capsaicin reduce postherpetic neuralgia.

(i) **Please visit www.clinicalevidence.bmj.com for full text and references**

What are the effects of interventions during an acute attack of herpes zoster aimed at preventing postherpetic neuralgia?

Likely To Be Beneficial	● Oral antiviral agents (aciclovir, famciclovir, valaciclovir, netivudine)
Unknown Effectiveness	● Dressings ● Topical antiviral agents (idoxuridine) for pain at 6 months ● TCAs (amitriptyline) to prevent postherpetic neuralgia
Likely To Be Ineffective Or Harmful	● Corticosteroids

What are the effects of interventions to relieve established postherpetic neuralgia after the rash has healed?

Beneficial	• Gabapentin • TCAs to treat postherpetic neuralgia
Likely To Be Beneficial	• Oral opioid analgesic drugs (oxycodone, morphine, methadone, tramadol)
Unknown Effectiveness	• Dextromethorphan • Topical anaesthesia • Topical counterirritants (capsaicin)

Search date December 2006

DEFINITION Postherpetic neuralgia is pain that sometimes follows resolution of acute herpes zoster and healing of the zoster rash. It can be severe, accompanied by itching, and follows the distribution of the original infection. Herpes zoster is caused by activation of latentVZV (human herpes virus 3) in people who have been rendered partially immune by a previous attack of chickenpox. Herpes zoster infects the sensory ganglia and their areas of innervation. It is characterised by pain in the distribution of the affected nerve, and crops of clustered vesicles over the area.

INCIDENCE/PREVALENCE In a UK general practice survey of 3600–3800 people, the annual incidence of herpes zoster was 3.4/1000. Incidence varied with age. Herpes zoster was relatively uncommon in people under the age of 50 years (under 2/1000 a year), but rose to 5–7/1000 a year in people aged 50–79 years, and 11/1000 in people aged 80 years or older. A population-based study in the Netherlands reported a similar incidence (3.4/1000 a year) and a similar increase of incidence with age (3–10/1000 a year in people over 50 years). Prevalence of postherpetic neuralgia depends on when it is measured after acute infection. There is no agreed time point for diagnosis.

AETIOLOGY/RISK FACTORS The main risk factor for postherpetic neuralgia is increasing age. In a UK general practice study (involving 3600–3800 people, 321 cases of acute herpes zoster) there was little risk in those under the age of 50 years, but postherpetic neuralgia developed in over 20% of people who had had acute herpes zoster aged 60–65 years, and in 34% of those aged over 80 years. No other risk factor has been found to predict consistently which people with herpes zoster will experience continued pain. In a general practice study in Iceland (421 people followed for up to 7 years after an initial episode of herpes zoster), the risk of postherpetic neuralgia was 1.8% (95% CI 0.6% to 4.2%) for people under 60 years of age, and the pain was mild in all cases. The risk of severe pain after 3 months in people aged over 60 years was 1.7% (95% CI 0% to 6.2%).

PROGNOSIS About 2% of people with acute herpes zoster in the UK general practice survey had pain for more than 5 years. Prevalence of pain falls as time elapses after the initial episode. Among 183 people aged over 60 years in the placebo arm of a UK trial, the prevalence of pain was 61% at 1 month, 24% at 3 months, and 13% at 6 months after acute infection. In a more-recent RCT, the prevalence of postherpetic pain in the placebo arm at 6 months was 35% in 72 people over 60 years.

Lilia Ziganshina and Paul Garner

KEY POINTS

- About a third of the world's population has latent tuberculosis.

    Over 14 million people had active tuberculosis in 2004. Approximately 1.7 million people died from the infection.

    Over 80% of new cases diagnosed in 2004 were in people in Africa, South-East Asia, and Western Pacific regions.

- Most people who inhale *Mycobacterium tuberculosis* clear the infection and become skin-test positive.

    Active infection is more likely in people affected by social factors such as poverty, overcrowding, homelessness, and inadequate health care, or with reduced immune function — such as with HIV infection.

    Some people develop latent infection — persistent bacterial presence which is asymptomatic and not infectious.

- Drug treatments can reduce the risk of active tuberculosis in people at high risk of infection.

    Prophylactic isoniazid for 6 months can reduce the risk of tuberculosis infection in high-risk people without HIV, but increases the risk of hepatotoxicity.

    Rifampicin plus isoniazid for 3 months, or isoniazid for 6–12 months, are equally effective at reducing active infection rates in people with latent tuberculosis.

- Treatment requires chemotherapy with combination regimens.

    Adding rifampicin to isoniazid is more effective than isoniazid treatment alone, and more effective than ethambutol plus isoniazid regimens.

    Regimens including pyrazinamide improve short-term sputum clearance, but long-term effects are unclear.

    Quinolones such as ciprofloxacin have not been shown to improve outcomes compared with ethambutol, isoniazid, and pyrazinamide regimens, but the evidence is sparse.

- The optimal length of treatment seems to be 6 months, but evidence is not robust.

    Relapse rates are the same after 6 months' treatment compared with longer regimens.

    Intermittent chemotherapy, taken 2–3 times a week, may be as effective as daily treatment for 6 or more months, but the evidence is weak.

- Current practice in multidrug-resistant tuberculosis is to use at least three drugs to which the particular strain is sensitive.

- Direct observation of treatment (DOT) does not seem to increase cure rates compared with self-administered treatment.

    We don't know how different types of support mechanisms for DOT compare with each other.

 Please visit www.clinicalevidence.bmj.com for full text and references

What are the effects of interventions to prevent tuberculosis in people without HIV infection at high risk of developing tuberculosis?

Trade-off Between Benefits And Harms	• Isoniazid
	• Rifampicin plus isoniazid

What are the effects of interventions to prevent tuberculosis in people without HIV at high risk of developing multidrug-resistant tuberculosis?

Unknown Effectiveness	• Comparative benefits of different regimens for preventing multidrug-resistant tuberculosis in people at high risk of MDR-TB

What are the effects of different drug regimens in people with newly diagnosed pulmonary tuberculosis without HIV infection?

Beneficial	• Shorter-course chemotherapy (6-month regimen as good as longer courses in preventing relapse)
Likely To Be Beneficial	• Adding pyrazinamide in chemotherapy regimens lasting up to 6 months • Adding rifampicin to isoniazid (more effective at reducing relapse than isoniazid alone)
Unknown Effectiveness	• Intermittent chemotherapy for 6 months or longer (compared with daily chemotherapy) • Regimens containing quinolones
Unlikely To Be Beneficial	• Ethambutol in place of rifampicin in continuation phase
Likely To Be Ineffective Or Harmful	• Chemotherapy for less than 6 months

What are the effects of different drug regimens in people with multidrug-resistant tuberculosis without HIV infection?

Unknown Effectiveness	• Comparative benefits of different regimens in multidrug-resistant tuberculosis

What are the effects of low-level laser therapy in people with tuberculosis without HIV infection?

Unknown Effectiveness	• Low-level laser therapy

Which interventions improve adherence to treatment in people with tuberculosis without HIV infection?

Unknown Effectiveness	• Support mechanisms for directly observed treatment
Unlikely To Be Beneficial	• Direct observation treatment (compared with self-administered treatment)

Search date October 2006

DEFINITION Tuberculosis is caused by *Mycobacterium tuberculosis* and can affect many organs. Specific symptoms relate to site of infection, and are generally accompanied by fever, sweats, and weight loss.

INCIDENCE/PREVALENCE The *Mycobacterium tuberculosis* organism kills more people than any other infectious agent. The number of cases of tuberculosis was stable or falling in five of six WHO regions in 2004, but growing at 0.6% a year globally. Incidence is rising in Africa, where the tuberculosis epidemic is still driven by the spread of HIV. According to WHO data, there were 8.9 million new cases of tuberculosis worldwide in 2004 (140/100,000 population), of which 3.9 million (62/100,000) were smear positive, and 741,000 were in adults infected with HIV. There were 14.6 million prevalent cases (229/100,000), of which 6.1 million were smear positive (95/100,000). More than 80% of people newly diagnosed with tuberculosis in 2004 were in the African, South-East Asia, and Western Pacific regions. About a third of the world's population has latent tuberculosis (see aetiology).

AETIOLOGY/RISK FACTORS The chief route of infection is through inhalation of airborne bacteria released by people with active respiratory tuberculosis by cough, sneeze, or speech. Inhaled mycobacteria reach the lung, and grow slowly over several weeks. The immune systems of most healthy exposed people (80–90%) kill the bacteria, and they are removed from the body with only a positive skin test left as a marker of exposure. In a small proportion of people infected, a defensive barrier is built around the infection, but the tuberculosis bacteria are not killed and lie dormant. This is known as latent tuberculosis, where the person is asymptomatic and not infectious. In the rest of those infected, active tuberculosis develops immediately. **Risk factors:** Social factors include poverty, overcrowding, homelessness, and inadequate health services. Medical factors include HIV and immunosuppression.

PROGNOSIS Prognosis varies widely and depends on treatment. An estimated 1.7 million people (27/100,000) died from tuberculosis in 2004, including those coinfected with HIV (248,000).

John Kellum, Martine Leblanc, and Ramesh Venkataraman

KEY POINTS

- Acute renal failure is characterised by abrupt and sustained decline in glomerular filtration rate, which leads to accumulation of urea and other chemicals in the blood.

  It can be classified according to a change from baseline serum creatinine or urine output, with "Risk" being defined by either a 50% increase in serum creatinine or a urine output of less than 0.5 mL/kg/hour for at least 6 hours; and "Failure" being defined by a threefold increase in serum creatinine or a urine output of less than 0.3 mL/kg/hour for 24 hours.

- In people at high risk of developing acute renal failure, intravenous sodium chloride (0.9%) hydration reduces incidences of acute renal failure compared with unrestricted oral fluids or 0.45% iv sodium chloride solution.

  N-acetylcysteine plus hydration may reduce contrast nephropathy compared with hydration alone in people undergoing contrast nephrography, although data about prevention of renal failure are inconclusive.

  Low-osmolality contrast medium is less nephrotoxic compared with standard-osmolality media.

  Prophylactic renal replacement therapy with haemofiltration and dialysis is unlikely to be beneficial since it does not reduce the risk of contrast nephropathy.

  Single-dose aminoglycosides seem as beneficial as multiple doses for treating infections, but are less nephrotoxic.

  Lipid formulations of amphotericin B may cause less nephrotoxicity than standard formulations, although the evidence for this is somewhat sparse.

  Mannitol, theophylline, aminophylline, fenoldopam, and calcium channel blockers do not appear to be useful treatments for people at high risk of acute renal failure.

- In critically ill people, high-dose continuous renal replacement therapy seems to reduce mortality compared with low dose, although we don't know whether continuous therapy is any more effective than intermittent renal replacement therapy.

  We found insufficient evidence to establish whether synthetic dialysis membranes are any more effective than cellulose-based membranes for treating people with acute renal failure.

  Loop diuretics plus fluids seem to increase the risk of developing acute renal failure compared with fluids alone both in high-risk and critically ill people, and do not seem to improve renal function or mortality compared with placebo in people with acute renal failure, but may increase the risks of ototoxicity and volume depletion.

  We found no evidence that examined whether intravenous albumin supplementation improved the effects of loop diuretics, nor whether continuous infusion was any more effective than bolus injection in the treatment of people who are critically ill with acute renal failure.

- Neither natriuretic peptides nor dopamine seem beneficial in either high-risk or critically ill people, and both are associated with significant adverse effects.

(i) Please visit www.clinicalevidence.bmj.com for full text and references

What are the effects of interventions to prevent acute renal failure in people at high risk?

Beneficial	• Contrast media (low-osmolality more effective than high-osmolality contrast media)
Likely To Be Beneficial	• Aminoglycosides (single dose as effective as multiple doses for treating infection, but with reduced nephrotoxicity) • Amphotericin B (lipid formulations may cause less nephrotoxicity than standard formulations)* • Contrast media (iso-osmolar maybe more effective than low-osmolality contrast media) • N-Acetylcysteine • Sodium chloride-based fluids
Unknown Effectiveness	• Sodium bicarbonate-based fluids (limited evidence better than sodium chloride for the prevention of contrast nephropathy)
Unlikely To Be Beneficial	• Fenoldopam • Mannitol • Natriuretic peptides • Renal replacement therapy (Prophylactic haemofiltration/dialysis) • Theophylline or aminophylline
Likely To Be Ineffective Or Harmful	• Calcium channel blockers (for early allograft dysfunction) • Dopamine • Loop diuretics

What are the effects of treatments for critically ill people with acute renal failure?

Likely To Be Beneficial	• Renal replacement therapy (reduced mortality compared with low dose)
Unknown Effectiveness	• Albumin supplementation plus loop diuretics (intravenous) • Dialysis membranes (unclear if synthetic or cellulose-based membranes more effective) • Loop diuretics (unclear if continuous infusion more effective than bolus injection)

	• Renal replacement therapy (unclear whether continuous or intermittent renal replacement therapy more effective)
Unlikely To Be Beneficial	• Loop diuretics
Likely To Be Ineffective Or Harmful	• Dopamine • Natriuretic peptides

Search date April 2006

*Categorisation based on consensus.

DEFINITION Acute renal failure is characterised by abrupt and sustained decline in glomerular filtration rate, which leads to accumulation of urea and other chemicals in the blood. Most studies define it biochemically as a serum creatinine of 2–3 mg/dL (200–25 µmol/L), an elevation of more than 0.5 mg/dL (4 µmol/L) over a baseline creatinine below 2 mg/dL, or a twofold increase of baseline creatinine. A recent international, interdisciplinary consensus panel has classified acute renal failure according to a change from baseline serum creatinine or urine output. The three-level classification begins with "Risk", defined by either a 50% increase in serum creatinine or a urine output of less than 0.5 mL/kg/hour for at least 6 hours, and concludes with "Failure", defined by a threefold increase in serum creatinine or a urine output of less than 0.3 mL/kg/hour for 24 hours. Acute renal failure is usually additionally classified according to the location of the predominant primary pathology (prerenal, intrarenal, and postrenal failure). Critically ill people are clinically unstable and at imminent risk of death, which usually implies that they need to be in, or have been admitted to, the intensive-care unit (ICU).

INCIDENCE/PREVALENCE Two prospective observational studies (2576 people) found that established acute renal failure affected nearly 5% of people in hospital and as many as 15% of critically ill people, depending on the definitions used.

AETIOLOGY/RISK FACTORS General risk factors: Risk factors for acute renal failure that are consistent across multiple causes include age; hypovolaemia; hypotension; sepsis; pre-existing renal, hepatic, or cardiac dysfunction; diabetes mellitus; and exposure to nephrotoxins (e.g. aminoglycosides, amphotericin, immunosuppressive agents, NSAIDs, ACE inhibitors, intravenous contrast media). **Risk factors/aetiology in critically ill people:** Isolated episodes of acute renal failure are rarely seen in critically ill people, but are usually part of multiple-organ dysfunction syndromes. Acute renal failure requiring dialysis is rarely seen in isolation (less than 5% of people). The kidneys are often the first organs to fail. In the perioperative setting, acute renal failure risk factors include prolonged aortic clamping, emergency rather than elective surgery, and use of higher volumes (above 10 mL) of intravenous contrast media. One study (3695 people) using multiple logistic regression identified the following independent risk factors: baseline creatinine clearance below 47 mL/minute (OR 1.20, 95% CI 1.12 to 1.30), diabetes (OR 5.5, 95% CI 1.4 to 21.0), and a marginal effect for doses of contrast media above 100 mL (OR 1.01, 95% CI 1.00 to 1.01). Mortality of people with acute renal failure requiring dialysis was 36% while in hospital. Prerenal acute renal failure is caused by reduced blood flow to the kidney from renal artery disease, systemic hypotension, or maldistribution of blood flow. Intrarenal acute renal failure is caused by parenchymal injury (acute tubular necrosis, interstitial nephritis, embolic disease, glomerulonephritis, vasculitis, or small-vessel disease). Postrenal acute renal failure is caused by urinary tract obstruction. Observational studies (in several hundred people from Europe, North America, and West Africa with acute renal failure) found a prerenal cause in 40–80%, an intrarenal cause in 10–50%, and a postrenal cause in the remaining 10%. Prerenal acute renal failure is the most common type of acute renal failure in people who are critically ill. Intrarenal acute renal failure in this context is

(continued over)

(from previous page)

usually part of multisystem failure, and most frequently because of acute tubular necrosis resulting from ischaemic or nephrotoxic injury, or both.

PROGNOSIS One retrospective study (1347 people with acute renal failure) found that mortality was less than 15% in people with isolated acute renal failure. One recent prospective study (more than 700 people) found that, in people with acute renal failure, overall mortality (72% in ICU v 32% in non-ICU; P = 0.001) and the need for dialysis (71% in ICU v 18% in non-ICU; P less than 0.001) were higher in an ICU than in a non-ICU setting, despite no significant difference between the groups in mean maximal serum creatinine (5.21 ± 2.34 mg/dL in ICU v 5.82 ± 3.26 mg/dL in non-ICU). One large study (more than 17,000 people admitted to Austrian ICUs) found that acute renal failure was associated with a greater than fourfold increase in mortality. Even after controlling for underlying severity of illness, mortality was still significantly higher in people with acute renal failure (62.8% in people with acute renal failure v 38.5% in people with no acute renal failure), suggesting that acute renal failure is independently responsible for increased mortality, even if dialysis is used. However, the exact mechanism that leads to increased risk of death is uncertain. A systematic review including 80 articles and a total of 15,897 people with acute renal failure from 1970 to 2004 found mortality unchanged, at about 50%, and exceeding 30% in most studies. An observational study including 54 sites and 23 countries screened 29,269 people and found that 1738 (5.7%) had severe acute renal failure warranting renal replacement therapy. Overall hospital mortality among people with severe acute renal failure was 60.3% (95% CI, 58.0% to 62.6%).

Catherine M Clase

KEY POINTS

- Chronic renal failure is characterised by a gradual and sustained decline in renal clearance or GFR.

  Continued progression of renal failure will lead to renal function too low to sustain healthy life. In resource-rich countries, such people will be offered renal replacement therapy in the form of dialysis or renal transplantation. Requirement for dialysis or transplantation is termed end-stage renal disease (ESRD).

  Diabetes, glomerulonephritis, hypertension, pyelonephritis, renovascular disease, polycystic kidney disease, and certain drugs may cause chronic renal failure.

- Evidence suggests that, in people with chronic renal failure, ACE inhibitors may lower mortality and prevent or slow the progression with ESRD.

  We do not know whether angiotensin II receptor antagonists are beneficial for chronic renal failure. However, evidence suggests that the combination of ACE inhibitors and angiotensin II receptor antagonists is probably beneficial compared with either drug alone.

  Lowering blood pressure below usual targets (with any drug) is unlikely to be beneficial.

- We do not know whether nicotinates or statins are beneficial in chronic renal disease, and the evidence shows that fibrates may have nephrotoxic effects.

- We do not know whether targeted lowering of albuminuria or proteinuria is beneficial in chronic renal disease.

- We do not know whether lifestyle interventions such as dietary sodium, exercise, smoking, or structured programmes to achieve therapeutic goals have an effect on chronic renal disease. We do, however, know that psychoeducational interventions are likely to delay the need for renal replacement therapy.

(i) Please visit www.clinicalevidence.bmj.com for full text and references

What are the effects of drug treatments used to reduce rate of progression of chronic renal failure?

Likely To Be Beneficial	• ACE inhibitors • ACE inhibitors plus angiotensin II receptor antagonists
Unknown Effectiveness	• Angiotensin II receptor antagonists • Nicotinates • Statins • Targeted lowering of albuminuria/proteinuria
Unlikely To Be Beneficial	• Lowering blood pressure below usual targets
Likely To Be Ineffective Or Harmful	• Fibrates

What are the effects of lifestyle changes used to reduce rate of progression of chronic renal failure?

Likely To Be Beneficial	• Psychoeducational intervention
Unknown Effectiveness	• Exercise • Smoking cessation • Sodium (dietary) • Structured programmes to achieve therapeutic goals

Search date April 2006

DEFINITION Chronic renal failure is characterised by a gradual and sustained decline in renal clearance or glomerular filtration rate (GFR), leading to the accumulation of urea and other chemicals in the blood. There is no widely established definition. Based on limited data on healthy aging, the Kidney Disease Improving Global Outcomes (KDIGO) statement has defined GFR of less than 60 mL/minute/1.73 m² as indicative of chronic kidney disease. This corresponds to serum creatinine concentration greater than 137 µmol/L in men, and greater than 104 µmol/L in women. The KDIGO classification further classifies people with low GFR as follows: GFR 30–60 mL/minute is defined as stage 3 chronic kidney disease; GFR 15–30 mL/minute as stage 4 chronic kidney disease; and GFR less than 15 mL/minute or a need for dialysis as stage 5 chronic kidney disease. In contrast, the term chronic renal failure usually excludes people whose chronic renal failure is treated with dialysis or transplantation, for whom the term end-stage renal disease (ESRD) is commonly used. The term chronic renal insufficiency is also widespread in the literature, and also lacks a clear definition. **For the purposes of this review, chronic renal failure, chronic renal insufficiency, and chronic kidney failure will be considered synonymous.** Chronic kidney disease, as defined by the National Kidney Foundation Kidney Disease Outcomes Quality Initiative (NKF-KDOQI), is a broader concept that encompasses not only low GFR but any clinically important abnormality of kidney structure or abnormality on urine analysis (e.g. protein or blood). Progression of chronic renal failure refers to further decline in renal clearance or GFR over time. This is often assessed as an event (such as increase in serum creatinine to 50% or 100% more than previous values) or — less meaningfully from a clinical perspective — as the rate of decline of clearance (measured or estimated creatinine clearance or GFR). Continued progression of renal failure, in the absence of the competing event of death, will lead to renal function too low to sustain healthy life. In resource-rich countries, people with this problem will usually be offered renal replacement therapy in the form of dialysis or renal transplantation. **Diagnosis:** the diagnosis of chronic renal failure is established by the finding, on at least two occasions separated by weeks or months, of elevated serum creatinine, low GFR, or low creatinine clearance. GFR and creatinine clearance may be measured directly or calculated from clinical variables and serum creatinine. Normal values for creatinine or GFR are the subject of some controversy. In the Framingham study of predominantly Caucasian American men and women, a subset, consisting of 3241 people who were free of known renal disease, CVD, hypertension, and diabetes, was used to define a healthy reference sample. The upper 95th percentiles for serum creatinine levels in the healthy reference sample were 136 µmol/L for men and 120 µmol/L for women. In terms of GFR, on the basis of prospective longitudinal studies of healthy aging, normal kidney function had generally been considered as a creatinine clearance of 150 mL/minute (standard deviation 20 mL/minute) for men aged 20–30 years, and to decline by 0.75 mL/minute a year. Average clearances of 90–100 mL/minute were expected in healthy elderly people. However, in participants in the US third National Health and Nutrition Examination Survey (NHANES III), a large proportion of the elderly population had low GFR (e.g. 14.5% of people in their 80s without diabetes had GFR of 60–80 mL/minute/1.73 m², and a further 3.2% had GFR of 30–60 mL/minute/1.73 m²). The distinction between decline in GFR caused by aging and that caused by disease in elderly people remains controversial. KDIGO defines GFR less than 60 mL/minute/1.73 m² as indicative of disease. Creatinine calibration varies greatly between laboratories, further increasing the difficulty in setting absolute thresholds for the definition of chronic renal failure, either in terms of creatinine values, or in terms of estimates of GFR calculated from serum creatinine. Few studies have been conducted on the cost-effective assessment of people with a new diagnosis of chronic renal failure. The rate of change of renal function, and the presence of known risk factors for chronic renal failure (e.g. diabetes, hypertension, known autoimmune or connective tissue disease, urinary tract obstruction, and family history of specific renal diseases) can be helpful diagnostically. Proteinuria and haematuria on urinalysis make glomerular or inflammatory tubulointerstitial disease more likely. Ultrasound may be useful to exclude urinary tract obstruction. Direct evidence about the measurement properties of clinical features or diagnostic tests in the diagnosis of unselected people with chronic renal failure is lacking, and detailed discussion of this issue is beyond the scope of this review. An opinion-based account of an approach to this problem can be found within the National Kidney Foundation Kidney Disease Outcome Quality Initiative (NKF-KDOQI) guidelines.

INCIDENCE/PREVALENCE Few data are available on incidence of chronic renal failure. In a UK study of clinical laboratory serum creatinine values, the incidence of new chronic renal failure, defined as a single creatinine value of greater than 180 µmol/L in men, or greater than 135 µmol/L in women (corresponding to GFR of about 30 mL/minute/1.73 m^2), was 0.244% a year. Prevalence of low GFR in people without diabetes is available from the third National Health and Nutrition Survey conducted in the USA between 1986 and 1994.

AETIOLOGY/RISK FACTORS Little is known about the epidemiology of the underlying cause of chronic renal failure in people without diabetes in the community or in primary care. In referral centres, glomerulonephritis, hypertension or renovascular disease, and polycystic kidney disease are the most common diagnoses, with a smaller proportion of people having tubulointerstitial disease or vasculitis. In people with chronic renal failure who progress to ESRD in Canada, after diabetes (24%), the most common causes are glomerulonephritis (20%), unknown (14%), hypertension (10%), pyelonephritis (7%), renovascular disease (7%), polycystic kidney disease (6%), and drug-induced disease (commonly lithium, analgesics, and NSAIDs, 2%).

PROGNOSIS A 10-year community-based cohort study in Japan found that higher serum creatinine levels may lead to an increase in the risk of developing end-stage renal disease (ESRD). In a community-based cohort in Tromsø, Norway, the 10-year cumulative incidence of renal failure (identified through clinical laboratory screening as having GFR 30–60 mL/minute/1.73 m^2) was 4% (95% CI 3% to 6%), and mortality was 51% (95% CI 48% to 55%). In a 5-year follow-up of a cohort identified through the laboratories of a large managed care organisation in the USA, the rate of ESRD was 1% and mortality 24% for people with GFR of 30–60 mL/minute/1.73 m^2, and ESRD was 20% and mortality 46% for those with GFR of 15–30 mL/minute/1.73 m^2. In a cohort study of men with serum creatinine greater than 300 µmol/L, and women with serum creatinine greater than 250 µmol/L, identified through clinical laboratories, 80% reached ESRD at follow-up of 55–79 months. In a UK community-based study of clinical laboratory serum creatinine values, chronic renal failure was defined as a single creatinine value of greater than 180 µmol/L in men, or greater than 13 µmol/L in women (corresponding to a GFR of about 30 mL/minute/1.73 m^2). In those people meeting this definition, but who had not been referred to a nephrologist, and in whom repeat serum creatinine levels were obtained, the annual rate of decline in GFR was less than 2 mL/minute/year in 79% of people, and 5 mL/minute/year or greater in 8% of people. In the National Health and Nutrition Examination Survey (NHANES III, conducted between 1986 and 1994) 4.3% of the group had low GFR (30–60 mL/minute/1.73 m^2), and 0.2% had very low GFR (15–30 mL/minute/1.73 m^2). In addition, in the United States Renal Data Survey (USRDS) for 1990, 0.06% of the group required renal replacement therapy. The data from these two studies strongly suggest that many unreferred people with low GFR do not have progressive disease, or are either of an age, or carrying a burden of co-morbidity, such that the competing risk of death outweighs the risk of ESRD. Proteinuria is a consistent multivariable risk factor for progression of renal failure and for ESRD, and can be classified in many ways. Frequently used classification systems are: dipstick (0, 1+, 2+, and 3+); albuminuria (sometimes divided into microalbuminuria and macroalbuminuria depending on the degree of albumin excretion, the collection method, and units used); proteinuria (non-proteinuric [less than 300 mg/day], non-nephrotic range proteinuria [300–3000 mg/day], and nephrotic range proteinuria [greater than 3000 mg/day]).

(continued over)

(from previous page)

Hypertension and cigarette smoking have also been shown to be risk factors for progression to ESRD. People referred to nephrologists differ from those in primary care in both prognostic markers and rates of progression. For example, in the Modification of Diet in Renal Disease (MDRD) study A (GFR 25–55 mL/minute/1.73 m²), 27% of participating people had greater than 1000 mg/day proteinuria, whereas in NHANES III, only 3% of participants with a GFR of 30–60 mL/minute/1.73 m² showed greater than 288 mg/day of albuminuria. Rate of progression also seems to differ between referred and unreferred people. In a review summarising studies of mostly referred people, the weighted mean loss of GFR was 7.56 mL/minute/year. In contrast to this, in a community-based study of unreferred people conducted in the UK, only 21% of people showed evidence of progression of renal disease (defined as at least 2.0 mL/minute/1.73 m² a year), and the remaining 79% showed no evidence of progression.

Yoshio N Hall and Glenn M Chertow

KEY POINTS

- End-stage renal disease (ESRD) affects over 1500 people per million population in countries with a high prevalence, such as the USA and Japan. Approximately two thirds of people with ESRD receive haemodialysis, a quarter have kidney transplants, and a tenth receive peritoneal dialysis.

  Risk factors for ESRD include advanced age, hypertension, diabetes mellitus, obesity, a history of renal disease, and tobacco, heroin, or analgesic use.

  ESRD leads to fluid retention, anaemia, disturbances of bone and mineral metabolism, and increased risk of CVD.

- In people receiving peritoneal dialysis, 7.5% icodextrin solution may increase fluid loss compared with lower concentration dextrose solutions. Icodextrin may affect the accuracy of blood glucose measurement.

  Increasing the dose of peritoneal dialysis does not seem to reduce mortality.

- In people receiving haemodialysis, there seems to be no difference in mortality for high membrane flux compared with low membrane flux, or increased-dose haemodialysis compared with standard dose.

- Erythropoietin and darbepoetin may help maintain haemoglobin levels in people with ESRD, but are associated with mortality, and with serious cardiovascular, arterial, and venous thromboembolic events in people with kidney disease.

- Disorders of calcium and phosphate metabolism may contribute to the increased risk of CVD in people with ESRD.

  Phosphate binders (sevelamer) may slow down arterial calcification, and may reduce serum low-density lipoprotein cholesterol levels, but we don't yet know whether this reduces cardiovascular events or mortality.

(i) **Please visit www.clinicalevidence.bmj.com for full text and references**

What are the effects of different doses and osmotic agents for peritoneal dialysis?

Likely To Be Beneficial	• Icodextrin (reduces volume overload compared with 1.36%, 2.27%, or 4.25% dextrose solutions)
Unlikely To Be Beneficial	• Increased-dose peritoneal dialysis (no more effective than standard-dose dialysis in reducing overall mortality)

What are the effects of different doses and membrane fluxes for haemodialysis?

Unlikely To Be Beneficial	• High-membrane-flux haemodialysis (no more effective than low-membrane-flux haemodialysis in reducing all-cause mortality)
	• Increased-dose haemodialysis (no more effective than standard-dose haemodialysis in reducing all-cause mortality)

What are the effects of interventions aimed at preventing secondary complications?

Likely To Be Beneficial	• Cinacalcet (improves control of secondary hyperparathyroidism compared with placebo) • Mupirocin (reduces *Staphylococcus aureus* catheter infections compared with placebo or no treatment) • Sevelamer (reduces progression of coronary artery and aortic calcification compared with calcium salts)
Trade-off Between Benefits And Harms	• Erythropoietin or darbepoetin (maintains haemoglobin levels but associated with increased mortality and cardiovascular events)

Search date April 2007

DEFINITION End-stage renal (ESRD) is defined as irreversible decline in a person's own kidney function, which is severe enough to be fatal in the absence of dialysis or transplantation. ESRD is included under stage 5 of the National Kidney Foundation Kidney Disease Outcomes Quality Initiative classification of chronic kidney disease (CKD), where it refers to individuals with an estimated glomerular filtration (GFR) rate below 15 mL per minute per 1.73 m^2 body surface area, or those requiring dialysis irrespective of GFR. Reduction in or absence of kidney function leads to a host of maladaptive changes including fluid retention (extracellular volume overload), anaemia, disturbances of bone and mineral metabolism, dyslipidaemia, and protein energy malnutrition. This review deals with ESRD in adults only. **Fluid retention** in people with ESRD contributes significantly to the hypertension, ventricular dysfunction, and excess cardiovascular events observed in this population. **Anaemia** associated with CKD is normocytic and normochromic, and is most commonly attributed to reduced erythropoietin synthesis by the affected kidneys. Additional factors contribute to the anaemia, including: iron deficiency from frequent phlebotomy, blood retention in the dialyser and tubing, and gastrointestinal bleeding; severe secondary hyperparathyroidism; acute and chronic inflammatory conditions (e.g. infection); and shortened red blood cell survival. **Disturbances of bone and mineral metabolism** such as hyperparathyroidism, hyperphosphataemia, and hypo- or hypercalcaemia, are common in people with CKD. If untreated, these disturbances can cause pain, pruritus, anaemia, bone loss, and increased fracture risk, and can contribute to hypertension and CVD.

INCIDENCE/PREVALENCE The incidence and prevalence of ESRD continue to grow worldwide. According to data collected from 120 countries with dialysis programmes, at the end of 2005 about 1,900,000 people were receiving renal replacement therapy (RRT). Among these individuals, 1,297,000 (68%) received haemodialysis and 158,000 (8%) received peritoneal dialysis, although an additional 445,000 (23%) were living with a kidney transplant. Precise estimates of ESRD incidence and prevalence remain elusive, because international databases of renal registries exclude individuals with ESRD who do not receive RRT. International comparisons of RRT pose similar challenges because of differences in healthcare systems, government funding, acceptance of treatment, demographics, and access to care. Worldwide, the highest incidence and prevalence rates are reported from the USA, Taiwan, and Japan. Prevalence data from several countries are listed below, although this list is not exhaustive. According to the US Renal Data System 2006 annual report, there were 104,364 new cases of ESRD in 2004 — equivalent to an annual incidence of 342 cases per million population. The prevalence of ESRD in the USA in 2003 was 494,471 (1555 cases per million population). According to reports published by the Japanese Society for Dialysis Therapy, 267 people per million population started dialysis in 2004. In 2005, there were 2018 people per million population in Japan receiving dialysis — the highest reported prevalence for industrialised nations. According to Taiwanese government reports, the prevalence of ESRD in 2004 was 1706 cases per million population, and the incidence was 376 cases per million population. In comparison, based on data pooled from the European Renal Association–European Dialysis and Transplant Association Registry and UK Renal Registry, the incidence of treated ESRD (based on the incidence of RRT) in 2004 ranged from 75 cases per million population in Iceland to 195 cases per million population in Greece. The prevalence of treated ESRD in 2004 ranged from about 479 cases per million population in Iceland to 1022 cases per million population in Italy. In 2004, the Australia and New Zealand Dialysis and Transplant Registry reported an annual incidence of treated ESRD of 95 people per million population in Australia and 110 people per million population in New Zealand. The prevalence of treated ESRD in 2004 was 707 people per million population for Australia and 737 people per million population for New Zealand.

AETIOLOGY/RISK FACTORS The amount of daily proteinuria remains one of the strongest predictors of progression to ESRD. Hypertension is a strong independent risk factor for progression to ESRD, particularly in people with proteinuria. Age is also a predictor for ESRD; people over 65 years of age have a four- to fivefold increase in risk of ESRD compared with people under 65 years of age. Additional risk factors for developing ESRD include a history of chronic renal insufficiency, diabetes mellitus, heroin abuse, tobacco or analgesic use, non-white race or ethnicity, lower socioeconomic status, obesity, hyperuricaemia, and a family history of kidney disease.

PROGNOSIS The overall prognosis of untreated ESRD remains poor. Most people with ESRD eventually die from complications of CVD, infection, or, if dialysis is not provided, progressive uraemia (hyperkalaemia, acidosis, malnutrition, altered mental functioning). Precise mortality estimates, however, are unavailable because international renal registries omit individuals with ESRD who do not receive renal replacement therapy. Among people receiving renal replacement therapy, CVD is the leading cause of mortality, and accounts for more than 40% of deaths in this population. Extracellular volume overload and hypertension — which are common among people with chronic kidney disease — are known predictors of left ventricular hypertrophy and cardiovascular mortality in this population. Even after adjustment for age, sex, race, or ethnicity, and the presence of diabetes, annual cardiovascular mortality remains roughly an order of magnitude higher in people with ESRD than in the general population, particularly among younger individuals.

Robyn Webber, David Tolley, James Lingeman

KEY POINTS

- Kidney stones develop when crystals separate from the urine and aggregate within the kidney papillae, renal pelvis, or ureter.

  The peak incidence for stone disease occurs at the ages of 20–40 years, although stones are seen in all age groups. There is a male to female ratio of 3:1.

- The evidence is somewhat sparse with regard to the best treatments for people with asymptomatic kidney stones.

  Extracorporeal shockwave lithotripsy (ESWL) may reduce the need for further invasive surgery, although we don't know for certain.

  We found no evidence examining the effectiveness of percutaneous nephrolithotomy (PCNL) or ureteroscopy in people with asymptomatic kidney stones.

- PCNL seems to be as effective as ESWL in treating people with symptomatic kidney stones less than 30 mm in diameter, but it is more invasive and associated with more complications.

  People with larger stones are likely to take longer to pass stone fragments after ESWL, and so in these cases percutaneous nephrolithotomy may be a more suitable option. However, the field is advancing rapidly, so the evidence is not always applicable to current practice.

  We don't know whether ureteroscopy or open nephrolithotomy are useful treatments for the removal of symptomatic kidney stones as there are no suitable studies.

  Open nephrolithotomy has been largely superseded by PCNL in the Western world.

- For people with symptomatic ureteric stones, ureteroscopy seems to increase overall stone-free rates and decrease the time needed to become stone free compared with ESWL, although the latter is associated with lower failure and complication rates.

  We found no evidence examining the effectiveness of ureterolithotomy (either open or laparoscopic) in treating people with ureteric stones.

Please visit www.clinicalevidence.bmj.com for full text and references

What are the effects of interventions for stone removal in people with asymptomatic kidney stones?

Unknown Effectiveness	• ESWL in people with asymptomatic renal or ureteric stones
	• PCNL in people with asymptomatic renal or ureteric stones
	• Ureteroscopy in people with asymptomatic renal or ureteric stones

What are the effects of interventions for the removal of symptomatic renal stones?

Likely To Be Beneficial	• ESWL in people with renal stones less than 20 mm*
	• PCNL in people with renal stones
Unknown Effectiveness	• Open nephrolithotomy in people with renal stones

	• Ureteroscopy in people with renal stones

What are the effects of interventions to remove symptomatic ureteric stones?

Likely To Be Beneficial	• ESWL in people with mid- and distal ureteric stones
Trade-off Between Benefits And Harms	• Ureteroscopy in people with mid- and distal ureteric stones
Unknown Effectiveness	• ESWL in people with proximal ureteric stones • Ureterolithotomy (open or laparoscopic) in people with ureteric stones • Ureteroscopy in people with proximal ureteric stones

What are the effects of interventions for the management of acute renal colic?

Likely To Be Beneficial	• NSAIDs (indomethacin and diclofenac) • Opioid analgesics*
Unknown Effectiveness	• Fluids (intravenous or oral)
Unlikely To Be Beneficial	• Antispasmodic drugs

Search date April 2006

*Based on consensus opinion.

DEFINITION Nephrolithiasis is the presence of stones within the kidney; urolithiasis is a more general term for stones anywhere within the urinary tract. Urolithiasis is usually categorised according to the anatomical location of the stones (i.e. renal calyces, renal pelvis, ureteric, bladder, and urethra). Ureteric urolithiasis is described further by stating in which portion (proximal, middle, or distal) the stone is situated. This review assesses the effects of treatments only for the removal of asymptomatic or symptomatic renal and ureteric stones. It excludes pregnant women, in whom some forms of diagnostic procedures and treatments for stone removal are contraindicated, and people with significant comorbidities (including severe cardiovascular and respiratory conditions) who may be at increased risk when having general anaesthesia. **Diagnosis:** Diagnosis is usually based on clinical history, supported by investigations with diagnostic imaging. One third of all kidney stones become clinically evident; typically causing pain, often severe in nature; renal angle tenderness; haematuria; or digestive symptoms (e.g. nausea, vomiting, or diarrhoea). The onset of pain is usually sudden, typically felt in the loin, and radiating to the groin, and genitalia (scrotum or labia). People are typically restless, find the pain excruciating, and describe it as the worst pain ever experienced. The cause and chemical composition of a stone may have some bearing on its diagnosis, management, and particularly on prevention of recurrence. Although the choices for surgical management in general remain the same for all types of stone disease, the recognition of a specific cause, such as recurrent infection with a urease-producing organism for struvite stones, or cysteinuria for cysteine

(continued over)

(from previous page)

stones, will inform further management. **Differential diagnosis:** Bleeding within the urinary tract may present with identical symptoms to kidney stones, particularly if there are blood clots present within the renal pelvis or ureter. Several other conditions may also mimic a renal colic and need to be considered for differential diagnosis. These include urinary tract infection (and indeed the two conditions may coexist), and analgesic abuse (either renal damage from excessive ingestion of analgesics, or in people with a history of opiate abuse, who may feign a renal colic in an attempt to obtain opiate analgesia). Rarely, people with sickle cell disease may also present with severe abdominal pain, which needs to be distinguished from a renal colic.

INCIDENCE/PREVALENCE The peak incidence for stone disease occurs at the ages of 20–40 years, although stones are seen in all age groups. There is a male to female ratio of 3:1. Calcium oxalate stones, the most common variety, have a recurrence rate of 10% at 1 year, 35% at 5 years, and 50% at 5 years after the first episode of kidney stone disease in North America.

AETIOLOGY/RISK FACTORS Kidney stones develop when crystals separate from the urine and aggregate within the kidney papillae, renal pelvis, or ureter. The most common type of stone contains varying amounts of calcium and oxalate, whereas "struvite" stones contain a mixture of magnesium, ammonium, and phosphate. Struvite stones are associated almost exclusively with infection with urease-producing organisms, while calcium oxalate stones have several aetiologies. Rarer stones include those formed from uric acid, cysteine, and xanthine, although this list is not exhaustive. In many otherwise healthy people the cause is uncertain. However, incidence is higher in people with hyperparathyroidism and people with disorders including small bowel dysfunction, urinary tract infection (in particular caused by urease-producing organisms), and structural/anatomical abnormalities of the kidney and ureter (including obstruction of the pelviureteric junction, hydronephrotic renal pelvis or calyces, calyceal diverticulum, horseshoe kidney, ureterocele, vesicoureteral reflux, ureteric stricture, or medullary sponge kidney). Other conditions associated with the development of renal stones include gout (especially leading to uric acid calculi) and chronic metabolic acidosis (typically resulting in stones composed of calcium phosphate). Women with a history of surgical menopause are also at higher risk because of increased bone resorption, and urinary excretion of calcium. Drugs, including some decongestants, diuretics, and anticonvulsants are also associated with an increased risk of stone formation.

PROGNOSIS Most kidney stones pass within 48 hours with expectant treatment (including adequate fluid intake and analgesia). Others may take longer to pass and the observation period can be extended to 3–4 weeks where appropriate. Ureteric stones less than 5 mm in diameter will pass spontaneously in about 90% of people, compared with 50% of ureteric stones between 5 mm and 10 mm. Expectant (conservative) management is considered on a case-to-case basis, and only in people with stones which are asymptomatic or very small (although stone size may not correlate with symptom severity), or both, and in people with significant comorbidities (including severe cardiovascular and respiratory conditions, who may be at increased risk when having general anaesthesia), in whom the risks of treatment may outweigh the likely benefits. Stones may migrate regardless of treatment or after treatment for their removal, and may or may not present clinically once in the ureter. Stones blocking the urine flow may lead to hydronephrosis and renal atrophy. They may also result in life-threatening complications including urinary infection, perinephric abscess, or urosepsis. Infection may also occur after invasive procedures for stone removal. Some of these complications may cause kidney damage and compromised renal function. Eventually, 10–20% of all kidney stones need treatment.

Robyn Webber

KEY POINTS

- Symptomatic benign prostatic hyperplasia (BPH) may affect up to 30% of men in their early 70s, causing urinary symptoms of bladder outlet obstruction.

  Symptoms can improve without treatment, but the usual course is a slow progression of symptoms, with acute urinary retention occurring in 1–2% of men with BPH per year.

- Alpha-blockers improve symptoms compared with placebo and with finasteride, and may be most effective in men with more severe symptoms of BPH or with hypertension.

- CAUTION: Since the last update of this review, a drug safety alert has been issued on risk of intraoperative floppy iris syndrome during cataract surgery with tamsulosin (www.mhra.gov.uk).

- 5 alpha-reductase inhibitors (finasteride) improve symptoms and reduce complications compared with placebo, and may be more effective in men with larger prostates.

- Transurethral resection of the prostate (TURP) improves symptoms of BPH more than watchful waiting, and has not been shown to increase the risk of erectile dysfunction or incontinence.

  Less-invasive surgical techniques such as transurethral incision or laser ablation seem to be as effective as TURP at improving symptoms.

  TURP may be more effective at improving symptoms and preventing retreatment compared with transurethral microwave thermotherapy, but causes more complications.

  Transurethral microwave thermotherapy reduces symptoms compared with sham treatment or with alpha-blockers, but long-term effects are unknown.

  We don't know whether transurethral needle ablation is effective.

- Saw palmetto plant extracts may be as effective as alpha-blockers and 5 alpha-reductase inhibitors, but few studies have been done.

  Beta-sitosterol plant extract may improve symptoms of BPH compared with placebo in the short term.

  We don't know whether rye grass pollen extract or *Pygeum africanum* are also beneficial, as few studies were found.

Please visit www.clinicalevidence.bmj.com for full text and references

What are the effects of medical treatments?	
Beneficial	• 5 alpha-reductase inhibitors
	• Alpha-blockers

What are the effects of surgical treatments?	
Beneficial	• Transurethral microwave thermotherapy
	• TURP versus no surgery
Unknown Effectiveness	• TURP versus less-invasive surgical techniques
	• TURP versus transurethral needle ablation

What are the effects of herbal treatments?	
Likely To Be Beneficial	• Beta-sitosterol plant extract • Saw palmetto plant extracts
Unknown Effectiveness	• *Pygeum africanum* • Rye grass pollen extract

Search date May 2005

DEFINITION Benign prostatic hyperplasia is defined histologically. Clinically, it is characterised by lower urinary tract symptoms (urinary frequency, urgency, a weak and intermittent stream, needing to strain, a sense of incomplete emptying, and nocturia) and can lead to complications, including acute urinary retention.

INCIDENCE/PREVALENCE Estimates of the prevalence of symptomatic benign prostatic hyperplasia range from 10–30% for men in their early 70s, depending on how benign prostatic hyperplasia is defined.

AETIOLOGY/RISK FACTORS The mechanisms by which benign prostatic hyperplasia causes symptoms and complications are unclear, although bladder outlet obstruction is an important factor. The best documented risk factors are increasing age and normal testicular function.

PROGNOSIS Community- and practice-based studies suggest that men with lower urinary tract symptoms can expect slow progression of symptoms. However, symptoms can wax and wane without treatment. In men with symptoms of benign prostatic hyperplasia, rates of acute urinary retention range from 1–2% a year.

Bradley A Erickson, Thomas Jang and Anthony J Schaeffer

KEY POINTS

- Chronic prostatitis can cause pain and urinary symptoms, and usually occurs without positive bacterial cultures from prostatic secretions (known as chronic abacterial prostatitis or chronic pelvic pain syndrome, CP/CPPS).

  Bacterial infection can result from urinary tract instrumentation, but the cause and natural history of CP/CPPS are unknown.

- Chronic bacterial prostatitis has identifiable virulent micro-organisms in prostatic secretions.

  Oral antimicrobial drugs are likely to be beneficial, although studies comparing them with placebo or no treatment have not been found.

  Clinical success rates from oral antimicrobials have reached about 70–90% at 6 months in studies comparing different regimens.

  Trimethoprim–sulfamethoxazole (co-trimoxazole) and quinolones are most commonly used and seem to be the most beneficial.

  Alpha-blockers may reduce symptoms and reduce recurrence if added to antimicrobial treatment.

  We don't know whether local injections of antimicrobial drugs, NSAIDs, TURP, or radical prostatectomy improve symptoms compared with no treatment.

- Effective treatment regimens for CP/CPPS remain to be defined, and strategies are based on symptomatic control and anxiety relief.

  Alpha-blockers may improve quality of life and symptoms compared with no treatment, but studies have been small.

  Oral antimicrobial drugs have not been shown to improve symptoms.

  We don't know whether 5 alpha-reductase inhibitors, NSAIDs, pentosan polysulfate, allopurinol, transurethral microwave thermotherapy, prostatic massage, Sitz baths, biofeedback, mepartricin, or quercetin reduce symptoms in men with CP/CPPS.

- Caution: Since the last update of this review, a drug safety alert has been issued on risk of intraoperative floppy iris syndrome during cataract surgery with tamsulosin (www.mhra.gov.uk).

Please visit www.clinicalevidence.bmj.com for full text and references

What are the effects of treatments for chronic bacterial prostatitis?

Likely To Be Beneficial	• Oral antimicrobial drugs
Unknown Effectiveness	• Alpha-blockers
	• Local injection of antimicrobial drugs
	• NSAIDss
	• Radical prostatectomy
	• TURP

What are the effects of treatments for chronic abacterial prostatitis/chronic pelvic pain syndrome?

Likely To Be Beneficial	• Alpha-blockers
Unknown Effectiveness	• 5 alpha-reductase inhibitors • Allopurinol • Biofeedback • Mepartricin • NSAIDs • Pentosan polysulfate • Quercetin • Sitz baths • Transurethral microwave thermotherapy
Unlikely To Be Beneficial	• Oral antimicrobial drugs • Prostatic massage

Search date July 2006

DEFINITION Chronic bacterial prostatitis is characterised by a positive culture of expressed prostatic secretions. It may cause symptoms such as suprapubic, lower back, or perineal pain, with or without mild urgency and increased frequency of urination and dysuria, and may be associated with recurrent UTIs. However, it may also be asymptomatic between acute episodes/exacerbations. **Chronic abacterial prostatitis/chronic pelvic pain syndrome (CP/CPPS)**, is characterised by pelvic or perineal pain in the absence of pathogenic bacteria in expressed prostatic secretions. It is often associated with irritative and obstructive voiding symptoms including urgency, frequency, hesitancy, and poor interrupted flow. Symptoms can also include pain in the suprapubic region, lower back, penis, testes, or scrotum, and painful ejaculation. CP/CPPS may be inflammatory (white cells present in prostatic secretions) or non-inflammatory (white cells absent in prostatic secretions). A classification system for the prostatitis syndromes has been developed by the National Institutes of Health (NIH).

INCIDENCE/PREVALENCE One community-based study in the USA (cohort of 2115 men aged 40–79 years) estimated that 9% of men have a diagnosis of prostatitis at any one time. Another observational study found that, in men presenting with genitourinary symptoms, 8% of them presenting to urologists and 1% of them presenting to primary-care physicians were diagnosed as having chronic prostatitis. Most cases of chronic prostatitis are abacterial. Chronic bacterial prostatitis, although easy to diagnose, is rare.

AETIOLOGY/RISK FACTORS Organisms commonly implicated in bacterial prostatitis include *Escherichia coli*, other Gram-negative enterobacteriaceae, occasionally *Pseudomonas* species, and rarely Gram-positive enterococci. Risk factors for bacterial prostatitis include urethral catheterisation or instrumentation, condom drainage, dysfunctional voiding (high-pressure urination), and unprotected anal intercourse. The cause of chronic abacterial prostatitis/chronic pelvic pain syndrome (CP/CPPS) is unclear, although it has been suggested that it may be caused by undocumented infections with *Chlamydia trachomatis*, *Ureaplasma urealyticum*, *Mycoplasma hominis*, and *Trichomonas vaginalis*. Viruses, *Candida* (in immunosuppressed people), and parasites have also rarely been implicated. Non-infectious factors might also be involved, including inflammation, autoimmunity, hormonal imbalances, pelvic floor tension myalgia, intraprostatic urinary reflux, and psychological disturbances. In one case-control study (463 men with CP/CPPS, 121 asymptomatic age matched controls), when compared with controls, men with CP/CPPS reported a significantly higher lifetime prevalence of non-specific urethritis (12% with CP/CPPS v 4% with no CP/CPPS; P = 0.008), CVD (11% with CP/CPPS v 2% with no CP/CPPS; P = 0.004), neurological disease (41% with CP/CPPS v 14% with no CP/CPPS; P less than 0.001), psychiatric conditions (29% with CP/CPPS v 11% with no CP/CPPS; P less than 0.001), and haematopoietic, lymphatic, or infectious disease (41% with CP/CPPS v 20% with no CP/CPPS; P less than 0.001). Further studies are necessary to determine whether these factors play a role in the pathogenesis of CP/CPPS.

PROGNOSIS The natural history of untreated chronic bacterial and abacterial prostatitis/ chronic pelvic pain syndrome (CP/CPPS) remains ill-defined. Chronic bacterial prostatitis may cause recurrent urinary tract infections in men whereas CP/CPPS does not. Several investigators have reported an association between chronic bacterial prostatitis, CP/CPPS, and infertility. One study found that CP/CPPS had an impact on quality of life similar to that of angina, Crohn's disease, or a previous MI.

Prathap Tharyan and Ganesh Gopalakrishanan

KEY POINTS

- Erectile dysfunction may affect 30–50% of men aged 40–70 years, with age, smoking and obesity being the main risk factors, although 20% of cases have psychological causes.

- Sildenafil improves erections and increases the likelihood of successful intercourse overall and in men with diabetes mellitus, heart disease, spinal-cord injury, prostate cancer or after radical prostatectomy.

    Tadalafil and vardenafil are also effective overall and in men with diabetes, and vardenafil may be effective after prostatectomy.

- CAUTION: sildenafil, tadalafil, and vardenafil are contraindicated in men who are taking nitrates as combined treatment has been associated with severe hypotension and death.

- Intracavernosal alprostadil improves erections compared with placebo, intraurethral alprostadil, and intracavernosal papaverine, but can cause penile pain in up to 40% of men.

    Intracavernosal alprostadil may be as effective as sildenafil and bimix, while topical alprostadil may also be effective.

    Adding phentoloamine to intracavernosal papaverine (bimix) may increase effectiveness compared with papaverine alone, and adding alprostadil to bimix (trimix) may be more effective again. However, papaverine injections may cause altered liver function, and penile bruising and fibrosis.

    Sublingual apomorphine, ginseng, and yohimbine may increase successful erections and intercourse compared with placebo.

- Vacuum devices may be as effective as intracavernosal alprostadil at increasing rigidity, but less effective for orgasm, and may block ejaculation.

    There is consensus that penile prostheses may be beneficial, but they can cause infections and are only used if less invasive treatments have failed.

- Psychosexual counselling and CBT may improve sexual functioning in men with psychological erectile dysfunction, but few good-quality studies have been found.

(i) **Please visit www.clinicalevidence.bmj.com for full text and references**

What are the effects of treatments in men with erectile dysfunction?

Beneficial	• Alprostadil (intracavernosal)
	• Alprostadil (intraurethral)
	• Apomorphine
	• Sildenafil
	• Tadalafil
	• Vardenafil
Likely To Be Beneficial	• Ginseng
	• Penile prosthesis*
	• Psychosexual counselling
	• Vacuum devices

	• Yohimbine
Trade-off Between Benefits And Harms	• Alprostadil (topical) • Papaverine • Papaverine plus phentolamine (bimix) • Papaverine plus phentolamine plus alprostadil (trimix)
Unknown Effectiveness	• CBT

Search date August 2005

*Categorisation based on consensus; RCTs unlikely to be conducted.

DEFINITION Erectile dysfunction is defined as the persistent inability to obtain or maintain sufficient rigidity of the penis to allow satisfactory sexual performance. The term erectile dysfunction has largely replaced the term "impotence". For the purposes of this review we included only men with normal testosterone and gonadotrophin levels, who could gain an erection while asleep. We also included men with comorbid conditions such as cardiovascular disorders, prostate cancer, diabetes, and spinal-cord injury. We excluded men with drug-induced sexual dysfunction. Because the cause of erectile dysfunction in men with CVD is unclear (the disease or treatment drugs), we included them.

INCIDENCE/PREVALENCE Cross-sectional epidemiological studies from around the world reveal that 30–50% of men aged 40–70 years report some degree of erectile dysfunction. About 150 million men worldwide are unable to achieve and maintain an erection adequate for satisfactory sexual intercourse. Age is the variable most strongly associated with erectile dysfunction; between the ages of 40 to 70 years, the incidence of moderate erectile dysfunction doubles from 17% to 34%, whereas that of severe erectile dysfunction triples from 5% to 15%.

AETIOLOGY/RISK FACTORS About 80% of cases are believed to have an organic cause, the rest being psychogenic in origin. Most cases of erectile dysfunction are believed to be multifactorial and secondary to disease, stress, trauma (such as spinal-cord injury, pelvic and prostate surgery), or drug adverse effects that interfere with the coordinated psychological, neurological, endocrine, vascular, and muscular factors necessary for normal erections. Risk factors include increasing age, smoking, and obesity. The prevalence of erectile dysfunction also increases in people with diabetes mellitus, hypertension, heart disease, anxiety, and depression.

PROGNOSIS We found no good evidence on prognosis in untreated organic erectile dysfunction.

Melissa L James

KEY POINTS

- Prostate cancer is the sixth most common cancer in the world and 85% of cases are diagnosed in men over the age of 65 years.

  Subclinical prostate cancer is common and increases with age, with an estimated prevalence of 30% in men aged 30–39 years, increasing to over 75% in men aged over 85 years.

  Risk factors include black ethnic origin, family history of prostate cancer, and diet.

  In men with well to moderately differentiated prostate cancer that remains within the capsule, clinical progression-free survival is 70% at 5 years and 40% at 10 years.

  Age-adjusted mortality rates for prostate cancer do not seem to be affected by national PSA screening and treatment rates.

- Radical prostatectomy may reduce mortality compared with watchful waiting in men with clinically localised prostate cancer, but the benefits in quality-adjusted life expectancy seem to be moderate.

  Radical prostatectomy may reduce overall and prostate-cancer mortality and metastasis, but increases the risk of urinary and sexual dysfunction.

- The benefits of external beam radiation therapy (EBRT) or brachytherapy compared with watchful waiting or radical prostatectomy are unknown. EBRT increases the risk of erectile dysfunction and toxicity to the surrounding tissues.

  Long-term survival after EBRT depends on pre-treatment PSA level and tumour differentiation.

- Hormone therapy may be used as neoadjuvant therapy before surgery or radiotherapy, concurrently with radiation therapy, or as an adjuvant to usual care. Evidence of benefit from hormone therapy in early prostate cancer is limited.

  Neoadjuvant hormone therapy may improve biochemical-free survival when used with EBRT, but not when given before surgery plus adjuvant hormonal therapy.

  Immediate hormone therapy in men with clinically localised prostate cancer may reduce disease progression, but may not reduce overall mortality, although few adequate studies have been found.

  Adjuvant hormonal therapy may reduce disease progression, but may not improve overall survival compared with placebo.

  Hormone therapy is associated with increased rates of gynaecomastia and breast pain.

(i) **Please visit www.clinicalevidence.bmj.com for full text and references**

What are the effects of treatments for early prostate cancer?

Trade-off Between Benefits And Harms	• Radical prostatectomy • Watchful waiting
Unknown Effectiveness	• Adding hormone therapy to external beam radiation therapy (to increase overall survival) • Brachytherapy • External beam radiation therapy

	• Hormone therapy plus brachytherapy
	• Hormone therapy plus standard care
	• Immediate hormone therapy for asymptomatic disease
	• Immediate hormone therapy for symptomatic disease
Unlikely To Be Beneficial	• Adding neoadjuvant hormone therapy to surgery plus adjuvant hormonal therapy
	• Neoadjuvant hormone therapy plus surgery

Search date February 2006

DEFINITION Prostatic cancer is staged according to two systems: the tumour, node, metastasis (TNM) classification system (where scores of T0, T1, T2, T3, T4, N0; M0 apply to non-metastatic prostate cancer) and the American Urologic Staging system (where stages A, B, and C apply to non-metastatic prostate cancer) Non-metastatic prostate cancer can be divided into clinically localised disease and advanced disease. Clinically localised disease (T0, T1, T2) is prostate cancer thought to be confined to the prostate gland by clinical examination. Locally advanced disease (T3 and T4) is prostate cancer which has spread beyond the capsule of, but is still connected to, the prostate gland. Metastatic disease is prostate cancer which has spread outside the prostate gland with no remaining connection. This review focuses on clinically localised disease that has not extended beyond the prostate capsule (TNM classification system T0, T1, T2, and American Urologic Staging system stages A and B).

INCIDENCE/PREVALENCE Prostate cancer is the sixth most common cancer in the world and the third most common cancer in men. In 2000, an estimated 513,000 new cases of prostate cancer were diagnosed, and about 250,000 deaths were attributed to prostate cancers worldwide. The estimated number of new cases of prostate cancer in the United States in 2005 was 232,090. Prostate cancer is uncommon under the age of 50 years. About 85% of men with prostate cancer are diagnosed after 65 years of age. Autopsy studies suggest that the prevalence of subclinical prostate cancer is high at all ages: 30% for men aged 30–39 years, 50% for men aged 50–59 years, and more than 75% for men over 85 years. Incidence varies widely by ethnic group and around the world.

AETIOLOGY/RISK FACTORS Risk factors for prostate cancer include increasing age, family history of prostate cancer, black ethnic group, and possibly higher dietary consumption of fat and meat, low intake of lycopene (from tomato products), low intake of fruit, and high dietary calcium. In the USA, black men have about a 60% higher incidence than white men. The prostate cancer incidence for black men living in the USA is about 90/100,000 in men aged under 65 years and about 1300/100,000 in men aged 65–74 years. For white men, incidence is about 44/100,000 in men aged under 65 years and 900/100,000 in men aged 65–74 years.

PROGNOSIS The chance that men with well to moderately differentiated, palpable, clinically localised prostate cancer will remain free of symptomatic progression is 70% at 5 years and 40% at 10 years. The risk of symptomatic disease progression is higher in men with poorly differentiated prostate cancer. One retrospective analysis of a large surgical series in men with clinically localised prostate cancer found that the median time from the increase in prostate specific antigen (PSA) concentration to the development of metastatic disease was 8 years. PSA doubling time and Gleason score were predictive of the probability and time to development of metastatic disease. Once men developed metastatic disease, the median actuarial time to death was less than 5 years. Morbidity from local or regional disease progression includes haematuria, bladder obstruction, and lower extremity oedema. The age-adjusted prostate cancer-specific mortality in the USA for all men aged 65 years and older has decreased by about 15% (244 deaths/100,000 to 207 deaths/ 100,000) from 1991–1997. The reasons for this are unclear, although inaccurate death

(continued over)

(from previous page)

certification, PSA screening, and earlier, more intensive treatment, including radical prostatectomy, radiotherapy, and androgen suppression, have been suggested. However, regions of the USA and Canada where PSA testing and early treatment are more common have similar prostate cancer mortality to regions with lower rates of both testing and early treatment. Similarly, countries with low rates of PSA testing and treatment, such as the UK, have similar age-adjusted prostate cancer mortality to countries with high rates of testing and treatment, such as the USA.

Richard Neal, Nicholas Stuart and Clare Wilkinson

KEY POINTS

- More than half of painless solid swellings of the body of the testis are malignant, with a peak incidence in men aged 25–35 years.

  About half of testicular cancers are seminomas, which tend to affect older men, and have a good prognosis.

- In men with seminoma confined to the testis (stage 1), standard treatment is orchidectomy followed by radiotherapy to infradiaphragmatic lymph nodes, which is associated with cure rates approaching 100%.

  Adjuvant chemotherapy and radiotherapy reduce the risk of relapse after orchidectomy compared with surveillance, but both reduce fertility and may increase the risk of secondary malignancy in the long term.

  We do not know which is the most effective chemotherapy regimen, or the optimum number of cycles to use. The high cure rate with standard therapy makes it difficult to show that any alternative therapy is superior.

  Toxicity is lower, but efficacy the same, with adjuvant irradiation of 20 Gy in 10 fractions compared with 30 Gy in 15 fractions, or with irradiation to para-aortic nodes compared with ipsilateral iliac nodes.

- In men with good prognosis non-stage 1 seminoma who have had orchidectomy, radiotherapy may improve survival and be less toxic than chemotherapy, except in men with large volume disease, in whom chemotherapy may be more effective.

  Combined chemotherapy may be more effective than single agents, but three cycles seem to be as effective as four and with less toxicity.

  Standard radiotherapy treatment comprises 30–36 Gy in 15–18 fractions, although we do not know whether this is more effective than other regimens.

- In men who are in remission after orchidectomy plus chemotherapy for good prognosis non-stage 1 seminoma, further chemotherapy is unlikely to reduce relapse rates or increase survival.

  We do not know whether chemotherapy increases survival in men with intermediate prognosis seminomas who have had orchidectomy.

(i) **Please visit www.clinicalevidence.bmj.com for full text and references**

What are the effects of treatments in men with stage 1 seminoma (confined to testis) who have undergone orchidectomy?

Beneficial	• Adjuvant irradiation of 20 Gy in 10 fractions to para-aortic area compared with 30 Gy in 15 fractions to para-aortic area and iliac nodes (similarly effective but less toxicity)
Trade-off Between Benefits And Harms	• Adjuvant chemotherapy (reduced risk of relapse compared with surveillance, increased immediate toxicity, and possible long-term fertility problems and development of secondary malignancies)*
	• Adjuvant radiotherapy (reduced risk of relapse compared with surveillance, increased immediate toxicity, and possible long-term fertility problems and development of secondary malignancies)*

	• Surveillance (avoids toxicity associated with adjuvant radiotherapy or chemotherapy, increased risk of relapse)*
Unknown Effectiveness	• Comparative effects of different drug combinations for adjuvant chemotherapy • Comparative effects of different number of cycles of adjuvant chemotherapy

What are the effects of treatments in men with good-prognosis non-stage 1 seminoma who have undergone orchidectomy?

Likely To Be Beneficial	• Chemotherapy using bleomycin added to vinblastine plus cisplatin (reduced relapse rates and mortality compared with two-drug regimen of vinblastine plus cisplatin alone) • Chemotherapy using etoposide plus cisplatin with or without bleomycin (increased relapse-free survival compared with other combined regimens) • Radiotherapy (30–36 Gy in 15–18 fractions)* • Three cycles of chemotherapy compared with four cycles (no significant difference in survival; reduced toxicity)
Trade-off Between Benefits And Harms	• Radiotherapy versus chemotherapy (less toxicity with radiotherapy compared with chemotherapy; higher risk of relapse)*
Unknown Effectiveness	• Adding higher compared with lower doses of cisplatin or vinblastine to a two-drug chemotherapy regimen
Unlikely To Be Beneficial	• Chemotherapy using single-agent carboplatin (may be less effective than combined chemotherapy in increasing relapse-free survival)

What are the effects of maintenance chemotherapy in men who are in remission after orchidectomy and chemotherapy for good-prognosis non-stage 1 seminoma?

Unlikely To Be Beneficial	• Maintenance chemotherapy

What are the effects of treatments in men with intermediate-prognosis seminomas who have undergone orchidectomy?

Unknown Effectiveness	• Chemotherapy

Search date April 2006

*No RCTs. Based on observational evidence and consensus.

DEFINITION Although testicular symptoms are common, testicular cancer is relatively rare. Solid swellings affecting the body of the testis have a high probability (over 50%) of being caused by cancer. The most common presenting symptom of cancer is a painless lump or swelling (over 85%). About 10% of men present with acute pain, and 20–30% experience a heavy dragging feeling or general ache. These symptoms may lead the cancer to be initially wrongly diagnosed as epididymitis or acute testicular torsion. A small percentage present with symptoms of metastatic disease and infertility. Testicular cancers are divided into **seminomas**, which make up about half of all testicular tumours, and which occur in older patients; and **non-seminomatous tumours**, comprising teratomas, mixed tumours, and other cell types, which tend to occur in younger patients. Several staging systems for testicular cancer have been developed. The most commonly used system in current practice is the International Germ Cell Consensus Classification, which classifies testicular tumours as good prognosis, intermediate prognosis, or poor prognosis. Because 90% of seminomas are classified as good prognosis, this system is less useful for seminomas, and so we have further divided good-prognosis seminoma into stage 1 (confined to testis) and non-stage 1 (with nodal but no non-visceral metastases), based on the Royal Marsden and TNM staging systems.

INCIDENCE/PREVALENCE There are about 1400 new cases of testicular cancer (semi-nona, teratoma, or mixed seminoma/teratoma) annually in the UK, with the peak incidence in men aged 25–35 years. It comprises 1% of all cancers in men and is the most common tumour in young men. Incidence varies markedly with geography; a study among 10 cancer registries in Northern Europe identified a 10-fold variation, with the highest incidence rate in Denmark (7.8 per 100,000) and lowest in Lithuania (0.9 per 100,000). Recent reviews of the incidence of testicular cancer have reported a clear trend toward increased incidence during the past 30 years in the majority of industrialised countries in North America, Europe, and Oceania.

AETIOLOGY/RISK FACTORS There appear to be both individual and environmental risk factors for testicular cancer. Having a close relative who has had testicular cancer increases the risk of getting the disease. Inherited genetic factors may play a role in up to one in five cancers. Men are more at risk of developing testicular cancer if they have a history of developmental abnormality (e.g. maldescent or gonadal dysgenesis), previous cancer in the opposite testis, HIV infection or AIDS, torsion, trauma (although this may be coincidental), and Klinefelter's syndrome. The wide geographical variation and changes over time in incidence rates imply that there are likely to be important environmental factors, because the individual risk factors described above do not explain global disease patterns.

PROGNOSIS Testicular tumours generally have a good prognosis. The International Germ Cell Consensus Classification classifies 90% of all seminomas as "good prognosis". These include those confined to the testis (stage 1 of the Royal Marsden or TNM system) as well as tumours with nodal but no non-pulmonary visceral metastases. The remaining 10% of seminomas, including those with non-pulmonary visceral metastases, are classified as "intermediate prognosis". No seminomas are classified as "poor prognosis". Untreated disease will progress over time, leading to large local tumours and distant spread. The first site of spread is the lymphatic system, particularly the pelvic and para-aortic lymph nodes. Haematological spread leading to lung, liver, and brain metastases is less common in seminomas; 75% of men present with stage 1 disease. From the perspective of the International Germ Cell Cancer Collaborative Group prognostic classification, 90% of

(continued over)

(from previous page)

seminomas present as "good prognosis" with a 5-year survival of 86%, and 10% present as "intermediate prognosis" with a 5-year survival of 73%. Seminoma is a radio-sensitive tumour, and the standard treatment for stage I seminoma is orchidectomy followed by infradiaphragmatic lymph node irradiation. Clinical observation suggests that, with this approach, cure rates are nearly 100%.

Chandra Shekhar Biyani, Jon Cartledge, and Günter Janetschek

KEY POINTS

- Varicocele is estimated to affect 10–15% of men and adolescent boys, usually occurs only on the left side, and is often asymptomatic. If symptoms do occur, they may include testicular ache or distress about cosmetic appearance.

  There is little evidence that varicocele reduces male fertility, although it is found in 12% of male partners of couples presenting with infertility, and in 25% of men with abnormal semen analysis.

- Varicocele is caused by dysfunction of the valves in the spermatic vein.

- We don't know what the outcomes are for expectant management of men with varicocele compared with surgical treatments, because studies have been of poor quality.

  We don't know whether surgical ligation or embolisation of the spermatic vein increase pregnancy rates or reduce symptoms of varicocele.

  Sclerotherapy may not improve fertility compared with no treatment. We don't know whether it reduces symptoms of varicocele.

Please visit www.clinicalevidence.bmj.com for full text and references

What are the effects of treatments in men with varicocele?

Unknown Effectiveness	• Embolisation
	• Expectant management
	• Sclerotherapy
	• Surgical ligation

Search date September 2006

DEFINITION Varicocele is a dilation of the pampiniform plexus of the spermatic cord. Severity is commonly graded as follows: **grade 0:** only demonstrable by technical investigation; **grade 1:** palpable or visible only on Valsalva manoeuvre (straining); **grade 2:** palpable but not visible when standing upright at room temperature; and **grade 3:** visible when standing upright at room temperature. Varicocele is unilateral and left sided in at least 85% of cases. In most of the remaining cases, the condition is bilateral. Unilateral right-sided varicocele is rare. Many men who have a varicocele have no symptoms. Symptoms may include testicular ache or discomfort, and distress about cosmetic appearance. This review deals with varicocele in adult men only.

INCIDENCE/PREVALENCE We found few data on the prevalence of varicocele. Anecdotally, it has been estimated that about 10–15% of men and adolescent boys in the general population have varicocele. One multicentre study found that, in couples with subfertility, the prevalence of varicocele in male partners was about 12%. In men with abnormal semen analysis, the prevalence of varicocele was about 25%.

AETIOLOGY/RISK FACTORS We found no reliable data on epidemiological risk factors for varicocele, such as a family history or environmental exposures. Anatomically, varicoceles are caused by dysfunction of the valves in the spermatic vein, which allows pooling of blood in the pampiniform plexus. This is more likely to occur in the left spermatic vein than in the right because of normal anatomical asymmetry.

PROGNOSIS Varicocele is believed to be associated with subfertility, although reliable evidence is sparse. The natural history of varicocele is unclear.

Anorexia nervosa

Janet Treasure and Ulrike Schmidt

KEY POINTS

- Anorexia nervosa is characterised by a low BMI, fear of gaining weight, denial of current low weight, and its impact on health and amenorrhoea.

  Estimated prevalence is highest in teenage girls and may affect up to 0.7% of this age group.

  Anorexia nervosa is related to biological, family, and socio-cultural factors. Psychiatric and personality disorders, such as depression, anxiety disorders, obsessive compulsive disorder, and perfectionism are commonly found in anorexia nervosa.

  While most people with anorexia nervosa recover completely or partially, approximately 5% will die of the condition and 20% develop a chronic eating disorder.

  Young women with anorexia nervosa are at increased risk of fractures later in life.

- There is no strong evidence that any treatments work well for anorexia nervosa. However, there is a gradual accumulation of evidence which suggests that early intervention is effective. Working with the family may also interrupt the development of a persistent form of the illness.

- Evidence on the benefit of psychotherapy is unclear.

- Refeeding is a necessary and effective component of treatment, but is not sufficient alone.

  Limited evidence from a quasi-experimental study suggests that a lenient approach to refeeding is as effective and more acceptable compared with a more strict approach.

  Refeeding may be as effective in an outpatient setting as during hospital admission.

  Nasogastric feeding is rarely required and can lead to problems due to hypophosphataemia.

- Limited evidence from two small RCTs has failed to show significant weight gain from antidepressants, which may cause serious adverse effects.

  TCAs may cause drowsiness, a dry mouth, blurred vision, and a prolonged QT interval in people with anorexia nervosa.

  SSRIs have not been shown to be beneficial, but the evidence is limited because the three RCTs we found were all small and had high withdrawal rates.

  Anxiolytic drugs may prolong the QT interval, increasing the risk of ventricular tachycardia, torsades de pointes, and sudden death.

- We found insufficient evidence to assess cyproheptadine for treating anorexia, or to assess whether oestrogen treatment could reduce the negative effects on bone mineral density associated with anorexia nervosa.

(i) **Please visit www.clinicalevidence.bmj.com for full text and references**

What are the effects of treatments in anorexia nervosa?

Likely To Be Beneficial	• Refeeding*
Unknown Effectiveness	• Cyproheptadine
	• Inpatient versus outpatient treatment setting
	• Psychotherapy

	• Selective serotonin reuptake inhibitors
Likely To Be Ineffective Or Harmful	• Anxiolytic drugs • TCAs

What are the effects of interventions to prevent or treat complications of anorexia nervosa?

Unknown Effectiveness	• Oestrogen treatment

Search date December 2005

*Not based on RCT evidence; RCTs unlikely to be conducted.

DEFINITION Anorexia nervosa is characterised by a refusal to maintain weight at or above a minimally normal weight (less than 85% of expected weight for age and height, or BMI of less than 17.5 kg/m²), or a failure to show the expected weight gain during growth. In association with this, there is often an intense fear of gaining weight, preoccupation with weight, denial of the current low weight and its adverse impact on health, and amenorrhoea. Two subtypes of anorexia nervosa, binge–purge and restricting, have been defined.

INCIDENCE/PREVALENCE One population-based study using consultation data from the General Practitioner database in the UK found a mean incidence of anorexia nervosa of 4/100,000 in people aged 10–39 years. One systematic review (5 studies) assessing prevalence in Europe in people aged over 19 years found a 12-month prevalence of 0.2–0.7%. Little is known of the incidence or prevalence in Asia, South America, or Africa.

AETIOLOGY/RISK FACTORS Anorexia nervosa has been related to family, biological, social, and cultural factors. Studies have found that anorexia nervosa is associated with a family history of anorexia nervosa (adjusted HR 11.4, 95% CI 1.1 to 89.0), bulimia nervosa (adjusted HR 3.5, 95% CI 1.1 to 14.0), depression, generalised anxiety disorder, obsessive compulsive disorder, or obsessive compulsive personality disorder (adjusted RR 3.6, 95% CI 1.6 to 8.0). A twin study suggested that anorexia nervosa may be related to genetic factors, but it was unable to estimate reliably how non-shared environmental factors contributed. Specific aspects of childhood temperament thought to be related include perfectionism, negative self-evaluation, and extreme compliance. Perinatal factors include prematurity, particularly if the baby was small for gestational age (prematurity: OR 3.2, 95% CI 1.6 to 6.2; prematurity and small for gestational age: OR 5.7, 95% CI 1.1 to 28.7). In a prospective cohort study (51 adolescents with anorexia nervosa), people with anorexia nervosa were significantly more likely to have an affective disorder than were controls matched for sex, age, and school (lifetime risk of affective disorder 96% in people with anorexia nervosa v 23% in controls; ARI 73%, 95% CI 60% to 85%). It is unclear whether affective disorders precede anorexia nervosa or occur as a consequence of starvation. Obsessive compulsive disorder was, similarly, significantly more likely to be present in people with anorexia nervosa compared with controls (30% v 10%; ARI 20%, 95% CI 10% to 41%). However, in two thirds of people with obsessive compulsive disorder and anorexia nervosa, obsessive compulsive disorder preceded the anorexia nervosa.

PROGNOSIS One prospective study followed up 51 people with teenage onset anorexia nervosa, about half of whom received no or minimal treatment (fewer than 8 sessions). After 10 years, 14/51 people (27.5%) had a persistent eating disorder, three (5.9%) had ongoing anorexia nervosa, and six (11.8%) had experienced a period of bulimia nervosa. About half of all participants in the study continued to have poor psychosocial functioning at 10 years (assessed using the Morgan Russell scale and Global Assessment of Functioning Scale). A summary of treatment studies (119 studies published between 1953–1999, 5590 people, length of follow-up 1–29 years) found that 47% of people recover completely from anorexia nervosa (range 0–92%), 34% improve (range 0–75%), 21% develop a chronic

(continued over)

(from previous page)

eating disorder (range 0–79%), and 5% die from anorexia nervosa (range 0–22%). Favourable prognostic factors include an early age at onset and a short interval between onset of symptoms and the beginning of treatment. Unfavourable prognostic factors include vomiting, bulimia, profound weight loss, chronicity, psychiatric comorbidity, psychosocial problems, and a history of premorbid developmental or clinical abnormalities. The all-cause standardised mortality ratio of eating disorders (anorexia nervosa and bulimia nervosa) has been estimated at 538, about three times higher than that of other psychiatric illnesses. In studies published between 1970 and 1996, the average annual mortality was 0.59% a year in females in 10 eating disorder populations (1322 people), with a minimum follow-up of 6 years. Mortality was higher for people with lower weight and with older age at presentation. Young women with anorexia nervosa are at an increased risk of fractures later in life.

John Geddes and David Briess

KEY POINTS

- Bipolar disorder, with mood swings between depression and mania, may affect up to 1.5% of adults, and increases the risk of suicide and disability.

  Most people improve over time, but two thirds may have residual dysfunction, and at least 40% may have recurrent episodes.

- Lithium reduces symptoms of mania compared with placebo, and seems as effective as haloperidol, carbamazepine, and clonazepam, but can cause adverse effects including hypothyroidism.

- Older antipsychotic drugs, such as chlorpromazine and haloperidol, are widely used to treat mania, but few studies have been done to confirm their efficacy.

  Olanzapine, valproate, carbamazepine, and risperidone increase the likelihood of response in people with mania compared with placebo, and seem to have similar efficacy as each other, with different adverse-effect profiles.

  Ziprasidone, quetiapine, and clonazepam may also be beneficial, but few studies have been done to assess the effects of lamotrigine or gabapentin in mania.

  Topiramate is unlikely to be beneficial in mania.

  Antidepressants increase treatment response compared with placebo in people with bipolar depression. It is possible that SSRIs are more effective, and less likely to induce mania, compared with TCAs.

  Lamotrigine may increase response rates in people with depression compared with placebo, but can cause headache.

  Quetiapine may also improve depression compared with placebo.

  We don't know whether lithium, carbamazepine, valproate, or topiramate improve depression in people with bipolar disorder.

  We don't know whether psychological treatments are effective for people with bipolar depression, as we found no studies.

- Lithium reduces relapse in bipolar disorder compared with placebo.

  Valproate, carbamazepine, and lamotrigine seem as effective as lithium in reducing relapse.

  Cognitive therapy and patient or family education may reduce the risk of relapse, but studies have given conflicting results.

  We don't know whether antidepressants can prevent relapse, and they may induce mood instability or manic episodes.

  Olanzapine may reduce relapse, but long-term use may be associated with weight gain.

(i) **Please visit www.clinicalevidence.bmj.com for full text and references**

What are the effects of treatments in people with mania associated with bipolar disorder?

Beneficial	• Lithium in mania
	• Olanzapine in mania
	• Risperidone in mania

	• Valproate in mania
Likely To Be Beneficial	• Carbamazepine in mania
	• Clonazepam in mania
	• Haloperidol in mania
	• Quetiapine in mania
	• Ziprasidone in mania
Unknown Effectiveness	• Chlorpromazine in mania
	• Gabapentin in mania
	• Lamotrigine in mania
Unlikely To Be Beneficial	• Topiramate in mania

What are the effects of treatments in bipolar depression?

Likely To Be Beneficial	• Antidepressants in bipolar depression
	• Lamotrigine in bipolar depression
	• Quetiapine in bipolar depression
Unknown Effectiveness	• Carbamazepine in bipolar depression
	• Lithium in bipolar depression
	• Psychological treatments in bipolar depression
	• Topiramate in bipolar depression
	• Valproate in bipolar depression

What are the effects of interventions to prevent relapse of mania or bipolar depression?

Beneficial	• Lithium to prevent relapse
Likely To Be Beneficial	• Carbamazepine to prevent relapse
	• Cognitive therapy to prevent relapse
	• Education to recognise symptoms of relapse
	• Family-focused psychoeducation to prevent relapse
	• Lamotrigine to prevent relapse
	• Valproate to prevent relapse
Trade-off Between Benefits And Harms	• Olanzapine to prevent relapse
Unknown Effectiveness	• Antidepressant drugs to prevent relapse

Search date July 2006

DEFINITION Bipolar disorder (bipolar affective disorder, manic depressive disorder) is characterised by marked mood swings between mania (mood elevation) and bipolar depression that cause significant personal distress or social dysfunction, and are not caused by drugs or known physical disorders. **Bipolar type I disorder** is diagnosed when episodes of depression are interspersed with mania or mixed episodes. **Bipolar type II disorder** is diagnosed when depression is interspersed with less severe episodes of elevated mood that do not lead to dysfunction or disability (hypomania). Bipolar disorder has been subdivided in several further ways.

INCIDENCE/PREVALENCE One 1996 cross-national community-based study (38,000 people) found lifetime prevalence rates of bipolar type I disorder ranging from 0.3% in Taiwan to 1.5% in New Zealand. It found that men and women were at similar risk, and that the mean age at first onset ranged from 19–29 years (average of 6 years earlier than first onset of major depression).

AETIOLOGY/RISK FACTORS The cause of bipolar disorder is uncertain, although family and twin studies suggest a genetic basis. The lifetime risk of bipolar disorder is increased in first-degree relatives of a person with bipolar disorder (40–70% for a monozygotic twin; 5–10% for other first-degree relatives). If the first episode of mania occurs in an older adult, it may be secondary mania caused by underlying medical or substance-induced factors.

PROGNOSIS Bipolar disorder is a recurring illness, and one of the leading causes of worldwide disability, especially in the 15–44 years age group. One 4-year inception cohort study (173 people treated for a first episode of mania or mixed affective disorder) found that 93% of people no longer met criteria for mania at 2 years (median time to recover from a syndrome 4.6 weeks), but that only 36% had recovered to premorbid function. It found that 40% of people had a recurrent manic (20%) or depressive (20%) episode within 2 years of recovering from the first episode. A meta-analysis, comparing observed versus expected rates of suicide in an age- and sex-matched sample of the general population, found that the lifetime prevalence of suicide in people with bipolar disorder was about 2% — or 15 times greater than expected.

Bulimia nervosa

Phillipa J Hay and Josue Bacaltchuk

KEY POINTS

- Up to 1% of young women may have bulimia nervosa, characterised by an intense preoccupation with body weight, uncontrolled binge-eating episodes and use of extreme measures to counteract the feared effects of overeating.

  People with bulimia nervosa may be of normal weight, making it difficult to diagnose.

  Obesity has been associated with both an increased risk of bulimia nervosa and a worse prognosis, as have personality disorders and substance misuse.

  After ten years, about half of people with bulimia nervosa will have recovered fully, a third will have made a partial recovery, and 10–20% will still have symptoms.

- CBT may improve clinical problems of bulimia nervosa compared with no treatment, and may be as effective as interpersonal psychotherapy, other psychological treatments, or antidepressants in reducing symptoms.

  We don't know whether other psychological therapies, such as cognitive orientation therapy, hypnobehavioural therapy, dialectical behavioural therapy, or motivational enhancement therapy, are more effective than a waiting list control in improving symptoms, as few studies have been found.

- Some antidepressant drugs (fluoxetine, citalopram, desipramine, and imipramine) may improve symptoms in people with bulimia nervosa compared with placebo.

  MAOIs may increase remission rates compared with placebo but may not reduce bulimic symptoms or depression scores.

  We don't know whether other antidepressants can improve symptoms or remission in people with bulimia nervosa.

- In people who are in remission, continuation of antidepressant treatment may maintain a reduction in vomiting frequency compared with withdrawing treatment.

(i) **Please visit www.clinicalevidence.bmj.com for full text and references**

What are the effects of treatments for bulimia nervosa in adults?

Likely To Be Beneficial	• CBT for bulimia nervosa
	• Combination treatment (antidepressants plus CBT as effective as either treatment alone)
	• MAOIs
	• SSRIs (evidence limited to fluoxetine and citalopram)
	• Topiramate
	• TCAs
Unknown Effectiveness	• CBT plus exposure response prevention enhancement
	• Cognitive orientation therapy
	• Dialectical behavioural therapy
	• Guided self-help CBT

- Hypnobehavioural therapy
- Interpersonal psychotherapy
- Mirtazapine
- Motivational enhancement therapy
- Pure or unguided self-help CBT
- Reboxetine
- Venlafaxine

What are the effects of discontinuing treatment in people with remission?

Unlikely To Be Beneficial	• Discontinuing fluoxetine

Search date June 2006

DEFINITION Bulimia nervosa is an intense preoccupation with body weight and shape, with regular episodes of uncontrolled overeating of large amounts of food (binge eating) associated with use of extreme methods to counteract the feared effects of overeating. If a person also meets the diagnostic criteria for anorexia nervosa, then the diagnosis of anorexia nervosa takes precedence. Bulimia nervosa can be difficult to identify because of extreme secrecy about binge eating and purgative behaviour. Weight may be normal but there is often a history of anorexia nervosa or restrictive dieting. Some people alternate between anorexia nervosa and bulimia nervosa. Some RCTs included people with sub-threshold bulimia nervosa or a related eating disorder, binge eating disorder. Where possible, only results relevant to bulimia nervosa are reported in this review.

INCIDENCE/PREVALENCE In community-based studies, the prevalence of bulimia nervosa is between 0.5% and 1.0% in young women, with an even social-class distribution. About 90% of people diagnosed with bulimia nervosa are women. The numbers presenting with bulimia nervosa in industrialised countries increased during the decade that followed its recognition in the late 1970s, and "a cohort effect" was reported in community surveys, implying an increase in incidence. Since that time, it is likely that the incidence has plateaued or even fallen, with an incidence of 6.6 per 100,000 reported in the UK in 2000. The prevalence of eating disorders, such as bulimia nervosa, is lower in non-industrialised populations, and varies across ethnic groups. African-American women have a lower rate of restrictive dieting than do white American women, but they have a similar rate of recurrent binge eating.

AETIOLOGY/RISK FACTORS The aetiology of bulimia nervosa is complex, but sociocultural pressures to be thin and the promotion of dieting does appear to increase risk. One community-based case-control study compared 102 people with bulimia nervosa versus 204 healthy controls and found higher rates of the following in people with the eating disorder: obesity, mood disorder, sexual and physical abuse, parental obesity, substance misuse, low self-esteem, perfectionism, disturbed family dynamics, parental weight/shape concern, and early menarche. Compared with a control group of 102 women who had other psychiatric disorders, women with bulimia nervosa had higher rates of parental problems and obesity.

PROGNOSIS A 10-year follow-up study (50 people with bulimia nervosa from a placebo-controlled trial of mianserin treatment) found that 52% receiving placebo had fully recovered, and only 9% continued to experience full symptoms of bulimia nervosa. A larger study (222 people from a trial of antidepressants and structured, intensive group psychotherapy) found that, after a mean follow-up of 11.5 years, 11% still met criteria for bulimia nervosa, whereas 70% were in full or partial remission. Short-term studies found similar results: about 50% of people made a full recovery, 30% made a partial recovery, and

(continued over)

(from previous page)

20% continued to be symptomatic. There are few consistent predictors of longer-term outcome. Good prognosis has been associated with shorter illness duration, a younger age of onset, higher social class, and a family history of alcohol abuse. Poor prognosis has been associated with a history of substance misuse, premorbid and paternal obesity, and, in some studies, personality disorder. One study (102 women) of the natural course of bulimia nervosa found that 31% and 15% still had the disorder at 15 months and 5 years, respectively. Only 28% received treatment during the follow-up period. In an evaluation of the response to CBT, early progress (reduction in purging of over 70% by session 6) best predicted outcome. A subsequent systematic review of the outcome literature found no consistent evidence to support early intervention and a better prognosis. A more recent systematic review evaluating the cost-effectiveness of treatments and prognostic indicators found only four consistent pretreatment predictors of poorer outcome for treatment of bulimia nervosa: features of borderline personality disorder, concurrent substance misuse, low motivation for change, and a history of obesity.

Deliberate self-harm (and attempted suicide)

G Mustafa Soomro

KEY POINTS

- Deliberate self-harm involves acts such as self-cutting or self-poisoning that are carried out deliberately, with or without the intention of committing suicide.

    The lifetime prevalence of deliberate self-harm is around 3–5% of the population of Europe or the USA, and prevalence has been increasing.

    Familial, biological, and psychosocial factors may contribute. Risks are higher in women and young adults, those who are socially isolated or deprived, and those with psychiatric or personality disorders.

- Around a quarter of people will repeat the self-harm within 4 years, and the long-term suicide risk is 3–7%.

    Younger adults are more likely to repeat non-fatal self harm, while adults aged over 45 years are more likely to commit suicide, especially if the previous self-harm involved a violent method.

- No pharmaceutical treatments have been clearly shown to be of benefit in reducing recurrent self-harm.

    It is possible that flupentixol depot injections may reduce the recurrence of self-harm, but with associated adverse effects.

    Mianserin seems not to reduce recurrence rates, but we don't know this for certain.

- CAUTION: Paroxetine has not been shown to reduce the risks of repeated deliberate self-harm and may increase suicidal ideation and congenital malformations.

- The effects of psychological treatments are also unclear.

    Problem-solving therapy may reduce depression and anxiety, but may not be effective in preventing recurrence of self-harm.

    Evidence for benefit from cognitive therapy or psychodynamic interpersonal therapy compared with usual care is unclear.

- Intensive follow-up plus outreach, nurse-led management, or hospital admission have not been shown to reduce recurrent self-harm compared with usual care.

(i) **Please visit www.clinicalevidence.bmj.com for full text and references**

What are the effects of treatments for deliberate self-harm in adolescents and adults?

Unknown Effectiveness	
	• Cognitive therapy
	• Continuity of care
	• Dialectical behavioural therapy
	• Emergency card
	• Flupentixol depot injection
	• Hospital admission
	• Mianserin
	• Nurse-led case management
	• Oral antipsychotics
	• Paroxetine

	• Problem-solving therapy
	• Psychodynamic interpersonal therapy
	• Telephone contact
Unlikely To Be Beneficial	• General practice-based guidelines
	• Intensive outpatient follow-up plus outreach

Search date October 2005

DEFINITION Deliberate self-harm is an acute non-fatal act of self-harm carried out deliberately in the form of an acute episode of behaviour by an individual with variable motivation. The intention to end life may be absent or present to a variable degree. Other terms used to describe this phenomenon are "attempted suicide" and "parasuicide". For the purpose of this review the term deliberate self-harm will be used throughout. Common methods of deliberate self-harm include self-cutting and self-poisoning, such as overdosing on medicines. Some acts of deliberate self-harm are characterised by high suicidal intent, meticulous planning (including precautions against being found out), and severe lethality of the method used. Other acts of deliberate self-harm are characterised by no or low intention of suicide, lack of planning and concealing the act, and low lethality of the method used. The related term of "suicide" is defined as an act with a fatal outcome that is deliberately initiated and performed by the person with the knowledge or expectation of its fatal outcome. This review focuses on the literature with recent deliberate self-harm (in people aged 15 years or over) as the main presenting problem, and main selection criterion for the RCTs. It excludes RCTs in which deliberate self-harm is an outcome in studies of others disorders, such as depression or borderline personality disorder, rather than the primary presenting problem. Deliberate self-harm is not defined in the DSM-IV or the ICD-10.

INCIDENCE/PREVALENCE Based on data from 16 European countries between 1989 and 1992, the lifetime prevalence of deliberate self-harm in people treated in hospital and other medical facilities, including general-practice settings, is estimated at about 3% for women and 2% for men. Over the last 50 years there has been a rise in the incidence of deliberate self-harm in the UK. A reasonable current estimate is about 400/100,000 population a year. In two community studies in the USA, 3–5% of responders said that they had made an attempt at deliberate self-harm at some time. Self-poisoning using organophosphates is particularly common in resource-poor countries. A large hospital (catering for 900,000 people) in Sri Lanka reported 2559 adult hospital admissions and 41% occupancy of medical intensive-care beds for deliberate self-harm with organophosphates over 2 years. An international survey using representative community samples of adults (aged 18–64 years) reported lifetime prevalence of self-reported deliberate self-harm of 3.82% in Canada, 5.93% in Puerto Rico, 4.95% in France, 3.44% in West Germany, 0.72% in Lebanon, 0.75% in Taiwan, 3.2% in Korea, and 4.43% in New Zealand.

AETIOLOGY/RISK FACTORS Familial, biological, and psychosocial factors may contribute to deliberate self-harm. Evidence for genetic factors includes a higher risk of familial suicide and greater concordance in monozygotic than dizygotic twins for deliberate self-harm. Evidence for biological factors includes reduced cerebrospinal fluid 5-hydroxyindoleacetic acid levels and a blunted prolactin response to the fenfluramine challenge test, indicating a reduction in the function of serotonin in the central nervous system. People who deliberately self-harm also show traits of impulsiveness and aggression, inflexible and impulsive cognitive style, and impaired decision making and problem solving. Deliberate self-harm is more likely to occur in women, young adults, and people who are single or divorced, of low education level, unemployed, disabled, or suffering from a psychiatric disorder, particularly depression, substance misuse, borderline and antisocial personality disorders, severe anxiety disorders, and physical illness.

PROGNOSIS Suicide is highest during the first year after deliberate self-harm. One systematic review found median rates of repetition of 16% (interquartile range [IQR] 12% to 25%) within the first year, 21% (IQR 12% to 30%) within 1–4 years, and 23% (IQR 11% to 32%) within 4 years or longer. It found median mortality from suicide after deliberate self-harm of 1.8% (IQR 0.8% to 2.6%) within the first year, 3.0% (IQR 2.0% to 4.4%) within 1–4 years, 3.4% (IQR 2.5% to 6.0%) within 5–10 years, and 6.7% (IQR 5.0% to 11.0%) within 9 years or longer. Repetition of deliberate self-harm is more likely in people aged 25–49 years who are unemployed, divorced, from lower social class, or who suffer from substance misuse, depression, hopelessness, powerlessness, personality disorders, have unstable living conditions or live alone, have a criminal record, previous psychiatric treatment, a history of stressful traumatic life events, or a history of coming from a broken home or of family violence. Factors associated with risk of suicide after deliberate self-harm are being aged over 45 years, male sex, being unemployed, retired, separated, divorced, or widowed, living alone, having poor physical health, psychiatric disorder (particularly depression, alcoholism, schizophrenia, and sociopathic personality disorder), high suicidal intent in current episode including leaving a written note, violent method used in current episode, and history of previous deliberate self-harm.

Dementia

James Warner, Rob Butler, and Balaji Wuntakal

KEY POINTS

- Dementia is characterised by chronic, global, non-reversible deterioration in memory, executive function, and personality. Speech and motor function may also be impaired.

- Median life expectancy for people with Alzheimer's and Lewy body dementia is around 6 years after diagnosis.

- Cognitive symptoms of dementia can be improved by donepezil, galantamine, and memantine.

  Donepezil improves cognitive function and global state in people with Alzheimer's disease over 2 years, and improves cognitive function in people with vascular dementia compared with placebo over 6 months.

  Galantamine improves cognitive function and global state over 6 months in people with both Alzheimer's disease and vascular dementia.

  Memantine improves cognition, global state, and activities of daily living in people with Alzheimer's disease over 28 weeks, and improves cognitive function in people with vascular dementia over 28 weeks.

- Rivastigmine and tacrine can improve cognitive function in people with dementia, but have high rates of adverse effects.

  Rivastigmine improves cognitive function and global state in people with Alzheimer's disease and Lewy body dementia, but increases gastro-intestinal adverse effects.

  Tacrine may improve cognitive function and global state in people with Alzheimer's disease.

- Ginkgo biloba may improve cognitive function in people with Alzheimer's disease or vascular dementia, but preparations are inconsistent.

- Carbamazepine and haloperidol may reduce agitation and aggression in the short term in people with dementia.

  However, haloperidol increases extrapyramidal adverse effects and may not be tolerated in people with dementia.

- CAUTION: Olanzapine and risperidone are associated with an increased risk of stroke, and should not be used in people with psychosis associated with dementia.

ⓘ Please visit www.clinicalevidence.bmj.com for full text and references

What are the effects of treatments on cognitive symptoms of dementia?

Beneficial	• Donepezil
	• Galantamine
Likely To Be Beneficial	• Ginkgo biloba
	• Memantine
Trade-off Between Benefits And Harms	• Rivastigmine
	• Tacrine
Unknown Effectiveness	• Music therapy
	• NSAIDs
	• Omega 3 (fish oil)

	• Physostigmine
	• Reminiscence therapy
	• Selegiline
	• Statins
Unlikely To Be Beneficial	• Oestrogen

What are the effects of treatments on behavioural and psychological symptoms of dementia?

Likely To Be Beneficial	• Carbamazepine
Trade-off Between Benefits And Harms	• Haloperidol • Olanzapine • Risperidone
Unknown Effectiveness	• Benzodiazepines • Donepezil • Galantamine • Quetiapine • Rivastigmine • Sodium valproate/Valproic acid • Trazodone

Search date February 2006

DEFINITION Dementia is characterised by chronic, global, non-reversible impairment in cerebral function. It usually results in loss of memory (initially of recent events), loss of executive function (such as the ability to make decisions or sequence complex tasks), and changes in personality. **Alzheimer's disease** is a type of dementia characterised by an insidious onset and slow deterioration, and involves impairments in speech, motor, personality, and executive function. It should be diagnosed after other systemic, psychiatric, and neurological causes of dementia have been excluded clinically and by laboratory investigation. **Vascular dementia** is often caused by multiple infarcts or generalised small vessel disease. It often presents with a stepwise deterioration in cognitive function with or without language and motor dysfunction. It usually occurs in the presence of vascular risk factors (diabetes, hypertension, arteriosclerosis, and smoking). Characteristically, it has a more sudden onset and stepwise progression than Alzheimer's disease. **Lewy body dementia** is a type of dementia that involves insidious impairment of executive function with Parkinsonism, visual hallucinations, fluctuating cognitive abilities, and increased risk of falls or autonomic failure. Careful clinical examination of people with mild to moderate dementia and the use of established diagnostic criteria accurately identifies 70–90% of causes confirmed at post mortem. In all types of dementia, people will experience problems with cognitive functioning, and are likely to experience behavioural and psychological symptoms of dementia. Where possible, we have divided outcomes into cognitive or behavioural/psychological, although there is often considerable crossover between these outcomes, both clinically and in research.

(continued over)

(from previous page)

INCIDENCE/PREVALENCE About 6% of people aged over 65 years and 30% of people aged over 90 years have some form of dementia. Dementia is rare before the age of 60 years. Alzheimer's disease and vascular dementia (including mixed dementia) are each estimated to account for 35–50% of dementia, and Lewy body dementia is estimated to account for up to 20% of dementia in the elderly, varying with geographical, cultural, and racial factors. There are numerous other causes of dementia, all of which are relatively rare, including frontotemporal dementia, alcohol-related dementia, Huntington's disease, normal pressure hydrocephalus, HIV infection, syphilis, subdural haematoma, and some cerebral tumours.

AETIOLOGY/RISK FACTORS Alzheimer's disease: The cause of Alzheimer's disease is unclear. A key pathological process is deposition of abnormal amyloid in the central nervous system. Most people with the relatively rare condition of early onset Alzheimer's disease (before age 60 years) exhibit an autosomal dominant inheritance owing to mutations in presenilin or amyloid precursor protein genes. Several gene mutations (on *APP*, *PS-1*, and *PS-2* genes) have been identified. Later onset dementia is sometimes clustered in families, but specific gene mutations have not been identified. Head injury, Down's syndrome, and lower premorbid intellect may be risk factors for Alzheimer's disease. **Vascular dementia:** Vascular dementia is related to cardiovascular risk factors, such as smoking, arteriosclerosis, hypertension, and diabetes. **Lewy body dementia:** The cause of Lewy body dementia is unknown. Brain acetylcholine activity is reduced in many forms of dementia, and the level of reduction correlates with cognitive impairment. Many treatments for Alzheimer's disease enhance cholinergic activity.

PROGNOSIS Alzheimer's disease: Alzheimer's disease usually has an insidious onset with progressive reduction in cerebral function. Diagnosis is difficult in the early stages. Median life expectancy after diagnosis is 5–6 years. **Vascular dementia:** We found no reliable data on prognosis. **Lewy body dementia:** People with Lewy body dementia have an average life expectancy of about 6 years after diagnosis. Behavioural problems, depression, and psychotic symptoms are common in all types of dementia. Eventually, most people with dementia find it difficult to perform simple tasks without help.

Depression in adults: drug and other physical treatments | 343

Corrado Barbui, Rob Butler, Andrea Cipriani, John Geddes, and Simon Hatcher

KEY POINTS

- Depression may affect up to 10% of the population, with half of affected people having recurrence of their symptoms.

- In mild to moderate depression, there is no reliable evidence that any one treatment is superior in improving symptoms, but the strength of evidence supporting different treatments varies.

  In severe depression, only prescription antidepressants and electroconvulsive treatment are known to improve symptoms.

- TCAs, SSRIs, MAOIs, reboxetine, and venlafaxine improve symptoms in the short term. However, long-term studies are lacking.

  No one class or individual antidepressant has been shown to be more effective than the others in the short term, but adverse effects vary between classes.

  St John's Wort may have similar efficacy compared with antidepressants, but preparations vary and drug interactions can occur.

  We don't know if exercise is beneficial in people with mild to moderate depression.

- CAUTION: TCAs and SSRIs may induce or worsen suicidal ideation and behaviour, and agitation after initiation of treatment.

- We don't know whether adding lithium or pindolol to other antidepressant drugs reduces symptoms in people with treatment-resistant depression.

- Continuing prescription antidepressant drugs reduces the risk of relapse after recovery.

Please visit www.clinicalevidence.bmj.com for full text and references

What are the effects of treatments in mild to moderate or severe depression?

Beneficial	• Electroconvulsive therapy (in severe depression)
	• MAOIs versus other prescription antidepressant drugs in atypical depressive disorders
	• Prescription antidepressant drugs (tricyclic antidepressants [including low-dose TCAs], SSRIs, MAOIs, reboxetine, or venlafaxine) (improved symptoms compared with placebo in mild to moderate and severe depression)
	• SSRIs and related drugs versus each other and other prescription antidepressant drugs
	• TCAs versus each other and other prescription antidepressant drugs
	• Venlafaxine versus other prescription antidepressant drugs
Likely To Be Beneficial	• Reboxetine versus other antidepressant drugs (in mild to moderate or severe depression)

	• St John's Wort (more effective than placebo, as effective as other antidepressants in mild to moderate depression)
Unknown Effectiveness	• Exercise (in mild to moderate depression)

What are the effects of interventions in treatment-resistant depression?

Unknown Effectiveness	• Lithium augmentation • Pindolol augmentation

Which interventions reduce relapse rates?

Beneficial	• Continuing prescription antidepressant drugs (reduced risk of relapse after recovery in people with mild to moderate depression)

Search date April 2006

DEFINITION Depressive disorders are characterised by persistent low mood, loss of interest and enjoyment, and reduced energy. They often impair day-to-day functioning. Most RCTs assessed in this review classify depression using the DSM-IV or the ICD-10. DSM-IV divides depression into major depressive disorder or dysthymic disorder. **Major depressive disorder** is characterised by one or more major depressive episodes (i.e. at least 2 weeks of depressed mood or loss of interest, accompanied by at least 4 additional symptoms of depression). **Dysthymic disorder** is characterised by at least 2 years of depressed mood for more days than not, accompanied by additional symptoms that do not reach the criteria for major depressive disorder. ICD-10 divides depression into mild to moderate or severe depressive episodes. Mild to moderate depression is characterised by depressive symptoms and some functional impairment. Severe depression is characterised by additional agitation or psychomotor retardation with marked somatic symptoms. **Treatment-resistant depression** is defined as an absence of clinical response to treatment with a TCA at a minimum dose of 150 mg daily of imipramine (or equivalent drug) for 4–6 weeks. In this review, we use both DSM-IV and ICD-10 classifications, but treatments are considered to have been assessed in severe depression if the RCT included inpatients. **Older adults:** Older adults are generally defined as people aged 65 years or older. However, some of the RCTs of older people in this review included people aged 55 years or over. The presentation of depression in older adults may be atypical: low mood may be masked, and anxiety or memory impairment may be the principal presenting symptoms. Dementia should be considered in the differential diagnosis of depression in older adults. **Treating depressive disorders in adults:** Depressive disorders are generally treated with a range of drug, physical, and psychological treatments. For coverage of psychological treatments (including drug treatments v psychological treatments) and for coverage of combined drug and psychological treatment, see review on depression in adults: psychological treatments and care pathways, p 344. **Population:** This review does not cover intervention in women with postnatal depression (see review on postnatal depression, p 473), seasonal affective disorder, or depression owing to a physical illness, such as stroke or substance abuse.

INCIDENCE/PREVALENCE Depressive disorders are common, with a prevalence of major depression between 5% and 10% of people seen in primary-care settings. Two to three times as many people may have depressive symptoms, but do not meet DSM-IV criteria for major depression. Women are affected twice as often as men. Depressive disorders are the fourth most important cause of disability worldwide, and are expected to become the second most important by 2020. **Older adults:** Between 10% and 15% of older people have depressive symptoms, although major depression is relatively rare in older adults.

AETIOLOGY/RISK FACTORS The causes of depression are uncertain, but are thought to include both childhood events and current psychosocial adversity. Recent studies suggest that genetic factors may also be important, indicating that several chromosomal regions may be involved. Phenotypes, however, do not seem to exhibit classic Mendelian inheritance. Psychiatric research has also focused on the role that psychosocial factors, such as social context and personality dimensions, have in depression. Many theories emphasise the importance of temperament (differences in the adaptive systems), which can increase vulnerability to mood disturbances. Impairment in social relationships, gender, socioeconomic status, and dysfunctional cognition may also have a role. It seems that integrative models, which take into account the interaction of biological and social variables, offer the most reliable way to approach the complex aetiology of depression.

PROGNOSIS About half of people suffering a first episode of major depressive disorder experience further symptoms in the next 10 years. **Older adults:** One systematic review (search date 1996, 12 prospective cohort studies, 1268 people, mean age 60 years) found that the prognosis may be especially poor in elderly people with a chronic or relapsing course of depression. Another systematic review (search date 1999, 23 prospective cohort studies in people aged at least 65 years, including 5 identified by the first review) found that depression in older people was associated with increased mortality (15 studies; pooled OR 1.73, 95% CI 1.53 to 1.95).

Depression in adults: psychological treatments and care pathways

Rob Butler, Simon Hatcher, Jonathan Price, and Michael Von Korff

KEY POINTS

- Depression may affect up to 10% of the population, with symptoms recurring in half of affected people.

- In mild to moderate depression, there is no reliable evidence that any one treatment is superior in improving symptoms of depression, but the strength of evidence supporting different treatments varies.

- CBT and interpersonal psychotherapy reduce symptoms of mild to moderate depression, although many of the trials have been small.

  Combining psychological treatment with antidepressant drugs may be more effective than either treatment alone.

  Non-directive counselling may also be effective, but we don't know whether problem-solving therapy or befriending are beneficial.

  Care pathways may improve the effectiveness of treatment for depression.

- We don't know whether CBT or relapse prevention programmes are beneficial in reducing the risk of relapse after recovery.

(i) **Please visit www.clinicalevidence.bmj.com for full text and references**

What are the effects of psychological treatments in mild to moderate or severe depression?

Beneficial	• Cognitive therapy (improves symptoms in mild to moderate depression) • Interpersonal psychotherapy (improves symptoms in mild to moderate depression)
Likely To Be Beneficial	• Combining prescription antidepressant drugs and psychological treatments (improves symptoms in mild to moderate and severe depression) • Non-directive counselling (improves symptoms in mild to moderate depression)
Unknown Effectiveness	• Befriending (in mild to moderate depression) • Problem-solving therapy (in mild to moderate depression)

What are the effects of psychological interventions to reduce relapse rates in mild to moderate or severe depression?

Unknown Effectiveness	• Cognitive therapy (weak evidence that may reduce relapse over 1–2 years after stopping treatment in people with mild to moderate depression compared with antidepressant drugs or usual clinical management) • Relapse prevention programme (improved symptoms over 1 year after recovery in people with mild to moderate depression but no significant difference in relapse rates)

What are the effects of psychological interventions to improve delivery of treatments in mild to moderate or severe depression?

Likely To Be Beneficial	• Care pathways (reduces relapse in mild to moderate depression)

Search date April 2006

DEFINITION Depressive disorders are characterised by persistent low mood, loss of interest and enjoyment, and reduced energy. They often impair day to day functioning. Most of the RCTs assessed in this review classify depression using the DSM-IV or the ICD-10. DSM-IV divides depression into major depressive disorder or dysthymic disorder. **Major depressive disorder** is characterised by one or more major depressive episodes (i.e. at least 2 weeks of depressed mood or loss of interest accompanied by at least 4 additional symptoms of depression). **Dysthymic disorder** is characterised by at least 2 years of depressed mood for more days than not, accompanied by additional symptoms that do not reach the criteria for major depressive disorder. ICD-10 divides depression into mild to moderate or severe depressive episodes. Mild to moderate depression is characterised by depressive symptoms and some functional impairment. Severe depression is characterised by additional agitation or psychomotor retardation with marked somatic symptoms. **Treatment-resistant depression** is defined as an absence of clinical response to treatment with a tricyclic antidepressant at a minimum dose of 150 mg daily of imipramine (or equivalent drug) for 4–6 weeks. In this review, we use both DSM-IV and ICD-10 classifications, but treatments are considered to have been assessed in severe depression if the RCT included inpatients. **Older adults:** Older adults are generally defined as people aged 65 years or older. However, some of the RCTs of older people in this review included people aged 55 years or over. The presentation of depression in older adults may be atypical: low mood may be masked, and anxiety or memory impairment may be the principal presenting symptoms. Dementia should be considered in the differential diagnosis of depression in older adults. **Treating depressive disorders in adults:** Depressive disorders are generally treated with a range of drug, physical, and psychological treatments. For coverage of drug and other physical treatments, see review on depression adults: drug and physical treatments, p 343. Combined drug and psychological treatment and comparisons of psychological versus drug treatment are covered in this review. **Population:** This review does not cover intervention in women with postnatal depression (see review on postnatal depression, p 473), seasonal affective disorder, or depression because of a physical illness, such as stroke or substance abuse.

INCIDENCE/PREVALENCE Depressive disorders are common, with a prevalence of major depression between 5% and 10% of people seen in primary-care settings. Two to three times as many people may have depressive symptoms but do not meet DSM-IV criteria for major depression. Women are affected twice as often as men. Depressive disorders are the fourth most important cause of disability worldwide, and are expected to become the second most important cause by 2020. **Older adults:** Between 10% and 15% of older people have depressive symptoms, although major depression is less common among older adults.

AETIOLOGY/RISK FACTORS The causes of depression are uncertain, but are thought to include both childhood events and current psychosocial adversity. Recent studies suggest that genetic factors may also be important, indicating that several chromosomal regions may be involved. However, phenotypes do not seem to exhibit classic Mendelian inheritance. Psychiatric research has also focused on the role that psychosocial factors, such as social context and personality dimensions, have in depression. Many theories emphasise the importance of temperament (differences in the adaptive systems), which can increase vulnerability to mood disturbances. Impairment in social relationships, gender, socioeconomic status, and dysfunctional cognition may also be involved. It seems that integrative models, which take into account the interaction of biological and social variables, offer the most reliable way to approach the complex causes of depression.

(continued over)

(from previous page)

PROGNOSIS About half of people suffering a first episode of major depressive disorder experience further symptoms in the subsequent 10 years. **Older adults:** One systematic review (search date 1996, 12 prospective cohort studies, 1268 people, mean age 60 years) found that the prognosis may be especially poor in elderly people with a chronic or relapsing course of depression. Another systematic review (search date 1999, 23 prospective cohort studies in people aged 65 years or over, including 5 identified by the first review) found that depression in older people was associated with increased mortality (15 studies; pooled OR 1.73, 95% CI 1.53 to 1.95).

Christopher Gale and Jane Millichamp

KEY POINTS

- Generalised anxiety disorder (GAD) is excessive worry and tension about everyday events, on most days, for at least 6 months, to the extent that there is distress or difficulty in performing day-to-day tasks. However, diagnosing GAD accurately can be difficult.

  Up to one in twenty people may have GAD at any one time, and most have other health problems. Less than half of people have full remission after 5 years.

  GAD may have a genetic component, and has also been linked to previous psychological or other trauma.

- In adults: CBT (including exposure, relaxation, and cognitive restructuring) improves anxiety and depression compared with waiting list control or treatment as usual.

  It is unclear whether CBT is more effective than supportive therapy.

- Various drug treatments, such as benzodiazepines, buspirone, hydroxyzine, antidepressants, and pregabalin may all reduce symptoms of anxiety in people with GAD, but they can have unpleasant adverse effects, and most studies have been short term.

  Benzodiazepines increase the risk of dependence, sedation, and accidents, and can cause adverse effects in neonates if used during pregnancy.

  Buspirone may be less effective if used in people who have recently been taking benzodiazepines.

  Antidepressants (imipramine, paroxetine, sertraline, escitalopram, venlafaxine, and opipramol) have been shown to reduce symptoms compared with placebo, but antidepressants can cause a variety of adverse effects including sedation, dizziness, falls, nausea, and sexual dysfunction.

  In general, comparisons between different antidepressants have shown similar effectiveness in reducing anxiety, although one study found limited evidence of an increased benefit with escitalopram compared with paroxetine.

- Antipsychotic drugs may reduce anxiety in people who have not responded to other treatments, but these drugs may have serious adverse effects (e.g. drowsiness, movement disorders).

- We don't know whether abecarnil reduces anxiety.

- In children and adolescents: CBT improves symptoms compared with waiting list control.

  Most studies of CBT in children and adolescents have included other anxiety disorders. We found no studies in participants with GAD alone, or in children aged less than 6 years.

- There is limited evidence regarding the efficacy of antidepressants for childhood GAD. SSRIs (fluvoxamine, fluoxetine, sertraline) have shown some promise, but antidepressants are associated with adverse effects such as abdominal pain and nausea, and other well-documented adverse effects.

- We found no evidence on the effects of applied relaxation, benzodiazepines, buspirone, hydroxyzine, abecarnil, pregabalin, or antipsychotics in children and adolescents.

(i) **Please visit www.clinicalevidence.bmj.com for full text and references**

What are the effects of treatments for generalised anxiety disorder in adults?

Beneficial	• CBT in adults
Likely To Be Beneficial	• Antidepressants in adults (imipramine, paroxetine, sertraline, escitalopram, venlafaxine, and opipramol) • Applied relaxation in adults • Buspirone in adults • Hydroxyzine in adults • Pregabalin in adults
Trade-off Between Benefits And Harms	• Antipsychotics in adults • Benzodiazepines in adults
Unknown Effectiveness	• Abecarnil in adults

What are the effects of treatments for generalised anxiety disorder in children and adolescents?

Beneficial	• CBT in children and adolescents
Trade-off Between Benefits And Harms	• Antidepressants in children and adolescents (sertraline, fluvoxamine, fluoxetine)
Unknown Effectiveness	• Abecarnil in children and adolescents • Antipsychotics in children and adolescents • Applied relaxation in children and adolescents • Benzodiazepines in children and adolescents • Buspirone in children and adolescents • Hydroxyzine in children and adolescents • Pregabalin in children and adolescents

Search date March 2007

DEFINITION Generalised anxiety disorder (GAD) is defined as excessive worry and tension about every day events and problems, on most days, for at least 6 months, to the point where the person experiences distress or has marked difficulty in performing day-to-day tasks. It may be characterised by the following symptoms and signs: increased motor tension (fatigability, trembling, restlessness, and muscle tension); autonomic hyperactivity (shortness of breath, rapid heart rate, dry mouth, cold hands, and dizziness); and increased vigilance and scanning (feeling keyed up, increased startling, and impaired concentration), but not by panic attacks. One non-systematic review of epidemiological and clinical studies found marked reduction in quality of life and psychosocial functioning in people with anxiety disorders, including GAD. It also found that people with GAD had low overall life satisfaction, and some impairment in ability to fulfil roles, social tasks, or both.

INCIDENCE/PREVALENCE The most recent community surveys have used a newer version of the Composite International Diagnostic Interview (CIDI) that allows direct comparisons between different surveys. One observational survey in Europe completed in 2003, which included people from Belgium, France, Germany, Italy, the Netherlands, and Spain, estimated the 12-month prevalence of GAD at 1.0% (0.5% males, 1.3% females). An observational survey in New Zealand (12,800 people) estimated the 12-month prevalence of GAD at 2.0%, 95% CI 1.7% to 2.3% (men: 1.4%, 95% CI 1.1% to 1.8%; women: 2.6%, 95% CI 2.2% to 3.1%). In this survey, people over the age of 65 years had a markedly lower 12-month prevalence of GAD (1.0%, 95% CI 0.6% to 1.5%). The lifetime prevalence of GAD was estimated to be 6.0%, 95% CI 5.5% to 6.6%. An observational survey in the UK in 2000 of people aged 16–74 years used the CIS-R, followed by a Schedules for Clinical Assessment in Neuropsychiatry (SCAN) interview of a stratified sample. The survey estimated that 4.7% of people had GAD (men: 4.6%; women: 4.8%). A survey of children and adolescents aged 5–16 years in the UK in 2004, which used a similar methodology, estimated that 0.7% had GAD (boys: 0.6%; girls: 0.8%). In the European survey of adults, 76% of those people who had more than one mental disorder for 12 months had GAD. Those people who had GAD were significantly more likely to have other mental disorders which included (odds ratio to have the disorder): major depression (OR 37.1, 95% CI 23.2 to 59.1), social phobia (OR 13.5, 95% CI 7.8 to 23.6), specific phobia (OR 7.4, 95% CI 4.6 to 12.0), post-traumatic stress disorder (OR 16.4, 95% CI 9.1 to 29.8), agoraphobia (OR 26.6, 95% CI 10.8 to 65.1), panic disorder (OR 21.8, 95% CI 11.5 to 41.2), and alcohol dependence (OR 18.9, 95% CI 4.8 to 74.4). Another observational survey in 2004 found that individuals with GAD were also more likely to have physical health problems. A non-systematic review (20 observational studies in younger and older adults) suggested that autonomic arousal to stressful tasks was decreased in older people, and that older people became accustomed to stressful tasks more quickly than younger people.

AETIOLOGY/RISK FACTORS GAD is believed to be associated with an increase in the number of minor life events, independent of demographic factors; however, this finding is also common in people with other diagnoses. One non-systematic review (5 case control studies) of psychological sequelae to civilian trauma found that rates of GAD reported in four of the five studies were significantly increased compared with a control population (RR 3.3, 95% CI 2.0 to 5.5). One systematic review (search date 1997) of cross-sectional studies found that bullying (or peer victimisation) was associated with a significant increase in the incidence of GAD (effect size 0.21, CI not reported). One systematic review (search date not reported, 2 family studies, 45 index cases, 225 first-degree relatives) found a significant association between GAD in the index cases and in their first-degree relatives (OR 6.1, 95% CI 2.5 to 14.9). One systematic review of twin and family studies (search date 2003, 23 twin studies, 12 family studies) found an association between GAD, other anxiety disorders, and depression, and postulated that a common genetic factor was implicated.

PROGNOSIS One systematic review found that 25% of adults with GAD will be in full remission after 2 years, and 38% will have a remission after 5 years. The Harvard–Brown anxiety research program reported 5-year follow-up of 167 people with GAD. During this period, the weighted probability for full remission was 38% and for at least partial remission was 47%; the probability of relapse from full remission was 27%, and of relapse from partial remission was 39%.

G Mustafa Soomro

KEY POINTS

- Obsessions or compulsions that cause personal distress or social dysfunction affect about 1% of men and 2% of women.

  About half of people with obsessive compulsive disorder (OCD) have an episodic course, whereas the other half have continuous problems. Up to half of people show improvement of symptoms over time.

- CBT improves symptoms of OCD compared with a waiting list control.

  Behavioural therapy seems to be as effective at improving symptoms as CBT, but we don't know how it compares with SRIs. Behavioural therapy is more effective than relaxation.

  We don't know whether combining SRIs and cognitive therapy or behavioural therapy improves symptoms compared with each treatment alone.

- Selective and non-SRIs inhibitors improve symptoms of OCD compared with placebo, but increase the risk of adverse effects.

  Selective and non-selective SRIs seem to be more effective at reducing symptoms compared with TCAs or MAOIs.

  Venlafaxine may be as effective as SSRIs, but sertraline has not been consistently shown to be beneficial.

  We don't know which is the most effective drug to use, or for how long maintenance treatment should continue.

- CAUTION: SSRIs have been associated with an increase in suicidal ideation.

- Adding antipsychotic drugs to SSRIs may improve symptoms in people who did not respond to SSRIs, although studies have given conflicting results.

- We do not know whether electroconvulsive therapy improves symptoms in people with OCD.

(i) **Please visit www.clinicalevidence.bmj.com for full text and references**

What are the effects of initial treatments for obsessive compulsive disorder in adults?

Beneficial	• Behavioural therapy
	• Cognitive therapy or CBT
	• SRIs (citalopram, clomipramine, fluoxetine, fluvoxamine, paroxetine, sertraline)
Unknown Effectiveness	• Behavioural therapy or cognitive therapy plus SRIs (unclear if the combination more effective than behavioural therapy or cognitive therapy alone)
	• Electroconvulsive therapy

What are the best forms of maintenance treatment for obsessive compulsive disorder in adults?

Unknown Effectiveness	• Optimum duration of maintenance treatment with SRIs

What are the effects of treatments for obsessive compulsive disorder in adults who have not responded to initial treatment with SRIs?

Likely To Be Beneficial	• Addition of antipsychotics to SRIs

Search date July 2006

DEFINITION Obsessive compulsive disorder (OCD) involves obsessions, compulsions, or both, that are not caused by drugs or by a physical disorder, and which cause significant personal distress or social dysfunction. The disorder may have a chronic or an episodic course. **Obsessions** are recurrent and persistent ideas, images, or impulses that cause pronounced anxiety and that the person perceives to be self-produced. **Compulsions** are repetitive behaviours or mental acts performed in response to obsessions or according to certain rules, which are aimed at reducing distress or preventing certain imagined dreaded events. People with OCD may have insight into their condition, in that obsessions and compulsions are usually recognised and resisted. There are minor differences in the criteria for OCD between the DSM-III, DSM-III-R, DSM-IV, and IDC-10.

INCIDENCE/PREVALENCE One national, community-based survey of OCD in the UK (1993, 10,000 people) found that 1.0% of men and 1.5% of women reported symptoms in the previous month. A survey of a random sample of people living in private households in the UK (2000, 8580 adults aged 16–74 years) found that 1.1% of those surveyed reported symptoms of OCD during the previous week. An epidemiological catchment area survey carried out in the USA in 1984 (about 10,000 people) found an age- and sex-standardised annual prevalence of OCD in people aged 26–64 years of 1.3%, and a lifetime prevalence of 2.3%. Subsequent national surveys used a similar methodology to the survey in the USA, and found broadly similar age and sex standardised annual and lifetime prevalence rates in Canada, Puerto Rico, Germany, Korea, and New Zealand, but a slightly lower prevalence in Taiwan.

AETIOLOGY/RISK FACTORS The cause of OCD is uncertain. Behavioural, cognitive, genetic, and neurobiological factors have been implicated. Limited evidence from genetic studies in families, and in twins, suggests that genetic factors may be involved, at least in some groups. Risk factors include a family history of OCD, being single (which could be a consequence of the disorder), and belonging to a higher socioeconomic class. The risk of OCD in women is higher than in men in most countries. Other risk factors include cocaine abuse, not being in paid employment, past history of alcohol dependence, affective disorder, and phobic disorder.

PROGNOSIS One study (144 people followed for a mean of 47 years) found that an episodic course of OCD was more common during the initial years (about 1–9 years), but that a chronic course was more common afterwards. Over time, the study found that 39–48% of people had symptomatic improvement. A 1-year prospective cohort study found that 46% of people had an episodic course and 54% had a chronic course.

Opioid dependence

Jacinta O'Shea, Fergus Law, and Jan Melichar.

KEY POINTS

- Dependence on opioids is a multifactorial condition involving genetic and psychosocial factors.

- There are three approaches to treating opioid dependence.

  Stabilisation is usually by opioid substitution treatments, and aims to ensure that the drug use becomes independent of mental state, such as craving and mood, and independent of circumstances, such as finance and physical location.

  The next stage is to withdraw (detox) from opioids.

  The final aim is relapse prevention.

- Methadone and buprenorphine help to stabilise opioid use, in that they decrease heroin use and help to keep people in treatment programmes.

  We don't know which of methadone or buprenorphine is better at stabilising opioid use.

- Methadone, buprenorphine, and alpha$_2$-adrenoceptor agonists (lofexidine/clonidine) can all help people withdraw from dependence on illicit opioids.

  Lofexidine and clonidine may be less effective than methadone and buprenorphine in withdrawal, although evidence is weak.

  Ultra-rapid withdrawal can help in detoxification, although there are important safety risks in keeping people heavily sedated or under general anaesthesia for a day, and outcomes are no better.

- Naltrexone can help prevent relapse of heroin use if combined with psychosocial treatment.

(i) **Please visit www.clinicalevidence.bmj.com for full text and references**

What are the effects of drug treatments for stabilisation (maintenance) in people with opioid dependence?	
Beneficial	• Buprenorphine for stabilisation
	• Methadone for stabilisation

What are the effects of drug treatments for withdrawal in people with opioid dependence?	
Beneficial	• Buprenorphine for withdrawal
	• Methadone for withdrawal
Likely To Be Beneficial	• Lofexidine/clonidine for withdrawal
Unknown Effectiveness	• Ultra-rapid (antagonist assisted — naltrexone and naloxone only) withdrawal

What are the effects of drug treatments for relapse prevention in people with opioid dependence?	
Likely To Be Beneficial	• Naltrexone for relapse prevention

Search date June 2006

DEFINITION Opioids (opiates) are highly addictive, and opioid dependence is a chronic relapsing disorder. Heroin is the most commonly abused opioid; others include morphine, buprenorphine, codeine, and methadone. Dependence is a cluster of physiological, behavioural, and cognitive phenomena in which the use of a substance takes on a much higher priority for a given individual than other behaviours that once had a greater value. **Diagnosis:** Diagnosis of dependence syndrome is usually made from a combination of history and urinalysis, looking for the presence of opioid metabolites (e.g. morphine) in the urine. A definite diagnosis of dependence should usually be made only if three or more of the following have been present together at some stage during the previous year: (1) a strong desire or compulsion to take opioids; (2) difficulties in controlling substance-taking behaviour in terms of its onset, termination, and levels of use; (3) a physiological withdrawal state; (4) evidence of tolerance; (5) progressive neglect of alternative pleasures or interests because of opioid use, (6) persisting with substance use despite clear evidence of overtly harmful consequences. Physical examination can also provide evidence of acute intoxication, withdrawal, and chronic or physical consequences of drug administration, such as abscesses, malnutrition, poor dentition, DVT, etc. When commencing treatment, urinalysis should confirm the use of opioids, and a number of samples should be taken, several days apart, to confirm ongoing use. However, with continuing treatment, regular urinalysis might not be necessary, because studies report that, in situations where there is no coercion, self-reports of drug users are sufficiently reliable and valid to provide descriptions of drug use, drug-related problems, and the natural history of drug use.

INCIDENCE/PREVALENCE Opioid use/intravenous drug use rose substantially in the 1990s. New notifications to the Addicts Index (a register held by the UK Home Office) by physicians of people dependent on opioids increased over 30-fold, from approximately 600 in 1966 to more than 18,000 in 1996, and nearly threefold during the 1990s. The UK drug strategy reported in the mid-1990s that there were 100,000–200,000 problem drug users. A pilot study of national estimation methods suggested that there were 143,000–266,000 problem drug users, with about 75,000–150,000 opioid users in England and Wales in 1996. More recently, the number of people becoming dependent on opioids in 2000 ranged from 13,000 (0.06/100 adults aged 15–44 years) to over 26,000 (0.13/100 adults aged 15–44 years). A reduction in the supply of heroin in Australia has also led to a halving in the prevalence of opioid abuse and dependence between the late 1990s and the present.

AETIOLOGY/RISK FACTORS Opioid dependence is a multifactorial condition involving genetic and psychosocial factors. Studies in twins report that both the genetic and shared environmental effects on risk for use and misuse are usually entirely non-specific in their effects. Environmental experiences unique to the person largely determine whether predisposed individuals will use or misuse opioids.

PROGNOSIS Addictive disorders are chronic relapsing conditions with no known "cure".

Shailesh Kumar and Mark Oakley-Browne

KEY POINTS

- Panic disorder is characterised by recurrent, unpredictable panic attacks, making people worry about, or change their behaviour to avert subsequent panic attacks or their consequences.

    Panic disorder occurs in up to 3% of the adult population at some stage, and is associated with other psychiatric and personality disorders, and drug and alcohol abuse.

    The risk of suicide and attempted suicide has been found to be higher in people with panic disorder than in people with other psychiatric illness, including depression.

- CBT is effective in reducing symptoms of panic disorder over 6 months or longer, but we don't know whether it is more effective than other psychological treatments.

    CBT is more effective than waiting list and other controls in reducing symptoms in panic disorder with or without mild-to-moderate agoraphobia. Self-help CBT treatments may be as effective as more intensive CBT treatments.

    There is some suggestion that CBT alone may be more effective than antidepressants alone, with a longer duration of benefit. Combined treatment with CBT plus antidepressants has been shown to be more effective in reducing symptoms than CBT alone or antidepressants alone in the short term.

- Other forms of psychotherapy can also be beneficial in reducing symptoms associated with panic disorder, with or without drug treatments.

    Applied relaxation, client-centred therapy, cognitive restructuring, and exposure to the panic-inducing stimulus are all likely to be effective in reducing symptoms.

    Self-help using CBT techniques may be as effective as therapist-based CBT.

    Breathing retraining, couple therapy, insight-orientated therapy, psychoeducation, and brief dynamic psychotherapy may be beneficial, but there is not enough evidence to be sure.

- SSRIs and TCAs are also effective at reducing the symptoms of panic disorder.

    Benzodiazepines can be effective in reducing symptoms in panic disorder, but their adverse effect profile makes them unsuitable for long-term treatment.

    We don't know whether buspirone or MAOIs are effective.

ⓘ **Please visit www.clinicalevidence.bmj.com for full text and references**

What are the effects of non-drug treatments for panic disorder?	
Beneficial	• CBT versus no treatment
Likely To Be Beneficial	• Applied relaxation
	• Client-centred therapy
	• CBT (may be more effective than drug treatments)
	• Cognitive restructuring
	• Exposure (external or interoceptive)

	• Self-help (may be as effective as other forms of CBT)
Unknown Effectiveness	• Breathing retraining • Brief dynamic psychotherapy • CBT (unclear how CBT compares with other psychological treatments) • Couple therapy • Insight-orientated therapy • Psychoeducation

What are the effects of drug treatments for panic disorder?

Beneficial	• SSRIs • TCAs (imipramine)
Trade-off Between Benefits And Harms	• Benzodiazepines
Unknown Effectiveness	• Buspirone • MAOIs

What are the effects of combined drug and psychological treatments for panic disorder?

Beneficial	• CBT plus drug treatments (more effective than drugs alone)
Likely To Be Beneficial	• CBT plus drug treatments (unclear if more effective than CBT alone)

Search date May 2006

DEFINITION A panic attack is a period in which there is sudden onset of intense apprehension, fearfulness, or terror, often associated with feelings of impending doom. Panic disorder is classified by the DSM-IV as recurrent, unpredictable panic attacks followed by at least 1 month of persistent concern about having another panic attack, worry about the possible implications or consequences of the panic attacks, or a significant behavioural change related to the attacks. The term "panic disorder" excludes panic attacks attributable to the direct physiological effects of a general medical condition, a substance, or another mental disorder. The ICD-10 classifies panic disorder as recurrent, unpredictable panic attacks, with sudden onset of palpitations, chest pain, choking sensations, dizziness, and feelings of unreality, often with associated fear of dying, losing control, or going mad, but without the requirement for the symptoms to have persisted for 1 month or longer. The DSM-IV classifies these conditions as primarily panic disorder with or without agoraphobia, whereas the ICD-10 classifies them as primarily agoraphobia with or without panic disorder. The diagnosis should not be made in people with comorbid depression, when the panic is considered to be secondary to depression. **Diagnosis:** Although panic attacks are a necessary feature of panic disorder, panic attacks alone are not enough to make the diagnosis. Panic attacks may happen in the context of specific situations such as social or specific phobia which are different from panic disorder. A

(continued over)

(from previous page)

diagnosis of panic disorder is made in the presence of recurrent unexpected panic attacks followed by at least 1 month of persistent concern about having another panic attack.

INCIDENCE/PREVALENCE Panic disorder often starts at about 20 years of age (between late adolescence and the mid-30s). Lifetime prevalence is 1–3%, and panic disorder is more common in women than in men. An Australian community study found 1-month prevalence rates for panic disorder (with or without agoraphobia) of 0.4% using ICD-10 diagnostic criteria, and of 0.5% using DSM-IV diagnostic criteria.

AETIOLOGY/RISK FACTORS The onset of panic disorder tends to be preceded by stressful life events, although a negative interpretation of these events, in addition to their occurrence, has been suggested as an important causal factor. Panic disorder is associated with major depression, social phobia, generalised anxiety disorder, obsessive compulsive disorder, and a substantial risk of drug and alcohol abuse. It is also associated with avoidant, histrionic, and dependent personality disorders.

PROGNOSIS The severity of symptoms in people with panic disorder fluctuates considerably, and people commonly experience periods of no attacks, or only mild attacks with few symptoms. There is often a long delay between the initial onset of symptoms and presentation for treatment. Recurrent attacks may continue for several years, especially if associated with agoraphobia. Reduced social or occupational functioning varies among people with panic disorder and is worse in people with associated agoraphobia. Panic disorder is also associated with an increased rate of attempted suicide, found in one study to occur in 20% of people with panic disorder, compared with 12% of those with panic attacks alone, 6% of those with other psychiatric disorder, and 1% of those with no disorders. The odds ratio for attempted suicide was increased if there were co-morbid conditions. One study analysing data from RCTs and systematic reviews found that co-existence of anxiety and depressive features adversely affected treatment response at 12 years compared with treatment of panic disorder alone.

KEY POINTS

- Post-traumatic stress disorder (PTSD) is characterised by disabling symptoms of re-experiencing a traumatic event, avoidance behaviour, and hyperarousal (e.g. irritability or hypervigilance), lasting at least 1 month.

    PTSD may affect 10% of women and 5% of men at some stage, and symptoms may persist for several years.

    Risk factors include major trauma, lack of social support, peritraumatic dissociation, and psychiatric or personality factors.

- Multiple-session CBT may reduce PTSD symptoms in people with psychological distress after a traumatic event.

- We don't know whether antiepileptic drugs, antihypertensive drugs, hydrocortisone, multiple-session collaborative trauma support, multiple-session education, propranolol, single-session debriefing, supportive counselling, or temazepam are beneficial in preventing PTSD.

    Single-session individual debriefing may increase the rate of PTSD compared with no debriefing after a traumatic event.

- In people with PTSD, CBT improves PTSD symptoms compared with no treatment or with other interventions, and eye-movement desensitisation and reprocessing is also likely to be beneficial.

    We don't know whether other psychological treatments (affect management, drama therapy, group therapy, hypnotherapy, inpatient treatment regimens, internet-based psychotherapy, psychodynamic psychotherapy, or supportive psychotherapy) are beneficial in people with PTSD.

- Fluoxetine and paroxetine may improve symptoms in people with PTSD. We found insufficient good evidence to assess other antidepressants, with the exception of venlafaxine, which does not seem to improve symptoms.

    We don't know whether antiepileptic drugs, antihypertensive drugs, benzodiazepines, carbamazepine, olanzapine, propranolol, or risperidone are beneficial in people with PTSD.

(i) Please visit www.clinicalevidence.bmj.com for full text and references

What are the effects of interventions to prevent post-traumatic stress disorder?

Likely To Be Beneficial	• Multiple-session CBT to prevent PTSD in people with acute stress disorder (reduced PTSD compared with supportive counselling)
Unknown Effectiveness	• Antiepileptic drugs to prevent PTSD
	• Antihypertensive drugs to prevent PTSD
	• Hydrocortisone to prevent PTSD
	• Multiple-session CBT to prevent PTSD in all people exposed to a traumatic event
	• Multiple-session collaborative trauma support to prevent PTSD
	• Multiple-session education to prevent PTSD
	• Propranolol to prevent PTSD
	• Single-session group debriefing to prevent PTSD

	• Temazepam to prevent PTSD
Unlikely To Be Beneficial	• Single-session individual debriefing to prevent PTSD
	• Supportive counselling to prevent PTSD

What are the effects of interventions to treat post-traumatic stress disorder?

Beneficial	• CBT to treat PTSD
	• Eye-movement desensitisation and reprocessing to treat PTSD
Likely To Be Beneficial	• Fluoxetine to treat PTSD
	• Paroxetine to treat PTSD
Unknown Effectiveness	• Affect management to treat PTSD
	• Antiepileptic drugs to treat PTSD
	• Antihypertensive drugs to treat PTSD
	• Benzodiazepines to treat PTSD
	• Brofaromine to treat PTSD
	• Carbamazepine to treat PTSD
	• Drama therapy to treat PTSD
	• Group therapy to treat PTSD
	• Hypnotherapy to treat PTSD
	• Inpatient treatment programmes to treat PTSD
	• Internet-based psychotherapy to treat PTSD
	• Mirtazapine to treat PTSD
	• Nefazodone to treat PTSD
	• Olanzapine to treat PTSD
	• Phenelzine to treat PTSD
	• Propranolol to treat PTSD
	• Psychodynamic psychotherapy to treat PTSD
	• Risperidone to treat PTSD
	• Sertraline to treat PTSD
	• SSRIs versus each other to treat PTSD
	• Supportive psychotherapy to treat PTSD
	• TCAs to treat PTSD
Unlikely To Be Beneficial	• Venlafaxine to treat PTSD

Search date December 2006

DEFINITION Post-traumatic stress disorder (PTSD) can occur after any major traumatic event. Symptoms include upsetting thoughts and nightmares about the traumatic event, avoidance behaviour, numbing of general responsiveness, increased irritability, and hyper-vigilance. To fulfil the DSM-IV criteria for PTSD, an individual must have been exposed to a traumatic event; have at least one re-experiencing, three avoidance, and two hyperarousal phenomena; have had the symptoms for at least 1 month; and the symptoms must cause clinically important distress or reduced day-to-day functioning. People with subsyndromal PTSD have all the criteria for PTSD except one of the re-experiencing, avoidance, or hyperarousal phenomena. **Acute stress disorder** occurs within the first month after a major traumatic event and requires the presence of symptoms for at least 2 days. It is similar to PTSD but dissociative symptoms are required to make the diagnosis. Treatments for PTSD may have similar effects, regardless of the traumatic event that precipitated PTSD. However, great caution should be applied when generalising from one type of trauma to another.

INCIDENCE/PREVALENCE One large cross-sectional study in the USA found that 1/10 (10%) women and 1/20 (5%) men experience PTSD at some stage in their lives.

AETIOLOGY/RISK FACTORS Risk factors include major trauma, such as rape, a history of psychiatric disorders, acute distress and depression after the trauma, lack of social support, and personality factors.

PROGNOSIS One large cross-sectional study in the USA found that over a third of people with previous PTSD continued to satisfy the criteria for PTSD 6 years after initial diagnosis. However, cross-sectional studies provide weak evidence about prognosis.

Schizophrenia

Zia Nadeem, Andrew McIntosh, and Stephen Lawrie

KEY POINTS

- One in a hundred people will develop schizophrenia, about 75% of people have relapses and continued disability, and a third fail to respond to standard treatment.

  Positive symptoms include auditory hallucinations, delusions and thought disorder. Negative symptoms (demotivation, self-neglect, and reduced emotion) have not been consistently improved by any treatment.

- Standard treatment of schizophrenia is with antipsychotic drugs, such as chlorpromazine and haloperidol, but these can all cause adverse effects such as parkinsonism, acute dystonia, and sedation.

  Amisulpride, clozapine, olanzapine, and risperidone may all be more effective at reducing symptoms compared with standard drugs but cause similar adverse effects.

  Loxapine, molindone, pimozide, quetiapine, risperidone, sulpiride, ziprasidone, and zotepine seem to be as effective as standard antipsychotic drugs in improving symptoms, but we don't know whether perazine is also effective. Again, these drugs cause similar adverse effects to antipsychotic drugs.

- CAUTION: Pimozide has been associated with sudden cardiac death at doses above 20 mg daily.

- Depot injections of bromperidol decanoate, haloperidol, or fluphenazine decanoate seem to be equally effective as each other, but we don't know whether they are more effective than oral treatments at improving symptoms or preventing relapse, and they cause similar adverse effects.

  Continuation of antipsychotic drugs for at least 6 months after an acute attack reduces the risk of relapse compared with no treatment, although no one drug seems to be more effective than the others at preventing relapse.

  Where available, multiple sessions of family interventions or psychoeducational interventions can reduce relapse rates compared with usual care. We don't know whether CBT or social-skills training are also beneficial.

  In people resistant to standard antipsychotic drugs, clozapine may improve symptoms, but we don't know whether olanzapine is also beneficial.

- Behavioural interventions, compliance therapy, and psychoeducational interventions may improve adherence to antipsychotic medication compared with usual care.

Please visit www.clinicalevidence.bmj.com for full text and references

What are the effects of drug treatments for positive and negative symptoms?

Trade-off Between Benefits And Harms	
	• Amisulpride
	• Chlorpromazine
	• Clozapine
	• Depot bromperidol decanoate
	• Depot haloperidol decanoate
	• Haloperidol
	• Loxapine
	• Molindone

	• Olanzapine
	• Pimozide
	• Quetiapine
	• Risperidone
	• Sulpiride
	• Ziprasidone
	• Zotepine
Unknown Effectiveness	• Perazine

Which interventions reduce relapse rates?

Beneficial	• Continuation of antipsychotic drugs for at least 6 months after an acute episode
	• Multiple-session family interventions
	• Psychoeducational interventions
Unknown Effectiveness	• CBT
	• Social-skills training

Which interventions are effective in people who are resistant to standard antipsychotic drugs?

Beneficial	• Clozapine (compared with standard antipsychotic drugs)
Unknown Effectiveness	• Olanzapine (compared with standard antipyschotic drugs)

Which interventions improve adherence to antipsychotic medication?

Likely To Be Beneficial	• Behavioural therapy
	• Compliance therapy
	• Psychoeducational interventions
Unknown Effectiveness	• Multiple-session family interventions

Search date September 2005

DEFINITION Schizophrenia is characterised by the positive symptoms of auditory hallucinations, delusions, and thought disorder, and by the negative symptoms of demotivation, self-neglect, and reduced emotion. People are defined as being resistant to standard antipsychotic drugs if, over the preceding 5 years, they have not had a clinically important improvement in symptoms after 2–3 regimens of treatment with standard antipsychotic drugs for at least 6 weeks (from at least 2 classes at doses of at least 1000 mg/day of

(continued over)

(from previous page)

chlorpromazine) and they have had no period of good functioning. About 30% (10–45%) of people with schizophrenia meet these criteria.

INCIDENCE/PREVALENCE Onset of symptoms typically occurs in early adult life (average age 25 years) and is earlier in men than in women. Prevalence worldwide is 2–4/1000. One in 100 people will develop schizophrenia in their lifetime.

AETIOLOGY/RISK FACTORS Risk factors include a family history (although no major genes have been identified), obstetric complications, developmental difficulties, central nervous system infections in childhood, cannabis use, and acute life events. The precise contributions of these factors, and ways in which they may interact, are unclear.

PROGNOSIS About three quarters of people suffer recurrent relapse and continued disability, although the proportion of people who improved significantly increased after the mid-1950s (mean: 48.5% from 1956–1985 v 35.4% from 1895–1956). Outcome may be worse in people with insidious onset and delayed initial treatment, social isolation, or a strong family history; in people living in industrialised countries; in men; and in people who misuse drugs. Drug treatment is generally successful in treating positive symptoms, but up to a third of people derive little benefit, and negative symptoms are notoriously difficult to treat. About half of people with schizophrenia do not adhere to treatment in the short term. The figure is even higher in the longer term.

Peter Struijs and Gino Kerkhoffs

KEY POINTS

- Injury of the lateral ligament complex of the ankle joint occurs in about one per 10,000 people a day, accounting for a quarter of all sports injuries.

  Pain may be localised to the lateral side of the ankle.

  Residual complaints include joint instability, stiffness, and intermittent swelling, and are more likely to occur after more extensive cartilage damage.

  Recurrent sprains can add new damage and increase the risk of long-term degeneration of the joint.

- Despite consensus views that immobilisation is more effective than no treatment, studies have shown that immobilisation worsens function and symptoms in the short- and long-term compared with functional treatment.

  Surgery and immobility may have similar outcomes in terms of pain, swelling, and recurrence, but surgery may lead to increased joint stability.

- Functional treatment, consisting of early mobilisation and an external support, improves function and stability of the ankle compared with minimal treatment, or immobilisation.

  We don't know which is the most effective functional treatment, or how functional treatments compare with surgery.

- Ultrasound has not been shown to improve symptoms or function compared with sham ultrasound.

  Cold treatment may reduce oedema compared with heat or a contrast bath, but has not been shown to improve symptoms compared with placebo.

  We don't know whether diathermy, homeopathic ointment, or physiotherapy improve function compared with placebo, as few studies have been found.

(i) **Please visit www.clinicalevidence.bmj.com for full text and references**

What are the effects of treatment strategies for acute ankle ligament ruptures?

Beneficial	• Functional treatment (early mobilisation with use of an external support)
Likely To Be Beneficial	• Immobilisation
Trade-off Between Benefits And Harms	• Surgery
Unknown Effectiveness	• Cold treatment • Diathermy • Homeopathic ointment • Physiotherapy
Unlikely To Be Beneficial	• Ultrasound

Search date March 2007

DEFINITION Ankle sprain is an injury of the lateral ligament complex of the ankle joint. The injury is graded on the basis of severity. Grade I is a mild stretching of the ligament complex without joint instability; grade II is a partial rupture of the ligament complex with mild instability of the joint (such as isolated rupture of the anterior talofibular ligament); and grade III involves complete rupture of the ligament complex with instability of the joint. This gradation has limited practical consequences since both grade II and III injuries are treated similarly, and grade I injuries need no specific treatment after diagnosis. Unless otherwise stated, studies included in this review did not specify the grades of injury included, or included both grade II and III.

INCIDENCE/PREVALENCE Ankle sprain is a common problem in acute medical care, occurring at a rate of about one injury per 10,000 people a day. Injuries of the lateral ligament complex of the ankle form a quarter of all sports injuries.

AETIOLOGY/RISK FACTORS The usual mechanism of injury is inversion and adduction (usually referred to as supination) of the plantar flexed foot. Predisposing factors are a history of ankle sprains, ligament hyperlaxity syndrome, and specific malalignment, such as crus varum and pes cavo-varus.

PROGNOSIS Some sports (e.g. basketball, football/soccer, and volleyball) are associated with a particularly high incidence of ankle injuries. Pain and intermittent swelling are the most frequent residual problems, often localised on the lateral side of the ankle. Other residual complaints include mechanical instability and stiffness. People with more extensive cartilage damage have a higher incidence of residual complaints. In the long term, the initial traumatic cartilage damage can lead to degenerative changes, especially if there is persistent or recurrent instability. Every further sprain has the potential to add new damage.

KEY POINTS

- Bunions are prominent and often inflamed metatarsal heads and overlying bursae, usually associated with hallux valgus, which cause pain and problems with walking and wearing normal shoes.

  Hallux valgus, where the great toe moves towards the second toe, is found in at least 2% of children aged 9–10 years, and almost half of adults, with greater prevalence in women.

  We don't know what role footwear plays in the development of hallux valgus or bunions.

- We don't know whether night splints or orthoses prevent deterioration of hallux valgus.

- Distal chevron osteotomy may be more effective than orthoses or no treatment at reducing pain and improving function, but we don't know whether it is more or less effective than other surgical procedures.

  We don't know whether other surgical procedures, such as arthrodesis, Keller's arthroplasty, phalangeal osteotomy, proximal osteotomy, or bone fixation methods are beneficial in improving outcomes.

- We don't know whether continuous passive motion, early weight bearing, or slipper casts are effective in improving recovery and outcomes post-operatively.

(i) **Please visit www.clinicalevidence.bmj.com for full text and references**

What are the effects of conservative treatments for bunions?	
Unknown Effectiveness	• Antipronatory orthoses in children
	• Night splints
	• Orthoses to treat hallux valgus in adults

What are the effects of surgery for bunions?	
Likely To Be Beneficial	• Distal chevron osteotomy (more effective than no treatment or orthoses, but insufficient evidence to compare with other osteotomies or arthrodesis)
Unknown Effectiveness	• Arthrodesis (Lapidus procedure)
	• Arthrodesis (versus no treatment)
	• Chevron osteotomy plus adductor tenotomy versus chevron osteotomy alone (relative benefits unclear)
	• Different methods of bone fixation (standard fixation, absorbable-pin fixation, screw fixation plus early weight bearing, suture fixation plus delayed weight bearing)
	• Keller's arthroplasty
	• Keller–Lelievre arthroplasty
	• Phalangeal (Akin) osteotomy plus distal chevron osteotomy

	• Proximal chevron osteotomy versus other types of proximal osteotomy (relative benefits unclear)
	• Proximal osteotomy versus distal chevron osteotomy (relative benefits unclear)

What are the effects of postoperative care after surgery for bunions?

Unknown Effectiveness	• Continuous passive motion
	• Early weight bearing
	• Slipper casts

Search date June 2006

DEFINITION Hallux valgus is a deformity of the great toe, whereby the hallux (great toe) moves towards the second toe, overlying it in severe cases. This abduction (movement away from the midline of the body) is usually accompanied by some rotation of the toe so that the nail is facing the midline of the body (valgus rotation). With the deformity, the metatarsal head becomes more prominent, and the metatarsal is said to be in an adducted position as it moves towards the midline of the body. Radiological criteria for hallux valgus vary, but a commonly accepted criterion is to measure the angle formed between the metatarsal and the abducted hallux. This is called the metatarsophalangeal joint angle, or hallux abductus angle, and it is considered abnormal when greater than 14.5 °. **Bunion** is the lay term used to describe a prominent and often inflamed metatarsal head and overlying bursa. Symptoms include pain, limitation in walking, and problems with wearing normal shoes.

INCIDENCE/PREVALENCE The prevalence of hallux valgus varies in different populations. In a recent study of 6000 UK school children aged 9–10 years, 2.5% had clinical evidence of hallux valgus, and 2% met both clinical and radiological criteria for hallux valgus. An earlier study found hallux valgus in 48% of adults. Differences in prevalence may result from different methods of measurement, varying age groups, or different diagnostic criteria (e.g. metatarsal joint angle more than 10 ° or more than 15 °).

AETIOLOGY/RISK FACTORS Nearly all population studies have found that hallux valgus is more common in women. Footwear may contribute to the deformity, but studies comparing people who wear shoes with those who do not have found contradictory results. Hypermobility of the first ray and excessive foot pronation are associated with hallux valgus.

PROGNOSIS We found no studies that looked at the progression of hallux valgus. While progression of deformity and symptoms is rapid in some people, others remain asymptomatic. One study found that hallux valgus is often unilateral initially, but usually progresses to bilateral deformity.

Nigel Ashworth

KEY POINTS

- Carpal tunnel syndrome is a neuropathy caused by compression of the median nerve within the carpal tunnel.

  Classic symptoms include numbness, tingling, burning, or pain in at least two of the three digits supplied by the median nerve (i.e. the thumb, and index and middle fingers).

  Symptoms can resolve within six months in about a third of people — particularly younger people — whereas poor prognosis is often indicated by bilateral symptoms and a positive Phalen's test. However, the severity of symptoms and signs does not often correlate well with the extent of nerve damage.

- Corticosteroid treatment (either local injection or systemic) appears to be beneficial in treating carpal tunnel syndrome, although the evidence suggests that there is greater improvement in long-term outcomes with local injections compared with systemic administration.

  Risks associated with local corticosteroid injections into the carpal tunnel include tendon rupture and injection into the median nerve.

- We do not know whether NSAIDs or pyridoxine are effective in treating carpal tunnel syndrome, because the RCTs identified have been too small to draw reliable conclusions.

- Diuretics seem unlikely to be beneficial in the treatment of carpal tunnel syndrome.

- We do not know whether nerve and tendon gliding exercises, therapeutic ultrasound, or wrist splints are effective in relieving symptoms of carpal tunnel syndrome.

- Surgery seems to improve clinical outcomes compared with wrist splints, but is not as effective as local corticosteroid injections.

  Both endoscopic and open carpal tunnel release seem to improve symptoms, although the data are unclear as to which is more beneficial. Both are associated with several adverse effects.

  Internal neurolysis in conjunction with open carpal tunnel release does not appear to relieve symptoms compared with open carpal tunnel release alone.

- Wrist splinting after carpal tunnel release has no effect on improving motor function, and seems to increase pain compared with surgery alone.

(i) **Please visit www.clinicalevidence.bmj.com for full text and references**

What are the effects of drug treatments for carpal tunnel syndrome?	
Likely To Be Beneficial	• Corticosteroids (local injection) • Corticosteroids (systemic)
Unknown Effectiveness	• Diuretics • NSAIDs • Pyridoxine

What are the effects of non-drug treatments for carpal tunnel syndrome?	
Unknown Effectiveness	• Acupuncture • Massage therapy

- Nerve and tendon gliding exercises
- Therapeutic ultrasound
- Wrist splints

What are the effects of surgical treatments for carpal tunnel syndrome?

Trade-off Between Benefits And Harms	• Endoscopic carpal tunnel release versus open carpal-tunnel release (seem to be equally effective in improving symptoms but both associated with adverse effects)
	• Surgery versus local corticosteroid injection (unclear which is most effective; both associated with adverse effects)
	• Surgery versus wrist splint (surgery more effective but associated with adverse effects)
Unknown Effectiveness	• Surgery (versus no treatment or placebo)
Unlikely To Be Beneficial	• Internal neurolysis in conjunction with open carpal tunnel release

What are the effects of postoperative treatments for carpal tunnel syndrome?

Unlikely To Be Beneficial	• Wrist splints after carpal tunnel release surgery

Search date December 2006

DEFINITION Carpal tunnel syndrome (CTS) is a neuropathy caused by compression of the median nerve within the carpal tunnel. Classical symptoms of CTS include numbness, tingling, burning, or pain in at least two of the three digits supplied by the median nerve (i.e. the thumb, index, and middle fingers). The American Academy of Neurology has described diagnostic criteria that rely on a combination of symptoms and physical examination findings. Other diagnostic criteria include results from electrophysiological studies.

INCIDENCE/PREVALENCE A general population survey in Rochester, Minnesota, found the age-adjusted incidence of CTS to be 105 (95% CI 99 to 112) cases per 100,000 person years. Age-adjusted incidence rates were 52 (95% CI 45 to 59) cases per 100,000 person-years for men and 149 (95% CI 138 to 159) cases per 100,000 person-years for women. The study found that incidence rates increased from 88 (95% CI 75 to 101) cases per 100,000 person-years in 1961–1965 to 125 (95% CI 112 to 138) cases per 100,000 person-years in 1976–1980. Incidence rates of CTS increased with age for men, whereas for women they peaked at the ages of 45–54 years. A general population survey in the Netherlands found prevalence to be 1% for men and 7% for women. A more comprehensive study in southern Sweden found that the general population prevalence for CTS was 3% (95% CI 2% to 3%). As in other studies, the overall prevalence in women was higher than in men (male to female ratio 1.0:1.4); however, among older people, the prevalence in women was almost four times that in men (age group 65–74 years: men 1%, 95% CI 0% to 4%; women 5%, 95% CI 3% to 8%). Over 50% of pregnant women develop symptoms of CTS. However, many trials exclude pregnant women, and we have not identified any RCTs assessing the treatment of pregnancy-induced CTS. The pathophysiology of idiopathic and pregnancy-induced CTS are likely to differ, with one key consideration in pregnancy-induced CTS being fluid retention. Therefore, strategies to reduce fluid retention will probably be of more benefit in pregnancy-induced CTS than they have been shown to be in idiopathic CTS.

AETIOLOGY/RISK FACTORS Most cases of CTS have no easily identifiable cause (idiopathic). Secondary causes of CTS include the following: space-occupying lesions (tumours, hypertrophic synovial tissue, fracture callus, and osteophytes); metabolic and physiological (pregnancy, hypothyroidism, and rheumatoid arthritis); infections; neuropathies (associated with diabetes mellitus or alcoholism); and familial disorders. One case-control study found that risk factors in the general population included repetitive activities requiring wrist extension or flexion, obesity, rapid dieting, shorter height, hysterectomy without oophorectomy, and recent menopause.

PROGNOSIS One observational study (CTS defined by symptoms and electrophysiological study results) found that 34% of people with idiopathic CTS without treatment had complete resolution of symptoms (remission) within six months of diagnosis. Remission rates were higher for younger age groups, and for women. One observational study in pregnant women found that, in most cases, pregnancy-induced CTS spontaneously improved after delivery. However, some women complained of symptoms of CTS one year after delivery. A more recent observational study of untreated idiopathic CTS also showed that symptoms can spontaneously resolve in some people. The main positive prognostic indicators were short duration of symptoms and young age, whereas bilateral symptoms and a positive Phalen's test were indicators of a poorer prognosis.

Steven Reid, Trudie Chalder, Anthony Cleare, Matthew Hotopf, and Simon Wessely

KEY POINTS

- Chronic fatigue syndrome (CFS) is characterised by severe, disabling fatigue and other symptoms including musculoskeletal pain, sleep disturbance, impaired concentration, and headaches.

   CFS affects between 0.006% and 3% of the population depending on the criteria used, with women being at higher risk than men.

- Graded exercise therapy has been shown to effectively improve measures of fatigue and physical functioning.

   Educational interventions with encouragement of graded exercise (treatment sessions, telephone follow-ups, and an educational package explaining symptoms and encouraging home-based exercise) improve symptoms more effectively than written information alone.

- CBT is also effective in treating chronic fatigue syndrome.

   CBT may also be beneficial when administered by therapists with no specific experience of chronic fatigue syndrome, but who are adequately supervised.

   In adolescents, CBT can reduce fatigue severity and improve school attendance compared with no treatment.

- We don't know how effective antidepressants, corticosteroids, and intramuscular magnesium are in treating CFS.

   Antidepressants should be considered in people with affective disorders, and TCAs in particular have potential therapeutic value because of their analgesic properties.

- Interventions such as dietary supplements, evening primrose oil, oral nicotinamide adenine dinucleotide, homeopathy, and prolonged rest have not been studied in enough detail for us to be able to draw conclusions on their efficacy.

- A large study has found that galantamine is no better than placebo at improving symptoms of CFS.

- Although there is some evidence that immunotherapy can improve symptoms compared with placebo, it is associated with considerable adverse effects and should therefore probably not be offered as a treatment for chronic fatigue.

(i) **Please visit www.clinicalevidence.bmj.com for full text and references**

What are the effects of treatments for chronic fatigue syndrome?

Beneficial	• CBT
	• Graded exercise therapy
Unknown Effectiveness	• Antidepressants
	• Corticosteroids
	• Dietary supplements
	• Evening primrose oil
	• Homeopathy
	• Magnesium (intramuscular)
	• Oral nicotinamide adenine dinucleotide

	• Prolonged rest
Unlikely To Be Beneficial	• Galantamine
Likely To Be Ineffective Or Harmful	• Immunotherapy

Search date September 2006

DEFINITION Chronic fatigue syndrome (CFS) is characterised by severe, disabling fatigue, and other symptoms, including musculoskeletal pain, sleep disturbance, impaired concentration, and headaches. Two widely used definitions of CFS, from the US Centers for Disease Control and Prevention (CDC) (current criteria issued in 1994, which superseded the CDC criteria issued in 1988) and from Oxford, UK, were developed as operational criteria for research. The principal difference between these definitions is the number and severity of symptoms, other than fatigue, that must be present. A third operational definition, the Australian criteria, is similar to the CDC diagnostic criteria and has also been used in treatment trials. The 1994 CDC criteria were recently reviewed with the aim of improving case ascertainment for research. The exclusion criteria were clarified, and the use of specific instruments for the assessment of symptoms was recommended.

INCIDENCE/PREVALENCE Community- and primary care-based studies have reported the prevalence of CFS to be from 0.007% to 2.8% in the general adult population and from 0.006% to 3.0% in primary care depending on the criteria used.

AETIOLOGY/RISK FACTORS Despite considerable research effort and several hypotheses, the cause of CFS remains poorly understood. Endocrine and immunological abnormalities have been found in many people, although it is unclear whether these changes are causal or part of the course of the syndrome. Certain infectious illnesses, such as Epstein–Barr virus, Q fever, and viral meningitis, are associated with a greater risk of developing CFS, but many people have no evidence of viral infection, and there is no evidence of persistent infection. Women are at higher risk than men (RR 1.3–1.7, depending on diagnostic criteria used; CIs not reported). Population surveys in the USA have found that white individuals have a lower risk of CFS compared with Latin Americans, African Americans, and Native Americans.

PROGNOSIS Studies have focused on people attending specialist clinics. A systematic review of studies of prognosis (search date 1996) found that children with CFS had better outcomes than adults: 54–94% of children showed definite improvement in symptoms (after up to 6 years' follow-up), whereas 20–50% of adults showed some improvement in the medium term (12–39 months) and only 6% returned to premorbid levels of functioning. Despite the considerable burden of morbidity associated with CFS, we found no evidence of increased mortality. The systematic review found that a longer duration of illness, fatigue severity, comorbid depression and anxiety, and a physical attribution for CFS are factors associated with a poorer prognosis.

Fracture prevention in postmenopausal women

Leif Mosekilde, Peter Vestergaard, Bente Langdahl

KEY POINTS

- The lifetime risk of fracture in white women is 20% for the spine, 15% for the wrist, and 18% for the hip, with an exponential increase in risk beyond the age of 50 years.

  About 13% of people die in the year after a hip fracture, and most survivors lose some or all of their previous independence.

- Alendronate, risedronate, and parathyroid hormone reduce vertebral and non-vertebral fractures compared with placebo.

  Etidronate, ibandronate, pamidronate, and raloxifene reduce vertebral fractures, but have not been shown to reduce non-vertebral fractures.

  Raloxifene protects against breast cancer, but increases venous thromboembolic events and stroke compared with placebo.

  Strontium ranelate reduces vertebral and, to some extent, non-vertebral fractures.

  Calcitonin may reduce vertebral fractures over 1–5 years, but has not been shown to reduce non-vertebral fractures.

  Clodronate has been shown in one large RCT to reduce non-vertebral but not vertebral fracture risk. One small RCT showed a decrease in vertebral but not non-vertebral fracture risk.

- CAUTION: HRT may reduce fractures, but it increases the risk of breast cancer and cardiovascular events.

- Combined calcium plus vitamin D, or vitamin D analogues alone, may reduce vertebral and non-vertebral fractures, but studies have given inconclusive results.

  Monotherapy with calcium or vitamin D has not been shown to reduce fractures.

- We don't know whether multifactorial non-pharmacological interventions, including environmental manipulation, or regular exercise reduce the risk of fractures.

  Hip protectors may reduce the risk of hip fractures in nursing home residents, but compliance tends to be low.

(i) **Please visit www.clinicalevidence.bmj.com for full text and references**

What are the effects of treatments to prevent fractures in postmenopausal women?

Beneficial	• Alendronate
	• Parathyroid hormone
	• Risedronate
	• Strontium ranelate
Likely To Be Beneficial	• Calcitonin
	• Calcium plus vitamin D
	• Clodronate
	• Etidronate
	• Hip protectors
	• Ibandronate
	• Pamidronate

	• Vitamin D analogues (alfacalcidol or calcitriol)
Trade-off Between Benefits And Harms	• Raloxifene
Unknown Effectiveness	• Exercise • Multifactorial non-pharmacological interventions
Unlikely To Be Beneficial	• Calcium alone • Vitamin D alone
Likely To Be Ineffective Or Harmful	• HRT

Search date January 2007

DEFINITION This review covers interventions to prevent fractures in postmenopausal women. A fracture is a break or disruption of bone or cartilage, and may be symptomatic or asymptomatic. Symptoms and signs may include immobility, pain, tenderness, numbness, bruising, joint deformity, joint swelling, limb deformity, and limb shortening. **Diagnosis:** Fracture is usually diagnosed on the basis of a typical clinical picture (see above) combined with results from an appropriate imaging technique. Usually, in trials dealing with osteoporosis, menopause is considered to be present 12 months after the last menstruation.

INCIDENCE/PREVALENCE The lifetime risk of fracture in white women is 20% for the spine, 15% for the wrist, and 18% for the hip. The incidence of postmenopausal fracture increases with age. Observational studies found that age-specific incidence rates for postmenopausal fracture of the hip increased exponentially beyond the age of 50 years. The incidence of fractures varies by ethnic group. The incidence of hip fractures is highest in white people, and then decreases successively in Hispanic, Asian, and African-American people.

AETIOLOGY/RISK FACTORS A fracture arises when load to the bone exceeds bone biomechanical competence (strength). Fractures usually arise from trauma, but may arise without any apparent injury. Risk factors are those factors that increase the risk of trauma and decrease bone biomechanical competence. An increased risk of trauma exists when the risk of falls is increased, such as in people with impaired vision, decreased postural balance, or neurological disorders (e.g. ataxia, stroke, epilepsy). Factors that decrease bone biomechanical competence, and so induce osteoporosis, include increasing age, low BMI or weight, genetic predisposition, diseases (e.g. hyperthyroidism, hyperparathyroidism, and rheumatoid arthritis), drugs (e.g. corticosteroids), and environmental factors (e.g. smoking). Postmenopausal women are at increased risk of fracture compared with premenopausal women and men of all ages because of hormone-related bone loss.

PROGNOSIS Fractures may result in pain, short- or long-term disability, haemorrhage, thromboembolic disease (see thromboembolism, p 53), shock, and death. Vertebral fractures are associated with pain, physical impairment, muscular atrophy, changes in body shape, loss of physical function, and lower quality of life. About 13% of people die in the first year after a hip fracture, representing a doubling of mortality compared to people of similar age and no hip fracture. Half of all elderly women who have previously been independent become partly dependent after hip fracture. A third become totally dependent.

Martin Underwood

KEY POINTS

- Gout is characterised by deposition of urate crystals, causing acute monoarthritis and crystal deposits (tophi) in the skin.

  Gout affects about 5% of men and 1% of women with up to 80% of people experiencing a recurrent attack within 3 years.

  Diagnosis is usually clinical, supported by signs of hyperuricaemia.

  Risk factors are those which are associated with increased serum urate concentrations, including older age, non-white ethnicity, obesity, consumption of alcohol, meat and fish, and use of diuretics.

  Hyperuricaemia may be associated with an increased risk of cardiovascular events; we do not know whether it is an independent risk factor.

- We don't know whether NSAIDs reduce pain and tenderness in an acute attack of gout, although they are commonly used in clinical practice. They are associated with increased risks of gastrointestinal, and possible cardiovascular, adverse effects.

  Indometacin is widely used to treat acute gout, despite the absence of RCT evidence of benefit. Etoricoxib is as effective as indometacin with reduced risks of gastrointestinal adverse effects.

- Although it has been widely used for many years, we don't know whether oral colchicine improves symptoms in acute gout. Its use is limited by the high incidence of adverse effects.

- We don't know whether intra-articular, parenteral or oral corticosteroids, or corticotropin (ACTH), improve symptoms in acute gout.

- We don't know whether colchicine prevents attacks of gout in people with prior episodes, but it may reduce the risk of an attack in a person starting allopurinol treatment.

  We don't know whether advice to lose weight or reduce alcohol or dietary purine intake prevents further attacks of gout.

  We don't know whether allopurinol or sulfinpyrazone reduce the risk of recurrent attacks compared with placebo or other treatments.

(i) **Please visit www.clinicalevidence.bmj.com for full text and references**

What are the effects of treatments for acute gout?

Unknown Effectiveness	• Colchicine (oral)
	• Corticosteroids
	• Corticotropin (adrenocorticotrophic hormone)
	• NSAIDs

What are the effects of treatments to prevent gout in people with prior acute episodes?

Unknown Effectiveness	• Advice to lose weight
	• Advice to reduce alcohol intake
	• Advice to reduce dietary intake of purines
	• Colchicine for preventing recurrence
	• Sulfinpyrazone

• Xanthine oxidase inhibitors

Search date June 2006

DEFINITION Gout is a syndrome caused by deposition of urate crystals. It typically presents as an acute monoarthritis of rapid onset. The first metatarsophalangeal joint is the most commonly affected joint (podagra). Gout also affects other joints: joints in the foot, ankle, knee, wrist, finger, and elbow are the most frequently affected. Crystal deposits (tophi) may develop around hands, feet, elbows, and ears. **Diagnosis:** This is usually made clinically. The American College of Rheumatology (ACR) criteria for diagnosing gout are as follows: (1) characteristic urate crystals in joint fluid; (2) a tophus proved to contain urate crystals; or (3) the presence of six or more defined clinical laboratory and x ray phenomena. We have included studies of people meeting the ACR criteria, studies in which the diagnosis was made clinically, and studies that used other criteria.

INCIDENCE/PREVALENCE Gout is more common in older people and men. In people aged 65–74 years in the UK, the prevalence is about 50/1000 in men and about 9/1000 in women. The annual incidence of gout in people aged over 50 years in the USA is 1.6/1000 in men and 0.3/1000 in women. One 12-year longitudinal study of 47,150 male health professionals with no previous history of gout estimated that annual incidence of gout ranged from 1.0/1000 for those aged 40–44 years, to 1.8/1000 for those aged 55–64 years. Gout may become more common because of increasing longevity, obesity, meat and fish consumption, and use of diuretics. Gout may be more common in some non-white ethnic groups. A pooled analysis of two cohort studies of former medical students found the annual incidence of gout to be 3.1/1000 in black men and 1.8/1000 in white men. After correcting for the higher prevalence of hypertension among black men, which is a risk factor for gout, the relative risk of gout in black men compared with white men was 1.30 (95% CI 0.77 to 2.19). A cross-sectional survey of 657 people aged 15 years and over in New Zealand found a higher prevalence of gout in Maoris than in people of a European background (6.4% in Maoris v 2.9% in people with European background; age-adjusted RR 3.2, 95% CI 1.6 to 6.6).

AETIOLOGY/RISK FACTORS Urate crystals form when serum urate concentration exceeds 0.42 mmol/L. Serum urate concentration is the principal risk factor for a first attack of gout, although 40% of people have normal serum urate concentration during an attack of gout. A cohort study of 2046 men followed for about 15 years found that the annual incidence was about 0.4% in men with a urate concentration of 0.42–0.47 mmol/L, rising to 4.3% when serum urate concentration was 0.45–0.59 mmol/L. One 5-year longitudinal study of 223 asymptomatic men with hyperuricaemia estimated the 5-year cumulative incidence of gout to be 10.8% for those with baseline serum urate of 0.42–0.47 mmol/L, 27.7% for baseline urate of 0.48–0.53 mmol/L, and 61.1% for baseline urate levels of 0.54 mmol/L or more. The study found that a 0.6 mmol/L difference in baseline serum urate increased the odds of an attack of gout by a factor of 1.8 (OR adjusted for other risk factors for gout: 1.84, 95% CI 1.24 to 2.72). One 12-year longitudinal study (47,150 male health professionals with no history of gout) estimated that the relative risks of gout associated with one additional daily serving of various foods (weekly for seafood) were as follows: meat 1.21 (95% CI 1.04 to 1.41), seafood (fish, lobster, and shellfish) 1.07 (95% CI 1.01 to 1.12), purine rich vegetables 0.97 (95% CI 0.79 to 1.19), low-fat dairy products 0.79 (95% CI 0.71 to 0.87), and high-fat dairy products 0.99 (95% CI 0.89 to 1.10). Alcohol consumption of greater than 14.9 g daily significantly increased the risk of gout compared with no alcohol consumption (RR for 15.0–29.9 g/day: 1.49, 95% CI 1.14 to 1.94; RR for 30.0–49.9 g/day: 1.96, 95% CI 1.48 to 2.60; RR for 50 g/day or more: 2.53, 95% CI 1.73 to 3.70). The longitudinal study also estimated the relative risk of gout associated with an additional serving of beer (355 mL, 12.8 g alcohol), wine (118 mL, 11.0 g alcohol), and spirits (44 mL, 14.0 g alcohol). It found that an extra daily serving of beer or spirits was significantly associated with gout, but an extra daily serving of wine was not (RR for 355 mL/day beer: 1.49, 95% CI 1.32 to 1.70; RR for 44 mL/day spirits: 1.15, 95% CI 1.04 to 1.28; RR for 118 mL/day wine: 1.04, 95% CI 0.88 to 1.22). Other suggested risk factors for gout include obesity, insulin resistance, dyslipidaemia, hypertension, and CVD.

PROGNOSIS We found few reliable data about prognosis or complications of gout. One study found that 3/11 (27%) people with untreated gout of the first metatarsophalangeal

(continued over)

(from previous page)

joint experienced spontaneous resolution after 7 days. A case series of 614 people with gout who had not received treatment to reduce urate levels, and could recall the interval between first and second attacks, reported recurrence rates of 62% after 1 year, 78% after 2 years, and 84% after 3 years. An analysis of two prospective cohort studies of 371 black and 1181 white male former medical students followed up for about 30 years found no significant difference in risk of CHD in men who had developed gout compared with men who had not (RR 0.85, 95% CI 0.40 to 1.81).

Jo Jordan, Kika Konstantinou, Tamara Shawver Morgan, and James Weinstein

KEY POINTS

- Herniated lumbar disc is a displacement of disc material (nucleus pulposus or annulus fibrosis) beyond the intervertebral disc space.

  The highest prevalence is among people aged 30–50 years, with a male to female ratio of 2:1.

- There is little evidence to suggest that drug treatments are effective in treating herniated discs.

  NSAIDs and cytokine inhibitors don't seem to improve symptoms of people with sciatica caused by disc herniation.

  We found no evidence examining the effectiveness of analgesics, antidepressants, or muscle relaxants in people with herniated discs.

  We found no evidence of sufficient quality to allow us to judge the effectiveness of epidural injections of corticosteroids.

- With regard to non-drug treatments, spinal manipulation seems to increase self-perceived improvement compared with placebo, although concerns exist regarding possible further herniation from spinal manipulation in people who are surgical candidates.

  Neither bed rest nor traction seems effective in treating people with sciatica caused by disc herniation.

  We found insufficient evidence about advice to stay active, acupuncture, massage, exercise, heat, or ice to be able to judge their efficacy in treating people with herniated discs.

- About 10% of people have sufficient pain after 6 weeks for surgery to become a consideration.

  Both standard discectomy and microdiscectomy seem to increase self-reported improvement to a similar extent.

  We found insufficient evidence to judge the effectiveness of automated percutaneous discectomy, laser discectomy, or percutaneous disc decompression.

(i) **Please visit www.clinicalevidence.bmj.com for full text and references**

What are the effects of drug treatments for herniated lumbar disc?	
Unknown Effectiveness	• Analgesics • Antidepressants • Corticosteroids (epidural injections) • Cytokine inhibitors (infliximab) • Muscle relaxants
Unlikely To Be Beneficial	• NSAIDs

What are the effects of non-drug treatments for herniated lumbar disc?	
Likely To Be Beneficial	• Spinal manipulation
Unknown Effectiveness	• Acupuncture • Advice to stay active

	• Exercise therapy
	• Heat
	• Ice
	• Massage
Unlikely To Be Beneficial	• Bed rest
	• Traction

What are the effects of surgery for herniated lumbar disc?

Likely To Be Beneficial	• Microdiscectomy (as effective as standard discectomy)
	• Standard discectomy (short-term benefit)
Unknown Effectiveness	• Automated percutaneous discectomy
	• Laser discectomy
	• Percutaneous disc decompression

Search date November 2006

DEFINITION Herniated lumbar disc is a displacement of disc material (nucleus pulposus or annulus fibrosis) beyond the intervertebral disc space. The diagnosis can be confirmed by radiological examination; however, magnetic resonance imaging findings of herniated disc are not always accompanied by clinical symptoms. This review covers treatment of people who have clinical symptoms relating to confirmed or suspected disc herniation. It does not include treatment of people with spinal cord compression, or people with cauda equina syndrome, which require emergency intervention. The management of non-specific acute low back pain, p 384 and chronic low back pain, p 387 are covered elsewhere in *BMJ Clinical Evidence*.

INCIDENCE/PREVALENCE The prevalence of symptomatic herniated lumbar disc is about 1–3% in Finland and Italy, depending on age and sex. The highest prevalence is among people aged 30–50 years, with a male to female ratio of 2:1. In people aged 25–55 years, about 95% of herniated discs occur at the lower lumbar spine (L4–L5 level); disc herniation above this level is more common in people aged over 55 years.

AETIOLOGY/RISK FACTORS Radiographical evidence of disc herniation does not reliably predict low back pain in the future, or correlate with symptoms; 19–27% of people without symptoms have disc herniation on imaging. Risk factors for disc herniation include smoking (OR 1.7, 95% CI 1.0 to 2.5), weight-bearing sports (e.g. weight lifting, hammer throw, etc), and certain work activities, such as repeated lifting. Driving a motor vehicle has been suggested to be a risk factor for disc herniation, although evidence is inconclusive (OR 1.7, 95% CI 0.2 to 2.7). This potential effect may be because the resonant frequency of the spine is similar to that of certain vehicles.

PROGNOSIS The natural history of disc herniation is difficult to determine, because most people take some form of treatment for their back pain, and a formal diagnosis is not always made. Clinical improvement is usual in most people, and only about 10% of people still have sufficient pain after 6 weeks to consider surgery. Sequential magnetic resonance images have shown that the herniated portion of the disc tends to regress over time, with partial to complete resolution after 6 months in two thirds of people.

David Oliver, Richard Griffiths, James Roche, and Opinder Sahota

KEY POINTS

- Between 12% and 37% of people will die in the year after a hip fracture, and 10–20% of survivors will move into a more dependent residence.

- Surgery is routinely used in the treatment of hip fracture.

  Surgical fixation leads to earlier mobilisation and less leg deformity compared with conservative treatment.

  In people with intracapsular hip fracture, internal fixation is associated with less operative trauma and deep-wound sepsis, but is more likely to require subsequent revision surgery, compared with arthroplasty. We don't know the best method for internal fixation, or the best method of arthroplasty for these fractures.

  In people with extracapsular hip fractures, short intramedullary cephalocondylic nails (such as the Gamma nail), Ender nails, and older fixed nail plates increase the risk of reoperation compared with extramedullary fixation with a sliding hip screw device, but we don't know whether other kinds of extramedullary devices are better than the sliding hip screw. We also don't know how different intramedullary devices compare with each other.

- Various perisurgical interventions may be used with the aim of improving surgical outcome and preventing complications.

  Routine preoperative traction to the injured limb has not been shown to relieve pain or to aid subsequent surgery.

  Antibiotic prophylaxis reduces wound infections, but we don't know which is the optimum regimen.

  Antiplatelet agents and heparin reduce the risk of DVT when used prophylactically, but both treatments increase the risk of bleeding. Cyclical compression devices also reduce the risk of DVT, but we don't know whether graduated elastic compression stockings are effective.

  Oral protein and energy multinutrient feeds may reduce unfavourable outcomes after surgery.

- Various rehabilitation interventions and programmes aim to improve recovery after a hip fracture, but we don't know how effective most of them are.

  Co-ordinated multidisciplinary care may improve outcomes compared with usual care, but we don't know which method is best.

(i) **Please visit www.clinicalevidence.bmj.com for full text and references**

What are the effects of surgical interventions in people with hip fracture?	
Trade-off Between Benefits And Harms	• Internal fixation versus arthroplasty for intracapsular hip fracture
Unknown Effectiveness	• Arthroplasty versus internal fixation for extracapsular fracture
	• Choice of implant for internal fixation of intracapsular hip fracture
	• Different types of arthroplasty for intracapsular hip fracture
	• External fixation for extracapsular fracture

	• Extramedullary implants other than older fixed nail plates versus sliding hip screw for extracapsular fracture • Type of intramedullary fixation for extracapsular hip fracture
Unlikely To Be Beneficial	• Conservative versus operative treatment for most types of hip fracture • Short cephalocondylic nail (e.g. Gamma nail) versus extramedullary fixation with sliding hip screw for extracapsular hip fracture
Likely To Be Ineffective Or Harmful	• Intramedullary fixation with condylocephalic nails (e.g. Ender nails) versus extramedullary fixation with sliding hip screw or fixed nail plate for extracapsular fracture • Older fixed nail plates for extramedullary fixation of extracapsular fracture (increased risk of fixation failure compared with sliding hip screws)

What are the effects of perisurgical medical interventions on surgical outcome and prevention of complications in people with hip fracture?

Beneficial	• Perioperative prophylaxis with antibiotics
Likely To Be Beneficial	• Cyclical compression of the foot or calf to reduce venous thromboembolism • Oral multinutrient feeds for nutritional supplementation after hip fracture • Perioperative prophylaxis with antiplatelet agents
Trade-off Between Benefits And Harms	• Perioperative prophylaxis with heparin to reduce venous thromboembolism
Unknown Effectiveness	• Graduated elastic compression to prevent venous thromboembolism • Low molecular weight versus unfractionated heparin to reduce venous thromboembolism after hip fracture surgery • Nasogastric feeds for nutritional supplementation after hip fracture • Nerve blocks for pain control before and after hip fracture • Operative-day (less than 24 hours) versus longer-duration multiple-dose antibiotic regimens • Regional versus general anaesthesia for hip fracture surgery

	• Single-dose (long-acting) versus multiple-dose antibiotic regimens
Unlikely To Be Beneficial	• Preoperative traction to the injured limb

What are the effects of rehabilitation interventions and programmes after hip fracture?

Likely To Be Beneficial	• Coordinated multidisciplinary approaches for inpatient rehabilitation of older people
Unknown Effectiveness	• Early supported discharge followed by home-based rehabilitation • Mobilisation strategies applied soon after hip fracture surgery • Systematic multicomponent home-based rehabilitation

Search date January 2007

DEFINITION A hip or proximal femoral fracture refers to any fracture of the femur between the hip joint articular cartilage to a point 5 cm below the distal part of the lesser trochanter. Femoral-head fractures are not included within this definition. Hip fractures are divided into two groups according to their relationship to the capsular attachments of the hip joint. **Intracapsular fractures** occur proximal to the point at which the hip joint capsule attaches to the femur, and can be subdivided into displaced and undisplaced fractures. Undisplaced fractures include impacted or adduction fractures. Displaced intracapsular fractures may be associated with disruption of the blood supply to the head of the femur leading to avascular necrosis. **Extracapsular fractures** occur distal to the hip joint capsule. In the most distal part of the proximal femoral segment (below the lesser trochanter), the term "subtrochanteric" fracture is used. Numerous further subclassifications of intracapsular and extracapsular fractures exist.

INCIDENCE/PREVALENCE Hip fractures may occur at any age, but are most common in older people (here defined as people aged over 65 years). In industrialised societies, the mean age of people with hip fracture is about 80 years, and about 80% are female. In the USA, the lifetime risk of hip fracture after age 50 years is about 17% in white women and 6% in white men. A study in the USA reported that prevalence increases from about 3/100 women aged 65–74 years to 12.6/100 women aged 85 years and above. The age-stratified incidence has also increased in some societies — not only are people living longer, but the incidence of fracture in each age group may have increased. An estimated 1.26 million hip fractures occurred in adults in 1990, with predictions of numbers rising to 7.3–21.3 million by 2050.

AETIOLOGY/RISK FACTORS Hip fractures are usually sustained through a fall from standing height or less. The pattern of incidence is consistent with an increased risk of falling, loss of protective reflex mechanisms, and loss of skeletal strength from osteoporosis. All these increased risks are associated with aging.

PROGNOSIS Reported figures for mortality after a hip fracture in adults vary considerably. One-year mortality figures vary from 12% to 37%, with about 9% of these deaths directly attributed to the hip fracture. After a hip fracture, a 15–25% decline in the ability to perform daily activities is to be expected, and about 10–20% of the survivors will require a change to a more dependent residential status.

Gavin Young

KEY POINTS

- **Involuntary, localised leg cramps are very common and typically affect the calf muscles at night.**

  The causes of leg cramps are unclear, but risk factors include pregnancy, exercise, salt and electrolyte imbalances, disorders affecting peripheral nerves, blood vessels or muscles, renal dialysis, and some drugs.

- **Quinine reduces the frequency of idiopathic leg cramps at night compared with placebo, but we don't know what is the optimal dose or length of treatment.**

  Adding theophylline to quinine may reduce the frequency of nocturnal leg cramps compared with quinine alone.

- **CAUTION: Quinine is a known teratogen and the risks are not outweighed by any potential benefits of its use in pregnancy.**

  We don't know whether analgesics, antiepileptic drugs, magnesium salts, vitamin E, stretching exercises, or compression hosiery reduce leg cramps.

  We don't know whether calcium salts, sodium chloride, or multivitamins and mineral supplements reduce leg cramps in pregnant women.

(i) **Please visit www.clinicalevidence.bmj.com for full text and references**

What are the effects of treatments for idiopathic leg cramps?

Beneficial	• Quinine
Likely To Be Beneficial	• Quinine plus theophylline
Unknown Effectiveness	• Analgesics
	• Antiepileptic drugs
	• Compression hosiery
	• Magnesium salts
	• Stretching exercises
	• Vitamin E

What are the effects of treatments for leg cramps in pregnancy?

Likely To Be Beneficial	• Magnesium salts
Unknown Effectiveness	• Calcium salts
	• Multivitamins and mineral supplements
	• Sodium chloride

Search date January 2006

DEFINITION Leg cramps are involuntary, localised, and usually painful skeletal muscle contractions, which commonly affect calf muscles. Leg cramps typically occur at night and usually last only seconds to minutes. Leg cramps may be idiopathic (of unknown cause) or may be associated with a definable process or condition such as pregnancy, renal dialysis, or venous insufficiency. This review does not currently cover leg cramps associated with renal dialysis or venous insufficiency.

INCIDENCE/PREVALENCE Leg cramps are common and their incidence increases with age. About half of people attending a general medicine clinic have had leg cramps within 1 month of their visit, and over two thirds of people over 50 years of age have experienced leg cramps.

AETIOLOGY/RISK FACTORS Very little is known about the causes of leg cramps. Risk factors include pregnancy, exercise, electrolyte imbalances, salt depletion, renal dialysis, PVD (both venous and arterial), peripheral nerve injury, polyneuropathies, motor neurone disease, muscle diseases, and certain drugs. Other causes of acute calf pain include, for example, trauma, DVT (see thromboembolism review, p 53), and ruptured Baker's cyst.

PROGNOSIS Leg cramps may cause severe pain and sleep disturbance.

Bart Koes and Maurits van Tulder

KEY POINTS

- Low back pain is pain, muscle tension, or stiffness localised below the costal margin and above the inferior gluteal folds, with or without leg pain (sciatica), and is defined as acute when it persists for less than 12 weeks.

  It affects about 70% of people in resource-rich countries at some point in their lives.

  Acute low back pain is usually self-limiting (90% of people recover within 6 weeks), although 2–7% develop chronic pain. It has a high recurrence rate with symptoms recurring, to a lesser degree, in 50–80% of people within a year.

- NSAIDs have been shown to effectively improve symptoms compared with placebo.

  Muscle relaxants may also reduce pain and improve overall clinical assessment, but are associated with some severe adverse effects, including drowsiness, dizziness, and nausea.

  The studies examining the effects of analgesics, such as paracetamol or opioids, were generally too small to detect any clinically important differences.

- We found no studies examining whether epidural injections of steroids were effective in treating people with acute low back pain.

- With regard to non-drug treatments, advice to stay active, be it as a single treatment or in combination with other interventions (such as back schools, a graded activity programme, or behavioural counselling), appears to be the most effective.

  Spinal manipulation (in the short term) also appears to reduce pain, but not functional outcomes, compared with sham treatments.

  We found no sufficient evidence to allow us to judge the effectiveness of acupuncture, back schools, behavioural therapy, or massage in treating people with acute low back pain.

  We found no evidence examining the effectiveness of electromyographic biofeedback, lumbar supports, temperature treatments, traction, or TENS in the treatment of acute low back pain.

  Back exercises do not seem to increase recovery time compared with no treatment, although the studies have been heterogeneous in their definitions of back exercise.

  Bed rest does not seem to improve symptoms any more effectively than other treatments, but does produce a number of adverse effects, including joint stiffness, muscle wasting, loss of bone mineral density, pressure sores, and venous thromboembolism.

(i) **Please visit www.clinicalevidence.bmj.com for full text and references**

What are the effects of oral drug treatments?	
Beneficial	• NSAIDs
Trade-off Between Benefits And Harms	• Muscle relaxants
Unknown Effectiveness	• Analgesics (paracetamol, opioids)

What are the effects of local injections?

Unknown Effectiveness	• Epidural steroid injections

What are the effects of non-drug treatments?

Beneficial	• Advice to stay active
Likely To Be Beneficial	• Multidisciplinary treatment programmes (for subacute low back pain) • Spinal manipulation (in the short term)
Unknown Effectiveness	• Acupuncture • Back schools • Behavioural therapy • Electromyographic biofeedback • Lumbar supports • Massage • Multidisciplinary treatment programmes (for acute low back pain) • Temperature treatments (short-wave diathermy, ultrasound, ice, heat) • Traction • TENS
Unlikely To Be Beneficial	• Back exercises
Likely To Be Ineffective Or Harmful	• Bed rest

Search date November 2004

DEFINITION Low back pain is pain, muscle tension, or stiffness localised below the costal margin and above the inferior gluteal folds, with or without leg pain (sciatica), and is defined as acute when it persists for less than 12 weeks. Non-specific low back pain is low back pain not attributed to a recognisable pathology (such as infection, tumour, osteoporosis, rheumatoid arthritis, fracture, or inflammation). This review excludes acute low back pain with symptoms or signs at presentation that suggest a specific underlying condition. People with sciatica (lumbosacral radicular syndrome) and herniated discs are also excluded. Unless otherwise stated, people included in this review have acute back pain (i.e. of less than 12 weeks' duration). Some included RCTs further subdivided acute low back pain of less than 12 weeks' duration into acute (less than 6 weeks' duration) or subacute (6–12 weeks' duration).

INCIDENCE/PREVALENCE Over 70% of people in resource-rich countries will experience low back pain at some time in their lives. Each year, 15–45% of adults suffer low back pain, and 1/20 (5%) people present to a health care professional with a new episode. Low back pain is most common between the ages of 35–55 years. About 30% of European workers

(continued over)

(from previous page)

reported that their work caused low back pain. Prevalence rates from different countries range from 13% to 44%. About 70% of people with sick leave due to low back pain return to work within 1 week, and 90% return within 2 months. However, the longer the period of sick leave, the less likely return to work becomes. Less than half of people with low back pain who have been off work for 6 months will return to work.

AETIOLOGY/RISK FACTORS Symptoms, pathology, and radiological appearances are poorly correlated. Pain is non-specific in about 85% of people. About 4% of people with low back pain in primary care have compression fractures and about 1% have a tumour. The prevalence of prolapsed intervertebral disc is about 1–3%. Ankylosing spondylitis and spinal infections are less common. Risk factors for the development of back pain include heavy physical work, frequent bending, twisting, lifting, and prolonged static postures. Psychosocial risk factors include anxiety, depression, and mental stress at work.

PROGNOSIS Acute low back pain is usually self-limiting (90% of people recover within 6 weeks), although 2–7% develop chronic pain. Acute low back pain has a high recurrence rate with symptoms recurring, to a lesser degree, in 50–80% of people within a year.

Maurits van Tulder and Bart Koes

KEY POINTS

- Over 70% of people in resource-rich countries develop low back pain at some time, which usually improves within 2 weeks, but up to 7% of affected people develop chronic low back pain.

- Opioid analgesics, with or without paracetamol, and NSAIDs may improve pain and function compared with placebo.

  Antidepressants decrease chronic low back pain compared with placebo in people with or without depression, but their effects on function are unclear.

  Muscle relaxants may improve pain, but studies have given conflicting results.

- CAUTION: Since the last update of this review, a drug safety alert has been issued on increased suicidal behaviour with antidepressants, and on major congenital malformations with paroxetine (www.fda.gov/medwatch).

- We don't know whether epidural steroid injections, or local injections with corticosteroids and local anaesthetic improve chronic low back pain in people without sciatica.

  Facet-joint corticosteroid injections may be no more effective than placebo at reducing pain.

- Exercise improves pain and function compared with other conservative treatments.

  Intensive multidisciplinary treatment programmes improve pain and function compared with usual care, but less-intensive programmes do not seem to be beneficial.

  Acupuncture, back schools, behavioural therapy, and spinal manipulation may all reduce pain in the short term, but we don't know how they compare with other active treatments.

  We don't know whether electromyographic biofeedback, lumbar supports, massage, traction, or TENS improve pain relief.

Please visit www.clinicalevidence.bmj.com for full text and references

What are the effects of oral drug treatments?	
Likely To Be Beneficial	• Analgesics
	• Antidepressants
	• NSAIDs
Trade-off Between Benefits And Harms	• Muscle relaxants

What are the effects of injection therapy?	
Unknown Effectiveness	• Epidural steroid injections
	• Local injections
Likely To Be Ineffective Or Harmful	• Facet-joint injections

What are the effects of non-drug treatments?

Beneficial	• Exercise • Intensive multidisciplinary treatment programmes (evidence of benefit for intensive programmes but none for less-intensive programmes)
Likely To Be Beneficial	• Acupuncture • Back schools • Behavioural therapy • Spinal manipulative therapy
Unknown Effectiveness	• Electromyographic biofeedback • Lumbar supports • Massage • Traction • TENS

Search date November 2004

DEFINITION Low back pain is pain, muscle tension, or stiffness localised below the costal margin and above the inferior gluteal folds, with or without leg pain (sciatica), and is defined as chronic when it persists for 12 weeks or more (see definition of low back pain [acute], p 386). Non-specific low back pain is low back pain not attributed to a recognisable pathology (such as infection, tumour, osteoporosis, rheumatoid arthritis, fracture, or inflammation). This review excludes low back pain with symptoms or signs at presentation that suggest a specific underlying condition. People with sciatica (lumbosacral radicular syndrome) or pain due to herniated discs are also excluded.

INCIDENCE/PREVALENCE Over 70% of people in resource-rich countries will experience low back pain at some time in their lives. Each year, 15–45% of adults suffer low back pain, and 1/20 people present to hospital with a new episode. About 2–7% of people with acute low back pain will go on to become chronic. Low back pain is most common between the ages of 35 and 55 years.

AETIOLOGY/RISK FACTORS Symptoms, pathology, and radiological appearances are poorly correlated. Pain is non-specific in about 85% of people. About 4% of people with low back pain in primary care have compression fractures and about 1% have a tumour. The prevalence of prolapsed intervertebral disc among people with low back pain in primary care is about 1–3%. Ankylosing spondylitis and spinal infections are less common. This review only covers non-specific chronic low back pain. Risk factors for the development of non-specific low back pain include heavy physical work, frequent bending, twisting, lifting, and prolonged static postures. Psychosocial risk factors include anxiety, depression, and mental stress at work. Having a previous history of low back pain and a longer duration of the present episode are significant risk factors for chronicity. A recently published systematic review of prospective cohort studies found that some psychological factors (distress, depressive mood, and somatisation) are associated with an increased risk of chronic low back pain. Individual and workplace factors have also been reported to be associated with the transition to chronic low back pain.

PROGNOSIS Generally, the clinical course of an episode of low back pain seems to be favourable, and most pain will resolve within 2 weeks. Back pain among people in a primary-care setting typically has a recurrent course characterised by variation and change, rather than an acute, self-limiting course. Most people with back pain have experienced a previous episode, and acute attacks often occur as exacerbations of chronic low back pain.

In general, recurrences will occur more frequently and be more severe if people have had frequent or long-lasting low back pain complaints in the past. The course of sick leave because of low back pain is similarly favourable. One study reported that 67% of people with sick leave because of low back pain returned to work within 1 week, and 90% within 2 months. However, the longer the period of sick leave, the less likely the return to work becomes. Less than 50% of people with low back pain who have been off work for 6 months will return to work. After 2 years of work absenteeism, the chance of returning to work is almost zero.

Allan Binder

KEY POINTS

- Uncomplicated neck pain has a postural or mechanical basis and affects about two thirds of people at some stage, especially in middle age.

  Acute neck pain resolves within days or weeks, but becomes chronic in about 10% of people.

  Whiplash injuries follow sudden acceleration-deceleration of the neck such as in road traffic or sporting accidents. Up to 40% of people still report symptoms 15 years after the accident.

- The evidence about the effects of individual interventions for neck pain is often contradictory because of the poor quality of the RCTs, the tendency for interventions to be given in combination, and for RCTs to be conducted in diverse groups. This lack of consistency in study design makes it difficult to isolate which intervention may be of use in which type of neck pain.

- Stretching and strengthening exercise reduces chronic neck pain compared with usual care, either alone or in combination with manipulation, mobilisation, or infrared.

  Manipulation and mobilisation may reduce chronic pain more than usual care or less active exercise. They seem likely to be as effective as each other or exercise, and more effective than PEMF treatment or heat treatment.

- Analgesics, NSAIDs, antidepressants, and muscle relaxants are widely used to treat chronic neck pain, but we don't know whether they are effective.

- We don't know whether traction, PEMF treatment, acupuncture, TENS, heat or cold, biofeedback, spray and stretch, multimodal treatment, patient education, soft collars, or special pillows are better or worse than other treatments at reducing chronic neck pain.

- Early mobilisation and return to normal activity may reduce pain in people with acute whiplash injury more than immobilisation or rest with a collar.

  We don't know whether exercise, PEMF treatment, multimodal treatment, or drug treatment can reduce pain in people with acute whiplash injury.

- We don't know whether percutaneous radiofrequency neurotomy, multimodal treatment, or physical treatment reduce pain in people with chronic whiplash injury.

- We don't know whether surgery, analgesics, NSAIDs, muscle relaxants, or cervical epidural steroid injections reduce pain in people with neck pain plus radiculopathy.

(i) **Please visit www.clinicalevidence.bmj.com for full text and references**

What are the effects of treatments for people with uncomplicated neck pain without severe neurological deficit?	
Likely To Be Beneficial	• Exercise
	• Manipulation
	• Manipulation plus exercise
	• Mobilisation
Unknown Effectiveness	• Acupuncture
	• Biofeedback

- Drug treatments (analgesics, NSAIDs, anti-depressants, muscle relaxants)
- Heat or cold
- Multimodal treatment
- Patient education
- PEMF treatment
- Soft collars and special pillows
- Spray and stretch
- Traction
- TENS

What are the effects of treatments for acute whiplash injury?

Likely To Be Beneficial	• Early mobilisation • Early return to normal activity
Unknown Effectiveness	• Drug treatments (analgesics, NSAIDs, anti-depressant drugs, or muscle relaxants) • Exercise • Multimodal treatment • PEMF treatment

What are the effects of treatments for chronic whiplash injury?

Unknown Effectiveness	• Multimodal treatment • Percutaneous radiofrequency neurotomy • Physical treatments

What are the effects of treatments for neck pain with radiculopathy?

Unknown Effectiveness	• Drug treatments (epidural steroid injections, analgesics, NSAIDs, or muscle relaxants) • Surgery versus conservative treatment

Search date May 2006

DEFINITION In this review, we have differentiated uncomplicated neck pain from whiplash, although many studies, particularly in people with chronic pain (more than 3 months' duration), do not specify which types of people are included. Most studies of acute pain (less than 3 months' duration) are confined to whiplash. Uncomplicated neck pain is defined as pain with a postural or mechanical basis, often called cervical spondylosis. It does not include pain associated with fibromyalgia. Uncomplicated neck pain may include some people with a traumatic basis for their symptoms, but not people for whom pain is specifically stated to have followed sudden acceleration–deceleration injuries to the neck,

(continued over)

(from previous page)

that is, whiplash. Whiplash is commonly seen in road-traffic accidents or sports injuries. It is not accompanied by radiographic abnormalities or clinical signs of nerve root damage. Neck pain often occurs in combination with limited movement and poorly defined neurological symptoms affecting the upper limbs. The pain can be severe and intractable, and can occur with radiculopathy or myelopathy. We have included under radiculopathy those studies involving people with predominantly radicular symptoms arising in the cervical spine.

INCIDENCE/PREVALENCE About two thirds of people will experience neck pain at some time in their lives. Prevalence is highest in middle age. Neck pain accounts for about 15% of hospital-based physiotherapy in the UK, and about 30% of chiropractic referrals in Canada. In the Netherlands, neck pain contributes up to 2% of general practitioner consultations.

AETIOLOGY/RISK FACTORS The aetiology of uncomplicated neck pain is unclear. Most uncomplicated neck pain is associated with poor posture, anxiety and depression, neck strain, occupational injuries, or sporting injuries. With chronic pain, mechanical and degenerative factors (often referred to as cervical spondylosis) are more likely. Some neck pain results from soft-tissue trauma, most typically seen in whiplash injuries. Rarely, disc prolapse and inflammatory, infective, or malignant conditions affect the cervical spine, and present with neck pain with or without neurological features.

PROGNOSIS Neck pain usually resolves within days or weeks but can recur or become chronic. In some industries, neck-related disorders account for as much time off work as low back pain (see review on low back pain [acute], p 386). The proportion of people in whom neck pain becomes chronic depends on the cause, but is thought to be about 10%, similar to low back pain. Neck pain causes severe disability in 5% of affected people. Whiplash injuries are more likely to cause disability than neck pain because of other causes; up to 40% of sufferers reported symptoms even after 15 years' follow-up. Factors associated with a poorer outcome after whiplash are not well defined. The incidence of chronic disability after whiplash varies among countries, although reasons for this variation are unclear.

Peter C Gøtzsche

KEY POINTS

- NSAIDs inhibit the cyclo-oxygenase (COX) enzyme to exert their anti-inflammatory, analgesic, and antipyretic effects.

- No important differences in efficacy have been demonstrated between different NSAIDs in the management of musculoskeletal disorders.

    There seems to be a plateau for effectiveness, with recommended doses close to those required for maximal effectiveness. However, the risk of adverse effects increases with increasing dose, with no plateau.

    NSAIDs that selectively inhibit COX-2 have a reduced risk of causing gastrointestinal ulcers compared with less selective NSAIDs. However, COX-2 inhibitors increase the risk of MI and other cardiovascular events.

    Paracetamol is less effective than NSAIDs at reducing pain in osteoarthritis, but similarly effective for acute musculoskeletal pain.

- Misoprostol reduces serious NSAID-related gastrointestinal complications and symptomatic ulcers compared with placebo, but is itself associated with adverse effects including diarrhoea, abdominal pain, and nausea.

    Proton pump inhibitors and H_2 antagonists have been shown to reduce endoscopic ulcers in people taking NSAIDs, but their clinical benefits are less clear.

    We don't know which treatment is the most effective at reducing gastrointestinal adverse effects from NSAIDs.

- We don't know whether topical NSAIDs are beneficial.

Please visit www.clinicalevidence.bmj.com for full text and references

Are there any important differences between systemic NSAIDs?	
Trade-off Between Benefits And Harms	• Differences in efficacy between NSAIDs
Unlikely To Be Beneficial	• Dose-response relationship of NSAIDs

What are the effects of co-treatments to reduce the risk of gastrointestinal adverse effects of NSAIDs?	
Trade-off Between Benefits And Harms	• Misoprostol in people who cannot avoid NSAIDs
Unknown Effectiveness	• H_2 blockers in people who cannot avoid NSAIDs • Proton pump inhibitors in people who cannot avoid NSAIDs

What are the effects of topical NSAIDs?	
Unknown Effectiveness	• NSAIDs (topical) • Topical versus systemic NSAIDs or alternative analgesics

Search date December 2006

DEFINITION NSAIDs have anti-inflammatory, analgesic, and antipyretic effects, and they inhibit platelet aggregation. This review deals specifically with the use of NSAIDs for the treatment of the symptoms of musculoskeletal conditions. NSAIDs have no documented effect on the course of musculoskeletal diseases. NSAIDs inhibit the enzyme cyclo-oxygenase (COX), which has two known isoforms: COX-1 and COX-2. NSAIDS are often categorised according to their ability to inhibit the individual isoforms, with newer NSAIDs often predominantly inhibiting the COX-2 isoform and older NSAIDs often being less specific inhibitors.

INCIDENCE/PREVALENCE NSAIDs are widely used. Almost 10% of people in The Netherlands used a non-aspirin NSAID in 1987, and the overall use was 11 defined daily doses per 1000 population per day. In Australia in 1994, overall use was 35 defined daily doses per 1000 population a day, with 36% of the people receiving NSAIDs for osteoarthritis, 42% for sprain and strain or low back pain, and 4% for rheumatoid arthritis; 35% of the people receiving NSAIDs were aged over 60 years.

Jiri Chard, Claire Smith, Stefan Lohmander and David Scott

KEY POINTS

- The hip is the second most common large joint to be affected with osteoarthritis, affecting about 5% of people aged over 60 years, although few will need surgery.

  Osteoarthritis is characterised by focal areas of damage to the cartilage surface of the bone, with remodelling of the underlying bone and mild synovitis, leading to pain, bony tenderness, and crepitus.

  Osteoarthritis of the hip seems to be more likely in people who are obese, who participate in sporting activities such as running, or who have occupations requiring a heavy physical workload, such as farming or lifting heavy loads.

- Oral NSAIDs and COX-2 inhibitors reduce short-term pain in people with osteoarthritis of the hip compared with placebo.

  Long-term benefits of NSAIDs are not known, and they increase the risk of serious gastrointestinal adverse effects including haemorrhage.

  Paracetamol may be less effective than NSAIDs, although we do not know this for sure. It is less likely than NSAIDs to cause gastrointestinal damage.

  Combined NSAIDs plus paracetamol may be more effective than NSAIDs alone.

- Chondroitin may reduce pain and improve function in people with osteoarthritis of the hip, but glucosamine may not be effective in improving pain and function. However, few studies have been performed on these treatments.

  The benefits of opioid analgesics, acupuncture, education to aid self-management, exercise, and physical aids remain unclear.

- Total hip replacement is an effective treatment for osteoarthritis of the hip, although we don't know which individuals are likely to respond.

  We don't know whether osteotomy is beneficial in reducing pain.

(i) **Please visit www.clinicalevidence.bmj.com for full text and references**

What are the effects of non-drug treatments for osteoarthritis of the hip?	
Unknown Effectiveness	• Acupuncture
	• Education to aid self-management
	• Exercise
	• Physical aids

What are the effects of drug treatments for osteoarthritis of the hip?	
Trade-off Between Benefits And Harms	• Oral NSAIDs (including COX-2 inhibitors)
Unknown Effectiveness	• Capsaicin
	• Chondroitin
	• Glucosamine
	• Opioid analgesics

- Oral NSAIDs plus simple oral or opioid analgesics
- Simple oral analgesics (versus placebo — less effective versus NSAIDs)

What are the effects of surgical treatments for osteoarthritis of the hip?

Beneficial	• Hip replacement
Unknown Effectiveness	• Osteotomy

Search date November 2005

DEFINITION Osteoarthritis is a heterogeneous condition for which the prevalence, risk factors, clinical manifestations, and prognosis vary according to the joints affected. It most commonly affects knees, hips, hands, and spinal apophyseal joints. It is characterised by focal areas of damage to the cartilage surfaces of synovial joints, and is associated with remodelling of the underlying bone and mild synovitis. It is variously defined by a number of clinical or radiological features, or both. Clinical features include pain, bony tenderness, and crepitus. When severe, there is often characteristic joint-space narrowing and osteophyte formation, with visible subchondral bone changes on radiography. The hip is the second most common large joint to be affected by osteoarthritis. It is associated with significant pain, disability, and impaired quality of life.

INCIDENCE/PREVALENCE Osteoarthritis is a common and important cause of pain and disability in older adults. Radiographic features are practically universal in at least some joints in people aged over 60 years, but significant clinical disease probably affects 10–20% of people. Hip disease is not as prevalent as knee disease in people aged over 60 years (about 5% v 10%). The actual impact that osteoarthritis has on an individual person is the result of a combination of physical (including comorbidities), psychological, cultural, and social factors, and this may influence outcomes found in research — for example, if comorbidities are not accounted for in analysis.

AETIOLOGY/RISK FACTORS There is moderate evidence for a positive association between osteoarthritis of the hip and obesity; participation in sporting activities, including running; and vocational activity, particularly involving a heavy physical workload, as characterised by farming (especially for more than 10 years) or lifting heavy loads (25 kg or more). Only limited evidence exists for a positive association between the occurrence of osteoarthritis of the hip and participation in athletics or presence of hip dysplasia in older persons.

PROGNOSIS The natural history of osteoarthritis of the hip is poorly understood. Only a minority of people with clinical disease of the hip will progress to requiring surgery.

David Scott and Anna Kowalczyk

KEY POINTS

- Osteoarthritis of the knee affects about 10% of adults aged over 60 years, with increased risk in those with obesity, and joint damage or abnormalities.

  Progression of disease on x rays is commonplace, but x ray changes don't correlate well with clinical symptoms.

  We don't know the long-term effectiveness of any non-surgical treatment in reducing pain and improving function.

- Exercise and physiotherapy, and joint bracing or taping reduce pain and disability in people with knee osteoarthritis, but we don't know whether patient education or insoles are beneficial.

- Oral and topical NSAIDs reduce pain in the short term compared with placebo, but can cause gastrointestinal, renal, and cardiac adverse effects.

  Paracetamol reduces pain in the short term compared with placebo, but may be less effective than NSAIDs.

  Opioid analgesics reduce pain in knee osteoarthritis, but they are associated with serious adverse effects, so are not recommended for first-line treatment.

- Intra-articular corticosteroids and intra-articular hyaluronan may improve pain, although most studies are of poor quality.

  We don't know whether acupuncture, capsaicin, glucosamine, or oral or intramuscular chondroitin improve symptoms in knee osteoarthritis.

- Consensus is that total knee replacement is the most clinically effective treatment for severe osteoarthritis of the knee.

  Unicompartmental knee replacement may be more effective than tricompartmental knee replacement in the long term.

  Tibial osteotomy may be as effective as unicompartmental knee replacement in reducing symptoms of medial compartment knee osteoarthritis.

(i) **Please visit www.clinicalevidence.bmj.com for full text and references**

What are the effects of non-surgical treatments for osteoarthritis of the knee?

Beneficial	• Exercise and physiotherapy (pain relief and improved function) • NSAIDs (oral) for short-term pain relief
Likely To Be Beneficial	• Corticosteroids (intra-articular — short-term pain relief) • Hyaluronan (intra-articular) • Joint bracing • NSAIDs (topical) for short-term pain relief • Simple oral analgesics (short-term pain relief only) • Taping
Trade-off Between Benefits And Harms	• Opioid analgesics
Unknown Effectiveness	• Acupuncture • Capsaicin

- Chondroitin
- Education (to aid self-management)
- Glucosamine
- Insoles

What are the effects of surgical treatments for osteoarthritis of the knee?

| Likely To Be Beneficial | • Knee replacement |
| | • Osteotomy |

Search date October 2006

DEFINITION Osteoarthritis is a heterogeneous condition for which the prevalence, risk factors, clinical manifestations, and prognosis vary according to the joints affected. It most commonly affects knees, hips, hands, and spinal apophyseal joints. It is characterised by focal areas of damage to the cartilage surfaces of synovial joints, and is associated with remodelling of the underlying bone, and mild synovitis. It is variously defined by a number of clinical or radiological features, or both. Clinical features include pain, bony tenderness, and crepitus. When severe, there is often characteristic joint-space narrowing and osteophyte formation, with visible subchondral bone changes on radiography. Osteoarthritis of the knee is common, causes considerable pain and frequent instability, and, consequently, often results in physical disability. x Ray changes are not strongly associated with disability.

INCIDENCE/PREVALENCE Osteoarthritis is a common and important cause of pain and disability in older adults. Radiographical features are practically universal in people aged over 60 years in at least some joints, but significant clinical disease probably affects 10–20% of people. Knee disease is about twice as prevalent as hip disease in people aged over 60 years (about 10% knee v 5% hip). In a general practice setting. 1% of people aged over 45 years have a currently-recorded clinical diagnosis of knee osteoarthritis; 5% will have had the clinical diagnosis made at some point. A community-based cohort study showed that radiological features of knee osteoarthritis were very common: 13% of women aged 45–65 years developed new knee osteophytes — an incidence of 3% per year.

AETIOLOGY/RISK FACTORS Risk factors for osteoarthritis include abnormalities in joint shape, injury, and previous joint inflammation. Obesity is a major risk factor for osteoarthritis of the knee. Genetic factors modulate obesity and other risks.

PROGNOSIS The natural history of osteoarthritis of the knee is poorly understood. Radiological progression is commonplace, with 25% of osteoarthritic knees with initially normal joint space showing major damage after 10 years, although x ray progression is not related to clinical features. People with peripheral-joint osteoarthritis of sufficient severity to lead to hospital referral generally have bad outcomes, with high levels of physical disability, anxiety, and depression; they also have high levels of healthcare resources utilisation, including joint replacement, drugs, and walking aids.

Karl B Landorf and Hylton B Menz

KEY POINTS

- Plantar heel pain causes soreness or tenderness of the sole of the foot under the heel, which sometimes extends into the medial arch.

    The prevalence and prognosis are unclear, but in most people the symptoms seem to resolve over time.

- Casted orthoses (custom-made insoles) may improve function (but not pain) at 3 months in people with plantar heel pain compared with a sham orthosis, but they may be no better than appropriate prefabricated orthoses.

- Supportive taping may improve pain in the short term at 1 week, but we found no evidence on its effectiveness beyond 1 week.

- We don't know whether heel pads, heel cups, or night splints reduce pain.

- Corticosteroid injections are commonly used to treat plantar heel pain, but we don't know whether they reduce pain compared with placebo or other treatments.

    Corticosteroid injections have been associated with long-term complications.

    We don't know whether local anaesthetic injections, alone or added to corticosteroids, improve pain relief compared with corticosteroids alone.

- Extracorporeal shock-wave therapy may reduce pain, but we don't know for sure that it is beneficial.

- We don't know whether laser treatment, ultrasound, or surgery reduce symptoms compared with sham treatment or no treatment.

- We don't know whether stretching exercises reduce pain compared with no treatment or other treatments.

Please visit www.clinicalevidence.bmj.com for full text and references

What are the effects of treatments for plantar heel pain?	
Likely To Be Beneficial	• Casted orthoses (custom-made insoles) (improved function [but not pain] at 3 months compared with sham orthosis, but no difference between casted [custom] orthosis and prefabricated orthosis at 3 months)
	• Taping (limited evidence of reduced pain at 1 week; no evidence beyond 1 week)
Unknown Effectiveness	• Corticosteroid injection (in the short term)
	• Corticosteroid injection plus local anaesthetic injection in the short term (with or without NSAIDs or heel pads)
	• Extracorporeal shock-wave therapy (ESWT)
	• Heel pads and heel cups
	• Lasers
	• Local anaesthetic injection
	• Night splints plus NSAIDs
	• Stretching exercises

	• Surgery
	• Ultrasound
Likely To Be Ineffective Or Harmful	• Corticosteroid injection in the medium to long term (with or without heel pad)
	• Corticosteroid injection plus local anaesthetic injection in the medium to long term (with or without NSAIDs or heel pads)

Search date January 2007

DEFINITION Plantar heel pain is soreness or tenderness of the heel that is restricted to the sole of the foot. It often radiates from the central part of the heel pad or the medial tubercle of the calcaneum, but may extend along the plantar fascia into the medial longitudinal arch of the foot. Severity may range from an irritation at the origin of the plantar fascia, which is noticeable on rising after rest, to an incapacitating pain. This review excludes clinically evident underlying disorders; for example, calcaneal fracture, and calcaneal-nerve entrapment, which may be distinguished clinically — a calcaneal fracture may present after trauma, and calcaneal nerve entrapment gives rise to shooting pains and feelings of "pins and needles" on the medial aspect of the heel.

INCIDENCE/PREVALENCE The incidence and prevalence of plantar heel pain are uncertain. However, it has been estimated that 7% of people aged over 65 years report tenderness in the region of the heel, that plantar heel pain accounts for a quarter of all foot injuries relating to running, and that the diagnosis and treatment of plantar heel pain accounts for over 1 million visits a year to physicians in the USA. The condition affects both athletic and sedentary people, and does not seem to be influenced by gender.

AETIOLOGY/RISK FACTORS Unknown. Suggested risk factors include overweight, prolonged standing, and having a reduced range of motion in the ankle and 1st metatarsophalangeal joint.

PROGNOSIS One systematic review found that almost all of the included trials reported an improvement in discomfort regardless of the intervention received (including placebo), suggesting that the condition is at least partially self-limiting. A telephone survey of 100 people treated conservatively (average follow-up 47 months) found that 82 people had resolution of symptoms, 15 had continued symptoms but no limitations of activity or work, and three had persistent bilateral symptoms that limited activity or changed work status. Thirty-one people said that they would have seriously considered surgical treatment at the time that medical attention was sought. In addition, one recent RCT has observed marked improvement in pain and function over time in 45 people randomised to a sham intervention.

Janet Pope

KEY POINTS

- Raynaud's phenomenon is episodic vasospasm of the peripheral arteries, causing pallor followed by cyanosis and redness with pain and sometimes paraesthesia. On rare occasions it can lead to ulceration of the fingers and toes (and in some cases of the ears or nose).

  Prevalence varies by sex and country, affecting around 3–5% of people in most population studies, and is slightly more common in women than in men.

  Attacks may last from several minutes to a few hours, and long-term sufferers can go on to display features of underlying disorders, such as scleroderma.

- Nifedipine seems to reduce the frequency and severity of Raynaud's attacks, although it is associated with high rates of adverse effects, such as tachycardia, headache, and flushing.

  We found no evidence of sufficient quality to judge the effectiveness of amlodipine, diltiazem, or moxisylyte in treating Raynaud's phenomenon.

- Other drug treatments, such as nicardipine, naftidrofuryl oxalate, inositol nicotinate, and prazosin may successfully treat Raynaud's phenomenon, but the studies have all been too small for us to draw conclusions.

- We found no evidence examining the efficacy of lifestyle changes, such as keeping warm, smoking cessation, and exercise, in treating and preventing Raynaud's phenomenon.

(i) **Please visit www.clinicalevidence.bmj.com for full text and references**

What are the effects of treatments for primary Raynaud's phenomenon?	
Trade-off Between Benefits And Harms	• Nifedipine
Unknown Effectiveness	• Amlodipine • Diltiazem • Exercise • Inositol nicotinate • Keeping warm • Moxisylyte (thymoxamine) • Naftidrofuryl oxalate • Nicardipine • Prazosin • Smoking cessation

Search date October 2006

DEFINITION Raynaud's phenomenon is episodic vasospasm of the peripheral arteries, causing pallor followed by cyanosis or erythema, or both, which can cause pain and sometimes paraesthesia, and, rarely, ulceration of the fingers and toes (and in some cases of the ears or nose). Primary or idiopathic Raynaud's phenomenon (Raynaud's disease)

(continued over)

(from previous page)

occurs without an underlying disease. Secondary Raynaud's phenomenon (Raynaud's syndrome) occurs in association with an underlying disease — usually connective tissue disorders, such as scleroderma, systemic lupus erythematosus, rheumatoid arthritis, Sjogren's syndrome, or polymyositis. This review excludes secondary Raynaud's phenomenon. **Diagnosis:** The diagnosis of Raynauds phenomenon is by a history of clearly demarcated pallor of digit(s), followed by at least one other colour change (cyanosis, erythema), which is usually precipitated by cold. A good history, physical examination, and laboratory results can help rule out secondary Raynaud's phenomenon. Review of symptoms or signs for connective tissue disease should be done. Laboratory testing may include CBC, ESR, and ANA with pattern, if connective tissue diseases are suspected. Magnification of the nailbeds to observe abnormal capillaries is also important in order to rule out Raynaud's phenomenon associated with connective tissue diseases.

INCIDENCE/PREVALENCE The prevalence of primary Raynaud's phenomenon varies by sex, country, and exposure to workplace vibration. One large US cohort study (4182 people) found symptoms in 9.6% of women and 8.1% of men, of whom 81% had primary Raynaud's phenomenon. Smaller cohort studies in Spain have estimated the prevalence of Raynaud's phenomenon to be 3.7–4.0%, of which 90% is primary Raynaud's phenomenon. One study in Japan (332 men, 731 women) found symptoms of primary Raynaud's phenomenon in 3.4% of women and 3.0% of men. A study of 12,907 people in Great Britain reported that 4.6% of people had demarcated finger blanching with cold exposure.

AETIOLOGY/RISK FACTORS The cause of primary Raynaud's phenomenon is unknown. There is evidence for genetic predisposition, usually in those people with early onset Raynaud's phenomenon (aged under 40 years). One prospective observational study (424 people with Raynaud's phenomenon) found that 73% of sufferers first developed symptoms before the age of 40 years. Women are more at risk than men (OR 3.0, 95% CI 1.2 to 7.8, in 1 US case control study [235 people]). The other known risk factor is occupational exposure to vibration from tools (symptoms developed in about 8% with exposure v 2.7% with no exposure in 2 cohorts from Japan). People who are obese may be less at risk. Symptoms are often worsened by cold, or by heightened emotion. Rarely, primary Raynaud's phenomenon may progress to secondary. This most commonly occurs in people with auto-antibodies (e.g. anti-nuclear antibodies), increased ESR, or abnormal nailbed capillaries, or both, and occurs at a rate of 2% for suspected secondary Raynaud's phenomenon and 1% for secondary Raynaud's phenomenon annually.

PROGNOSIS Attacks may last from several minutes to a few hours. One systematic review (search date 1996, 10 prospective observational studies, 639 people with primary Raynaud's phenomenon) found that 13% of long-term sufferers later manifested an underlying disorder such as scleroderma. Complications such as digital ulcers are extremely rare in primary Raynaud's phenomenon.

Karen Walker-Bone and Sarah Fallow

KEY POINTS

- Rheumatoid arthritis is a chronic inflammatory disorder that mainly affects the peripheral joints and surrounding tissue.

  It usually starts as a symmetrical polyarthritis, and its course is marked by flares and remissions.

  The aims of treatment are to relieve pain and swelling, and to improve function. In addition, DMARDs may reduce disease progression.

- The DMARD methotrexate is widely used as first-line treatment in people with rheumatoid arthritis because of consensus about its effectiveness in practice.

  Sulfasalazine and combined treatment with methotrexate and sulfasalazine are as effective as methotrexate in improving pain, joint swelling, and function in people with early rheumatoid arthritis who have not previously received DMARDs.

  Antimalarials may improve symptoms and function in DMARD-naïve people, and are reasonably well tolerated, but radiological evidence of erosion is more marked with antimalarials than with sulfasalazine.

- There is a variety of DMARDs available for second-line treatment of rheumatoid arthritis, and we found no clear evidence that one is superior.

  Methotrexate, sulfasalazine, penicillamine, and leflunomide cause similar improvements in symptoms and function when given to people as second-line DMARD treatment, although methotrexate causes fewer adverse effects.

  The combination of methotrexate plus sulfasalazine plus hydroxychloroquine is more effective in reducing measures of disease activity in people receiving second-line treatment than any of the drugs used alone. Adding the cytokine inhibitors infliximab or etanercept to methotrexate is more effective than using methotrexate alone.

  Although antimalarials and oral gold seem to improve clinical disease activity when given as second-line treatment, they are not as effective as methotrexate or sulfasalazine. Although parenteral gold is more effective than oral gold, it leads to higher levels of toxicity than most of the other commonly used DMARDs.

  Ciclosporin offers short-term control of rheumatoid arthritis when used as second-line treatment, but is associated with nephrotoxicity.

  We don't know whether cyclophosphamide is as effective as other DMARDs for second-line treatment.

  Cytokine inhibitors may offer an alternative to traditional DMARDs for second-line treatment of rheumatoid arthritis, but more research is needed.

  Etanercept may be as effective as methotrexate in improving symptoms, function, and radiological evidence of progression, but more evidence for its effect is needed.

  Azathioprine is less effective and not as well tolerated as methotrexate.

  We don't know whether anakinra or adalimumab are as effective as other DMARDs for second-line treatment.

  Although widely used for the initial short-term relief of clinical disease activity in rheumatoid arthritis, we don't know how corticosteroids compare with other drugs for first- or second-line treatment.

Please visit www.clinicalevidence.bmj.com for full text and references

What are the effects of drug treatments in people with rheumatoid arthritis who have not previously received any disease-modifying antirheumatic drug treatment?

Beneficial	• Methotrexate (first-line treatment) • Sulfasalazine (first-line treatment)
Likely To Be Beneficial	• Antimalarial drugs (first-line treatment)
Unknown Effectiveness	• Corticosteroids (first-line treatment)

How do different drug treatments compare in people with rheumatoid arthritis who have either not responded or are intolerant of first-line disease-modifying antirheumatic drugs?

Beneficial	• Infliximab plus methotrexate (second-line treatment) • Leflunomide (second-line treatment) • Methotrexate (second-line treatment) • Methotrexate plus sulfasalazine plus hydroxychloroquine (second-line treatment) • Penicillamine (second-line treatment) • Sulfasalazine (second-line treatment)
Likely To Be Beneficial	• Antimalarial drugs (second-line treatment) • Azathioprine (second-line treatment) • Ciclosporin (second-line treatment) • Etanercept (second-line treatment) • Gold (oral) (second-line treatment)
Trade-off Between Benefits And Harms	• Gold (parenteral) (second-line treatment)
Unknown Effectiveness	• Adalimumab (second-line treatment) • Anakinra (second-line treatment) • Corticosteroids (second-line treatment) • Cyclophosphamide (second-line treatment)

Search date June 2005

DEFINITION Rheumatoid arthritis is a chronic inflammatory disorder. It is characterised by chronic pain and swelling that primarily affects the peripheral joints and related periarticular tissues. It usually starts as an insidious symmetrical polyarthritis, often with non-specific symptoms such as malaise and fatigue.

INCIDENCE/PREVALENCE Studies from the USA have suggested age-adjusted incidence rates of between 0.7 and 0.4 per 1000 person-years at risk, but data from European studies suggest a slightly lower incidence rate (0.25/1000 person-years). With the exception of some Native-American populations where incidence is higher, there is marked consistency in the prevalence of rheumatoid arthritis worldwide. All studies suggest a female incidence rate between two and three times higher than the male rate, and that incidence rates increase progressively with age.

AETIOLOGY/RISK FACTORS The cause of rheumatoid arthritis is, as yet, unknown. Genetic factors, hormonal influences, obesity, diet, and cigarette smoking have all been implicated as risk factors. The most widely accepted cause of rheumatoid arthritis is an infection with a micro-organism in a genetically susceptible host.

PROGNOSIS Rheumatoid arthritis is a chronic condition. In most cases, it follows a course of relapses and remissions (polycyclic pattern). Relapses ("flares") are associated with generalised pain, swelling, and stiffness, which may affect most joints simultaneously. People with rheumatoid arthritis have reduced life expectancy compared with healthy controls, as shown by a longitudinal cohort study undertaken in the UK including 1010 people with rheumatoid arthritis (standardised all-cause mortality among men: 1.45, 95% CI 1.22 to 1.71; standardised all-cause mortality among women: 1.84, 95% CI 1.64 to 2.05). People with rheumatoid arthritis also have excess CVD mortality (standardised cardiovascular mortality among men: 1.36, 95% CI 1.04 to 1.75; standardised cardiovascular mortality among women: 1.93, 95% CI 1.65 to 2.26).

Shoulder pain

Cathy Speed

KEY POINTS

- Shoulder pain covers a wide range of problems and affects up to 20% of the population. It is not a specific diagnosis.

  Shoulder pain can be caused by problems with the acromioclavicular joint, shoulder muscles, or referred pain from the neck.

- Rotator cuff problems account for 65–70% of cases of shoulder pain.

  Rotator cuff disorders are associated with musculoskeletal problems that affect the joints and muscles of the shoulder, cuff degeneration due to ageing and ischaemia, and overloading of the shoulder.

- Adhesive capsulitis (frozen shoulder) accounts for 2% of cases of shoulder pain.

  Risk factors for frozen shoulder include female sex, older age, shoulder trauma and surgery, diabetes, and cardiovascular, cerebrovascular, and thyroid disease.

- In many people, the cornerstone of treatment is achieving pain control to allow appropriate physiotherapy to proceed. In people with acute post-traumatic tear, an early surgical option is warranted.

- We don't know whether oral or topical NSAIDs, oral paracetamol, opioid analgesics or transdermal glyceryl trinitrate improve shoulder pain. If pain control fails, the diagnosis should be reviewed and other interventions considered.

- Physiotherapy improves pain and function in people with mixed shoulder disorders compared with placebo or sham laser treatment.

  Physiotherapy seems to be of similar efficacy to intra-articular or sub-acromial corticosteroid injections or surgical arthroscopic decompression over 6–12 months.

- Intra-articular injections may be beneficial, but only if accurately sited.

  Intra-articular corticosteroid injections may reduce pain in the short term compared with physiotherapy, but their benefit compared with placebo or local anaesthetic is unclear.

  Clinical outcome correlates with accuracy of injection, but even experienced clinicians may fail to locate the correct site in the majority of cases.

- Suprascapular nerve blocks improve pain at 1 month in people with adhesive capsulitis and degenerative disease, but we don't know whether it improves shoulder pain from other causes.

- Extracorporeal shock-wave therapy may improve pain in calcific tendonitis, and manipulation under anaesthesia may reduce symptoms of adhesive capsulitis, but neither intervention is beneficial in rotator cuff lesions.

(i) **Please visit www.clinicalevidence.bmj.com for full text and references**

What are the effects of oral drug treatment?	
Likely To Be Beneficial	• Oral NSAIDs (reduce pain in people with acute tendonitis or subacromial bursistis, or both)
Unknown Effectiveness	• Corticosteroids (oral) • Opioid analgesics • Paracetamol

What are the effects of topical drug treatment

Unknown Effectiveness	• NSAIDs (topical) • Phonophoresis • Transdermal glyceryl trinitrate

What are the effects of local injections?

Likely To Be Beneficial	• Nerve block
Unknown Effectiveness	• Intra-articular corticosteroid injections • Intra-articular guanethidine • Intra-articular NSAID injections • Subacromial corticosteroid injections

What are the effects of non-drug treatment

Likely To Be Beneficial	• Extracorporeal shock wave therapy (in people with calcific tendinitis) • Laser treatment • Physiotherapy (manual treatment, exercises)
Unknown Effectiveness	• Electrical stimulation • Ice • Multidisciplinary biopsychosocial rehabilitation • Ultrasound

What are the effects of surgical treatment?

Likely To Be Beneficial	• Manipulation under anaesthesia plus intra-articular injection in people with frozen shoulder • Surgical arthroscopic decompression
Unknown Effectiveness	• Arthroscopic laser subacromial decompression

Search date February 2006

DEFINITION Shoulder pain arises in or around the shoulder from its joints and surrounding soft tissues. Joints include the glenohumeral, acromioclavicular, sternoclavicular, "subacromial", and scapulothoracic. Regardless of the disorder, pain is the most common reason for consulting a practitioner. In adhesive capsulitis (frozen shoulder), pain is associated with pronounced restriction of movement. Rotator cuff disorders may affect one or more portions of the rotator cuff and can be further defined as rotator cuff tear (partial/full thickness), non-calcific tendinosis (previously termed tendinitis), or calcific tendinitis. A subacromial/subdeltoid bursitis may be associated with any of these disorders, or may occur in isolation. For most shoulder disorders, diagnosis is based on clinical features, with

(continued over)

(from previous page)

imaging studies playing a role in some people. Post-stroke shoulder pain and pain referred from the cervical spine are not addressed in this review.

INCIDENCE/PREVALENCE Each year in primary care in the UK, about 1% of adults aged over 45 years present with a new episode of shoulder pain. Prevalence is uncertain, with estimates from 4–20%. One community survey (392 people) in the UK found a 1-month prevalence of shoulder pain of 34%. A second survey (644 people aged 70 years or over) in a communiy-based rheumatology clinic in the UK reported a point prevalence of 21%, with a higher frequency in women than men (25% v 17%). Seventy per cent of cases involved the rotator cuff. Further analysis of 134 people included in the survey found that 65% of cases were rotator cuff lesions; 11% were caused by localised tenderness in the pericapsular musculature; 10% involved acromioclavicular-joint pain; 3% involved glenohumeral-joint arthritis; and 5% were referred pain from the neck. Another survey in Sweden found that, in adults, the annual incidence of frozen shoulder was about 2%, with those aged 40–70 years most commonly affected. The age distribution of specific shoulder disorders in the community is unknown.

AETIOLOGY/RISK FACTORS Rotator cuff disorders are associated with excessive overloading, instability of the glenohumeral and acromioclavicular joints, muscle imbalance, adverse anatomical features (narrow coracoacromial arch and a hooked acromion), cuff degeneration with ageing, ischaemia, and musculoskeletal diseases that result in wasting of the cuff muscles. Risk factors for adhesive capsulitis (frozen shoulder) include female sex, older age, shoulder trauma, surgery, diabetes, cardiorespiratory disorders, cerebrovascular events, thyroid disease, and hemiplegia. Arthritis of the glenohumeral joint can occur in numerous forms, including primary and secondary osteoarthritis, rheumatoid arthritis, and crystal arthritides. Shoulder pain can also be referred from other sites, in particular the cervical spine. It can also arise after stroke. Post-stroke shoulder pain and referred pain are not addressed in this review.

PROGNOSIS One survey in an elderly community found that most people with shoulder pain were still affected 3 years after the initial survey. One prospective cohort study of 122 adults in primary care found that 25% of people with shoulder pain reported previous episodes and 49% reported full recovery at 18 months' follow-up.

Rajan Madhok and Olivia Wu

KEY POINTS

- Systemic lupus erythematosus (SLE) is a chronic, multisystem, inflammatory connective tissue disorder of unknown cause that can involve joints, kidneys, serous surfaces, skin, and vessel walls. It occurs predominantly in young women, but also in children. The course of SLE is highly variable, involving non-organ-threatening symptoms such as arthritis, arthralgia, and rashes, organ-threatening symptoms, such as lupus nephritis, and neuropsychiatric disorders, such as seizures and cognitive dysfunction.

  The prevalence of SLE varies widely worldwide, ranging from about 1 in 3500 women (regardless of race) in the UK, to 1 in 1000 women in China, to 1 in 250 black women in the USA.

- There is consensus that NSAIDs and corticosteroids are useful in relieving pain caused by arthralgia/arthritis, and pleuritis and pericarditis associated with SLE. We found no evidence that the well-documented adverse effects of NSAIDS differ in people with SLE.

  There is also consensus that corticosteroids and sunscreens are effective in reducing cutaneous manifestations of SLE.

- Hydroxychloroquine or chloroquine are likely to be effective in reducing arthritis, pleuritis, and pericarditis. They may also improve cutaneous symptoms.

  Methotrexate may also be effective for both joint and cutaneous symptoms, but are associated with adverse effects.

- Combining immunosuppressants plus corticosteroids may be more effective than corticosteroids alone in people with lupus nephritis, but with an increase in adverse effects.

  We don't know how corticosteroids alone compare with immunosuppressants alone in people with proliferative lupus nephritis.

- We don't know if corticosteroids, immunosuppressants, plasmapheresis, or intravenous immunoglobulin are effective in people with neuropsychiatric symptoms of lupus.

  Most people with neuropsychiatric lupus and psychotic symptoms will be offered antipsychotic drugs to control symptoms unless there are contraindications, despite the lack of RCTs assessing their effectiveness.

(i) **Please visit www.clinicalevidence.bmj.com for full text and references**

What are the effects of treatments on joint (arthralgia/arthritis) symptoms and other non-organ-threatening symptoms, such as serositis and fatigue, in people with systemic lupus erythematosus?	
Likely To Be Beneficial	• Hydroxychloroquine or chloroquine
Trade-off Between Benefits And Harms	• Corticosteroids (oral)* • Methotrexate • NSAIDs*

What are the effects of interventions for cutaneous involvement in people with systemic lupus erythematosus?

Likely To Be Beneficial	• Hydroxychloroquine or chloroquine • Sun block*
Trade-off Between Benefits And Harms	• Corticosteroids* • Methotrexate
Unknown Effectiveness	• Acitretin

What are the effects of treatments in people with proliferative (WHO grades 3–5) lupus nephritis?

Trade-off Between Benefits And Harms	• Combination corticosteroids plus immunosuppressants (may be more effective than corticosteroids alone but increase adverse effects)
Unknown Effectiveness	• Corticosteroids (unclear how they compare with immunosuppressants)

What are the effects of treatments for neuropsychiatric involvement in people with systemic lupus nephritis?

Unknown Effectiveness	• Antipsychotic drugs • Corticosteroids (unclear how they compare with immunosuppressants) • Intravenous immunoglobulin • Plasmapheresis

Search date April 2006

*Based on consensus; RCTs unlikely to be conducted.

DEFINITION Systemic lupus erythematosus (SLE) is a chronic, multisystem, inflammatory connective tissue disorder of unknown cause that can involve joints, kidneys, serous surfaces, and vessel walls. It occurs predominantly in young women, but also in children. The course of SLE is highly variable, and may be characterised by exacerbations. **Non-organ-threatening symptoms** occur in most people with SLE during the course of active disease. These include: arthritis or arthralgia (84%), oral ulcers (24%), fever (52%), and serositis (pleuritis or pericarditis; 36%). **Lupus glomerulonephritis (lupus nephritis)** is the diagnosis applied to people with renal inflammation occurring in the context of SLE. It occurs in 39% of people. The WHO graded the disease in 1982, based on histological features, as follows: grade 1 = normal kidney or minor abnormalities, grade 2 = mesangial proliferation, grade 3 = focal proliferative glomerulonephritis, grade 4 = diffuse proliferative glomerulonephritis, grade 5 = membranous disease, and grade 6 = sclerosing glomerulonephritis. This review covers treatments of WHO grade 3–5. **Cutaneous involvement** may include malar rash (which occurs in 58% of people), photosensitivity (45%), discoid rash (10%), livedo reticularis (14%), and subacute cutaneous lesions (6%). **Neuropsychiatric involvement** occurs in 27% of people and has a wide variety of clinical presentations, including seizures, chronic headache, transverse myelitis, vascular brain disease, psychosis, and neural cognitive dysfunction. SLE is also characterised by haematological features, such as haemolytic anaemia (8%), thrombocytopenia (22%), and lymphadenopathy (12%), and cardiovascular complications such as thrombosis (14%) and Raynaud's phenomenon (34%). Prevention and treatment of haematological and cardiovascular complications is not currently covered by this review. **Diagnosis:** The American College of Rheumatology (ACR) has developed classification criteria for SLE. For a diagnosis to be made, four of the 11 criteria must be met: malar rash, discoid rash, photosensitivity, oral ulcers, arthritis, serositis, renal disorder, neuropsychiatric disorder, haematologic disorder, immunologic disorder, and antinuclear antibody.

INCIDENCE/PREVALENCE The prevalence of SLE worldwide varies greatly. From population based epidemiological studies, it has been estimated that 1 in 3450 women (independent of race) in the UK, 1 in 250 black women in the USA, 1 in 1000 Chinese women, and 1 in 4200 white women in New Zealand may have SLE. Although the prevalence of SLE is higher in black people than in white people in the USA and UK, the prevalence of lupus is low in most African countries.

AETIOLOGY/RISK FACTORS Although the exact cause of SLE remains unclear, genetic, environmental, and hormonal influences are all thought to play a role.

PROGNOSIS The manifestations of SLE that determine survival include lupus nephritis, cardiovascular complications, and neuropsychiatric involvement. In cohort studies performed since 1980, survival at 5 years has exceeded 90%, a higher survival rate than in studies performed earlier than 1980. One multicentre study performed in Europe found a survival probability of 92% at 10 years after diagnosis. A lower survival probability was detected in those people who presented at the beginning of the study with nephropathy (88% in people with nephropathy v 94% in people without nephropathy; P = 0.045). When the causes of death during the initial 5 years of follow up (1990–1995) were compared with those during the ensuing 5 years (1995–2000), active SLE and infections (29% each) seemed to be the most common causes during the initial 5 years, although thromboses (26%) became the most common cause of death during the last 5 years. Race is an independent predictor of mortality; black people in the USA have a worse prognosis than white people, as do Asian people in the UK compared with white people in the UK.

Rachelle Buchbinder, Sally Green, and Peter Struijs

KEY POINTS

- Lateral pain in the elbow affects up to 3% of the population and is usually an overload injury that often follows minor trauma to extensor forearm muscles.

  Although usually self-limiting, symptoms may persist in up to 20% of people for over 1 year.

- Corticosteroid injections improve pain from tennis elbow in the short term compared with placebo, local anaesthetic, orthoses, physiotherapy, or oral NSAIDs.

  We don't know which corticosteroid regimen leads to greatest pain relief.

  In the long term, physiotherapy or oral NSAIDs may be more effective than corticosteroid injections at reducing pain.

  Topical NSAIDs lead to short-term pain relief, but long-term effects are unknown.

- Extracorporeal shock-wave therapy is unlikely to be more effective at improving pain compared with placebo, and may be less effective than injected corticosteroids.

  We don't know whether acupuncture, exercise, and mobilisation reduce symptoms of tennis elbow, as few studies have been found and they gave conflicting results.

  We don't know whether orthoses (braces) reduce symptoms compared with no treatment or other treatments, as few studies have been found.

  We don't know whether open or percutaneous surgical techniques improve pain and function, as no good-quality studies have been found.

(i) **Please visit www.clinicalevidence.bmj.com for full text and references**

What are the effects of treatments for tennis elbow?	
Likely To Be Beneficial	• Corticosteroid injections (for short-term pain relief)
Unknown Effectiveness	• Acupuncture (for short-term pain relief) • Exercise and mobilisation • Oral NSAIDs (for longer-term pain relief) • Orthoses (bracing) • Surgery • Topical NSAIDs (for longer-term pain relief)
Unlikely To Be Beneficial	• Extracorporeal shock-wave therapy

Search date August 2006

DEFINITION Tennis elbow has many analogous terms, including lateral elbow pain, lateral epicondylitis, rowing elbow, tendonitis of the common extensor origin, and peritendinitis of the elbow. Tennis elbow is characterised by pain and tenderness over the lateral epicondyle of the humerus and pain on resisted dorsiflexion of the wrist, middle finger, or both. For the purposes of this review, tennis elbow is restricted to lateral elbow pain or lateral epicondylitis.

INCIDENCE/PREVALENCE Lateral elbow pain is common (population prevalence 1–3%), with peak incidence occurring at 40–50 years of age. In women aged 42–46 years, incidence increases to 10%. In the UK, the Netherlands, and Scandinavia the incidence of lateral elbow pain in general practice is 4–7/1000 people a year.

AETIOLOGY/RISK FACTORS Tennis elbow is considered to be an overload injury, typically after minor and often unrecognised trauma of the extensor muscles of the forearm. Despite the title tennis elbow, tennis is a direct cause in only 5% of those with lateral epicondylitis.

PROGNOSIS Although lateral elbow pain is generally self-limiting, in a minority of people symptoms persist for 18 months to 2 years, and in some cases for much longer. The cost is therefore high, both in terms of lost productivity and healthcare use. In a general practice trial of an expectant waiting policy, 80% of the people with elbow pain of already greater than 4 weeks' duration had recovered after 1 year.

David Murdoch

KEY POINTS

- Up to half of people who ascend to heights above 2500 m may develop acute mountain sickness, pulmonary oedema, or cerebral oedema, with the risk being greater at higher altitudes, and faster rates of ascent.

  Symptoms of acute mountain sickness include headache, weakness, fatigue, nausea, insomnia, and decreased appetite.

  It is generally thought that symptoms resolve over a few days if no further ascent is attempted, but little is known about the long-term prognosis.

- Little good-quality research has been done on the prevention or treatment of this condition. The consensus is that slow ascent reduces the risk of acute mountain sickness.

- Acetazolamide and dexamethasone reduce the risk of acute mountain sickness compared with placebo, although we don't know whether they are more or less effective than each other, or than other prophylactic treatments.

  Acetazolamide causes polyuria and paraesthesia in a high proportion of people while, in some people, dexamethasone may cause depression following withdrawal.

- We don't know whether ginkgo biloba reduces the risk of acute mountain sickness compared with placebo, but it may be less effective than acetazolamide.

- Dexamethasone may reduce symptom scores in people with acute mountain sickness compared with placebo.

- The consensus is that people who develop acute mountain sickness should descend if possible, but we don't know of any RCTs showing that this improves symptoms compared with resting at the same altitude.

(i) **Please visit www.clinicalevidence.bmj.com for full text and references**

What are the effects of interventions to prevent acute mountain sickness?	
Beneficial	• Acetazolamide • Dexamethasone • Slow ascent (or acclimatisation)*
Unknown Effectiveness	• Ginkgo biloba

What are the effects of treatments for acute mountain sickness?	
Likely To Be Beneficial	• Descent compared with resting at the same altitude* • Dexamethasone
Unknown Effectiveness	• Acetazolamide

Search date January 2007

*Although we found no RCTs on the effects of these interventions, there is a general consensus that they are effective.

DEFINITION Altitude sickness (or high-altitude illness) includes acute mountain sickness, high-altitude pulmonary oedema, and high-altitude cerebral oedema. **Acute mountain sickness** typically occurs at altitudes greater than 2500 m (about 8000 feet), and is characterised by the development of some or all of the symptoms of headache, weakness, fatigue, listlessness, nausea, insomnia, and suppressed appetite. Symptoms may take days to develop or may occur within hours, depending on the rate of ascent and the altitude attained. More severe forms of altitude sickness have been identified. **High-altitude pulmonary oedema** is characterised by symptoms and signs typical of pulmonary oedema, such as shortness of breath, coughing, and production of frothy or blood stained sputum. **High-altitude cerebral oedema** is characterised by confusion, ataxia, and a decreasing level of consciousness. This review covers only acute mountain sickness.

INCIDENCE/PREVALENCE The incidence of acute mountain sickness increases with absolute height attained and with the rate of ascent. One survey in Taiwan (93 people ascending above 3000 m) found that 27% of people experienced acute mountain sickness. One survey in the Himalayas (278 unacclimatised hikers at 4243 m) found that 53% of people developed acute mountain sickness. One survey in the Swiss Alps (466 climbers at 4 altitudes between 2850 m and 4559 m) found the prevalence of two or more symptoms of acute mountain sickness to be 9% of people at 2850 m; 13% of people at 3050 m; 34% of people at 3650 m; and 53% of people at 4559 m.

AETIOLOGY/RISK FACTORS One survey in the Himalayas identified the rate of ascent and absolute height attained as the only risk factors for acute mountain sickness. It found no evidence of a difference in risk between men and women, or that previous episodes of altitude experience, load carried, or recent respiratory infections affected risk. However, the study was too small to exclude these as risk factors, or to quantify risks reliably. One systematic review (search date 1999) comparing prophylactic agents versus placebo found that, among people receiving placebo, the incidence of acute mountain sickness was higher with a faster rate of ascent (54% of people at a mean ascent rate of 91 m/hour; 73% at a mean ascent rate of 1268 m/hour; 89% at a simulated ascent rate in a hypobaric chamber of 1647 m/hour). One survey in Switzerland (827 mountaineers ascending to 4559 m) examined the effects of susceptibility, pre-exposure, and ascent rate on acute mountain sickness. In this study, pre-exposure was defined as having spent more than 4 days above 3000 m in the preceding 2 months, and slow ascent was defined as ascending in more than 3 days. It found that, in susceptible people (who had previously had acute mountain sickness at high altitude), the prevalence of acute mountain sickness was 58% with rapid ascent and no pre-exposure, 29% with pre-exposure only, 33% with slow ascent only, and 7% with both pre-exposure and slow ascent. In non-susceptible people, the corresponding values were 31%, 16%, 11%, and 4%. The overall odds ratio for developing acute mountain sickness in susceptible compared with non-susceptible people was 2.9 (95% CI 2.1 to 4.1).

PROGNOSIS We found no reliable data on prognosis. It is widely held that if no further ascent is attempted, then the symptoms of acute mountain sickness tend to resolve over a few days. We found no reliable data about long-term sequelae in people whose symptoms have completely resolved.

Bell's palsy

Julian Holland

KEY POINTS

- Bell's palsy is characterised by unilateral, acute paresis or acute paralysis of the face, which may occur with mild pain, numbness, increased sensitivity to noise, and altered taste.

  Up to 30% of people with acute peripheral facial palsy have other identifiable causes, including stroke, tumours, middle-ear disease, or Lyme disease. Severe pain is more consistent with Ramsay Hunt syndrome caused by herpes zoster infection, which has a worse prognosis than Bell's palsy.

  Bell's palsy is most common in people aged 15–40 years, and pregnant women may be at higher risk.

  Bell's palsy may be caused by reactivation of herpes viruses in the cranial nerve ganglia. Most people make a spontaneous recovery within 3 weeks, but up to 30% may have residual problems.

- We don't know whether corticosteroids or antiviral treatment improve recovery of motor function, or cosmetically-disabling sequelae compared with placebo or with other treatments.

  Combined treatment with aciclovir plus corticosteroids may be more effective than steroids alone.

  In pregnant women, antiviral treatments such as aciclovir should only be prescribed under guidance of an obstetrician.

  There is some consensus that valaciclovir may be more effective than aciclovir, as it has improved bioavailability and compliance.

- We don't know whether facial nerve decompression surgery is beneficial in Bell's palsy, as no studies of adequate quality have been found.

- Mime therapy may improve facial stiffness and lip mobility in Bell's palsy, but the evidence is too weak to draw conclusions.

Please visit www.clinicalevidence.bmj.com for full text and references

What are the effects of drug treatments for Bell's palsy in adults and children?	
Likely To Be Beneficial	• Corticosteroids plus antiviral treatment
Unknown Effectiveness	• Antiviral agents • Corticosteroids

What are the effects of surgical treatments for Bell's palsy in adults and children?	
Unknown Effectiveness	• Facial nerve decompression surgery

What are the effects of physical treatments for Bell's palsy in adults and children?	
Unknown Effectiveness	• Mime therapy

Search date February 2007

DEFINITION Bell's palsy is an idiopathic, acute, unilateral paresis or paralysis of the face in a pattern consistent with peripheral facial nerve dysfunction, and may be partial or complete, occurring with equal frequency on the right and left sides of the face. While other possible causes need to be excluded, there is increasing evidence that Bell's palsy is caused by herpes viruses. Additional symptoms of Bell's palsy may include mild pain in or behind the ear, oropharyngeal or facial numbness, impaired tolerance to ordinary levels of noise, and disturbed taste on the anterior part of the tongue. Severe pain is more suggestive of herpes zoster virus infection (shingles) and possible progression to a Ramsay Hunt syndrome, but another cause should be carefully excluded. Up to 30% of people with an acute peripheral facial palsy will not have Bell's palsy; other causes may include stroke, tumour, trauma, middle-ear disease, and Lyme disease. Features such as sparing of movement in the upper face (central pattern), or weakness of a specific branch of the facial nerve (segmental pattern), suggest an alternative cause. Bell's palsy is less commonly the cause of facial palsy in children under 10 (under 40%), so an alternative cause should be carefully excluded. The assessment should identify acute suppurative ear disease (including mastoiditis), a parotid mass or Lyme disease in endemic areas.

INCIDENCE/PREVALENCE The incidence is about 20/100,000 people a year, or about 1/60 people in a lifetime. Bell's palsy has a peak incidence between the ages of 15 and 40 years. Men and women are equally affected, although the incidence may be increased in pregnant women.

AETIOLOGY/RISK FACTORS The cause of Bell's palsy is unknown, but it is thought that reactivated herpes viruses from the cranial nerve ganglia have a key role in the development of this condition. HSV-1 has been detected in up to 50% of cases by some researchers, and herpes zoster virus in approximately 13% of cases. Herpes-zoster-associated facial palsy more frequently presents as zoster sine herpete (without vesicles), although 6% of people will subsequently develop vesicles (Ramsay Hunt syndrome). Thus, treatment plans for the management of Bell's palsy should recognise the high incidence of herpes zoster virus, which is associated with worse outcomes. Inflammation of the facial nerve initially results in reversible neuropraxia, but ultimately Wallerian degeneration ensues.

PROGNOSIS Overall, Bell's palsy has a fair prognosis without treatment. Clinically important improvement occurs within 3 weeks in 85% of people, and within 3–5 months in the remaining 15%. People failing to show signs of improvement by 3 weeks may have suffered severe degeneration of the facial nerve, or have an alternative diagnosis that requires identification by specialist examination or investigations, such as computed tomography or magnetic resonance imaging. Overall, 71% of people will fully recover facial muscle function (61% of people with complete palsy, 94% of people with partial palsy). The remaining 29% are left with mild to severe residual facial-muscle weakness, 17% with contracture and 16% with hemifacial spasm or synkinesis. Incomplete recovery of facial expression may have a long-term impact on quality of life. The prognosis for children with Bell's palsy is generally good, with a high rate (more than 90%) of spontaneous recovery, in part because of the high frequency of partial paralysis. However, children with complete palsies may suffer poor outcomes as frequently as adults.

Cluster headache

Manjit Matharu and Nicholas Silver

KEY POINTS

- The revised International Headache Society (IHS) criteria for cluster headache are: attacks of severe or very severe, strictly unilateral pain, which is orbital, supraorbital, or temporal pain, lasting 15–180 minutes and occurring from once every other day to eight times daily. The attacks are associated with one or more of the following, all of which are ipsilateral: conjunctival injection, lacrimation, nasal congestion, rhinorrhoea, forehead and facial sweating, miosis, ptosis, and eyelid oedema. Most people are restless or agitated during an attack. Cluster headache may be episodic or chronic.

  Cluster headache is rare, but the exact prevalence remains a matter of debate.

- The main focus of intervention is to abort attacks once they have begun and to prevent future attacks.

- Sumatriptan, used subcutaneously or intranasally, reduces the severity and duration of episodic or chronic cluster headache attacks once they have begun. We don't know whether oral sumatriptan is effective.

  Oral zolmitriptan reduces severity of attacks in people with episodic cluster headache. We don't know how effective it is in people with chronic cluster headache.

  There is consensus that high-dose and high-flow-rate oxygen is effective for abortive treatment of episodic or chronic cluster headache. We don't know whether this consensus can be applied to hyperbaric oxygen, as little research has been conducted.

  There is also consensus that subcutaneous octreotide is effective for abortive treatment of cluster headache.

  We don't know whether intranasal lidocaine is effective for abortive treatment of cluster headache.

- There is consensus that both verapamil and lithium prevent cluster headache, but that verapamil is more effective than lithium, and causes fewer adverse effects.

  There is also consensus that corticosteroids and greater occipital nerve injections (betamethasone plus xylocaine) are effective for preventive treatment.

  We don't know whether baclofen, botulinum toxin, capsaicin, chlorpromazine, civamide, clonidine, ergotamine or dihydroergotamine, gabapentin, leuprolide, melatonin, methysergide, pizotifen, sodium valproate, topiramate, or TCAs are effective for prevention of cluster headache. Some of these interventions are not routinely used in clinical practice.

(i) **Please visit www.clinicalevidence.bmj.com for full text and references**

What are the effects of interventions to abort cluster headache?	
Beneficial	• Sumatriptan (subcutaneous and intranasal) for episodic or chronic cluster headache
Likely To Be Beneficial	• High-dose and high-flow-rate oxygen for episodic or chronic cluster headache* • Octreotide (subcutaneous)*

	• Zolmitriptan (oral) for episodic cluster headache (unknown effectiveness for chronic cluster headache)
Unknown Effectiveness	• Hyperbaric oxygen • Lidocaine (intranasal) • Sumatriptan (oral)

What are the effects of preventive interventions for cluster headache?

Likely To Be Beneficial	• Corticosteroids (oral)* • Greater occipital nerve injections (betamethasone plus xylocaine)* • Lithium (oral) (consensus that effective for preventing chronic cluster headache but less so than verapamil and more adverse effects)* • Verapamil (consensus that more effective than lithium for preventing chronic cluster headache and fewer adverse effects)*
Unknown Effectiveness	• Baclofen (oral) • Botulinum toxin (intramuscular) • Capsaicin (intranasal) • Chlorpromazine • Civamide (intranasal) • Clonidine (transdermal) • Ergotamine and dihydroergotamine (oral or intranasal) • Gabapentin (oral) • Leuprolide • Melatonin • Methysergide (oral) • Pizotifen (oral) • Sodium valproate (oral) • Sumatriptan (oral) • Topiramate (oral) • TCAs

Search date September 2006

*Categorisation based on consensus.

DEFINITION The revised International Headache Society (IHS) criteria for cluster headache are: attacks of severe or very severe, strictly unilateral pain, which is orbital, supraorbital or

(continued over)

(from previous page)

temporal pain, lasting 15–180 minutes and occurring from once every other day to eight times daily. The attacks are associated with at least one of the following cranial autonomic features, all of which are ipsilateral: conjunctival injection, lacrimation, nasal congestion, rhinorrhoea, forehead and facial sweating, miosis, ptosis, and eyelid oedema. The revised IHS criteria allow the diagnosis of cluster headache to be made in the absence of ipsilateral cranial autonomic features, provided the person reports a sense of restlessness or agitation. Attacks usually occur in series (cluster periods) lasting for weeks or months separated by remission periods usually lasting months or years. However, about 10–15% of people have chronic symptoms without remissions. Cluster headache is further subclassified according to the duration of the bout. Episodic cluster headache (ECH) is diagnosed when cluster headache attacks occur in periods lasting 7 days to 1 year separated by remissions lasting 1 month or longer. Chronic cluster headache (CCH) is diagnosed when cluster headache attacks occur for more than 1 year without remission, or with remissions lasting less than 1 month. The term cluster headache is now widely accepted, although historically the condition has been known by several different names, including: migrainous neuralgia, Horton's headache, histaminic cephalalgia, spheno-palatine neuralgia, Sluder's neuralgia, petrosal neuralgia, red migraine, erythroprosopalgia of Bing, ciliary neuralgia, erythromelalgia of the head, Vidian neuralgia, hemicrania angioparalytica, Hemicrania periodic neuralgiforms, syndrome of hemicephalic vasodilation of sympathetic origin, and autonomic faciocephalalgia.

INCIDENCE/PREVALENCE Cluster headache is rare, but the exact prevalence remains a matter of debate because of the remarkable variation of the estimated prevalence — between 56 and 401 per 100,000 population — in the various studies. Recent studies suggest that the prevalence of cluster headache is likely to be at least one person per 500. Cluster headache is more prevalent in men. The gender ratio in the various case series varies between 2.5:1 and 7.2:1.

AETIOLOGY/RISK FACTORS There is a small increased familial risk of cluster headache, suggesting a genetic role in causation. People with cluster headache may over indulge in non-essential consumption habits including smoking, intake of alcohol, and consumption of coffee. There is an increased incidence of previous head trauma in cluster headache, ranging between 5% and 37%, although there is often a long interval between the head trauma and the onset of the headaches.

PROGNOSIS Onset of symptoms most commonly occurs between the second and fourth decades of life, although cluster headache has been reported in all age groups. Although there is a paucity of literature on the long-term prognosis of cluster headache, the available evidence suggests that it is a lifelong disorder in most people. In one study, ECH evolved into CCH in about 10% of people, whereas CCH transformed into ECH in a third of people. Furthermore, a substantial proportion of people with cluster headache can expect to develop longer remission periods with increasing age.

Ailsa Snaith and Derick Wade

KEY POINTS

- Dystonia is characterised by involuntary muscle contractions resulting in abnormal postures and twisting of body parts.

  It is usually a lifelong condition with persistent pain and disability.

  Focal dystonia affects a single part of the body; generalised dystonia can affect most or all of the body.

  It is more common in women, and some types of dystonia are more common in people of European Ashkenazi Jewish descent.

- Botulinum toxin is effective in relieving cervical dystonia symptoms in adults.

  Botulinum toxin A and botulinum toxin B are both effective.

  We found most evidence for botulinum toxin, and it is the mainstay of modern treatment for focal dystonia.

- We don't know if any other drug treatments are effective (benzodiazepines, GABA inhibitors, atypical antipsychotics, anticonvulsants, dopaminergic agonists and antagonists) for either focal or generalised dystonia.

- We don't know if any surgical interventions are effective (thalamotomy, pallidotomy, deep brain stimulation of thalamus and globus pallidus, selective peripheral denervation, myectomy, or microvascular decompression) for either focal or generalised dystonia.

- Most people will see a physiotherapist after diagnosis, but there is no consistent approach to treatment.

Please visit www.clinicalevidence.bmj.com for full text and references

What are the effects of drug treatments for focal dystonia?	
Beneficial	• Botulinum toxin (in cervical dystonia; both A and B toxin beneficial compared with placebo and similarly effective when compared with each other)
Unknown Effectiveness	• Anticholinergic drugs • Anticonvulsants • Atypical antipsychotic drugs • Benzodiazepines • Dopaminergic agonists and antagonists • GABA inhibitors

What are the effects of drug treatments for generalised dystonia?	
Unknown Effectiveness	• Acetylcholine receptor inhibitors • Anticholinergic drugs • Anticonvulsants • Atypical antipsychotic drugs • Benzodiazepines • Dopaminergic agonists and antagonists • GABA inhibitors

What are the effects of surgical treatments for focal dystonia?

Unknown Effectiveness	• Deep brain stimulation of thalamus and globus pallidus • Microvascular decompression • Myectomy • Pallidotomy • Selective peripheral denervation • Thalamotomy

What are the effects of surgical treatments for generalised dystonia?

Unknown Effectiveness	• Deep brain stimulation of thalamus and globus pallidus • Microvascular decompression • Myectomy • Pallidotomy • Selective peripheral denervation • Thalamotomy

What are the effects of physical treatments for focal dystonia?

Likely To Be Beneficial	• Physiotherapy for cervical dystonia in children (categorisation based on case series)
Unknown Effectiveness	• Acupuncture • Biofeedback • Chiropractic manipulation • Occupational therapy • Osteopathy • Speech therapy

What are the effects of physical treatments for generalised dystonia?

Unknown Effectiveness	• Acupuncture • Biofeedback • Chiropractic manipulation • Occupational therapy • Osteopathy • Physiotherapy

• Speech therapy

Search date May 2006

DEFINITION Dystonia is a neurological disorder characterised by involuntary, abnormal muscle contractions that result in sustained abnormal postures, twisting, or both, and repetitive movements of body parts. It arises from dysfunction of the motor control system within the central nervous system. Dystonia is most simply classified by location: **focal dystonia** involves a single body part; **multifocal dystonia** involves two or more unrelated body parts; **segmental dystonia** affects two or more adjacent parts of the body; **hemidystonia** involves the arm and leg on the same side of the body; and **generalised dystonia** affects most or all of the body. For the purpose of this review we have classified dystonia into focal dystonia and generalised/other dystonia. The central nervous system dysfunctions that cause dystonia are unknown. **Diagnosis:** The clinical diagnosis of dystonia is based on the hallmark features of the abnormal, involuntary, and prolonged muscle contractions that lead to an abnormal posture of the area affected. There is no definitive diagnostic test for of dystonia. Investigation typically involves history and physical examination, laboratory tests, and imaging to establish severity and potential cause. Laboratory tests and neuroimaging may help rule out metabolic or structural causes.

INCIDENCE/PREVALENCE Dystonia occurs worldwide. In the US, the prevalence of focal dystonia has been reported as 30 people per 100,000, and generalised dystonia as 0.2–6.7 people per 100,000 population. In Europe, the prevalence of primary dystonia has been estimated at 15.2 per 100,000 people. Cervical dystonia (torticollis or "wry neck") is the most common adult form of focal dystonia with a prevalence in Europe of 5.7 per 100,000, followed by blepharospasm (forceful eyelid closures) affecting 3.6 per 100,000, and limb dystonias (e.g. writer's cramp) affecting 1.4 per 100,000. Dystonia occurs with greater frequency in women, and generalised dystonia affects more people of European Ashkenazi Jewish descent.

AETIOLOGY/RISK FACTORS The pathophysiology of dystonia remains unclear. Dystonia may occur because of abnormal neurochemical transmission in the basal ganglia, brainstem, or both, resulting in abnormal execution of motor control. There is debate on the extent to which psychological factors cause dystonia, although they can undoubtedly exacerbate it. Dystonia can be classified as primary (where underlying cause is unknown) or secondary (related to known disorders). The primary disorders may be further classified as hereditary or sporadic. Currently, 13 types of dystonia can be distinguished on a genetic basis. Secondary dystonia may occur as part of a wide variety of neurological conditions, for example Huntington's Disease, Wilson's Disease, head injury, tumours, and Parkinsonism; or it may result from use of drugs, for example neuroleptic drugs and metoclopramide. We have not distinguished between primary and secondary dystonia in this review, although both are covered.

PROGNOSIS For most people dystonia is a lifelong disorder, although a small minority experience complete remission. Most people with dystonia have a normal life expectancy but with continued symptoms. The presence and severity of symptoms is unpredictable as symptoms may fluctuate over time (e.g. stressful situations may make symptoms worse) or they may disappear or stabilise for a period of time. Regardless of the cause, dystonic contractions may have a chronic course and may lead to severe persistent pain and disability. Furthermore, embarrassment (caused by the symptoms) may lead to social withdrawal. Prognosis seems to depend on a number of factors, including age of onset, distribution, and cause. Focal dystonia may become generalised over time. Dystonia with a later age of onset has a lower likelihood of spreading than dystonia beginning in childhood. Similarly, dystonia starting in the neck is less likely to spread than dystonia starting in the limbs.

Anthony Marson and Sridharan Ramaratnam

KEY POINTS

- During their lifetime, about 3% of people will be diagnosed with epilepsy, but about 70% of people with epilepsy eventually go into remission.

- After a first seizure, antiepileptic drugs may delay or prevent subsequent seizures, but they can cause adverse effects, and their long-term benefit is unknown.

- Carbamazepine, phenobarbital, phenytoin, and sodium valproate are widely considered to be effective in controlling seizures in partial or in newly-diagnosed generalised (tonic clonic) epilepsy, but we found no RCTs comparing them with placebo, and a placebo-controlled trial would now be considered unethical.

  Systematic reviews found no reliable evidence on which to base a choice among antiepileptic drugs; carbamazepine is considered to be the drug of choice for partial epilepsy.

  Adding second-line drugs to usual treatment reduces seizure frequency in people with drug-resistant partial epilepsy, but increases adverse effects, such as dizziness and somnolence. We don't know whether any one is more likely to reduce seizures compared with the others.

- In people who have been seizure free for at least 2 years on treatment, almost 60% of those who withdraw from antiepileptic treatment will remain seizure free, compared with almost 80% of people who continue treatment.

- Educational programmes may reduce seizure frequency and improve psycho-social functioning in people with epilepsy, but we don't know whether other behavioural or psychological treatments are beneficial.

- There is consensus that temporal lobectomy or amygdalohippocampectomy can improve seizure control and quality of life in people with drug-resistant temporal-lobe epilepsy, but they can cause neurological adverse effects.

- High-level vagus nerve stimulation may reduce seizure frequency in people with drug-resistant partial seizures, but it may cause hoarseness and dyspnoea, and long-term effects are unknown.

- CAUTION: Vigabatrin, which may be used as second-line treatment, causes concentric visual-field abnormalities, that are probably irreversible in about 40% of people.

(i) **Please visit www.clinicalevidence.bmj.com for full text and references**

What are the benefits and risks of starting antiepileptic drug treatment following a single seizure?	
Trade-off Between Benefits And Harms	• Antiepileptic drugs after a single seizure

What are the effects of monotherapy in newly diagnosed partial epilepsy?	
Beneficial	• Carbamazepine*
	• Phenobarbital*
	• Phenytoin*
	• Sodium valproate*

What are the effects of monotherapy in newly diagnosed generalised epilepsy (tonic clonic type)?

Beneficial	• Carbamazepine*
	• Phenobarbital*
	• Phenytoin*
	• Sodium valproate*

What are the effects of additional treatments in people with drug-resistant partial epilepsy?

Beneficial	• Addition of second-line drugs (gabapentin, levetiracetam, lamotrigine, oxcarbazepine, tiagabine, topiramate, vigabatrin, or zonisamide)

Which people in remission from seizures are at risk of relapse on withdrawal of drug treatment?

Trade-off Between Benefits And Harms	• Antiepileptic drug withdrawal for people in remission

What are the effects of behavioural and psychological treatments for people with epilepsy?

Likely To Be Beneficial	• Educational programmes
Unknown Effectiveness	• Biofeedback
	• CBT
	• Family counselling
	• Relaxation plus behavioural modification therapy
	• Relaxation therapy
	• Yoga

What are the effects of surgery in people with drug-resistant temporal-lobe epilepsy?

Beneficial	• Temporal lobectomy*
Likely To Be Beneficial	• Amygdalohippocampectomy*
	• Vagus nerve stimulation as adjunctive therapy for partial seizures
Unknown Effectiveness	• Lesionectomy

Search date November 2005

*Categorisation based on consensus.

DEFINITION Epilepsy is a group of disorders rather than a single disease. Seizures can be classified by type as partial or focal (categorised as simple partial, complex partial, and secondary generalised tonic clonic seizures) or generalised (categorised as generalised tonic clonic, absence, myoclonic, tonic, and atonic seizures). A person is considered to have epilepsy if they have had two or more unprovoked seizures.

INCIDENCE/PREVALENCE Epilepsy is common, with an estimated prevalence in the developed world of 5–10/1000, and an annual incidence of 50/100,000 people. About 3% of people will be given a diagnosis of epilepsy at some time in their lives.

AETIOLOGY/RISK FACTORS Epilepsy is a symptom rather than a disease, and it may be caused by various disorders involving the brain. The causes/risk factors include birth/neonatal injuries, congenital or metabolic disorders, head injuries, tumours, infections of the brain or meninges, genetic defects, degenerative disease of the brain, cerebrovascular disease, or demyelinating disease. Epilepsy can be classified by cause. **Idiopathic generalised** epilepsies (such as juvenile myoclonic epilepsy or childhood absence epilepsy) are largely genetic. **Symptomatic epilepsies** result from a known cerebral abnormality; for example, temporal-lobe epilepsy may result from a congenital defect, mesial temporal sclerosis, or a tumour. **Cryptogenic epilepsies** are those that cannot be classified as idiopathic or symptomatic.

PROGNOSIS About 60% of untreated people have no further seizures during the 2 years after their first seizure. For most people with epilepsy the prognosis is good. About 70% go into remission, defined as being seizure free for 5 years on or off treatment. This leaves 20–30% who develop chronic epilepsy, which is often treated with multiple antiepileptic drugs.

Joaquim Ferreira and Cristina Sampaio

KEY POINTS

- Essential tremor refers to a persistent bilateral oscillation of both hands and forearms, or an isolated tremor of the head, without abnormal posturing, and when there is no evidence that the tremor arises from another identifiable cause.

  Essential tremor is one of the most common movement disorders throughout the world, with a prevalence of 0.4–3.9% in the general population.

  Although most people with essential tremor are only mildly affected, those who seek medical care are disabled to some extent, and most are socially handicapped by the tremor.

- Overall, we found few RCTs that assessed the long-term effects of drug treatments for essential tremor of the hand.

- Propranolol seems to effectively improve clinical scores, tremor amplitude, and self-evaluation of severity compared with placebo in people with hand tremor.

  We found insufficient evidence to judge the efficacy of other beta-blockers such as atenolol, metoprolol, nadolol, pindolol, and sotalol in treating essential tremor of the hand.

- Barbiturates, such as phenobarbital (phenobarbitone) and primidone, may improve hand tremor in the short term, but are associated with depression, and with cognitive and behavioural adverse effects.

- Benzodiazepines may improve hand tremor and function in the short term, but we were unable to draw reliable conclusions because of the weakness of the studies.

  Benzodiazepines are also associated with adverse effects such as dependency, sedation, and cognitive and behavioural effects.

- We don't know whether carbonic anhydrase inhibitors, dihydropyridene calcium channel blockers, flunarizine, clonidine, isoniazid, or gabapentin are useful in treating essential tremor of the hand, because the studies have all been too small to detect clinically important differences in symptoms.

- Botulinum A toxin-haemagglutinin complex and topiramate both appear to improve clinical rating scales for hand tremor in the short term, but are associated with frequent adverse effects.

  Botulinum A toxin-haemagglutinin complex is associated with hand weakness which is dose dependent and transient.

  The most common adverse effects of topiramate are appetite suppression, weight loss, and paraesthesia.

- Adding mirtazapine to antitremor drugs such as propranolol does not seem to improve outcomes further in people with essential tremor of the hand, and leads to more frequent adverse effects, such as drowsiness, confusion, dry mouth, and weight gain.

Please visit www.clinicalevidence.bmj.com for full text and references

What are the effects of drug treatments in people with essential tremor of the hand?

Likely To Be Beneficial	• Propranolol
Trade-off Between Benefits And Harms	• Botulinum A toxin–haemagglutinin complex (improved clinical rating scales at 4–12 weeks, but associated with hand weakness)

	• Phenobarbital (may improve tremor at 5 weeks, but associated with depression and cognitive adverse effects) • Primidone (may improve tremor and function at 5 weeks compared with placebo and at 1 year compared with baseline, but associated with depression, and with cognitive adverse effects) • Topiramate (improved tremor scores after 24 weeks' treatment, but associated with appetite suppression, weight loss, and paraesthesia)
Unknown Effectiveness	• Benzodiazepines • Beta-blockers other than propranolol (atenolol, metoprolol, nadolol, pindolol, and sotalol) • Calcium channel blockers (dihydropyridine) • Carbonic anhydrase inhibitors • Clonidine • Flunarizine • Gabapentin • Isoniazid
Likely To Be Ineffective Or Harmful	• Mirtazapine added to other antitremor drugs

Search date December 2006

DEFINITION Tremor is a rhythmic, mechanical oscillation of at least one body region. The term essential tremor is used when there is either a persistent bilateral tremor of hands and forearms, or an isolated tremor of the head, without abnormal posturing, and when there is no evidence that the tremor arises from another identifiable cause. The diagnosis is not made if there are: abnormal neurological signs; known causes of enhanced physiological tremor; a history or signs of psychogenic tremor; sudden change in severity; primary orthostatic tremor; isolated voice tremor; isolated position-specific or task-specific tremors; and isolated tongue, chin, or leg tremor.

INCIDENCE/PREVALENCE Essential tremor is one of the most common movement disorders throughout the world, with a prevalence of 0.4–3.9% in the general population.

AETIOLOGY/RISK FACTORS Essential tremor is sometimes inherited with an autosomal dominant pattern. About 40% of people with essential tremor have no family history of the condition. Alcohol ingestion provides symptomatic benefit in 50–70% of people.

PROGNOSIS Essential tremor is a persistent and progressive condition. It usually begins during early adulthood and the severity of the tremor slowly increases. Only a small proportion of people with essential tremor seek medical advice, but the proportion in different surveys varies from 0.5% to 11%. Most people with essential tremor are only mildly affected. However, most of the people who seek medical care are disabled to some extent, and most are socially handicapped by the tremor. A quarter of people receiving medical care for the tremor change jobs or retire because of essential tremor-induced disability.

Nicholas Silver

KEY POINTS

- Chronic tension-type headache (CTTH) is a disorder that evolves from episodic tension-type headache, with daily or frequent episodes of headache lasting minutes to days.

    It affects 4.1% of the general population in the USA, and is more prevalent in women (up to 65% of cases).

- We found only limited evidence about the treatment of CTTH.

    Regular acute pain-relief medication may itself lead to chronic headache symptoms and reduce the effectiveness of prophylactic treatment.

- We found insufficient evidence to judge the effectiveness of benzodiazepines or SSRIs in treating CTTH, although both are commonly associated with significant adverse effects.

- Amitriptyline and mirtazapine are similarly effective in reducing the duration and frequency of CTTH, although amitriptyline is associated with a less favourable adverse-effect profile.

    We found no evidence examining the effectiveness of other tricyclic or noradrenergic and specific serotonergic antidepressants.

    Botulinum toxin does not seem to be a useful treatment for CTTH, and is associated with several adverse effects including facial weakness, difficulty in swallowing, and disturbed local sensation.

    CBT seems to reduce the symptoms of CTTH.

    We don't know whether other non-drug treatments, such as relaxation and electromyographic biofeedback, or acupuncture are effective in treating CTTH.

(i) **Please visit www.clinicalevidence.bmj.com for full text and references**

What are the effects of drug treatments for chronic tension-type headache?

Beneficial	• Amitriptyline
	• Mirtazapine (only short-term evidence)
Unknown Effectiveness	• SRIs
	• TCAs (other than amitriptyline)
Likely To Be Ineffective Or Harmful	• Benzodiazepines
	• Botulinum toxin
	• Regular acute pain-relief medication

What are the effects of non-drug treatments for chronic tension-type headache?

Likely To Be Beneficial	• CBT
Unknown Effectiveness	• Acupuncture
	• Indian head massage

● Relaxation and electromyographic biofeedback

Search date October 2005

DEFINITION Chronic tension-type headache (CTTH) is a disorder that evolves from episodic tension-type headache, with daily or frequent episodes of headache lasting minutes to days. The 2004 International Headache Society criteria for CTTH are headaches on 15 or more days a month (180 days/year) for at least 3 months; pain that is bilateral, pressing, or tightening in quality and non-pulsating, of mild or moderate intensity, which does not worsen with routine physical activity such as walking or climbing stairs; presence of no more than one additional clinical feature (mild nausea, photophobia, or phonophobia) and without moderate/severe nausea or vomiting. CTTH is generally regarded as a featureless headache. Not all experts agree that mild features more typically seen in migraine such as photophobia, phonophobia, etc, should be included in the operational definition of CTTH, and it is often difficult to distinguish mild migraine headache from tension-type headache. CTTH is to be distinguished from other causes of chronic daily headache that require different treatment strategies (e.g. new daily persistent headache, medication overuse headache, chronic migraine, and hemicrania continua). Many people who develop chronic daily headache owing to chronic migraine or medication overuse also develop mild migrainous "background" headaches that might be mistaken for coincidental CTTH. It is therefore extremely important to take a full headache history to elicit the individual features of the headache and look for prodromal or accompanying features that might indicate an alternative diagnosis. In contrast to CTTH, episodic tension-type headache can last for 30 minutes to 7 days and occurs for fewer than 180 days a year. The greatest obstacle to studying tension-type headache is the lack of any single proved specific or reliable, clinical, or biological defining characteristic of the disorder. Terms based on assumed mechanisms (muscle-contraction headache, tension headache) are not operationally defined. Old studies that used these terms may have included people with many different types of headache.

INCIDENCE/PREVALENCE The prevalence of chronic daily headache from a survey of the general population in the USA was 4.1%. Half of sufferers met the International Headache Society criteria for CTTH. In a survey of 2500 undergraduate students in the USA, the prevalence of CTTH was 2%. The prevalence of CTTH was 2.5% in a Danish population based survey of 975 individuals. One community-based survey in Singapore (2096 people from the general population) found that the prevalence was 1.8% in females and 0.9% in males.

AETIOLOGY/RISK FACTORS Tension-type headache is more prevalent in women (65% of cases in 1 survey). Symptoms begin before the age of 10 years in 15% of people with CTTH. Prevalence declines with age. There is a family history of some form of headache in 40% of people with CTTH, although a twin study found that the risk of CTTH was similar for identical and non-identical twins.

PROGNOSIS The prevalence of CTTH declines with age.

KEY POINTS

- Head injury in young adults is often associated with motor vehicle accidents, violence, and sports injuries. In older adults it is often associated with falls. This review covers moderate to severe head injury only.

  Severe head injury can lead to secondary brain damage from cerebral ischaemia resulting from hypotension, hypercapnia, and raised intracranial pressure.

  Poor outcome correlates with low post-resuscitation Glasgow Coma Scale (GCS) score, older age, eye pupil abnormalities, hypoxia or hypotension before definitive treatment, traumatic subarachnoid haemorrhage, and inability to control intracranial pressure.

  Severity of brain injury is assessed using the GCS. While about a quarter of people with severe brain injury (GCS score less than 8) will make a good recovery, about a third will die, and a fifth will have severe disability or be in a vegetative state.

- There is no strong evidence of benefit from any treatment in reducing the complications of moderate to severe head injury. Despite this, most clinicians implement various combinations of treatments discussed here.

- Hyperventilation and mannitol are frequently used to lower intracranial pressure. Anticonvulsants, barbiturates, antibiotics, and hypothermia are less commonly implemented.

  Evidence on hyperventilation, mild hypothermia, and mannitol has been inconclusive.

  Carbamazepine and phenytoin may reduce early seizures in people with head injury, but have not been shown to reduce late seizures, neurological disability, or death.

  Barbiturates have not been shown to be effective in reducing intracranial pressure or in preventing adverse neurological outcomes after head injury.

  Prophylactic antibiotics have not been shown to reduce the risks of death or meningitis in people with skull fracture.

- CAUTION: Corticosteroids have been shown to increase mortality when used acutely in people with head injury.

  One large RCT (the CRASH trial) found that death from all causes and severe disability at 6 months were more likely in people with head injury given methylprednisolone infusion than in those given placebo. Corticosteroids are no longer used in the treatment of head injuries.

(i) Please visit www.clinicalevidence.bmj.com for full text and references

What are the effects of interventions to reduce complications of moderate to severe head injury as defined by Glasgow Coma Scale?

Unknown Effectiveness	• Antibiotics
	• Hyperventilation
	• Hypothermia

	• Mannitol
Unlikely To Be Beneficial	• Anticonvulsants
Likely To Be Ineffective Or Harmful	• Corticosteroids

Search date April 2007

DEFINITION The basic operational components of a head injury are a history of blunt or penetrating trauma to the head, which may be followed by a period of altered consciousness, and the presence of physical evidence of trauma. The specific elements of a head injury are related to its severity. Some guidelines define head injury more broadly as any trauma to the head other than superficial injuries to the face. Head injuries are classified in a variety of ways: severity of injury as assessed by the Glasgow Coma Scale (GCS; mild, moderate, severe); mechanism (blunt or penetrating); or morphology (skull fractures or intracranial lesions). Since its introduction in 1974, the GCS has been widely used as an initial measure of the severity of brain injury. The scale incorporates neurological findings such as voluntary movements, speech, and eye movements, into a 3–15 point scale. GCS allows measurement of neurological findings, and has been used to predict immediate and long-term outcome after head injury. A GCS of 8 or lower is considered representative of a **severe** brain injury, 9–13 of a **moderate** head injury, and 14–15 a **mild** head injury. The GCS is complicated by difficulties of communication and cooperation in the younger child. In children over the age of 5 years, the adult GCS can be used. In younger children the verbal response is modified, and in very young children the motor response is also modified, because these children are unable to obey commands. In this review we cover only moderate to severe head injury as classified by GCS. **Diagnosis and monitoring:** The Advanced Trauma Life Support (ATLS) and Advanced Paediatric Life Support (APLS) guidelines contain standardised protocols for the initial assessment of traumatic head-injured adults and children, respectively. Most moderate to severe head injuries will require investigations after standard history and physical examination. Computed tomography (CT) scan is the investigation of choice in people with traumatic head injuries. Numerous organisations, including the NICE, the Scottish Intercollegiate Guidelines Network, and the Royal College of Paediatrics and Child Health, have developed evidence-based pathways to provide physicians with guidance regarding whether a CT scan is required, and how urgently it should be performed. Monitoring of people with head injury may range from monitoring of intracranial pressure (ICP) with ventricular drains in people with severe head injuries to regular clinical neurological observations in people with less severe head injuries.

INCIDENCE/PREVALENCE Head injury remains the leading cause of death in trauma cases in Europe and the USA, and accounts for a disproportionate amount of morbidity in trauma survivors. Worldwide, several million people, mostly children and young adults, are treated each year for severe head injury. In the UK, 1.4 million people, 50% of whom are children, present to emergency departments every year after a head injury. This represents 11% of all new emergency department presentations. About 80% of people presenting to emergency departments can be categorised as having mild head injury, 10% as moderate, and 10% as severe.

AETIOLOGY/RISK FACTORS The main causes of head injury include injuries incurred from motor vehicle accidents, falls, acts of violence, and sports injuries. Motor vehicle crashes account for most fatal and severe head injuries. Young adults (15–35 years old) are the most commonly affected group, reflecting increased risk-taking behaviour. A second peak occurs in the elderly (more than 70 years old), related to an increased frequency of falls. For most age groups, with the exception of extremes of age, there is a 2:1 male predominance. Severe head injury marks the beginning of a continuing encephalopathic process — secondary brain damage from ongoing cerebral ischaemia closely linked to factors such as hypotension, hypercapnia, and elevated ICP is a potential cause of morbidity and mortality.

PROGNOSIS Head injury can result in death or a lifelong impairment in physical, cognitive, and psychosocial functioning. Several factors have been shown to correlate with poor outcome — including low post-resuscitation GCS score, older age, eye pupil abnormalities, hypoxia or hypotension before definitive treatment, traumatic subarachnoid haemorrhage, and inability to control ICP. Data from the Traumatic Coma Data Bank found that people with an initial GCS score of 3 had 78% mortality, whereas those with a GCS score of 8 had 11% mortality. Overall, prognoses for people with severe head injury (GCS score 3–8) were: good recovery 27%, moderate disability 16%, severe disability 16%, vegetative 5%, and mortality 36%. Despite such data, the role of GCS in determining prognosis in head injury remains controversial. The impacts of head injury range from mild cognitive and psychosocial changes to severe physical disability and cognitive and sensory losses.

Richard Nicholas and Jeremy Chataway

KEY POINTS

- Multiple sclerosis is characterised by central nervous system lesions causing neurological dysfunction and other problems such as fatigue, pain, depression, and anxiety.

  Early disease is usually relapsing and remitting, but most people develop secondary progressive disease over time. No treatment has been shown to affect long-term outcome.

  Irreversible disability can occur, but life expectancy is generally not affected.

- In people with relapsing and remitting disease, parenteral glatiramer acetate and azathioprine may reduce relapse rates, but have not been shown to affect disease progression.

  Intravenous immunoglobulin may prevent relapse after a first demyelinating event, but we don't know whether it is effective in people with relapsing and remitting disease.

  Interferon beta and mitoxantrone may reduce both exacerbations and disease progression.

  Oral glatiramer acetate may not reduce relapse rates, or delay disease progression.

  Toxicity associated with azathioprine means that 10% of people cannot tolerate it at therapeutic doses.

- CAUTION: Interferon beta and mitoxantrone have been associated with serious adverse effects.

- We don't know whether interferon beta, intravenous immunoglobulin, or methotrexate delay disease progression in people with secondary progressive multiple sclerosis, as studies have given conflicting results.

- Corticosteroids may improve symptoms in people with an acute exacerbation of multiple sclerosis compared with placebo, but we don't know whether plasma exchange or intravenous immunoglobulin are beneficial. We don't know which is the most effective corticosteroid.

  We don't know whether amantadine, behavioural modification, modafinil, or exercise reduce fatigue. Exercise may help to maintain strength, fitness, and mobility, but studies have been difficult to compare.

  We don't know whether botulinum toxin, gabapentin, intrathecal baclofen, oral antispasmodic drugs, or physiotherapy improve spasticity.

- Inpatient rehabilitation may improve function in the short term, but we don't know whether outpatient rehabilitation is also of benefit.

(i) **Please visit www.clinicalevidence.bmj.com for full text and references**

What are the effects of interventions aimed at reducing relapse rates and disability in people with multiple sclerosis?

Likely To Be Beneficial	• Glatiramer acetate (parenteral) in people with relapsing and remitting multiple sclerosis
	• Interferon beta in people having a first demyelinating event or with relapsing and remitting multiple sclerosis

	• Intravenous immunoglobulin in people having a first demyelinating event
Trade-off Between Benefits And Harms	• Azathioprine • Mitoxantrone in people with relapsing and remitting multiple sclerosis
Unknown Effectiveness	• Interferon beta in people with secondary progressive multiple sclerosis • Intravenous immunoglobulin in people with relapsing and remitting or secondary progressive multiple sclerosis • Methotrexate
Unlikely To Be Beneficial	• Glatiramer acetate (oral) in people with relapsing and remitting multiple sclerosis

What are the effects of interventions to improve symptoms during acute relapse in people with multiple sclerosis?

Likely To Be Beneficial	• Corticosteroids (methylprednisolone, corticotrophin, or dexamethasone) versus placebo
Unknown Effectiveness	• Corticosteroids (methylprednisolone, corticotrophin, or dexamethasone) versus each other (insufficient evidence to compare effectiveness) • Intravenous immunoglobulin in people with acute relapse of multiple sclerosis • Plasma exchange

What are the effects of treatments for fatigue in people with multiple sclerosis?

Unknown Effectiveness	• Amantadine • Behaviour modification • Exercise • Modafinil

What are the effects of treatments for spasticity in people with multiple sclerosis?

Unknown Effectiveness	• Botulinum toxin • Drug treatments (oral) • Gabapentin • Intrathecal baclofen • Physiotherapy

What are the effects of multidisciplinary care on disability in people with multiple sclerosis?

Unknown Effectiveness	• Inpatient rehabilitation • Outpatient rehabilitation

Search date November 2006

DEFINITION Multiple sclerosis is a chronic inflammatory disease of the central nervous system. Diagnosis requires evidence of lesions that are separated in both time and space, and the exclusion of other inflammatory, structural, or hereditary conditions that might give a similar clinical picture. The disease takes three main forms: relapsing and remitting multiple sclerosis, characterised by episodes of neurological dysfunction interspersed with periods of stability; primary progressive multiple sclerosis, in which progressive neurological disability occurs from the outset; and secondary progressive multiple sclerosis, in which progressive neurological disability occurs later in the course of the disease. Axonal loss is the major determinant of the accumulation of irreversible (progressive) disability as a result of inflammation during both the relapsing and remitting and progressive phases of multiple sclerosis, but also because of possible neurodegeneration through loss of trophic support. The emergence of treatment for multiple sclerosis has led to the recognition of a first demyelinating event or "clinically isolated syndrome" (CIS), a single episode of neurological dysfunction lasting for greater than 24 hours, that can be a prelude to multiple sclerosis. Characteristic episodes include optic neuritis, solitary brainstem lesions, and transverse myelitis that, when associated with magnetic resonance imaging changes, result in 30–70% risk of developing multiple sclerosis. Increasingly recognised are other demyelinating syndromes thought to be distinct from multiple sclerosis. These include Devic's disease (neuromyelitis optica), relapsing optic neuritis, and relapsing myelitis. Apart from episodes of neurological dysfunction, chronic symptoms produce much of the disability in multiple sclerosis. Symptoms include fatigue (the main symptom in two thirds of people), spasticity, bladder/bowel problems, ataxia/tremor, visual problems, pain, depression/anxiety, dysphagia, and sexual dysfunction.

INCIDENCE/PREVALENCE Prevalence varies with geography and racial group. It is highest in white populations in temperate regions. In Europe and North America, prevalence is 1/800 people, with an annual incidence of 2–10/100,000, making multiple sclerosis the most common cause of neurological disability in young adults. Age of onset is broad, peaking at between 20 and 40 years.

AETIOLOGY/RISK FACTORS The cause remains unclear, although current evidence suggests that multiple sclerosis is an autoimmune disorder of the central nervous system resulting from an environmental stimulus in genetically susceptible individuals. Multiple sclerosis is currently regarded as a single disorder with clinical variants, but there is some evidence that it may consist of several related disorders with distinct immunological, pathological, and genetic features.

PROGNOSIS In 90% of people, early disease is relapsing and remitting. Although some people follow a relatively benign course over many years, most develop secondary progressive disease, usually 6–10 years after onset. In 10% of people, initial disease is primary progressive. Apart from a minority of people with "aggressive" multiple sclerosis, life expectancy is not greatly affected, and the disease course is often of more than 30 years' duration.

Carl E Clarke and A Peter Moore

KEY POINTS

- Around 1% of adults have Parkinson's disease, with a median time of 9 years between diagnosis and death.

- Levodopa is considered effective at reducing symptoms in early Parkinson's disease, but can cause irreversible dyskinesias and motor fluctuation in the long term. We don't know whether levodopa, or any other treatment, improves survival.

    Modified-release levodopa seems no more effective than immediate-release levodopa at improving symptoms, and delaying motor complications.

- MAOBIs may improve symptoms, reduce motor fluctuations, and delay the need for levodopa, but can cause adverse effects.

- We don't know whether amantadine is beneficial for people with early Parkinson's disease, although it is currently used to treat dyskinesia. People taking amantadine for dyskinesia in early Parkinson's may have a higher risk of psychiatric adverse effects in the later stages of the disease.

- Adding a catechol-O-methyl transferase (COMT) inhibitor or dopamine agonist to levodopa, or using dopamine agonists as monotherapy, may reduce 'off' time and improve symptoms compared with levodopa alone, but can cause adverse effects.

    The COMT inhibitor tolcapone can cause fatal hepatic toxicity.

- Surgery may be considered in people with later Parkinson's disease, but can cause fatalities. Postoperative complications include speech problems and apraxia.

    Although evidence is lacking, many clinicians feel that both pallidal deep brain stimulation and subthalamic nucleus deep brain stimulation improve symptoms of advanced Parkinson's disease.

    Bilateral subthalamic nucleus deep brain stimulation may lead to greater improvement in motor symptoms, but more cognitive impairment, than pallidal deep brain stimulation. Pallidal deep brain stimulation is associated with severe intraoperative complications.

    Adding subthalamic nucleus deep brain stimulation to medical treatment may improve quality of life and motor symptoms compared with medical treatment alone or other forms of surgery. It can, however, cause neurological complications, neuropsychological adverse effects, and fatal surgical complications.

    Unilateral pallidotomy may improve symptoms and function more than medical treatment, but may be less effective than bilateral subthalamic stimulation.

    We don't know whether subthalamotomy or thalamotomy are effective.

- Nurse-specialist interventions, occupational therapy, physiotherapy, speech and language therapy, and swallowing therapy are generally considered effective and safe in people with Parkinson's disease, although few studies have been found.

Please visit www.clinicalevidence.bmj.com for full text and references

What are the effects of drug treatments in people with early-stage Parkinson's disease?

Beneficial	• Immediate-release levodopa† (compared with placebo or no treatment)*
Trade-off Between Benefits And Harms	• Dopamine agonists (reduced dyskinesia and motor fluctuations compared with levodopa†, but were associated with increased treatment withdrawal and poorer motor scores) • Dopamine agonists plus levodopa† (reduced dyskinesia compared with levodopa alone, but increased disability) • MAOBIs
Unknown Effectiveness	• Amantadine
Unlikely To Be Beneficial	• Modified-release levodopa† (no more effective than immediate-release levodopa)

What are the effects of adding other treatments in people with Parkinson's disease who have motor complications from levodopa?

Likely To Be Beneficial	• Adding amantadine to reduce dyskinesia*
Trade-off Between Benefits And Harms	• Adding a catechol-O-methyl transferase (COMT) inhibitor to levodopa† • Adding a dopamine agonist to levodopa†

What are the effects of surgery in people with later Parkinson's disease?

Trade-off Between Benefits And Harms	• Pallidal deep brain stimulation • Pallidotomy • Subthalamic nucleus deep brain stimulation
Unknown Effectiveness	• Subthalamotomy • Thalamic deep brain stimulation • Thalamotomy

What are the effects of nursing and rehabilitation treatments in people with Parkinson's disease?

Likely To Be Beneficial	• Parkinson's disease nurse specialist interventions*
Unknown Effectiveness	• Occupational therapy • Physiotherapy

- Speech and language therapy for speech disturbance
- Swallowing therapy for dysphagia

Search date November 2006

*Categorisation based on consensus.
†We have used the term levodopa to refer to a combination of levodopa and a peripheral decarboxylase inhibitor.

DEFINITION Idiopathic Parkinson's disease is an age-related neurodegenerative disorder, which is associated with a combination of asymmetrical bradykinesia, hypokinesia, and rigidity, sometimes combined with rest tremor and postural changes. Clinical diagnostic criteria have a sensitivity of 80% and a specificity of 30% (likelihood ratio +ve test 1.14, −ve test 0.67) compared with the gold standard of diagnosis at autopsy. The primary pathology is progressive loss of cells that produce the neurotransmitter dopamine from the substantia nigra in the brainstem. Treatment aims to replace or compensate for the lost dopamine. A good response to treatment supports, but does not confirm, the diagnosis. Several other catecholaminergic neurotransmitter systems are also affected in Parkinson's disease. There is no consistent definition distinguishing early from late-stage Parkinson's disease. In this review, we consider people with early-stage disease to be those who have not yet developed motor complications associated with long-term levodopa treatment (such as dyskinesias and motor fluctuations, also known as "on/off" fluctuations). Late-stage Parkinson's disease is taken to mean that motor complications of long-term levodopa treatment are present.

INCIDENCE/PREVALENCE Parkinson's disease occurs worldwide, with equal incidence in both sexes. In 5–10% of people who develop Parkinson's disease, the condition appears before the age of 40 (young onset). The mean age of onset is about 65. Overall age-adjusted prevalence is 1% worldwide, and 1.6% in Europe, rising from 0.6% at age 60–64 to 3.5% at age 85–89.

AETIOLOGY/RISK FACTORS The cause is unknown. Parkinson's disease may represent different conditions with a final common pathway. People may be affected differently by a combination of genetic and environmental factors (viruses, toxins, 1-methyl-4-phenyl-1, 2, 3, 6-tetrahydropyridine, well water, vitamin E, and smoking). First-degree relatives of affected people may have twice the risk of developing Parkinson's disease (17% chance of developing the condition in their lifetime) compared with the general population. However, purely genetic varieties probably affect a small minority of people with Parkinson's disease. The parkin gene on chromosome 6 may be associated with Parkinson's disease in families with at least one member with young-onset Parkinson's disease; and multiple genetic factors, including the tau gene on chromosome 17q21, may be involved in idiopathic late-onset disease.

PROGNOSIS Parkinson's disease is currently incurable. Disability is progressive, and is associated with increased mortality (RR of death compared with matched control populations ranges from 1.6–3.0). Treatment can reduce symptoms and slow progression, but rarely achieves complete control. Whether treatment reduces mortality remains controversial. Levodopa seemed to reduce mortality in the UK for 5 years after its introduction, before a "catch-up" effect was noted, and overall mortality rose towards previous levels. This suggested a limited prolonging of life. An Australian cohort study followed 130 people treated for 10 years. The standardised mortality ratio was 1.58 (P less than 0.001). At 10 years, 25% had been admitted to a nursing home, and only four people were still employed. The mean duration of disease until death was 9.1 years. In a similar Italian cohort study conducted over 8 years, the relative risk of death for affected people compared with healthy controls was 2.3 (95% CI 1.60 to 3.39). Age at initial census date was the main predictor of outcome (for people aged under 75 years: RR of death 1.80, 95% CI 1.04 to 3.11; for people aged over 75 years: RR of death 5.61, 95% CI 2.13 to 14.80).

Trigeminal neuralgia

Joanna M Zakrzewska and Mark Linskey

KEY POINTS

- Trigeminal neuralgia is a sudden, unilateral, brief, stabbing, recurrent pain in the distribution of one or more branches of the fifth cranial nerve. The diagnosis is made on the history alone, based on characteristic features of the pain.

  Pain occurs in paroxysms which last between a few seconds to 2 minutes. The frequency of the paroxysms ranges from a few to hundreds of attacks a day.

  Periods of remission can last for months to years, but tend to get shorter over time.

  The annual incidence in the UK is 26.8/100,000.

- Carbamazepine is considered the gold standard in treatment for symptoms of trigeminal neuralgia.

  Carbamazepine has been shown to increase pain relief compared with placebo, but also increases adverse effects, such as drowsiness, dizziness, constipation, and ataxia.

  Long-term use may reduce the effectiveness of carbamazepine.

  There is consensus that oxcarbazepine is an effective treatment in people with trigeminal neuralgia, although there is a lack of RCT-based data to confirm this.

- We found insufficient evidence to judge the effectiveness of tizanidine, baclofen, or lamotrigine.

  Lamotrigine is often used in people who cannot tolerate carbamazepine, but the dose must be escalated slowly to avoid rashes, thus making it unsuitable for acute use.

  There is consensus that baclofen may be useful for people with multiple sclerosis who develop trigeminal neuralgia.

- We don't know the effectiveness of other antiepileptic drugs, such as phenytoin, clonazepam, sodium valproate, gabapentin, or topimirate, or of the antiarrhythmic drug mexiletine in people with trigeminal neuralgia.

- Despite a lack of RCT data, observational evidence has suggested that microvascular decompression may relieve symptoms of trigeminal neuralgia.

- We found no good-quality studies that examined the effectiveness of nerve treatments, such as cryotherapy, nerve block, radiosurgery, or acupuncture.

- Proparacaine eye drops (single application) do not seem to relieve pain in people with trigeminal neuralgia, despite initial open-label use that suggested they were helpful.

Please visit www.clinicalevidence.bmj.com for full text and references

What are the effects of treatments in people with trigeminal neuralgia?

Likely To Be Beneficial	• Baclofen (in people with multiple sclerosis who develop trigeminal neuralgia)* • Carbamazepine • Oxcarbazepine*
Unknown Effectiveness	• Cryotherapy of peripheral nerves • Lamotrigine

	• Mexiletine
	• Microvascular decompression
	• Nerve block
	• Other antiepileptics (phenytoin, clonazepam, sodium valproate, gabapentin, topiramate)
	• Peripheral acupuncture
	• Peripheral laser surgery
	• Stereotactic radiosurgery
	• Tizanidine
Unlikely To Be Beneficial	• Proparacaine eye drops (single application)

Search date August 2006

*Categorisation based on consensus.

DEFINITION Trigeminal neuralgia is a characteristic pain in the distribution of one or more branches of the fifth cranial nerve. The diagnosis is made on the history alone, based on characteristic features of the pain. It occurs in paroxysms, with each pain lasting a few seconds to 2 minutes. The frequency of paroxysms is highly variable, ranging from hundreds of attacks a day to long periods of remission that can last years. Between paroxysms, the person is asymptomatic. The pain is severe and described as intense, sharp, superficial, stabbing, shooting — often like an electric shock. In any individual, the pain has the same character in different attacks. It is triggered by light touch in a specific area or by eating, talking, washing the face, or cleaning the teeth. Other causes of facial pain may need to be excluded. In trigeminal neuralgia, the neurological examination is usually normal.

INCIDENCE/PREVALENCE Most evidence about the incidence and prevalence of trigeminal neuralgia is from the USA. The annual incidence (age adjusted to the 1980 age distribution of the USA) is 5.9/100,000 women and 3.4/100,000 men. The incidence tends to be slightly higher in women at all ages, and increases with age. In men aged over 80 years, the incidence is 45.2/100,000. One questionnaire survey of neurological disease in a single French village found one person with trigeminal neuralgia among 993 people. A retrospective cohort study in UK primary care, which examined the histories of 6.8 million people, found that 8268 people had trigeminal neuralgia, giving it an incidence of 26.8/100,000 person years.

AETIOLOGY/RISK FACTORS The cause of trigeminal neuralgia remains unclear. It is more common in people with multiple sclerosis (RR 20.0, 95% CI 4.1 to 59.0). Hypertension is a risk factor in women (RR 2.1, 95% CI 1.2 to 3.4) but the evidence is less clear for men (RR 1.53, 95% CI 0.30 to 4.50). One case control study in the USA found that people with trigeminal neuralgia smoked less, consumed less alcohol, had fewer tonsillectomies, and were less likely than matched controls to be Jewish or an immigrant.

PROGNOSIS One retrospective cohort study found no reduction in 10-year survival in people with trigeminal neuralgia. We found no evidence about the natural history of trigeminal neuralgia. The illness is characterised by recurrences and remissions. Many people have periods of remission with no pain for months or years. Anecdotal reports suggest that in many people it becomes more severe and less responsive to treatment with time. Most people with trigeminal neuralgia are initially managed medically, and a proportion eventually have a surgical procedure. We found no good evidence about the proportion of people who require surgical treatment for pain control. Anecdotal evidence indicates that pain relief is better after surgery than with medical treatment.

444 Aphthous ulcers (recurrent)

Stephen Porter and Crispian Scully CBE

KEY POINTS

- Most people with recurrent aphthous ulcers develop a few ulcers less than 1 cm in diameter, that heal after 5–14 days without scarring.

  The causes are unknown, but risks of recurrence may decrease if the person gives up smoking.

  Local physical trauma may trigger ulcers in susceptible people.

  In 10% of sufferers, lesions are more than 1 cm in diameter and can cause scarring.

- Chlorhexidine mouth rinses may reduce the severity and pain of ulceration, although studies have reported inconclusive results about whether the incidence of new ulcers is reduced.

- We don't know whether topical corticosteroids reduce the number of new ulcers, but they may reduce pain and increase healing of ulcers without causing notable adverse effects.

- We don't know whether carbenoxolone gel or mouthwash, local analgesics, or tetracycline mouthwash work, as we found few well-planned studies.

(i) **Please visit www.clinicalevidence.bmj.com for full text and references**

What are the effects of treatments for recurrent aphthous ulcers?

Likely To Be Beneficial	• Chlorhexidine and similar agents
Unknown Effectiveness	• Analgesics (Local) • Carbenoxolone mouthwash • Corticosteroids (topical) • Tetracycline antibiotic mouthwash

Search date August 2006

DEFINITION Recurrent aphthous ulcers are superficial, rounded, painful mouth ulcers usually occurring in recurrent bouts at intervals of a few days to a few months in otherwise well people.

INCIDENCE/PREVALENCE The point prevalence of recurrent aphthous ulcers in Swedish adults has been reported as 2%. Prevalence may be 5–10% in some groups of children. Up to 66% of young adults give a history consistent with recurrent aphthous ulceration.

AETIOLOGY/RISK FACTORS The cause of aphthous ulcers remains unknown. Associations with haematinic deficiency, infections, gluten-sensitive enteropathy, food sensitivities, and psychological stress have rarely been confirmed. Similar ulcers are seen in Behçet's syndrome. Local physical trauma may initiate ulcers in susceptible people. Recurrent aphthous ulcers are uncommon on keratinised oral mucosal surfaces, and the frequency of recurrent aphthous ulcers may fall if people cease any tobacco smoking habit.

PROGNOSIS About 80% of people with recurrent aphthous ulcers develop a few ulcers smaller than 1 cm in diameter that heal within 5–14 days without scarring (the pattern known as minor aphthous ulceration). The episodes recur typically after an interval of 1–4 months. One in 10 people with recurrent ulceration may have multiple minute ulcers (herpetiform ulceration). Likewise, one in 10 sufferers has a more severe form (major aphthous ulceration), with lesions larger than 1 cm that may recur after a shorter interval, which and can cause scarring. Most of the trials in this review have focused on the treatment of minor aphthous ulceration.

John Buchanan and Joanna Zakrzewska

KEY POINTS

- Burning mouth syndrome is characterised by discomfort or pain of the mouth, with no known medical or dental cause. It may affect up to a third of postmenopausal women and up to 15% of adults overall.

  Symptoms of burning mouth can also be caused by infections, allergies, vitamin deficiencies, and ill-fitting dentures, leading to problems identifying effective treatments.

  Psychogenic factors may be involved in some people, such as anxiety, depression, or personality disorders.

  People with burning mouth syndrome may show altered sensory and pain thresholds, or other signs of neuropathy.

  Long-term outcomes are unknown, but half of people may have spontaneous resolution of their symptoms over 6–7 years.

- CBT may improve symptom intensity compared with placebo, although no good-quality studies have been found.

- Topical clonazepam may reduce pain compared with placebo, but may be absorbed systemically, with increased risk of dependence over time.

  We don't know whether antidepressants, benzydamine hydrochloride, dietary supplements, or HRT in postmenopausal women can improve symptoms of burning mouth, as few studies have been found.

(i) **Please visit www.clinicalevidence.bmj.com for full text and references**

What are the effects of treatments for burning mouth syndrome?	
Likely To Be Beneficial	• CBT
Trade-off Between Benefits And Harms	• Benzodiazepines (topical clonazepam)
Unknown Effectiveness	• Anaesthetics (local)
	• Antidepressants
	• Benzydamine hydrochloride
	• Dietary supplements
	• HRT in postmenopausal women

Search date February 2007

DEFINITION Burning mouth syndrome is an idiopathic burning discomfort or pain affecting people with clinically normal oral mucosa, in whom a medical or dental cause has been excluded. Terms previously used to describe what is now called burning mouth syndrome include glossodynia, glossopyrosis, stomatodynia, stomatopyrosis, sore tongue, and oral dysaesthesia. A survey of 669 men and 758 women randomly selected from 48,500 people aged 20–69 years found that people with burning mouth also have subjective dryness (66%), take some form of medication (64%), report other systemic illnesses (57%), and have altered taste (11%). Many studies of people with symptoms of burning mouth do not distinguish those with burning mouth syndrome (i.e. idiopathic disease) from those with other conditions (such as vitamin B deficiency), making results unreliable. Local and

(continued over)

(from previous page)

systemic factors (such as infections, allergies, ill-fitting dentures, hypersensitivity reactions, and hormone and vitamin deficiencies) may cause the symptom of burning mouth, and should be excluded before diagnosing burning mouth syndrome. This review deals only with idiopathic burning mouth syndrome.

INCIDENCE/PREVALENCE Burning mouth syndrome mainly affects women, particularly after the menopause, when its prevalence may be 18–33%. One study in Sweden found a prevalence of 4% for the symptom of burning mouth without clinical abnormality of the oral mucosa (11/669 [2%] men, mean age 59 years; 42/758 [6%] women, mean age 57 years), with the highest prevalence (12%) in women aged 60–69 years. Reported prevalence in general populations varies from 1% to 15%. Incidence and prevalence vary according to diagnostic criteria, and many studies included people with the symptom of burning mouth, rather than with burning mouth syndrome as defined above.

AETIOLOGY/RISK FACTORS The cause is unknown, and we found no good aetiological studies. Possible causal factors include hormonal disturbances associated with the menopause, psychogenic factors (including anxiety, depression, stress, life events, personality disorders, and phobia of cancer), and neuropathy in so-called supertasters. Support for a neuropathic aetiology comes from studies that have shown altered sensory and pain thresholds in people with burning mouth syndrome. Two studies using blink reflex and thermal quantitative sensory tests have demonstrated signs of neuropathy in most people with burning mouth syndrome.

PROGNOSIS We found no prospective cohort studies describing the natural history of burning mouth syndrome. We found anecdotal reports of at least partial spontaneous remission in about 50% of people with burning mouth syndrome within 6–7 years. However, a recent retrospective study assessing 53 people with burning mouth syndrome (48 women and 5 men, mean duration of burning mouth syndrome 5.5 years, mean follow-up 56 months) found a complete spontaneous resolution of oral symptoms in 11% of people (2/19) who received no treatment. Overall, 30% of people (15/53) experienced a moderate improvement, with or without treatment.

Caroline L Pankhurst

KEY POINTS

- Opportunistic infection with Candida albicans causes painful red or white lesions of the oropharynx, which can affect taste, speech, and eating.

  Candida is present in the mouth of up to 60% of healthy people, but overt infection is associated with immunosuppression, diabetes, broad-spectrum antibiotics, and corticosteroid use.

- In people with immunosuppression following cancer treatment, absorbed or partially absorbed antifungal drugs (ketoconazole, itraconazole, fluconazole) prevent oropharyngeal candidiasis compared with placebo or non-absorbed antifungal drugs.

  Non-absorbed antifungal drugs (nystatin, amphotericin B) may be no more effective than placebo at preventing candidiasis.

  We don't know whether antifungal prophylaxis is effective in adults having radiotherapy or tissue transplants, as few studies have been found.

  We don't know whether any treatments are effective in preventing or treating oropharyngeal candidiasis in people with diabetes mellitus.

- Fluconazole is more effective than oral nystatin or amphotericin B at preventing candidiasis in immunocompromised infants and children, while fluconazole and miconazole increase cure rates compared with nystatin.

- Antifungal drugs may increase clinical improvement or cure in people with oropharyngeal candidiasis caused by wearing dentures.

  We don't know whether denture hygiene or removing dentures at night reduces the risk of developing oropharyngeal candidiasis.

- Daily or weekly prophylaxis with fluconazole, itraconazole, or nystatin reduces the incidence and relapse rates of candidiasis in people with HIV infection.

  Topical suspensions of miconazole, clotrimazole, and itraconazole, used in a swish-and-swallow mode, are as effective as oral tablets or pastilles at reducing symptoms of candidiasis in people with HIV infection.

- Continuous prophylaxis with antifungal agents has not been shown to increase the risk of developing antifungal resistance in people with HIV infection compared with intermittent prophylaxis, and is more likely to reduce the number of attacks.

(i) **Please visit www.clinicalevidence.bmj.com for full text and references**

What are the effects of interventions to prevent and treat oropharyngeal candidiasis in adults having treatment causing immunosuppression?

Beneficial	• Antifungal prophylaxis with absorbed or partially absorbed antifungal drugs in adults having anticancer drugs (more effective than placebo or non-absorbed drugs)
Unknown Effectiveness	• Antifungal prophylaxis in adults having tissue transplants (to prevent oropharyngeal candidiasis) • Antifungal treatment in adults having chemotherapy, radiotherapy, or both treatments for cancer

What are the effects of interventions to prevent and treat oropharyngeal candidiasis in infants and children?

Beneficial	• Antifungal treatment with miconazole or fluconazole in immunocompetent and immunocompromised infants and children (more effective than nystatin)
Likely To Be Beneficial	• Antifungal prophylaxis with fluconazole in immunocompromised infants and children (more effective than oral nystatin or amphotericin B)

What are the effects of interventions to prevent and treat oropharyngeal candidiasis in people with diabetes?

Unknown Effectiveness	• Antifungal prophylaxis or treatment in people with diabetes mellitus

What are the effects of interventions to prevent and treat oropharyngeal candidiasis in people with dentures?

Likely To Be Beneficial	• Antifungal treatment for denture stomatitis
Unknown Effectiveness	• Denture hygiene

What are the effects of interventions to prevent and treat oropharyngeal candidiasis in people with HIV infection?

Beneficial	• Antifungal prophylaxis with fluconazole, itraconazole, or nystatin in people with advanced HIV disease
	• Topical antifungal treatment (absorbed, partially absorbed, and non-absorbed antifungal drugs in people with HIV infection)

Which treatments reduce the risk of acquiring resistance to antifungal drugs?

Unlikely To Be Beneficial	• Intermittent treatment in people with HIV infection and acute episodes of oropharyngeal candidiasis (no difference in antifungal resistance and increased recurrence of oropharyngeal candidiasis compared with continuous prophylaxis)

Search date June 2006

DEFINITION Oropharyngeal candidiasis is an opportunistic mucosal infection caused, in most cases, by *Candida albicans*, but which can be caused by other species such as *C glabrata*, *C tropicalis*, and *C krusei*. The four main types of oropharyngeal candidiasis are: (1) pseudomembranous (thrush), consisting of white, curd-like, discrete plaques on an erythematous background, which is exposed after the removal of the plaque, and found on the buccal mucosa, throat, tongue, or gingivae; (2) erythematous, consisting of smooth red patches on the hard or soft palate, dorsum of tongue, or buccal mucosa; (3) hyperplastic, consisting of white, firmly adherent patches or plaques that cannot be removed, usually bilaterally distributed on the buccal mucosa, tongue, or palate; and (4) denture-induced stomatitis, presenting as either a smooth or granular erythema confined to the denture bearing area of the hard palate, and often associated with an angular cheilitis, which occurs as red, fissured lesions in the corners of the mouth. Symptoms vary, ranging from none to a sore and painful mouth with a burning tongue and altered taste. Oropharyngeal candidiasis can impair speech, nutritional intake, and quality of life. Oropharyngeal candidiasis is the most common oral manifestation of HIV infection. HIV-seropositive people with recurrent oropharyngeal candidiasis have overall lower levels of oral health as measured by a higher decayed, missing, and filled-teeth index, dry mouth, and taste problems.

INCIDENCE/PREVALENCE *Candida* species are commensals in the gastrointestinal tract. Most infections are endogenously acquired, although infections in neonates can be primary infections. Transmission can also occur directly from infected people or on fomites (objects that can harbour pathogenic organisms). *Candida* is found in the mouth of 18–60% of healthy people in high- and middle-income countries. One cross-sectional study in China (77 HIV-seropositive outpatients and 217 HIV-negative students) found no significant difference in the rates of asymptomatic *Candida* carriage reported in healthy and HIV-seropositive people (18.0% of healthy people v 28.6% of HIV-seropositive people; P = 0.07). Denture stomatitis associated with *Candida* is prevalent in 65% of denture wearers. Oropharyngeal candidiasis affects 15–60% of people with haematological or oncological malignancies during periods of immunosuppression. Oropharyngeal candidiasis occurs in 7–48% of people with HIV infection and in over 90% of those with advanced disease. In severely immunosuppressed people, relapse rates are high (30–50%) and relapse usually occurs within 14 days of stopping treatment.

AETIOLOGY/RISK FACTORS Risk factors associated with symptomatic oropharyngeal candidiasis include: local or systemic immunosuppression; haematological disorders; broad-spectrum antibiotic use; inhaled or systemic steroids; xerostomia; diabetes; wearing dentures, obturators, or orthodontic appliances; and smoking. Smoking predisposes to oral carriage of *Candida*. In one study of 2499 men with HIV and a baseline CD4+ cell count greater than 200 cells/μL, smoking increased the risk of pseudomembranous candidiasis by 40% (P less than or equal to 0.01). However, another study (139 people with HIV) suggested that smoking was not a risk factor for those with a baseline CD4+ cell count less than 200 cells/μL. The exact mechanism of action by which smoking predisposes to *Candida* is not known, but may involve the impairment of local immunity by inducing cytokine changes and reducing epithelial cell mediated anticandidal activity. The same *Candida* strain may persist for months or years in the absence of infection. In people with HIV infection, there is no direct correlation between the number of organisms and the presence of clinical disease. Candidal strains causing disease in people with HIV infection seem to be the same as those colonising people who are HIV negative, and in most people do not change over time. Symptomatic oropharyngeal candidiasis associated with *in vitro* resistance to fluconazole occurs in 5% of people with advanced HIV disease. Resistance to azole antifungal drugs is associated with severe immunosuppression (CD4+ cell count 50 cells/μL or less), more episodes treated with antifungal drugs, and longer median duration of systemic azole treatment.

PROGNOSIS In most people, untreated candidiasis persists for months or years unless associated risk factors are treated or eliminated. In neonates, spontaneous cure of oropharyngeal candidiasis usually occurs after 3–8 weeks.

Crispian Scully CBE and Stephen Porter

KEY POINTS

- **Halitosis can be caused by oral disease, or by respiratory-tract conditions such as sinusitis, tonsillitis, and bronchiectasis, but an estimated 40% of affected individuals have no underlying disease.**

  The main chemicals causing the odour seem to be volatile sulphur compounds, but little is known about the cause of physiological halitosis.

- **Regular use of a mouthwash may reduce breath odour compared with placebo, but single-use mouthwash may have only a short-term benefit.**

- **We don't know whether tongue cleaning, sugar-free chewing gums, zinc toothpastes, artificial saliva, or dietary modification reduce halitosis, as no studies of adequate quality have been found.**

Please visit www.clinicalevidence.bmj.com for full text and references

What are the effects of treatments in people with physiological halitosis?	
Likely To Be Beneficial	• Regular-use mouthwash • Single-use mouthwash (short-term benefit only)
Unknown Effectiveness	• Artificial saliva • Diet modification (drinking plenty of liquids; chewing herbs; eating fresh, fibrous vegetables such as carrots; avoiding coffee) • Sugar-free chewing gums • Tongue cleaning, brushing, or scraping • Zinc toothpastes

Search date December 2006

DEFINITION Halitosis is an unpleasant odour emitted from the mouth. It may be caused by oral conditions, including poor oral hygiene, and periodontal disease, or by respiratory-tract conditions, such as chronic sinusitis, tonsillitis, and bronchiectasis. In this review, we deal only with physiological halitosis (i.e. confirmed persistent bad breath in the absence of systemic, oral, or periodontal disease). We have excluded halitosis caused by underlying systemic disease which would require disease-specific treatment, pseudo-halitosis (in people who believe they have bad breath but whose breath is not considered malodorous by others), and artificially-induced halitosis (e.g. in studies requiring people to stop brushing their teeth). This review is only applicable, therefore, to people in whom such underlying causes have been ruled out, and in whom pseudo-halitosis has been excluded. There is no consensus regarding duration of bad breath for diagnosis of halitosis, although the standard organoleptic test for bad breath involves smelling the breath on at least two or three different days.

INCIDENCE/PREVALENCE We found no reliable estimate of prevalence, although several studies report the population prevalence of halitosis (physiological or because of underlying disease) to be about 50%. One cross-sectional study of 491 people found that about 5% of people with halitosis have pseudo-halitosis and about 40% have physiological bad breath not caused by underlying disease. We found no reliable data about age or sex distribution of physiological halitosis.

AETIOLOGY/RISK FACTORS We found no reliable data about risk factors for physiological bad breath. Mass spectrometric and gas chromatographic analysis of expelled air from the mouths of people with any type of halitosis have shown that the principal malodorants are volatile sulphur compounds, including hydrogen sulphide, methyl mercaptan, and dimethyl sulphide.

PROGNOSIS We found no evidence on the prognosis of halitosis.

Impacted wisdom teeth

Marco Esposito

KEY POINTS

- Impacted wisdom teeth occur because of a lack of space, obstruction, or abnormal position.

  They can cause pain, swelling, infection, and may destroy adjacent teeth and bone.

  The incidence is high, with some 72% of Swedish people between the ages of 20 and 30 having at least one impacted third molar.

- The surgical removal of impacted third molars (symptomatic and asymptomatic) is the most common procedure performed by oral and maxillofacial surgeons.

- While it is clear that symptomatic impacted wisdom teeth should be surgically removed, it appears that extracting asymptomatic, disease-free wisdom teeth is not advisable because of the risk of damage to the inferior alveolar nerve.

  Some non-RCT evidence suggests that extraction of the asymptomatic tooth may be beneficial if caries are present in the adjacent second molar, or if periodontal pockets are present distal to the second molar.

Please visit www.clinicalevidence.bmj.com for full text and references

Should asymptomatic and disease-free impacted wisdom teeth be removed prophylactically?

Likely To Be Ineffective Or Harmful	• Prophylactic extraction

Search date August 2005

DEFINITION Wisdom teeth are third molars that develop in the majority of adults and generally erupt between the ages of 18 and 24 years, although there is wide variation in the age of eruption. In some people, the teeth become partially or completely impacted below the gum line because of lack of space, obstruction, or abnormal position. Impacted wisdom teeth may be diagnosed because of pain and swelling or incidentally by routine dental radiography.

INCIDENCE/PREVALENCE Third molar impaction is common. Over 72% of Swedish people aged 20–30 have at least one impacted lower third molar. The surgical removal of impacted third molars (symptomatic and asymptomatic) is the most common procedure performed by oral and maxillofacial surgeons. It is performed on about 4/1000 people each year in England and Wales, making it one of the top 10 inpatient and day case procedures. Up to 90% of people on oral and maxillofacial surgery hospital waiting lists are awaiting removal of wisdom teeth.

AETIOLOGY/RISK FACTORS Retention and impaction of wisdom teeth may be more common than it was previously because the modern diet tends to be softer than in the past.

PROGNOSIS Impacted wisdom teeth can cause pain, swelling, and infection, and may destroy adjacent teeth and bone. The removal of diseased and symptomatic wisdom teeth alleviates pain and suffering and improves oral health and function. We found no good evidence on untreated prognosis in people with asymptomatic impacted wisdom teeth.

Michelle Conde and Valerie Lawrence

KEY POINTS

- Postoperative pulmonary infections are associated with cough, phlegm, shortness of breath, chest pain, temperature above 38 °C, and pulse rate above 100 a minute.

    Up to half of people may have asymptomatic chest signs after surgery, and up to a quarter develop symptomatic disease.

    The main risk factor is the type of surgery, with higher risks associated with surgery to the chest, abdomen, and head and neck compared with other operations.

    Other risk factors include age over 50 years, prior COPD, smoking, recent alcohol use, and being functionally dependent.

- Prophylactic lung-expansion techniques reduce the risk of pulmonary infection in people undergoing abdominal surgery, but we don't know whether they are of benefit in people undergoing cardiac surgery, or in people at low risk of infection.

    We don't know which is the most effective lung-expansion technique to use.

- Regional anaesthesia (epidural or spinal), either alone or with general anaesthesia, may reduce the risk of developing postoperative pulmonary infections compared with general anaesthesia alone, although studies have given conflicting results.

    It has been estimated that one infection would be prevented for every 50 people having regional anaesthesia.

    Regional anaesthesia is associated with a small risk (around 4 per 10,000 procedures in total) of seizures, cardiac arrest, respiratory depression, or neurological injury.

- We don't know whether advice to stop smoking before surgery reduces the risk of developing postoperative pulmonary infections.

    It is possible that people need to have stopped smoking at least 2 months before surgery in order to reduce the risks of chest infection.

(i) **Please visit www.clinicalevidence.bmj.com for full text and references**

What are the effects of interventions to prevent postoperative pulmonary infections?	
Beneficial	• Prophylactic lung expansion techniques
Likely To Be Beneficial	• Regional (epidural or spinal) anaesthesia
Unknown Effectiveness	• Advice to stop smoking preoperatively

Search date May 2006

DEFINITION A working diagnosis of postoperative pulmonary infection may be based on three or more new findings from: cough, phlegm, shortness of breath, chest pain, temperature above 38 °C, and pulse rate above 100 a minute. In this review, we are dealing strictly with pneumonia that is regarded to be a complication of the operation. We examine a selection of pre-, intra-, and postoperative techniques to reduce the risk of this

(continued over)

(from previous page)

complication. In this review, the diagnosis of pneumonia implies consolidation observed in a chest radiograph.

INCIDENCE/PREVALENCE Reported morbidity for chest complications depends on how carefully they are investigated and the type of surgery performed. One observational study found blood-gas and chest-radiograph abnormalities in about 50% of people after open cholecystectomy. However, less than 20% of these had abnormal clinical signs and only 10% had a clinically significant chest infection. One observational study found the incidence of pneumonia to be 17.5% after thoracic and abdominal surgeries. Another observational study found the incidence of pneumonia to be 2.8% (using a more restrictive definition of pneumonia) after laparotomy.

AETIOLOGY/RISK FACTORS Risk factors include increasing age (over 50 years), with the odds of developing postoperative pneumonia systematically increasing with each decile above the age of 50 years; functional dependency; a history of COPD; weight loss more than 10% in last 6 months; impaired sensorium (acute confusion / delirium associated with current illness); cigarette smoking; recent alcohol use; and blood urea nitrogen level above 7.5 mmol/L. Serum albumin level below 35 g/l is also a risk factor for the development of overall postoperative pulmonary complications. The strongest risk factor, however, is the type of surgery (particularly aortic aneurysm repair, thoracic surgery, abdominal surgery, neurosurgery, head and neck surgery, and vascular surgery). Interestingly, obesity was not found to be an independent risk factor in a recent systematic review of preoperative pulmonary risk stratification for non-cardiothoracic surgery.

PROGNOSIS In one large systematic review (search date 1997, 141 RCTs, 9559 people), 10% of people with postoperative pneumonia died. If systemic sepsis ensues, mortality is likely to be substantial. Pneumonia delays recovery from surgery and poor tissue oxygenation may contribute to delayed wound healing. In a cohort of 160,805 US veterans undergoing major non-cardiac surgery, 1.5% of people developed postoperative pneumonia, and the 30-day mortality rate was 10-fold higher in these people compared with those without postoperative pneumonia.

Nicholas Phin

KEY POINTS

- The main symptoms of carbon monoxide poisoning are non-specific in nature, and relate to effects on the brain and heart. The symptoms correlate poorly with serum carboxyhaemoglobin levels.

    People with comorbidity, the elderly or very young, and pregnant women are most susceptible.

    Carbon monoxide is produced by the incomplete combustion of carbon fuels, including inadequately ventilated heaters and car exhausts, or from chemicals such as methylene chloride paint stripper.

    Poisoning is considered to have occurred at carboxyhaemoglobin levels over 10%, with severe poisoning associated with levels over 20–25% plus symptoms associated with severe cerebral or cardiac ischaemia. However, people living in areas of pollution may have levels of 5%, and heavy smokers can tolerate levels up to 15%.

    Severe poisoning can be fatal, and up to a third of survivors have delayed neurological sequelae.

- Immediate care requires removal of the person from the source of carbon monoxide and giving oxygen through a non-re-breather mask.

    Normobaric 100% oxygen is considered to be effective, but studies proving benefit compared with air or lower concentrations of oxygen have not been found and would be unethical.

    28% oxygen is used by paramedics and is thought to be beneficial compared with air, but may be less effective than higher concentrations.

    We don't know what is the optimum duration of oxygen treatment, but it is usually continued for at least 6 hours, or until carboxyhaemoglobin levels fall below 5%.

- We don't know whether hyperbaric oxygen is more effective than normobaric 100% oxygen at preventing neurological complications in people with mild carbon monoxide poisoning, but it may be beneficial in more severe poisoning.

    Hyperbaric 100% oxygen reduces the half-life of carboxyhaemoglobin, but clinical benefit may depend on the treatment regimen used.

    The possible benefits of hyperbaric oxygen for an individual need to be weighed against the hazards of a long journey by ambulance.

(i) **Please visit www.clinicalevidence.bmj.com for full text and references**

What are the effects of oxygen treatments for acute carbon monoxide poisoning?	
Beneficial	• Oxygen 100% via non-re-breather mask (compared with air)*
Likely To Be Beneficial	• Hyperbaric oxygen 100% at 2–3 ATA (compared with normobaric oxygen 100% in moderate to severe poisoning) • Oxygen 28% (compared with air)*
Unknown Effectiveness	• Hyperbaric oxygen 100% (compared with oxygen 100% in mild poisoning)

Search date August 2004

*Categorisation is based on consensus and physiological studies.

DEFINITION Carbon monoxide is an odourless, colourless gas and poisoning causes hypoxia, cell damage, and death. **Diagnosis of carbon monoxide poisoning:** Exposure to carbon monoxide is measured either directly from blood samples, and expressed as a percentage of carboxyhaemoglobin or indirectly using the carbon monoxide in expired breath. Percentage carboxyhaemoglobin is the most frequently used biomarker of carbon monoxide exposure. Although the diagnosis of carbon monoxide poisoning can be confirmed by detecting elevated levels of blood carboxyhaemoglobin levels, the presence of clinical signs and symptoms after known exposure to carbon monoxide should not be ignored. The signs and symptoms of carbon monoxide poisoning are mainly associated with the brain and heart, which are most sensitive to hypoxia. The symptoms of carbon monoxide poisoning are non-specific and varied, and include headache, fatigue, malaise, "trouble thinking", confusion, nausea, dizziness, visual disturbances, chest pain, shortness of breath, loss of consciousness, and seizures. In people suffering from coexisting morbidities, symptoms such as shortness of breath or chest pain may be more evident. The classical signs of carbon monoxide, described as cherry-red lips, peripheral cyanosis, and retinal haemorrhages, are in reality rarely seen. **Interpretation of carboxyhaemoglobin levels:** Non-smokers living away from urban areas have carboxyhaemoglobin levels of between 0.4% and 1.0% reflecting endogenous carbon monoxide production, whereas levels of up to 5% may be considered normal in a busy urban or industrial setting. Smokers are exposed to increased levels of carbon monoxide in cigarettes and otherwise healthy heavy smokers can tolerate levels of carboxyhaemoglobin of up 15%. The use of percentage carboxyhaemoglobin as a measure of severity of carbon monoxide poisoning, or to predict treatment options, is limited because carboxyhaemoglobin levels are affected by the removal from the source of carbon monoxide, and any oxygen treatment given before measurement of percentage carboxyhaemoglobin. In addition, people with co-morbidities that make them more sensitive to the hypoxia associated with carbon monoxide can present with symptoms of poisoning at carboxyhaemoglobin levels that are either low or within the normal range. Attempts have been made in the literature to equate symptoms and signs to different carboxyhaemoglobin levels, but it is accepted that carboxyhaemoglobin levels in an acutely poisoned person only roughly correlate with the clinical signs and symptoms, especially those relating to neurological function. Earlier studies attempted to differentiate between smokers and non-smokers. Attempts have also been made in the literature to divide carbon monoxide poisoning into mild, moderate, and severe based on percentage carboxyhaemoglobin levels and clinical symptoms, but there is no clear clinical consensus or agreement on this issue. The degree of poisoning has been described in the literature as *mild carbon monoxide poisoning:* a carboxyhaemoglobin level of greater than 10% without clinical signs or symptoms of carbon monoxide poisoning; *moderate carbon monoxide poisoning:* a carboxyhaemoglobin level of greater than 10% and less than 20–25% with minor clinical signs and symptoms of poisoning such as headache, lethargy or fatigue; and *severe carbon monoxide poisoning:* a carboxyhaemoglobin level of greater than 20–25%, loss of consciousness and confusion or signs of cardiac ischaemia, or both. **Population:** For the purposes of this review, we have included adults presenting to healthcare professionals with suspected carbon monoxide poisoning. Although there is as yet no clear consensus on this issue, most studies examining carbon monoxide poisoning and its management use a carboxyhaemoglobin level of 10% or more or the presence of clinical signs and symptoms after known exposure to carbon monoxide to be indicative of acute carbon monoxide poisoning. Unless otherwise stated this is the definition of acute carbon monoxide poisoning that has been used throughout this review. Where appropriate, the terms mild, moderate, or severe have been used to reflect the descriptions of populations in individual studies.

INCIDENCE/PREVALENCE Carbon monoxide poisoning is considered to be one of the leading causes of death and injury worldwide and a major public health problem. In 2000, there were 521 deaths where carbon monoxide was the recorded cause of death (ICD-9 – E986) in England and Wales, compared with 1363 deaths recorded in 1985; a trend that has also been observed in the US. Of the 521 deaths attributed to carbon monoxide poisoning, 148 were accidental and the remaining 373 the result of suicide or self-inflicted injury. Poisoning by carbon monoxide is almost certainly underdiagnosed because of the varied ways in which it can present, and it has been estimated in the US that there are over 40,000 emergency department visits a year; many presenting with a flu-like illness. In 2003, there were 534 recorded medical episodes in English hospitals involving people suffering from the toxic effects of carbon monoxide. This may be a substantial underestimate if the US experience reflects the true morbidity associated with carbon monoxide poisoning. Studies in the US have shown that the incidence of accidental carbon monoxide poisoning peaks during the winter months, and is associated with increased use of indoor heating and petrol-powered generators and reduced external ventilation. This seasonal rise in numbers coincides with the annual increase in influenza notifications and, given the similarity in symptoms, many cases of mild carbon monoxide poisoning are probably misdiagnosed.

AETIOLOGY/RISK FACTORS People at high risk: People who are most at risk from carbon monoxide poisoning include those with CHD, vascular disease, or anaemia; pregnant women and their fetus; infants; and the elderly. In people with CHD, experimentally induced blood carboxyhaemoglobin levels of 4.5% shorten the period of exercise before the onset of anginal pain, and the duration of pain is prolonged. In people with anaemia, the oxygen-carrying capacity of the blood is already compromised and therefore they will be more sensitive to carbon monoxide. The elderly are at risk because of existing co-morbidities, such as heart disease or respiratory disease, and because of a reduced compensatory response to hypoxic situations. During pregnancy, a woman's oxygen-carrying capacity is reduced because of an increased endogenous carbon monoxide production and additional endogenous carbon monoxide from the developing fetus, leading to an increased carboxyhaemoglobin concentration. A higher ventilation rate during pregnancy will lead to increased uptake of carbon monoxide at any given carbon monoxide concentration. The fetus is also at risk, and there have been occasional fetal deaths in non-fatal maternal exposures. In the developing fetus, oxygen is released at a lower oxygen partial pressure, and fetal haemoglobin binds with carbon monoxide more quickly compared with adults. Carbon monoxide may be a teratogen where there is a significant increase in maternal carboxyhaemoglobin, or where there is moderate to severe maternal toxicity. Infants may be more susceptible to the effect of carbon monoxide because of their greater oxygen consumption in relation to adults and their response and symptoms are more variable. There are recorded instances of children travelling in the same car and having varying symptoms with similar carboxyhaemoglobin levels, or widely varying carboxyhaemoglobin levels with similar carbon monoxide exposure. **Sources of carbon monoxide:** Carbon monoxide is produced by the incomplete combustion of carbon containing fuel, such as gas (domestic or bottled), charcoal, coke, oil, and wood. Gas stoves, fires, and boilers; gas-powered water heaters; car exhaust fumes; charcoal barbeques; paraffin heaters; solid-fuel-powered stoves; boilers; and room heaters that are faulty or inadequately ventilated are all potential sources. A sometimes overlooked source of carbon monoxide is methylene chloride in some paint strippers and sprays. Methylene chloride is readily absorbed through the skin and lungs and once in the liver, is converted to carbon monoxide. Methylene chloride is stored in body tissues and released gradually; the carbon monoxide elimination half-life in people exposed to methylene chloride is more than twice that of inhaled carbon monoxide. Natural background levels of carbon monoxide in the outdoor environment range from 0.01–0.23 mg/m^3 (0.009–0.2 ppm), but in urban traffic in the UK the 8-hour mean concentrations are higher at about 20 mg/m^3 (17.5 ppm); exposure to this level for prolonged periods could result in a carboxyhaemoglobin level of about 3%.

PROGNOSIS The data regarding prognosis in carbon monoxide poisoning are inconclusive and contradictory. However, there is general agreement that outcome and prognosis are related to the level of carbon monoxide that a person is exposed to, the duration of exposure, and the presence of underlying risk factors. A poor outcome is predicted by lengthy carbon monoxide exposure, loss of consciousness, and advancing age. In addition, hypotension and cardiac arrest independently predict permanent disability and death. After acute carbon monoxide poisoning, the organs most sensitive to hypoxia will be most affected; i.e. the brain and the heart. Pre-existing co-morbidities that affect these organs will, to an extent, influence the clinical presentation and the prognosis; an individual with pre-existing heart disease may present with myocardial ischaemia that could lead to infarction and death. The prognosis for people resuscitated after experiencing cardiac arrest with carbon monoxide poisoning is poor. In a small retrospective study, 18 people with carboxyhaemoglobin levels of 31.7 ± 11.0% given hyperbaric oxygen after resuscitation after cardiac arrest all died. The effects on the brain are more subtle given that different sections of the brain are more sensitive to hypoxic insults, either as a consequence of reduced oxygen delivery or by direct effects on intracellular metabolism. Therefore, in

(continued over)

(from previous page)

addition to the acute neurological sequelae leading to loss of consciousness, coma and death, neurological sequelae such as poor concentration and memory problems may be apparent in people recovering from carbon monoxide poisoning (persistent neurological sequelae), or develop after a period of apparent normality (delayed neurological sequelae). Delayed neurological sequelae develop between 2 days to 240 days after exposure and are reported to affect 10–32% of people recovering from carbon monoxide poisoning. Symptoms include cognitive changes, personality changes, incontinence, psychosis, and Parkinsonism. Fortunately, 50–75% of people recover within 1 year.

Michael Eddleston, Surjit Singh, and Nick Buckley

KEY POINTS

- Acetylcholinesterase inhibition by organophosphorus pesticides or nerve gases can cause acute parasympathetic system dysfunction, muscle weakness, seizures, coma, and respiratory failure.

  Prognosis depends on the dose and relative toxicity of the specific compound, as well as pharmacokinetic factors.

- Initial resuscitation, followed by atropine and oxygen, are considered to be the mainstays of treatment, although no good-quality studies showing benefit have been found.

  We don't know the optimum dose of atropine, but common clinical practice is to administer sufficient to keep the heart rate greater than 80 beats per minute, systolic blood pressure above 80 mmHg, and the lungs clear.

  Glycopyrronium bromide may be as effective as atropine in preventing death, with fewer adverse effects, although no adequately powered studies have been done.

- Washing the poisoned person and removing contaminated clothes is a sensible approach, but no studies have been done to evaluate benefit.

  Healthcare workers should ensure that washing does not distract them from other treatment priorities, and should protect themselves from contamination.

- Benzodiazepines are considered standard treatment to control organophosphorus-induced seizures, although no studies have been found.

- We don't know whether activated charcoal, alpha$_2$ adrenergic receptor agonists (clonidine), butyrylcholinesterase-replacement therapy using fresh frozen plasma or plasmapheresis, magnesium sulphate, N-methyl-D-aspartate receptor antagonists, organophosphorus hydrolases, sodium bicarbonate, milk and other "home remedies" taken soon after ingestion, cathartics, or extracorporeal clearance improve outcomes.

  Oximes have not been shown to improve outcomes, but studies have been of poor quality so a definite conclusion cannot be made.

  Potential benefits from gastric lavage or ipecacuanha are likely to be outweighed by the risks of harm, such as aspiration.

Please visit www.clinicalevidence.bmj.com for full text and references

What are the effects of treatments for acute organophosphorus poisoning?

Likely To Be Beneficial	• Atropine*
	• Benzodiazepines to control organophosphorus-induced seizures*
	• Glycopyrronium bromide (glycopyrrolate)*
	• Washing the poisoned person and removing contaminated clothes*
Unknown Effectiveness	• Activated charcoal (single or multiple dose)
	• Alpha$_2$ adrenergic receptor agonists
	• Butyrylcholinesterase-replacement therapy

	• Extracorporeal clearance
	• Gastric lavage
	• Magnesium sulphate
	• Milk or other "home remedy" immediately after ingestion
	• N-methyl-D-aspartate receptor antagonists
	• Organophosphorus hydrolases
	• Oximes
	• Sodium bicarbonate
Unlikely To Be Beneficial	• Cathartics*
Likely To Be Ineffective Or Harmful	• Ipecacuanha (ipecac)*

Search date August 2006

*Based on consensus, RCTs would be considered unethical.

DEFINITION Acute organophosphorus poisoning occurs after dermal, respiratory, or oral exposure to either low volatility pesticides (e.g. chlorpyrifos, dimethoate) or high-volatility nerve gases (e.g. sarin, tabun). Inhibition of acetylcholinesterase at synapses results in accumulation of acetylcholine, and overactivation of acetylcholine receptors at the neuromuscular junction, and in the autonomic and central nervous systems. Early clinical features (the acute cholinergic crisis) reflect involvement of the parasympathetic system, and include bronchorrhoea, bronchospasm, miosis, salivation, defecation, urination, and hypotension. Features indicating involvement of the neuromuscular junction (muscle weakness and fasciculations) and central nervous system (seizures, coma, and respiratory failure) are common at this stage. Respiratory failure may also occur many hours later, either separated in time from the cholinergic crisis (intermediate syndrome) or merged into the acute cholinergic crisis. The pathophysiology of this late respiratory failure seems to involve downregulation of nicotinic acetylcholine receptors. Intermediate syndrome is particularly important since people who are apparently well can progress rapidly to respiratory arrest. A late motor or motor/sensory peripheral neuropathy can develop after recovery from acute poisoning with some organophosphorus pesticides. Acute poisoning may result in long-term neurological and psychiatric effects, but the evidence is still unclear. There are differences between pesticides in the clinical syndrome they produce and in the frequency and timing of respiratory failure and death.

INCIDENCE/PREVALENCE Most cases occur in resource-poor countries as a result of occupational or deliberate exposure to organophosphorus pesticides. Although data are sparse, organophosphorus pesticides seem to be the most important cause of death from deliberate self-poisoning worldwide, causing about 200,000 deaths each year. For example, in Sri Lanka, about 10,000–20,000 admissions to hospital for organophosphorus poisoning occur each year. Of these, at least 10% die. In most cases, the poisoning is intentional. Case mortality across resource-poor countries is commonly greater than 20%. In Central America, occupational poisoning is reported to be more common than intentional poisoning, and deaths are fewer. Deaths from organophosphorus nerve gases occurred during the Iran–Iraq war. Military or terrorist action with these chemical weapons remains possible. Twelve people died in a terrorist attack in Tokyo, and probably thousands died in Iran after military use.

AETIOLOGY/RISK FACTORS The widespread accessibility of pesticides in rural parts of resource-poor countries makes them an easy option for acts of self-harm. Occupational exposure is usually caused by insufficient or inappropriate protective equipment.

PROGNOSIS There are no validated scoring systems for categorising severity or predicting outcome of acute organophosphorus poisoning. The highly variable natural history and difficulty in determining the dose and specific organophosphorus compound ingested make predicting outcome for an individual person inaccurate and potentially hazardous, because people admitted in good condition can deteriorate rapidly and require intubation and mechanical ventilation. Prognosis in acute self-poisoning is likely to depend on dose and toxicity of the specific organophosphorus compound that has been ingested (e.g. neurotoxicity potential, half life, rate of aging, whether activation to the toxic compound is required (e.g. parathion to paraoxon [pro-poison]), and whether it is dimethylated or diethylated. Prognosis in occupational exposure is better because the dose is normally smaller and the route is dermal.

Paracetamol (acetaminophen) poisoning

Nick Buckley and Michael Eddleston

KEY POINTS

- **Paracetamol (acetaminophen) is a common means of self-poisoning in Europe and North America, often taken as an impulsive act of self-harm in young people.**

  Mortality from paracetamol overdose is now about 0.4%, although without treatment severe liver damage occurs in at least half of people with blood paracetamol levels above the UK standard treatment line.

  In adults, ingestion of less than 125 mg/kg is unlikely to lead to hepatotoxicity; even higher doses may be tolerated by children without causing liver damage.

- **Standard treatment of paracetamol overdose is acetylcysteine, which based on animal studies and clinical experience, is widely believed to reduce liver damage and mortality, although few studies have been done.**

  Adverse effects from acetylcysteine include rash, urticaria, vomiting, and anaphylaxis which can, rarely, be fatal.

  We don't know what the optimal dose, route, and duration of acetylcysteine treatment should be. However, liver damage is less likely to occur if treatment is started within 8–10 hours of ingestion.

- **It is possible that methionine reduces the risk of liver damage and mortality after paracetamol poisoning compared with supportive care, but we don't know for sure.**

- **We don't know whether activated charcoal, gastric lavage, or ipecacuanha reduce the risks of liver damage after paracetamol poisoning.**

  The rapid absorption of paracetamol suggests that a beneficial effect from treatments that reduce gastric absorption is unlikely in many cases.

- **Liver transplantation may increase survival rates in people with fulminant liver failure after paracetamol poisoning compared with waiting list controls, but long-term outcomes are unknown.**

Please visit www.clinicalevidence.bmj.com for full text and references

What are the effects of treatments for acute paracetamol poisoning?

Beneficial	• Acetylcysteine
Likely To Be Beneficial	• Methionine
Unknown Effectiveness	• Activated charcoal (single or multiple dose) • Gastric lavage • Ipecacuanha • Liver transplant

Search date March 2007

DEFINITION Paracetamol poisoning occurs as a result of either accidental or intentional overdose with paracetamol (acetaminophen).

INCIDENCE/PREVALENCE Paracetamol is the most common drug used for self-poisoning in the UK. It is also a common means of self-poisoning in the rest of Europe, North America, and Australasia. There has been an exponential rise in the number of hospital admissions caused by paracetamol poisoning in England and Wales from 150 in 1968 to a peak of 41,200 in 1989–1990, before falling to around 25,000 in 2001–2002. Overdoses from paracetamol alone result in an estimated 150–200 deaths and 15–20 liver transplants each year in England and Wales (data from routinely collected health and coronial statistics). Pack-size restrictions instituted in the UK in 1998 resulted in modest reductions in large overdoses, liver transplants, and deaths in England and Wales. In Scotland, the reduction in admissions and mortality from paracetamol overdose was short lived.

AETIOLOGY/RISK FACTORS Most cases in the UK are impulsive acts of self-harm in young people. In one cohort study of 80 people who had overdosed with paracetamol, 42 had obtained the tablets for the specific purpose of taking an overdose, and 33 had obtained them less than 1 hour before the act.

PROGNOSIS People with blood paracetamol concentrations above the standard treatment line (defined in the UK as a line joining 200 mg/L at 4 hours and 30 mg/L at 15 hours on a semilogarithmic plot) have a poor prognosis without treatment. In one cohort study of 57 untreated people with blood concentrations above this line, 33/57 (58%) developed severe liver damage and 3/57 (5%) died. People with a history of chronic alcohol misuse, use of enzyme inducing drugs, eating disorders, or multiple paracetamol overdoses may be at risk of liver damage with blood concentrations below this line. In the USA, a lower line is used as an indication for treatment, but we found no data relating this line to prognostic outcomes. More recently, a modified nomogram specifically designed to estimate prognosis (not need for treatment) has been developed by modelling data from a large cohort. This takes into account time to initiation of acetylcysteine treatment, and the effect of alcohol use. However, it has not yet been validated, and is not widely used. Reversible renal injury occurs in some people, most commonly (but not always) in association with hepatic injury. **Dose effect:** The dose ingested also indicates the risk of hepatotoxicity. One case series showed that people ingesting less than 125 mg/kg had no significant hepatotoxicity, with a sharp dose-dependent rise for higher doses. The threshold for toxicity after acute ingestion may be higher in children, where a single dose of less than 200 mg/kg has not been reported to lead to death and rarely causes hepatotoxicity. The higher threshold for toxicity in children may relate to different metabolic pathways or their larger relative liver size. For people who present later than 24 hours, or an unknown time after ingestion, several other prognostic indicators have been proposed, including prothrombin time, and abnormal liver function tests. These have not been validated prospectively. **Slow-release preparations:** Pharmacokinetic studies of small overdoses of slow-release paracetamol formulations in healthy volunteers showed that peak plasma concentrations usually still occur within 4 hours, and the apparent half-life is the same as or only slightly longer than that of conventional paracetamol preparations. The bioavailability was not increased. The nomogram has not specifically been validated for these formulations. However, only a small proportion of cases of slow release preparation ingestion have resulted in initial non-toxic levels and subsequent toxic levels on the usual nomograms. In just one case, with other risk factors, the use of the nomogram led to treatment being ceased, and this may have contributed to a fatal outcome. **Children and repeated supra-therapeutic doses:** There are reports of major dosing errors leading to severe hepatotoxicity in children. Of more concern are other cases of apparent toxicity with repeated doses only slightly above the current maximum recommended doses (around 75 mg/kg/day). There are possibly additional risk factors in these cases, but these have not been established.

Juan C Vazquez

KEY POINTS

- Constipation, heartburn, and haemorrhoids are common gastrointestinal complaints during pregnancy.

- Constipation occurs in 11–38% of pregnant women.

- Stimulant laxatives may be more effective than bulk laxatives in improving constipation in pregnancy, although adverse effects, such as abdominal pain and diarrhoea, could limit their use.

  Dietary fibre may improve constipation in pregnant women compared with placebo.

  We don't know whether increasing fluid intake improves constipation in pregnancy. However, because of other health benefits, increased fluid intake may be recommended as one of the first measures to relieve constipation.

  We have no good evidence to show that bulk-forming or osmotic laxatives are of benefit for constipation in pregnancy.

- Although the exact prevalence of haemorrhoids during pregnancy is unknown, the condition is common, and the prevalence of symptomatic haemorrhoids in pregnant women is higher than in non-pregnant women.

- Rutosides improve the symptoms of haemorrhoids compared with placebo. However, further studies are needed to assess their potential adverse effects.

  We don't know whether increased fibre and fluid intake are effective in relieving the symptoms of haemorrhoids in pregnancy, although it seems reasonable to encourage pregnant women to consume a fluid- and fibre-rich diet as a preventive measure.

  We don't know whether stimulant laxatives, bulk-forming laxatives, or osmotic laxatives are effective in relieving symptomatic haemorrhoids in pregnancy, although, if constipation is associated with haemorrhoids, treating constipation with stimulant laxatives may relieve straining, and thereby provide some symptomatic relief.

  We found no good evidence assessing the effects of topical anaesthetics, topical corticosteroids, or compound topical corticosteroids plus anaesthetics to treat symptomatic haemorrhoids in pregnancy. However, despite this, women who have painful complicated haemorrhoids may be offered topical anaesthetic agents unless contraindicated.

- The incidence of heartburn in pregnancy is reported to be 17–45%.

- Antacids may provide effective heartburn relief in pregnancy.

  We don't know whether dietary and lifestyle modifications are of benefit to prevent or treat heartburn in pregnancy. However, there is consensus that lifestyle and dietary modifications, including avoiding fatty foods and caffeine, should remain first-line treatment for heartburn in pregnant women.

  We also don't know whether acid-suppressing drugs such as ranitidine are of benefit to treat heartburn in pregnancy.

(i) **Please visit www.clinicalevidence.bmj.com for full text and references**

What are the effects of interventions to prevent or treat constipation in pregnancy?

Unknown Effectiveness	• Bulk-forming laxatives for constipation in pregnant women

- Increased fibre intake for constipation in pregnant women

- Increased fluid intake for constipation in pregnant women

- Osmotic laxatives for constipation in pregnant women

- Stimulant laxatives for constipation in pregnant women

What are the effects of interventions to prevent or treat haemorrhoids in pregnancy?

Likely To Be Beneficial	• Rutosides (improve symptoms of haemorrhoids but insufficient evidence about adverse effects)
Unknown Effectiveness	• Anaesthetics (topical) for haemorrhoids in pregnant women
	• Bulk-forming laxatives for haemorrhoids in pregnant women
	• Compound corticosteroids plus anaesthetics (topical) for haemorrhoids in pregnant women
	• Corticosteroids (topical) for haemorrhoids in pregnant women
	• Increased fibre intake for haemorrhoids in pregnant women
	• Increased fluid intake for haemorrhoids in pregnant women
	• Osmotic laxatives for haemorrhoids in pregnant women
	• Sitz baths for haemorrhoids in pregnant women
	• Stimulant laxatives for haemorrhoids in pregnant women

What are the effects of interventions to prevent or treat heartburn in pregnancy?

Likely To Be Beneficial	• Antacids with or without alginates for heartburn in pregnant women
Unknown Effectiveness	• Acid-suppressing drugs for heartburn in pregnant women
	• Raising the head of the bed for heartburn in pregnant women
	• Reducing caffeine intake for heartburn in pregnant women
	• Reducing the intake of fatty foods for heartburn in pregnant women

● Reducing the size and frequency of meals for heartburn in pregnant women

Search date July 2007

DEFINITION Constipation: Some women will have experienced chronic constipation prior to becoming pregnant, and in others constipation develops for the first time during pregnancy. For a full definition of constipation, see review on constipation in adults, p 166. The diagnosis of constipation is mainly clinical, based on a history of decreased frequency of defecation, as well as on the characteristics of the faeces. An extensive evaluation is usually unnecessary for women who present with chronic constipation, or if constipation develops for the first time during pregnancy. **Heartburn:** Heartburn is defined as a sensation of "burning" in the upper part of the digestive tract, including the throat. It can be associated with oesophagitis. One study reported the results of endoscopy on 73 pregnant women with heartburn, and found endoscopic and histological evidence of oesophagitis in most women. As complications associated with heartburn during pregnancy are rare (e.g. erosive oesophagitis), upper endoscopy and other diagnostic tests are infrequently needed. Therefore, the diagnosis of heartburn is mainly clinical, based on the history. **Haemorrhoids:** Haemorrhoids (piles) are swollen veins at or near the anus, which are usually asymptomatic. Haemorrhoids can become symptomatic if they prolapse (the forward or downward displacement of a part of the rectal mucosae through the anus) or because of other complications such as thrombosis. Associated anal fissures (a break or slit in the anal mucosa) can also lead to symptoms. Haemorrhoids can be classified by severity: first-degree haemorrhoids bleed but do not prolapse; second-degree haemorrhoids prolapse on straining and reduce spontaneously; third-degree haemorrhoids prolapse on straining and require manual reduction; and fourth-degree haemorrhoids are prolapsed and incarcerated. Diagnosis of haemorrhoids is based on history and examination. Symptoms include bleeding, mucosal or faecal soiling, itching, and occasionally pain. Fourth-degree haemorrhoids may become "strangulated" and present with acute severe pain. Progressive venous engorgement and incarceration of the acutely inflamed haemorrhoid leads to thrombosis and infarction. The diagnosis of haemorrhoids is confirmed by rectal examination, and inspection of the perianal area for skin tags, fissures, fistulae, polyps, or tumours. Prolapsing haemorrhoids may appear at the anal verge on straining. It is important to exclude more serious causes of rectal bleeding. Assessment should include anoscopy to view the haemorrhoidal cushions. Haemorrhoidal size, and severity of inflammation and bleeding should be assessed.

INCIDENCE/PREVALENCE Constipation: Constipation is common in pregnant women, and can develop during pregnancy or increase in severity during pregnancy. The prevalence of constipation in pregnancy is reported to be 11–38%. Parity or previous caesarean section have been associated with constipation. **Heartburn:** Heartburn is one of the most common gastrointestinal symptoms in pregnant women, with an incidence in pregnancy of 17–45%. In some studies, the prevalence of heartburn has been found to increase from 22% in the first trimester to 39% in the second trimester to 60–72% in the third trimester. However, one prospective cohort study found that, in most pregnant women, heartburn, acid regurgitation, or both began in the first trimester and disappeared during the second trimester; and another cohort study also found that gastrointestinal symptoms, such as heartburn and nausea, were more common in the first trimester. The study also found that primigravidae reported more gastrointestinal symptoms than multiparae. **Haemorrhoids:** Although the exact prevalence of haemorrhoids during pregnancy is unknown, the condition is common in pregnancy, and the prevalence of symptomatic haemorrhoids is higher in pregnant than in non-pregnant women. In a population of pregnant women in Serbia and Montenegro, haemorrhoids were present in 85% of women during the second and third pregnancy. Haemorrhoids are also a frequent complaint among women who have recently given birth, and they become more common with increased age and parity.

AETIOLOGY/RISK FACTORS Constipation: Constipation in pregnancy is probably caused by rising progesterone levels. Low fluid and fibre intake may also be contributing factors. There is some evidence that pregnant women consume less fibre than is currently recommended for the non-pregnant population. Low fluid intake has been linked to constipation in pregnancy, particularly in the third trimester. Some medications taken during pregnancy, such as iron salts and magnesium sulphate, have been also been linked to constipation. Hypothyroidism may also be a rare cause of constipation during pregnancy. **Heartburn:** The cause of heartburn during pregnancy is multifactorial. Increased amounts of progesterone or its metabolites cause relaxation of smooth muscle, which results in a reduction in gastric tone and motility, and a decrease in lower oesophageal sphincter pressure. It has also been found that, during pregnancy, the lower oesophageal sphincter is displaced into the thoracic cavity (an area of negative pressure), which allows food and gastric acid to pass from the stomach into the oesophagus, leading to oesophageal inflammation and a sensation of "burning". Pressure of the growing uterus on gastric contents as the pregnancy progresses may worsen heartburn, although some authors believe that mechanical factors have a smaller role. Heartburn may also be caused by medications taken during pregnancy, such as antiemetics. **Haemorrhoids:** Haemorrhoids result from impaired venous return in prolapsed anal cushions, with dilation of the venous plexus and venous stasis. Inflammation occurs with erosion of the anal cushion's epithelium, resulting in bleeding. Constipation with prolonged straining at stool, or raised intra-abdominal pressure as occurs in pregnancy, may result in symptomatic haemorrhoids. During pregnancy, delivery, and the puerperium, sphincteral muscles and pelvic floor structures could be modified in tone and position, leading to an alteration of the normal functioning of the haemorrhoidal cushion, which may predispose to symptoms.

PROGNOSIS Constipation: Constipation, if mild, is often self-treated with home remedies or non-prescription preparations. Primary-care providers usually are confident managing constipation in pregnancy, unless severe, refractory to conventional management, or if additional diagnostic studies are required. Therefore referral to a gastroenterologist is seldom necessary. **Heartburn:** Most cases of heartburn improve with lifestyle modifications and dietary changes, but in some cases severity may increase throughout the course of pregnancy. **Haemorrhoids:** In women with haemorrhoids, symptoms are usually mild and transient and include pain and intermittent bleeding from the anus. Depending on the degree of pain, quality of life can be affected, varying from mild discomfort to difficulty in dealing with the activities of everyday life. Treatment during pregnancy is mainly directed to the relief of symptoms, especially pain control. For many women, symptoms will resolve spontaneously soon after birth.

Ectopic pregnancy

Rajesh Varma and Janesh Gupta

KEY POINTS

- Approximately one in a hundred pregnancies are ectopic, with the conceptus usually implanting in the fallopian tube. Some ectopic pregnancies can resolve spontaneously, but others continue to grow and lead to rupture of the tube.

  Risks are higher in women with damage to the fallopian tubes due to pelvic infections, surgery, or previous ectopic pregnancy or abortion, and in smokers.

  The IUD does not increase the absolute risk, but a pregnancy that does occur with IUD use is more likely to be ectopic than intrauterine.

- Expectant management of unruptured ectopic pregnancies may lead to similar subsequent intrauterine-pregnancy rates compared with surgery, but few studies have been done.

  Ongoing surveillance is required as part of expectant management, but tubal rupture can occur despite falling beta hCG levels.

- The likelihood of subsequent intrauterine pregnancy seems to be similar after salpingectomy or salpingotomy.

  Salpingotomy by laparoscopy may lead to fewer complications and shorter recovery times compared with laparotomy, but may also be less likely to remove all the trophoblast.

- Methotrexate, as single- or multiple-dose regimens, seems as likely as salpingotomy to remove trophoblast material and leave a patent fallopian tube in women with non-invasive, small ectopic pregnancies with no tubal rupture or bleeding, no sign of fetal cardiac activity and low beta human chorionic gonadotrophin (hCG) levels.

  About 15–40% of ectopic pregnancies may be suitable for such non-surgical management.

  Systemic or intratubal methotrexate may also reduce persistent trophoblast after salpingotomy.

  Adding mifepristone to systemic methotrexate seems unlikely to increase treatment success compared with methotrexate alone, other than in women with higher progesterone levels.

(i) **Please visit www.clinicalevidence.bmj.com for full text and references**

What treatments improve outcomes in women with unruptured tubal ectopic pregnancy?	
Beneficial	• Salpingectomy (in women not desiring future fertility)
Likely To Be Beneficial	• Prophylactic methotrexate (systemic) following salpingotomy • Systemic methotrexate (single or multiple dose)
Unknown Effectiveness	• Expectant management of unruptured ectopic pregnancies • Salpingotomy (compared with laparoscopic salpingectomy)
Unlikely To Be Beneficial	• Systemic methotrexate plus mifepristone (versus systemic methotrexate alone)

Search date June 2006

DEFINITION Ectopic pregnancy is defined as a conceptus implanting outside the uterine endometrium. The most common implantation site is within the fallopian tube (95.5%), followed by ovarian (3.2%) and abdominal (1.3%) sites. The sites of tubal implantation in descending order of frequency are ampulla (73.3%), isthmus (12.5%), fimbrial (11.6%), and interstitial (2.6%). **Population:** In this systematic review, we will consider haemodynamically stable women with unruptured tubal ectopic pregnancy, diagnosed by non-invasive or invasive techniques.

INCIDENCE/PREVALENCE Around 10,000 ectopic pregnancies are diagnosed annually in the UK. The incidence of ectopic pregnancy in the UK (11.0/1000 pregnancies) is similar to that in other countries, such as Norway (14.9/1000) and Australia (16.2/1000). Since 1994, the overall rate of ectopic pregnancy and mortality rate (0.4/1000 ectopic pregnancies) have been static in the UK. Until recently, most epidemiological studies have failed to distinguish between ectopic pregnancies occurring in women who did not use contraception (reproductive failure) and women who used contraception (contraceptive failure). A French population study undertaken from 1992–2002 found that, over the duration of the study, the rate of reproductive-failure ectopic pregnancies increased by 17%, whereas the rate of contraceptive-failure ectopic pregnancies decreased by 29%. Increasing rates of chlamydia infection, smoking, and assisted reproductive-technology usage may have contributed to the disproportionate increase in reproductive failure ectopic pregnancy rate over contraceptive-failure ectopic pregnancy rate. Widespread use of dedicated early pregnancy assessment units and non-invasive diagnostic algorithms are likely to have contributed to increasing rates of ectopic pregnancy diagnosis.

AETIOLOGY/RISK FACTORS The aetiology of ectopic pregnancy is unclear. Ectopic pregnancy arising from reproductive failure or contraceptive failure should be considered as separate entities with differing aetiology, risk factors, and reproductive outcomes. The main risk factors for reproductive failure are a history of PID, previous ectopic pregnancy, pelvic and tubal surgery, infertility, smoking, and assisted conception. The main risk factor for contraceptive-failure ectopic pregnancy is IUD failure. IUDs do not increase the absolute risk of ectopic pregnancy, but a pregnancy occurring with IUD is more likely to be ectopic than intrauterine. Other risk factors for ectopic pregnancy include prior spontaneous abortion, prior induced abortion, endometriosis, uterotubal anomalies, and prior in utero exposure to diethylstilbestrol. However, fewer than half of the ectopic pregnancies diagnosed are associated with risk factors.

PROGNOSIS Ectopic pregnancies: As the pregnancy advances, tubal pregnancies may either diminish in size and spontaneously resolve, or increase in size and eventually lead to tubal rupture, with consequent maternal morbidity and mortality. There are no reliable clinical, sonographic, or biological markers (e.g. serum beta human chorionic gonadotrophin or serum progesterone) that can predict rupture of tubal ectopic pregnancy. Maternal mortality following ectopic pregnancy is an uncommon short-term outcome in resource-rich countries. The recent UK Confidential Enquiry into Maternal Deaths cited ectopic pregnancy as a cause of 11 maternal deaths (0.4/1000 ectopic pregnancies). Short-term maternal morbidity relates to pain, transfusion requirement, and operative complications. Primary treatment success and long-term fertility outcomes depend on the clinical characteristics of the ectopic pregnancy (e.g. whether the ectopic pregnancy occurred in a woman using contraception or not, tubal rupture or not, contralateral tubal disease) and the type of surgical or medical treatment chosen. A 10-year follow-up of ectopic pregnancies showed that the rate of repeat ectopic pregnancy was much higher in women with an IUD in place at the time of the index ectopic pregnancy compared with women whose ectopic pregnancy was not associated with IUD use. By contrast, the rate of intrauterine pregnancy was 1.7 times higher (fecundity rate ratio [FRR] 1.7, 95% CI 1.3 to 2.3) in women who had an IUD in place at the time of the index ectopic pregnancy compared with women whose index ectopic pregnancy was not associated with IUD use. Short- and long-term consequences on health-related quality of life and psychological issues (e.g. bereavement) are also important, but are rarely quantified. **Pregnancies of unknown location:** Pregnancy of unknown location is the absence of pregnancy localisation (either intrauterine or extrauterine) by transvaginal sonography when serum beta human chorionic gonadotrophin levels are below the discriminatory zone (1000–1500 IU/L). An observational study of pregnancies of unknown location has shown that 55% spontaneously resolve, 34% are subsequently diagnosed as viable, and 11% are subsequently diagnosed as ectopic pregnancies.

Nausea and vomiting in early pregnancy
Mario Festin

KEY POINTS

- More than half of pregnant women suffer from nausea and vomiting, which typically begins by the fourth week and disappears by the sixteenth week of pregnancy.

    The cause of nausea and vomiting in pregnancy is unknown, but may be due to the rise in human chorionic gonadotrophin concentration.

    In 1 in 200 women, the condition progresses to hyperemesis gravidarum, which is characterised by prolonged and severe nausea and vomiting, dehydration, and weight loss.

- Ginger may reduce nausea and vomiting in pregnancy compared with placebo, although studies have given inconclusive results.

    Pyridoxine may be as effective as ginger in reducing nausea, although studies have given inconsistent results about reduction of vomiting.

    We don't know whether dietary interventions other than ginger are beneficial.

- P6 acupressure may reduce nausea and vomiting compared with sham acupressure, but wristbands can be difficult to use.

    We don't know whether acupuncture is more effective than sham acupuncture at reducing nausea and vomiting.

- Antihistamines may reduce nausea and vomiting compared with placebo. One systematic review found that, compared with placebo, antihistamines did not increase the risk of teratogenicity.

    We don't know whether phenothiazines, metoclopramide, or domperidone reduce nausea or vomiting.

- We don't know whether acupuncture, intramuscular corticotrophin, corticosteroids, diazepam, ginger or other dietary interventions, or ondansetron are effective in treating hyperemesis gravidarum.

(i) **Please visit www.clinicalevidence.bmj.com for full text and references**

What are the effects of treatment for nausea and vomiting in early pregnancy?

Likely To Be Beneficial	• Acupressure • Antihistamines (H_1 antagonists) • Ginger • Pyridoxine (vitamin B_6)
Unknown Effectiveness	• Acupuncture • Dietary interventions (other than ginger) • Domperidone • Metoclopramide • Phenothiazines

What are the effects of treatments for hyperemesis gravidarum?

Unknown Effectiveness	• Acupuncture • Corticosteroids

- Corticotrophins
- Diazepam
- Dietary interventions (other than ginger)
- Ginger
- Ondansetron

Search date September 2006

DEFINITION Nausea and vomiting are common problems in early pregnancy. Although often called "morning sickness", nausea and vomiting can occur at any time of day and may persist throughout the day. Symptoms usually begin between 4 weeks' and 7 weeks' gestation (1 study found this to be the case in 70% of affected women) and disappear by 16 weeks' gestation in about 90% of women. One study found that less than 10% of affected women suffer nausea, vomiting, or both before the first missed period. Most women do not require treatment, and complete the pregnancy without any special intervention. However, if nausea and vomiting are severe and persistent, the condition can progress to hyperemesis, especially if the woman is unable to maintain adequate hydration, fluid and electrolyte balance, and nutrition. **Hyperemesis gravidarum** is a diagnosis of exclusion, characterised by prolonged and severe nausea and vomiting, dehydration, and weight loss. Laboratory investigation may show ketosis, hyponatraemia, hypokalaemia, hypouricaemia, metabolic hypochloraemic alkalosis, and ketonuria.

INCIDENCE/PREVALENCE Nausea affects about 70% and vomiting about 60% of pregnant women. The true incidence of hyperemesis gravidarum is not known. It has been documented to range from 3 in 1000 to 20 in 1000 pregnancies. However, most authors report an incidence of 1 in 200.

AETIOLOGY/RISK FACTORS The causes of nausea and vomiting in pregnancy are unknown. One theory, that they are caused by the rise in human chorionic gonadotrophin concentration, is compatible with the natural history of the condition, its severity in pregnancies affected by hydatidiform mole, and its good prognosis (see prognosis below). The cause of hyperemesis gravidarum is also uncertain. Again, endocrine and psychological factors are suspected, but evidence is inconclusive. Female fetal sex has been found to be a clinical indicator of hyperemesis. One prospective study found that *Helicobacter pylori* infection was more common in pregnant women with hyperemesis gravidarum than in pregnant women without hyperemesis gravidarum (number of women with positive serum *Helicobacter pylori* immunoglobulin G concentrations: 95/105 [91%] with hyperemesis gravidarum v 60/129 [47%] without hyperemesis gravidarum). However, it was not clear whether this link was causal.

PROGNOSIS One systematic review (search date 1988) found that nausea and vomiting were associated with a reduced risk of miscarriage (6 studies, 14,564 women; OR 0.36, 95% CI 0.32 to 0.42) but found no association with perinatal mortality. Hyperemesis gravidarum is thought by some to induce nutrient partitioning in favour of the fetus, which could explain the association with improved outcome in the fetus. Nausea and vomiting and hyperemesis usually improve over the course of pregnancy, but in one cross-sectional observational study 13% of women reported that nausea and vomiting persisted beyond 20 weeks' gestation. Although death from nausea and vomiting during pregnancy is rare, morbidities, including Wernicke's encephalopathy, splenic avulsion, oesophageal rupture, pneumothorax, and acute tubular necrosis, have been reported.

Perineal care

Chris Kettle

KEY POINTS

- Over 85% of women having a vaginal birth suffer some perineal trauma.

  Spontaneous tears requiring suturing are estimated to occur in at least a third of women in the UK and USA, with anal sphincter tears in 0.5% to 7% of women.

  Risk factors include first vaginal delivery, large or malpositioned baby, older or white mother, abnormal collagen synthesis, poor nutritional state, and forceps delivery.

- Perineal trauma can lead to long-term physical and psychological problems.

  Up to 10% of women continue to have long-term perineal pain; up to 25% will have dyspareunia or urinary problems, and up to 10% will report faecal incontinence.

- Restricting routine use of episiotomy reduces the risk of posterior perineal trauma.

  Using episiotomies only when there are clear maternal or fetal indications increases the likelihood of maintaining an intact perineum, and does not increase the risk of third-degree tears.

- We don't know whether pain or wound dehiscence are less likely to occur with midline episiotomy compared with mediolateral incision.

  Midline incisions may be more likely to result in severe tears, although we can't be sure about this.

- Instrumental delivery increases the risk of perineal trauma.

  The risk of instrumental delivery is increased after epidural analgesia. Vacuum extraction reduces the rate of severe perineal trauma compared with forceps delivery, but increases the risk of cephalhaematoma and retinal haemorrhage in the newborn.

- Continuous support during labour reduces the rate of assisted vaginal births, and thus the rate of perineal trauma.

- The "hands-poised" delivery method is associated with lower rates of episiotomy, but increased rates of short-term pain and manual removal of the placenta. Likewise an upright position during delivery is associated with lower rates of episiotomy, but no significant difference in overall rates of perineal trauma.

- Non-suturing of first- and second-degree tears (perineal skin and muscles) may be associated with reduced wound healing up to 3 months after birth. However, leaving the perineal skin alone un-sutured (vagina and perineal muscles sutured) reduces dyspareunia, and may reduce pain, up to 3 months.

- Absorbable synthetic sutures for repair of first- and second-degree tears and episiotomies are less likely to result in long-term pain compared with catgut sutures. Rapidly absorbed synthetic sutures reduces the need for suture removal. Continuous sutures reduce short-term pain.

- We don't know which is the best method to repair third- and fourth-degree anal sphincter tears.

(i) Please visit www.clinicalevidence.bmj.com for full text and references

What are the effects of intrapartum surgical interventions on rates of perineal trauma?

Beneficial	• Restrictive use of episiotomy (reduced risk of posterior trauma compared with routine use)
Trade-off Between Benefits And Harms	• Vacuum extraction (less perineal trauma than with forceps, but newborns have increased risk of cephalhaematoma)
Unlikely To Be Beneficial	• Midline episiotomy incision (associated with higher risk of third- or fourth-degree tears compared with mediolateral incision)
Likely To Be Ineffective Or Harmful	• Epidural analgesia (increased instrumental delivery, which is associated with increased rates of perineal trauma)

What are the effects of intrapartum non-surgical interventions on rates of perineal trauma?

Beneficial	• Continuous support during labour (reduced instrumental delivery, which is associated with increased perineal trauma)
Trade-off Between Benefits And Harms	• Upright position during delivery (fewer episiotomies but more second-degree tears than supine or lithotomy positions) • "Hands-poised" method of delivery (fewer episiotomies, but increased pain and need for manual delivery of placenta compared with "hands-on" method)
Unknown Effectiveness	• Passive descent in the second stage of labour (no difference in perineal trauma compared with active pushing) • Sustained breath holding (Valsalva) method of pushing (no difference in perineal trauma compared with spontaneous pushing)

What are the effects of different methods and materials for primary repair of first and second degree tears and episiotomies?

Beneficial	• Absorbable synthetic sutures for perineal repair of first- and second-degree tears and episiotomies (reduced short-term analgesic use compared with catgut sutures)

	• Continuous sutures for first- and second-degree tears and episiotomies (reduced short-term pain compared with interrupted sutures)
Likely To Be Beneficial	• Non-suturing of perineal skin alone in first- and second-degree tears and episiotomies (reduced dyspareunia compared with conventional suturing)
Likely To Be Ineffective Or Harmful	• Non-suturing of muscle and skin in first- and second-degree perineal tears (poorer wound-healing than with suturing)

What are the effects of different methods and materials for primary repair of obstetric anal sphincter injuries (third- and fourth-degree tears)?

Unknown Effectiveness	• Different methods and materials for primary repair of obstetric anal sphincter injuries (third- and fourth-degree tears)

Search date April 2006

DEFINITION Perineal trauma is any damage to the genitalia during childbirth that occurs spontaneously or intentionally by surgical incision (episiotomy). Anterior perineal trauma is injury to the labia, anterior vagina, urethra, or clitoris, and is usually associated with little morbidity. Posterior perineal trauma is any injury to the posterior vaginal wall, perineal muscles, or anal sphincter. First-degree spontaneous tears involve only skin; second-degree tears involve perineal muscles; third-degree tears partially or completely disrupt the anal sphincter; and fourth-degree tears completely disrupt the external and internal anal sphincter and epithelium.

INCIDENCE/PREVALENCE Over 85% of women having a vaginal birth sustain some form of perineal trauma, and 60–70% receive stitches — equivalent to 400,000 women a year in the UK in 1997. There are wide variations in rates of episiotomy: 8% in The Netherlands, 14% in England, 50% in the USA, and 99% in East-European countries. Sutured spontaneous tears are reported in about a third of women in the USA and the UK, but this is probably an underestimate because of inconsistencies in reporting and classification of perineal trauma. The incidence of anal-sphincter tears varies between 0.5% in the UK, 2.5% in Denmark, and 7% in Canada.

AETIOLOGY/RISK FACTORS Perineal trauma occurs during spontaneous or assisted vaginal delivery and is usually more extensive after the first vaginal delivery. Associated risk factors also include increased fetal size, mode of delivery, and malpresentation and malposition of the fetus. Other maternal factors that may increase the extent and degree of trauma are ethnicity (white women are probably at greater risk than black women), older age, abnormal collagen synthesis, and poor nutritional state. Clinicians' practices or preferences in terms of intrapartum interventions may influence the severity and rate of perineal trauma (e.g. use of ventouse v forceps).

PROGNOSIS Perineal trauma affects women's physical, psychological, and social wellbeing in the immediate postnatal period as well as in the long term. It can also disrupt breastfeeding, family life, and sexual relations. In the UK, about 23–42% of women continue to have pain and discomfort for 10–12 days postpartum, and 7–10% of women continue to have long term pain (3–18 months after delivery); 23% of women experience superficial dyspareunia at 3 months; 3–10% report faecal incontinence; and up to 24% have urinary problems. Complications depend on the severity of perineal trauma and on the effectiveness of treatment.

Louise Howard

KEY POINTS

- The differentiation between postnatal depression and other types of depression is often unclear, but there are treatment issues in nursing mothers that do not apply in other situations.

  Overall, the prevalence of depression in postpartum women is the same as the prevalence in women generally, at about 12–13%.

  Suicide is a major cause of maternal mortality in resource-rich countries, but rates are lower in women postpartum than in women who have not had a baby.

  Most episodes resolve spontaneously within 3–6 months, but a quarter of depressed mothers still have symptoms at 1 year. Depression can interfere with the mother–infant relationship.

- SSRIs may improve symptoms of postnatal depression, but few studies have been found that evaluate their effect specifically in postpartum women.

  We don't know whether other types of antidepressant are effective compared with placebo or psychological treatments.

  We don't know whether oestrogen treatment or St John's Wort improve symptoms compared with placebo.

- Psychological treatments such as individual CBT, non-directive counselling, interpersonal psychotherapy, and psychodynamic therapy are likely to improve symptoms compared with routine care, but long-term benefits are unclear.

  We don't know whether light therapy, group CBT, psychoeducation with the partner, mother–infant interaction coaching, telephone-based peer support, infant massage, or physical exercise improve symptoms of postnatal depression, as few studies have been found.

(i) **Please visit www.clinicalevidence.bmj.com for full text and references**

What are the effects of drug treatments for postnatal depression?	
Likely To Be Beneficial	• Antidepressants other than selective SSRIs*
	• SSRIs (fluoxetine, paroxetine, and sertraline)*
Unknown Effectiveness	• Hormones
	• St John's Wort (*Hypericum perforatum*)

What are the effects of non-drug treatments for postnatal depression?	
Likely To Be Beneficial	• CBT (individual)
	• Interpersonal psychotherapy
	• Non-directive counselling (effective in the short term although may not have long-term beneficial effects)
Unknown Effectiveness	• CBT (group)
	• Infant massage by mother

	• Light therapy
	• Physical exercise
	• Psychodynamic therapy
	• Psychoeducation with partner
	• Telephone-based peer support (mother to mother)
Unlikely To Be Beneficial	• Mother–infant interaction coaching (improved maternal responsiveness but no significant difference in depression scores)

Search date September 2006

*Antidepressants are categorised on the evidence of their effectiveness in the treatment of depression in general.

DEFINITION Postnatal depression (PND) has been variously defined as non-psychotic depression occurring during the first 6 months, the first 4 weeks postpartum, and the first 3 months postpartum, but recently 3 months postpartum was suggested in the UK as a useful clinical definition. Puerperal mental disorders have only recently been categorised separately in psychiatric classifications, but both the ICD-10 and the DSM-IV require certain qualifications to be met that limit their use: ICD-10 categorises mental disorders that occur postpartum as puerperal, but only if they cannot otherwise be classified, and DSM-IV allows "postpartum onset" to be specified for mood disorders starting within 4 weeks postpartum. In clinical practice and research, the broader definition above is often used, because whether or not PND is truly distinct from depression in general, depression in the postpartum period raises treatment issues for the nursing mother and has implications for the developing infant (see prognosis below). However, there is increased recognition that many PNDs start during pregnancy. The symptoms are similar to symptoms of depression at other times of life, but in addition to low mood, sleep disturbance, change in appetite, diurnal variation in mood, poor concentration, and irritability, women with PND also experience guilt about their inability to look after their new baby. In many countries, health visitors screen for PND using the EPDS, which identifies depressive symptoms, but does not include somatic symptoms such as appetite changes, which can be difficult to assess in most women in the postnatal period.

INCIDENCE/PREVALENCE The prevalence of depression in women postpartum is similar to that found in women generally. However, the incidence of depression in the first month after childbirth is three times the average monthly incidence in non-childbearing women. A meta-analysis of studies mainly based in resource-rich countries found the incidence of PND to be 12–13%, with higher incidence in resource-poor countries.

AETIOLOGY/RISK FACTORS Four systematic reviews have identified the following risk factors for PND: past history of any psychopathology (including history of previous PND), low social support, poor marital relationship, and recent life events. Recent studies from India also suggest that spousal disappointment with the sex of the newborn child, particularly if the child is a girl, is associated with the development of PND.

PROGNOSIS Most episodes of PND resolve spontaneously within 3–6 months, but about one in four affected mothers are still depressed by the child's first birthday. In resource-rich countries, suicide is now the main cause of maternal deaths in the first year postpartum, but the suicide rate is lower at this time than in age-matched non-postpartum women. PND is also associated with negative effects in the infant, including reduced likelihood of secure attachment, deficits in maternal–infant interactions, and impaired cognitive and emotional development of the child, particularly in boys living in areas of socioeconomic deprivation. These associations remain significant even after controlling for subsequent episodes of depression in the mother. However, there is also evidence to suggest that later effects on the child are related to chronic or recurrent maternal depression, rather than postpartum depression per se. Women whose depression persists beyond 6 months postpartum have been found to have fewer positive interactions with their infants than women who were depressed but whose depressive symptoms ended before 6 months, suggesting that the timing of depression is an important factor in determining its effect on the mother–infant relationship.

Postpartum haemorrhage: prevention

David Chelmow

KEY POINTS

- Loss of more than 500 mL of blood is usually caused by failure of the uterus to contract fully after delivery of the placenta, and occurs in over 10% of deliveries with a 1% mortality rate worldwide.

  Other causes of postpartum haemorrhage include retained placental tissue, lacerations to the genital tract, and coagulation disorders.

  Uterine atony is more likely in women who have had a general anaesthetic or oxytocin, an overdistended uterus, a prolonged or precipitous labour, or who are of high parity.

- Active management of the third stage of labour, with controlled cord traction, early cord clamping plus drainage, and prophylactic oxytocic agents, reduces the risk of postpartum haemorrhage and its complications.

  Active management increases nausea, vomiting, and headache, but generally improves maternal satisfaction.

  Controlled cord traction may reduce the risk of retained placenta and need for medical treatment, and can be used in any resource setting.

  Uterine massage and immediate breastfeeding are often used to prevent postpartum haemorrhage, but we found few studies that assessed their benefit.

- Oxytocin has been shown to effectively reduce the risk of postpartum haemorrhage compared with placebo.

  A combination of oxytocin plus ergometrine may be slightly more effective than oxytocin alone, although there are more adverse effects.

  Ergot alkaloids seem as effective as oxytocin, but are also associated with adverse effects, including nausea, placenta retention, and hypertension.

- Prostaglandin treatments vary in their efficacy, but are all associated with adverse effects.

  Carboprost and prostaglandin E2 compounds may be as effective as oxytocin and ergot compounds, but have gastrointestinal adverse effects such as diarrhoea.

  Misoprostol seems ineffective when administered orally, rectally, or vaginally, and is associated with adverse effects, including shivering and fever.

(i) **Please visit www.clinicalevidence.bmj.com for full text and references**

What are the effects of non-drug interventions to prevent primary postpartum haemorrhage?	
Beneficial	• Active management of the third stage of labour
Likely To Be Beneficial	• Controlled cord traction
Unknown Effectiveness	• Immediate breastfeeding • Uterine massage

What are the effects of drug interventions to prevent primary postpartum haemorrhage?	
Beneficial	• Oxytocin
Trade-off Between Benefits And Harms	• Carboprost injection

	• Ergot compounds (ergometrine/methylergotamine) • Oxytocin plus ergometrine combinations
Unknown Effectiveness	• Misoprostol (sublingual) • Prostaglandin E2 compounds
Unlikely To Be Beneficial	• Misoprostol (vaginal)
Likely To Be Ineffective Or Harmful	• Misoprostol (oral) • Misoprostol (rectal)

Search date July 2006

DEFINITION Postpartum haemorrhage is characterised by an estimated blood loss greater than 500 mL. The leading cause of postpartum haemorrhage is uterine atony: the failure of the uterus to contract fully after delivery of the placenta. Postpartum haemorrhage is divided into immediate (primary) and delayed (secondary). Primary postpartum haemorrhage occurs within the first 24 hours after delivery, whereas secondary postpartum haemorrhage occurs after 24 hours and before 6 weeks after delivery. This review will address the effects of strategies for prevention of postpartum haemorrhage after vaginal delivery in low- and high-risk women, specifically looking at strategies to prevent uterine atony. Future updates will examine strategies to prevent postpartum haemorrhage owing to other causes, as well as treatment strategies.

INCIDENCE/PREVALENCE Postpartum haemorrhage complicates 11% of deliveries world-wide, and is responsible for 132,000 deaths, with a case fatality of 1%. It is the leading direct cause of maternal mortality, with most maternal deaths occurring in the most resource-poor countries, particularly Africa and Asia. The imbalance between resource-rich and resource-poor areas probably stems from a combination of: increased prevalence of risk factors such as grand multiparity, safe blood-banking being unavailable, no routine use of prophylaxis against haemorrhage, and measures for drug and surgical management of atony not being available.

AETIOLOGY/RISK FACTORS In addition to uterine atony, immediate postpartum haemorrhage is frequently caused by retained placental tissue; trauma such as laceration of the perineum, vagina, or cervix; rupture of the uterus; or coagulopathy. Risk factors for uterine atony include use of general anaesthetics; an overdistended uterus, particularly from multiple gestations, a large fetus, or polyhydramnios; prolonged labour; precipitous labour; use of oxytocin for labour induction or augmentation; high parity; chorioamnionitis; or history of atony in a previous pregnancy.

PROGNOSIS Most postpartum haemorrhage, particularly in Europe and the USA, is well tolerated by women. However, in low-resource settings, where women may already be significantly anaemic during pregnancy, blood loss of 500 mL is significant. Although death from pregnancy is rare in the USA, postpartum haemorrhage accounts for 17% of deaths. Maternal death is 50–100 times more frequent in resource-poor countries, and postpartum haemorrhage is responsible for a similar proportion of deaths as in the USA. Other significant morbidities associated with postpartum haemorrhage include renal failure, respiratory failure, multiple organ failure, need for transfusion, need for surgery including dilatation and curettage, and, rarely, hysterectomy. Some women with large blood loss will later develop Sheehan's syndrome.

Pre-eclampsia and hypertension

Lelia Duley

KEY POINTS

- Pre-eclampsia (raised blood pressure and proteinuria) complicates 2–8% of pregnancies, and raises morbidity and mortality in the mother and child.

  Pre-eclampsia is more common in women with multiple pregnancy and those who have conditions associated with microvascular disease.

- Antiplatelet drugs (low-dose aspirin) reduce the risk of pre-eclampsia, death of the baby, and premature delivery, without increasing the risks of bleeding, in women at high risk of pre-eclampsia.

  Calcium supplementation reduces the risk of pre-eclampsia and low birthweight compared with placebo.

  We don't know whether fish oil, evening primrose oil, salt restriction, magnesium supplementation, antioxidants, or glyceryl trinitrate are beneficial in high-risk women, because there are insufficient data to draw reliable conclusions.

  We don't know whether atenolol improves pre-eclampsia, but it may worsen outcomes for babies.

- In women with mild to moderate hypertension in pregnancy, antihypertensive drugs reduce the risk of progression to severe hypertension, but may not improve other clinical outcomes.

  ACE inhibitors have been associated with fetal renal failure, and beta-blockers are associated with the baby being small for its gestational age.

  We don't know whether bed rest or hospital admission are also beneficial.

- The consensus is that women who develop severe hypertension in pregnancy should receive antihypertensive treatment, but we don't know which is the most effective antihypertensive agent to use.

  We don't know whether plasma volume expansion, antioxidants, epidural analgesia, or early delivery improve outcomes in women with severe pre-eclampsia.

- Magnesium sulphate reduces the risk of first or subsequent seizures in women with eclampsia compared with placebo, with fewer adverse effects for the mother or baby.

(i) Please visit www.clinicalevidence.bmj.com for full text and references

What are the effects of preventive interventions in women at risk of pre-eclampsia?

Beneficial	• Antiplatelet drugs
	• Calcium supplementation
Unknown Effectiveness	• Antioxidants
	• Fish oil, evening primrose oil, or both
	• Glyceryl trinitrate
	• Magnesium supplementation
	• Salt restriction
Unlikely To Be Beneficial	• Atenolol

What are the effects of interventions in women who develop mild–moderate hypertension during pregnancy?

Unknown Effectiveness	• Antihypertensive drugs for mild to moderate hypertension • Bed rest/admission v day care

What are the effects of interventions in women who develop severe pre-eclampsia or very high blood pressure during pregnancy?

Beneficial	• Prophylactic magnesium sulphate in severe pre-eclampsia
Likely To Be Beneficial	• Antihypertensive drugs for very high blood pressure*
Unknown Effectiveness	• Antioxidants in severe pre-eclampsia • Choice of analgesia during labour with severe pre-eclampsia • Early delivery for severe early-onset pre-eclampsia • Plasma volume expansion in severe pre-eclampsia

What is the best choice of anticonvulsant for women with eclampsia?

Beneficial	• Magnesium sulphate for eclampsia (better and safer than other anticonvulsants)

Search date November 2005

*Consensus opinion is that women with severe hypertension during pregnancy should have antihypertensive treatment. Placebo-controlled trials would therefore be unethical.

DEFINITION Hypertension during pregnancy may be associated with one of several conditions. **Pregnancy-induced hypertension** is a rise in blood pressure, without proteinuria, during the second half of pregnancy. **Pre-eclampsia** is a multisystem disorder, unique to pregnancy, which is usually associated with raised blood pressure and proteinuria. It rarely presents before 20 weeks' gestation. **Eclampsia** is one or more convulsions in association with the syndrome of pre-eclampsia. **Pre-existing hypertension** (not covered in this review) is known hypertension before pregnancy or raised blood pressure before 20 weeks' gestation. It may be essential hypertension or, less commonly, secondary to underlying disease.

INCIDENCE/PREVALENCE Pregnancy-induced hypertension affects 10% of pregnancies, and pre-eclampsia complicates 2–8% of pregnancies. Eclampsia occurs in about 1/2000 deliveries in resource-rich countries. In resource-poor countries, estimates of the incidence of eclampsia vary from 1/100–1/1700.

AETIOLOGY/RISK FACTORS The cause of pre-eclampsia is unknown. It is likely to be multifactorial, and may result from deficient placental implantation during the first half of pregnancy. Pre-eclampsia is more common among women likely to have a large placenta,

(continued over)

(from previous page)

such as those with multiple pregnancy, and among women with medical conditions associated with microvascular disease, such as diabetes, hypertension, and collagen vascular disease. Other risk factors include genetic susceptibility, increased parity, and older maternal age. Cigarette smoking seems to be associated with a lower risk of pre-eclampsia, but this potential benefit is outweighed by an increase in adverse outcomes, such as low birthweight, placental abruption, and perinatal death.

PROGNOSIS The outcome of pregnancy in women with pregnancy-induced hypertension alone is at least as good as that for normotensive pregnancies. However, once pre-eclampsia develops, morbidity and mortality rise for both mother and child. For example, perinatal mortality for women with severe pre-eclampsia is double that for normotensive women. Perinatal outcome is worse with early gestational hypertension. Perinatal mortality also increases in women with severe essential hypertension.

David M Haas

KEY POINTS

- Around 5–10% of all births in resource-rich countries occur before 37 weeks' gestation, leading to increased risks of neonatal and infant death and neurological disability in surviving infants.

- Progestogens and prophylactic cervical cerclage may reduce preterm birth when used in high-risk women, but enhanced antenatal-care programmes and bed rest have repeatedly been shown not to be beneficial.

   Prophylactic cervical cerclage may reduce preterm births in women with cervical changes or protruding membranes, but is unlikely to be effective, and may increase infection, in women with no cervical changes or with twin pregnancies.

- A single course of antenatal corticosteroids reduces respiratory distress syndrome, intraventricular haemorrhage, and neonatal mortality compared with placebo, with no long-term complications, in babies born before 37 weeks' gestation.

   Adding thyrotropin-releasing hormone to corticosteroids has not been shown to improve outcomes compared with corticosteroids alone, and increases the risk of adverse effects.

- Antibiotics may prolong the pregnancy and reduce infection after premature rupture of the membranes, but are not beneficial when the membranes are intact.

- Calcium channel blockers may be effective at delaying labour compared with other tocolytics.

   Beta$_2$ agonists and magnesium sulphate do not prevent premature birth and do increase fetal and maternal adverse effects compared with placebo.

   We cannot be sure whether oxytocin receptor antagonists (such as atosiban) or prostaglandin inhibitors (such as indometacin) prevent preterm delivery.

- Elective caesarean section increases maternal morbidity compared with selective caesarean sections, but neonatal morbidity and mortality seem to be the same.

 Please visit www.clinicalevidence.bmj.com for full text and references

What are the effects of preventive interventions in women at high risk of preterm delivery?

Likely To Be Beneficial	• Progesterone • Prophylactic cervical cerclage for women at risk of preterm labour with cervical changes
Unknown Effectiveness	• Prophylactic cervical cerclage in women at risk of preterm labour with protruding membranes
Unlikely To Be Beneficial	• Prophylactic cervical cerclage for women at risk of preterm labour with no cervical changes
Likely To Be Ineffective Or Harmful	• Bed rest • Enhanced antenatal-care programmes for socially deprived population groups/high-risk groups

What are the effects of interventions to improve outcome after preterm rupture of membranes?

Likely To Be Beneficial	• Antibiotic treatment for premature rupture of membranes (prolongs gestation and may reduce infection, but unknown effect on perinatal mortality; Co-amoxiclav significantly increases necrotising enterocolitis)
Unknown Effectiveness	• Amnioinfusion for preterm rupture of membranes

What are the effects of treatments to stop contractions in preterm labour?

Likely To Be Beneficial	• Calcium channel blockers
Unknown Effectiveness	• Oxytocin receptor antagonists (atosiban) • Prostaglandin inhibitors (indometacin)
Unlikely To Be Beneficial	• Beta mimetics
Likely To Be Ineffective Or Harmful	• Magnesium sulphate

What are the effects of elective compared with selective caesarean delivery for women in preterm labour?

Unlikely To Be Beneficial	• Elective rather than selective caesarean delivery in preterm labour

What are the effects of interventions to improve outcome in preterm delivery?

Beneficial	• Antenatal corticosteroids
Likely To Be Ineffective Or Harmful	• Antibiotic treatment for preterm labour with intact membranes • Thyrotropin-releasing hormone plus corticosteroids before preterm delivery

Search date June 2006

DEFINITION Preterm or premature birth is defined by the WHO as delivery of an infant before 37 completed weeks of gestation. Clinically, deliveries at less than 34 weeks' gestation may be a more relevant definition. There is no set lower limit to this definition, but 23–24 weeks' gestation is widely accepted, which approximates to an average fetal weight of 500 g.

INCIDENCE/PREVALENCE Preterm birth occurs in about 5–10% of all births in resource-rich countries, but in recent years the incidence seems to have increased in some countries, particularly the USA. We found little reliable evidence for incidence (using the definition of premature birth given above) in resource-poor countries. The rate in northwestern Ethiopia has been reported to vary from 11 to 22%, depending on the age group of mothers studied, and is highest in teenage mothers.

AETIOLOGY/RISK FACTORS About 30% of preterm births are unexplained and spontaneous. Multiple pregnancy accounts for about another 30% of cases. Other known risk factors include genital-tract infection, preterm rupture of the membranes, antepartum haemorrhage, cervical incompetence, and congenital uterine abnormalities, which collectively account for about 20–25% of cases. The remaining cases (15–20%) are attributed to elective preterm delivery secondary to hypertensive disorders of pregnancy, intrauterine fetal growth restriction, congenital abnormalities, trauma, and medical disorders of pregnancy. About 50% of women receiving placebo therapy do not give birth within 7 days from the start of treatment. This statistic could be interpreted as indicating either that a large proportion of preterm labour resolves spontaneously, or that there are inaccuracies in the diagnosis. The two strongest risk factors for idiopathic preterm labour are low socioeconomic status and previous preterm delivery. Women with a history of preterm birth had a significantly increased risk of subsequent preterm birth (less than 34 weeks) compared with women who had previously given birth after 35 weeks' gestation (OR 5.6, 95% CI 4.5 to 7.0).

PROGNOSIS Preterm birth is the leading cause of neonatal death and infant mortality, often as a result of respiratory distress syndrome as a consequence of immature lung development. Children who survive are also at high risk of neurological disability. Observational studies have found that one preterm birth significantly raises the risk of another in a subsequent pregnancy.

Recurrent miscarriage

Kirsten Duckitt and Aysha Qureshi

KEY POINTS

- Recurrent miscarriage is the spontaneous loss of three or more consecutive pregnancies with the same biological father in the first trimester, and affects 1–2% of women, in half of whom there is no identifiable cause.

  Overall, 75% of affected women will have a successful subsequent pregnancy, but this rate falls for older mothers and with increasing number of miscarriages.

  Antiphospholipid syndrome, with anticardiolipin or lupus anticoagulant antibodies, is present in 15% of women with recurrent first- and second-trimester miscarriage.

- We don't know whether bed rest, early scanning, lifestyle adaptation to stop smoking, reduce alcohol consumption and lose weight, low-dose aspirin, human chorionic gonadotrophin, trophoblastic membrane infusion, or vitamin supplementation increase the likelihood of a successful pregnancy in women with recurrent miscarriage.

- We don't know whether oestrogen supplementation increases the live-birth rate in women with recurrent miscarriage, but it may increase the miscarriage rate and cause abnormalities in the fetus.

  We don't know whether progesterone supplementation or corticosteroids reduce miscarriage rates compared with placebo.

- Paternal white-cell immunisation and intravenous immunoglobulin treatment do not seem likely to improve live-birth rates compared with placebo.

- We don't know whether low-dose aspirin, alone or combined with heparin, can increase the live-birth rate in women with antiphospholipid syndrome, compared with placebo.

  Prednisolone plus aspirin may not increase live-birth rates in women with antiphospholipid syndrome, and increases the risk of adverse effects compared with placebo.

(i) **Please visit www.clinicalevidence.bmj.com for full text and references**

What are the effects of treatments for unexplained recurrent miscarriage?	
Unknown Effectiveness	• Aspirin (low dose) in unexpected miscarriage
	• Bed rest
	• Corticosteroids
	• Early scanning in subsequent pregnancies
	• Human chorionic gonadotrophin
	• Lifestyle adaptation (smoking cessation, reducing alcohol consumption, losing weight)
	• Progesterone
	• Trophoblastic membrane infusion
	• Vitamin supplementation
Unlikely To Be Beneficial	• Intravenous immunoglobulin treatment
	• Paternal white-cell immunisation
Likely To Be Ineffective Or Harmful	• Oestrogen

What are the effects of treatments for recurrent miscarriage caused by antiphospholipid syndrome?

Unknown Effectiveness	• Aspirin (low dose) in antiphospholipid syndrome
	• Low-dose aspirin plus heparin
Likely To Be Ineffective Or Harmful	• Corticosteroids

Search date November 2005

DEFINITION Recurrent miscarriage is usually defined as three or more consecutive, spontaneous miscarriages occurring in the first trimester, with the same biological father. They may or may not follow a successful birth. About half of recurrent miscarriages are unexplained. This review covers unexplained recurrent miscarriage. **Antiphospholipid syndrome (APS)** is one of the known causes of first- and second-trimester recurrent miscarriage. APS is defined as the presence of anticardiolipin antibodies or lupus anticoagulant antibodies, in association with either three or more consecutive fetal losses before week 10 of gestation, one or more unexplained intrauterine deaths beyond 10 weeks of gestation, or one or more premature births before 34 weeks because of severe pre-eclampsia or impaired fetal growth. This review covers both and first- and second-trimester recurrent miscarriages in women with APS.

INCIDENCE/PREVALENCE In western populations, recurrent miscarriage affects 1–2% of women of childbearing age, and about half of these are unexplained. Antiphospholipid antibodies are present in 15% of women with recurrent miscarriage.

AETIOLOGY/RISK FACTORS Increasing maternal age and number of previous miscarriages increase the risk of further miscarriages. No separate risk factors for APS are known.

PROGNOSIS On average, the live-birth rate for women with unexplained recurrent miscarriage is 75% in a subsequent pregnancy, with a miscarriage rate of 20% up to 9 weeks and a 5% miscarriage rate after this period. However, prognosis varies depending on maternal age and number of previous miscarriages. The chance of a successful subsequent pregnancy after three previous unexplained miscarriages varies from about 54% in a 45-year-old woman to about 90% in a 20-year-old woman. A 30-year-old woman with two previous unexplained miscarriages has about an 84% chance of a successful subsequent pregnancy, whereas for a woman of the same age with five previous unexplained miscarriages the success rate drops to about 71%.

Sat Sharma

KEY POINTS

- Acute respiratory distress syndrome (ARDS) is characterised by lung inflammation with severe hypoxia, which usually develops over 4–48 hours and persists for days or weeks.

  The main causes of ARDS are infections, aspiration of gastric contents, and trauma.

  Between a third and a half of people with ARDS die, but mortality depends on the underlying cause. Some survivors have long-term respiratory or cognitive problems.

- Low tidal volume ventilation, at 6 mL/kg of predicted body weight, reduces mortality compared with high tidal volume ventilation, but can lead to respiratory acidosis.

  Protective ventilation (positive end expiratory pressure [PEEP]) that maintains PaO_2 above 60 mm Hg is considered effective in people with ARDS, but no difference in mortality has been found for high-PEEP compared with lower-PEEP strategies.

- People with ARDS may remain hypoxic despite mechanical ventilation. Nursing in the prone position may improve oxygenation, but has not been shown to reduce mortality, and can increase sedation and facial oedema.

  The prone position is contraindicated in people with spinal instability, and should be used with caution in people with haemodynamic and cardiac instability, or who have had recent thoracic or abdominal surgery.

- We found insufficient evidence to draw reliable conclusions on the effects of corticosteroids on mortality or reversal of ARDS.

  Corticosteroids have been used in late-phase ARDS when an exaggerated fibroproliferative response can occur. Despite improvement in cardiopulmonary physiology, corticosteroids did not affect survival, while late administration increased the risk of death.

- Nitric oxide has not been shown to improve survival or duration of ventilation, or hospital admission, compared with placebo. It may modestly improve oxygenation in the short term but the improvement is not sustained.

(i) **Please visit www.clinicalevidence.bmj.com for full text and references**

What are the effects of interventions in adults with acute respiratory distress syndrome?	
Beneficial	• Low tidal volume mechanical ventilation
Likely To Be Beneficial	• Protective ventilation
Trade-off Between Benefits And Harms	• Prone position
Unknown Effectiveness	• Corticosteroids
Unlikely To Be Beneficial	• Nitric oxide

Search date August 2006

DEFINITION Acute respiratory distress syndrome (ARDS), originally described by Ashbaugh et al in 1967, is a clinical syndrome that represents the severe end of the spectrum of acute lung injury (ALI). In 1994, the American–European Consensus Conference on ARDS made the following recommendations. Widespread acceptance of these definitions by clinicians and researchers has improved standardisation of clinical research. **Acute lung injury:** a syndrome of acute and persistent inflammatory disease of the lungs characterised by three clinical features: 1) bilateral pulmonary infiltrates on the chest radiograph; 2) a ratio of the partial pressure of arterial oxygen to the fraction of inspired oxygen (PaO_2/FiO_2) of less than 300; 3) absence of clinical evidence of left atrial hypertension (if measured, the pulmonary capillary wedge pressure is 18 mm Hg or less). **Acute respiratory distress syndrome:** The definition of ARDS is the same as that of ALI, except that the hypoxia is severe a PaO_2/FiO_2 ratio of 200 mm Hg or less. The distinction between ALI and ARDS is arbitrary, because the severity of hypoxia does not correlate reliably with the extent of the underlying pathology, and does not influence predictably clinical course or survival. ARDS is an acute disorder, which typically develops over 4–48 hours and persists for days to weeks. Subacute or chronic lung diseases, such as sarcoidosis and idiopathic pulmonary fibrosis, are excluded from the definition of ARDS. The early pathological features of ARDS are generally described as diffuse alveolar damage. Recognition of diffuse alveolar damage requires histological examination of the lung tissue, which is not necessary to make a clinical diagnosis. **Population:** For the purpose of this review, we have defined ARDS as including people with ALI and ARDS. It therefore includes adults with ALI and ARDS from any cause and with any level of severity. Neonates and children less than 12 years of age have been excluded.

INCIDENCE/PREVALENCE Ten to fifteen per cent of all people admitted to an intensive-care unit, and up to 20% of mechanically ventilated people meet the criteria for ARDS. The incidence of ALI in the USA (17–64/100,000 person-years) seems to be higher than in Europe, Australia, and other resource-rich countries (17–34/100,000 person-years). One prospective, population-based cohort study (1113 people in Washington State aged over 15 years) found the crude incidence of ALI to be 78.9/100,000 person years, and the age-adjusted incidence to be 86.2/100,000 person years. An annual incidence of 15.5 cases a year or 5.9 cases/100,000 people a year was reported in a recent epidemiological study from Iceland. An observational cohort reported that in Shanghai, China, of 5320 adults admitted to intensive care units in 1 year, 108 (2%) had symptoms that met with ARDS criteria.

AETIOLOGY/RISK FACTORS ARDS encompasses many distinct disorders that share common clinical and pathophysiological features. More than 60 causes of ARDS have been identified. Although the list of possible causes is long, most episodes of ARDS are associated with a few common causes or predisposing conditions, either individually or in combination. These include sepsis, aspiration of gastric contents, infectious pneumonia, severe trauma, surface burns, lung contusion, fat embolism syndrome, massive blood transfusion, lung and bone marrow transplantation, drugs, acute pancreatitis, near drowning, cardiopulmonary bypass, and neurogenic pulmonary oedema. The incidence of ALI in a large cohort of people with subarachnoid haemorrhage has been reported to be 27% (170/620 people; 95% CI, 24% to 31%). One or more of these predisposing conditions are often evident at the onset of ALI. When ARDS occurs in the absence of common risk factors such as trauma, sepsis, or aspiration, an effort should be made to identify a specific cause for lung injury. In such cases, a systematic review of the events that immediately preceded the onset of ARDS is normally undertaken to identify the predisposing factors.

PROGNOSIS Mortality: Survival for people with ARDS has improved remarkably in recent years, and cohort studies have found mortality to range from 34% to 58%. Mortality varies with the cause; however, by far the most common cause of death is multiorgan system failure rather than acute respiratory failure. In a prospective cohort study (207 people at risk of developing ARDS, of which 47 developed ARDS during the trial), only 16% of deaths were considered to have been caused by irreversible respiratory failure. Most deaths in the first 3 days of being diagnosed with ARDS could be attributed to the underlying illness or injury. Most late deaths (after 3 days, 16/22 [72.7%]) were related to sepsis syndrome. One prospective cohort study (902 mechanically ventilated people with ALI) found that an

(continued over)

(from previous page)

age of 70 years or younger significantly increased the proportion of people who survived at 28 days (74.6% aged up to 70 years v 50.3% aged at least 71 years; P less than 0.001). In a recent observational study (2004), the overall intensive-care-unit mortality was 10.3%. In-hospital mortality was 68.5%, and 90-day mortality was 70.4% in people with ARDS, and accounted for 13.5% of the overall intensive-care-unit mortality. **Lung function and morbidity:** One cohort study of 16 long-term survivors of severe ARDS (lung-injury score at least 2.5) found that only mild abnormalities in pulmonary function (and often none) were observed. Restrictive and obstructive ventilatory defects (each noted in 4/16 [25%] people) were observed in ARDS survivors treated with low or conventional tidal volumes. One cohort study of 109 people found no significant difference between various ventilatory strategies and long-term abnormalities in pulmonary function or health-related quality of life. However, it did find an association between abnormal pulmonary function and decreased quality of life at 1-year follow-up. One retrospective cohort study (41 people with ARDS) found that duration of mechanical ventilation and severity of ARDS were important determinants of persistent symptoms 1 year after recovery. Better lung function was observed when no illness was acquired during the intensive care unit stay, and with rapid resolution of multiple organ failure (e.g. pneumonia during ARDS: 7/41 [17.1%] people with long-term impairment v 2/41 [4.9%] with no long-term impairment; significance assessment not performed). Persistent disability 1 year after discharge from the intensive care unit in survivors of ARDS is secondary to extrapulmonary conditions, most importantly muscle wasting and weakness. **Cognitive morbidity:** One cohort study (55 people 1 year after ARDS) found that 17/55 (30.1%) exhibited generalised cognitive decline and 43/55 (78.2%) had all, or at least one, of the following: impaired memory, attention, concentration, and decreased mental processing speed. These deficits may be related to hypoxaemia, drug toxicity, or complications of critical illness. To date, no association between different ventilatory strategies and long-term neurological outcomes has been found.

Peter Wark

KEY POINTS

- Acute bronchitis, with transient inflammation of the trachea and major bronchi, affects over 40/1000 adults a year in the UK.

  The causes are usually considered to be infective, but only around half of people have identifiable pathogens.

  The role of smoking or environmental tobacco-smoke inhalation in predisposing to acute bronchitis is unclear.

  A third of people may have longer term symptoms or recurrence.

- Antibiotics have only a modest effect on the duration of cough compared with placebo, and increase the risks of adverse effects and drug resistance.

  We don't know for sure which antibiotic regimen is superior.

  There is no evidence to support the use of broad-spectrum antibiotics such as quinolones or amoxicillin plus clavulonic acid over amoxicillin alone in acute bronchitis.

  Smokers have not been shown to be more likely than non-smokers to benefit from antibiotics.

- We don't know whether antihistamines, antitussives, inhaled or oral beta$_2$ agonists, or expectorants improve symptoms of acute bronchitis compared with placebo, as few good-quality studies have been found.

(i)   **Please visit www.clinicalevidence.bmj.com for full text and references**

What are the effects of treatments for acute bronchitis in people without chronic respiratory disease?

Trade-off Between Benefits And Harms	• Antibiotics versus placebo and other treatments
Unknown Effectiveness	• Amoxicillin, cephalosporins, and macrolides versus each other (no significant difference in clinical cure among different antibiotics; insufficient evidence on adverse effects) • Antihistamines • Antitussives • Beta$_2$ agonists (inhaled) • Beta$_2$ agonists (oral) • Expectorants
Unlikely To Be Beneficial	• Amoxicillin plus clavulanic acid (no significant difference in clinical cure compared with cephalosporins but increased adverse effects)

Search date July 2006

DEFINITION Acute bronchitis is a transient inflammation of the trachea and major bronchi. Clinically, it is diagnosed on the basis of cough and occasionally sputum, dyspnoea, and wheeze. This review is limited to episodes of acute bronchitis in people (smokers and non-smokers) with no pre-existing respiratory disease such as a pre-existing diagnosis of asthma or chronic bronchitis, evidence of fixed airflow obstruction, or both, and excluding

(continued over)

(from previous page)

those with clinical or radiographic evidence of pneumonia. However, the reliance on a clinical definition for acute bronchitis implies that people with conditions such as transient/mild asthma or mild COPD may have been recruited in some of the reported studies.

INCIDENCE/PREVALENCE Acute bronchitis affects 44/1000 adults (over 16 years old) each year in the UK, with 82% of episodes occurring in autumn or winter. One survey found that acute bronchitis was the fifth most common reason for people of any age to present to a general practitioner in Australia.

AETIOLOGY/RISK FACTORS Infection is believed to be the trigger for acute bronchitis. However, pathogens have been identified in fewer than 55% of people. Community studies that attempted to isolate pathogens from the sputum of people with acute bronchitis found viruses in 8–23%, typical bacteria (*Streptococcus pneumoniae, Haemophilus influenzae, Moraxella catarrhalis*) in 45%, and atypical bacteria (*Mycobacterium pneumoniae, Chlamydia pneumoniae, Bordetella pertussis*) in 0–25%. It is unclear whether smoking affects the risk for developing acute bronchitis.

PROGNOSIS Acute bronchitis is regarded as a mild, self-limiting illness, but there are limited data on prognosis and rates of complications such as chronic cough or progression to chronic bronchitis or pneumonia. One prospective longitudinal study reviewed 653 previously well adults who presented to suburban general practices over a 12-month period with symptoms of acute lower respiratory tract infection. It found that, within the first month of the illness, 20% of people re-presented to their general practitioner with persistent or recurrent symptoms, mostly persistent cough. The no-treatment control group of one RCT (212 people; about 16% took antibiotics outside of the study protocol) found that participants had at least a slight problem with cough for a mean of 11.4 days, with "moderately bad" cough lasting for a mean of 5.7 days. Another prospective study of 138 previously well adults found that 34% had symptoms consistent with either chronic bronchitis or asthma 3 years after initial presentation with acute bronchitis. It is also unclear whether acute bronchitis plays a causal role in the progression to chronic bronchitis or is simply a marker of predisposition to chronic lung disease. Although smoking has been identified as the most important risk factor for chronic bronchitis, it is unclear whether the inflammatory effects of cigarette smoke and infection causing acute bronchitis have additive effects in leading to chronic inflammatory airway changes. In children, exposure to parental environmental tobacco smoke is associated with an increase in risk for community lower respiratory infection in children aged 0–2 years and an increase in symptoms of cough and phlegm in those aged 5–16 years.

Bruce Arroll

KEY POINTS

- Transmission of common cold infections is mostly through hand-to-hand contact rather than droplet spread. Several types of virus can cause symptoms of colds.

  Each year, children suffer up to 5 colds and adults have 2–3 infections, leading to time off school or work and considerable discomfort. Most symptoms resolve within a week, but coughs often persist for longer.

- Nasal and oral decongestants reduce nasal congestion over 3–10 hours, but we don't know whether they are effective in the longer term (more than 10 hours).

- Antibiotics don't reduce symptoms overall, and may cause adverse effects and increase antibiotic resistance.

  Antibiotics may improve symptoms after 5 days compared with placebo in people with nasopharyngeal culture-positive *Haemophilus influenzae*, *Moraxella catarrhalis*, or *Streptococcus pneumoniae*, but it is difficult to identify which people may have these infections.

- Vitamin C seems unlikely to reduce the duration or severity of cold symptoms compared with placebo.

  We don't know whether zinc gel or lozenges, Echinacea, steam inhalation, analgesics, or anti-inflammatory drugs reduce the duration of symptoms of colds.

- Antihistamines may slightly reduce runny nose and sneezing, but their overall effect seems to be small. Some antihistamines may cause sedation or arrhythmias.

Please visit www.clinicalevidence.bmj.com for full text and references

What are the effects of treatments?	
Likely To Be Beneficial	• Antihistamines (may improve runny nose and sneezing, no significant difference in overall symptoms) • Decongestants (norephedrine, oxymetazoline, or pseudoephedrine) provided short-term (3–10 hour) relief of congestive symptoms
Unknown Effectiveness	• Analgesics or anti-inflammatory drugs • Decongestants (insufficient evidence to assess longer-term [more than 10 hours] effects on congestive symptoms) • Echinacea • Steam inhalation • Zinc (intranasal gel or lozenges)
Unlikely To Be Beneficial	• Vitamin C
Likely To Be Ineffective Or Harmful	• Antibiotics

Search date May 2006

DEFINITION Common colds are defined as upper respiratory tract infections that affect the predominantly nasal part of the respiratory mucosa. Because upper respiratory tract infections can affect any part of the mucosa, it is often arbitrary whether an upper respiratory tract infection is called a "cold" or "sore throat" ("pharyngitis" or "tonsillitis"), "sinusitis", "acute otitis media", or "bronchitis". Sometimes all areas (simultaneously or at different times) are affected in one illness. Symptoms include sneezing, rhinorrhoea (runny nose), headache, and general malaise. In addition to nasal symptoms, half of sufferers experience sore throat, and 40% experience cough. This review does not include treatments for people with acute sinusitis (see acute sinusitis, p 203), acute bronchitis (see bronchitis (acute), p 491), or sore throat (see sore throat, p 496).

INCIDENCE/PREVALENCE Upper respiratory tract infections, nasal congestion, throat complaints, and cough are responsible for 11% of general practice consultations in Australia. Each year, children suffer about five such infections and adults 2–3 infections. One cross-sectional study in Norwegian children aged 4–5 years found that 48% experienced more than two common colds annually.

AETIOLOGY/RISK FACTORS Transmission of common cold infection is mostly through hand-to-hand contact with subsequent passage to the nostrils or eyes rather than, as commonly perceived, through droplets in the air. Common cold infections are mainly caused by viruses (typically rhinovirus, but also coronavirus and respiratory syncytial virus, or metapneumovirus and others). For many colds, no infecting organism can be identified.

PROGNOSIS Common colds are usually short lived, lasting a few days, with a few lingering symptoms lasting longer, especially cough. Symptoms peak within 1–3 days and generally clear by 1 week, although cough often persists. Although they cause no mortality or serious morbidity, common colds are responsible for considerable discomfort, lost work, and medical costs.

Mark Loeb

KEY POINTS

- In the northern hemisphere, about 12/1000 people a year on average contract pneumonia while living in the community, with most cases caused by *Streptococcus pneumoniae.*

  People at greatest risk include those at the extremes of age, smokers, alcoholics, and those with lung or heart disease, or immunosuppression.

  Mortality ranges from about 5–35% depending on severity of disease, with a worse prognosis in older people, men, and people with chronic diseases.

- Deaths from influenza are usually caused by pneumonia. Influenza vaccine reduces the risk of clinical influenza, and may reduce the risk of pneumonia and mortality in elderly people.

  Pneumococcal vaccine is unlikely to reduce all-cause pneumonia or mortality in immunocompetent adults, but may reduce pneumococcal pneumonia in this group.

- Antibiotics lead to clinical cure in 80% or more of people with pneumonia being treated in the community or in hospital, although no one regimen has been shown to be superior to the others in either setting.

  Early mobilisation may reduce hospital stay compared with usual care in people being treated with antibiotics.

  Intravenous antibiotics have not been shown to improve clinical cure rates or survival compared with oral antibiotics in people treated in hospital for non-severe community acquired pneumonia.

- Prompt administration of antibiotics may improve survival in people receiving intensive care for community-acquired pneumonia, compared with delayed treatment, although few studies have been done.

  We don't know which is the optimum antibiotic regimen to use in these people.

(i) **Please visit www.clinicalevidence.bmj.com for full text and references**

What are the effects of interventions to prevent community-acquired pneumonia?

Likely To Be Beneficial	• Influenza vaccine (in elderly people)†
Unlikely To Be Beneficial	• Pneumococcal vaccine (for all-cause pneumonia and mortality in immunocompetent adults)

What are the effects of treatments for community-acquired pneumonia in outpatient settings?

Beneficial	• Antibiotics in outpatient settings (compared with no antibiotics)*

What are the effects of treatments for community-acquired pneumonia in people admitted to hospital?

Beneficial	• Antibiotics in hospital (compared with no antibiotics)*
Likely To Be Beneficial	• Early mobilisation (reduced hospital stay compared with usual care)
Unlikely To Be Beneficial	• Intravenous antibiotics in immunocompetent people in hospital without life-threatening illness (compared with oral antibiotics)

What are the effects of treatments in people with community-acquired pneumonia receiving intensive care?

Likely To Be Beneficial	• Prompt administration of antibiotics in people admitted to intensive care with community-acquired pneumonia (improved outcomes compared with delayed antibiotic treatment)†
Unknown Effectiveness	• Different combinations of antibiotics in intensive-care settings

Search date April 2006

*Based on consensus, RCTs likely to be considered unethical.
† Based on observational data.

DEFINITION Community-acquired pneumonia is pneumonia contracted in the community rather than in hospital. It is defined by clinical symptoms (such as cough, sputum production, and pleuritic chest pain) and signs (such as fever, tachypnoea, and rales), with radiological confirmation.

INCIDENCE/PREVALENCE In the northern hemisphere, community-acquired pneumonia affects about 12/1000 people a year, particularly during winter and at the extremes of age (annual incidence in people under 1 year old: 30–50/1000; 15–45 years old: 1–5/1000; 60–70 years old: 10–20/1000; 71–85 years old: 50/1000).

AETIOLOGY/RISK FACTORS More than 100 microorganisms have been implicated in community-acquired pneumonia, but most cases are caused by *Streptococcus pneumoniae*. Case-control study data suggest that smoking is probably an important risk factor. One large cohort study conducted in Finland (4175 people aged at least 60 years) suggested that risk factors for pneumonia in older people included alcoholism (RR 9.0, 95% CI 5.1 to 16.2), bronchial asthma (RR 4.2, 95% CI 3.3 to 5.4), immunosuppression (RR 3.1, 95% CI 1.9 to 5.1), lung disease (RR 3.0, 95% CI 2.3 to 3.9), heart disease (RR 1.9, 95% CI 1.7 to 2.3), institutionalisation (RR 1.8, 95% CI 1.4 to 2.4), and increasing age (at least 70 years v 60–69 years; RR 1.5, 95% CI 1.3 to 1.7).

PROGNOSIS Severity varies from mild- to life-threatening illness within days of the onset of symptoms. A prospective cohort study (over 14,000 people) found that old age was an extremely important factor in determining prognosis. One systematic review of prognosis studies for community-acquired pneumonia (search date 1995, 33,148 people) found overall mortality to be 13.7%, ranging from 5.1% for ambulant people to 36.5% for people who required intensive care. The following prognostic factors were significantly associated with mortality: male sex (OR 1.3, 95% CI 1.2 to 1.4), absence of pleuritic chest pain (OR 2.00, 95% CI 1.25 to 3.30); hypothermia (OR 5.0, 95% CI 2.4 to 10.4); systolic hypotension (OR 4.8, 95% CI 2.8 to 8.3); tachypnoea (OR 2.9, 95% CI 1.7 to 4.9); diabetes mellitus (OR 1.3, 95% CI 1.1 to 1.5); neoplastic disease (OR 2.8, 95% CI 2.4 to 3.1); neurological disease (OR 4.6, 95% CI 2.3 to 8.9); bacteraemia (OR 2.8, 95% CI 2.3 to 3.6); leucopenia (OR 2.5, 95% CI 1.6 to 3.7); and multilobar radiographic pulmonary infiltrates (OR 3.1, 95% CI 1.9 to 5.1).

Tim Kenealy

KEY POINTS

- Sore throat is an acute upper respiratory tract infection that affects the respiratory mucosa of the throat.

- About 10% of people present to primary healthcare services with sore throat each year.

  The causative organisms of sore throat may be bacteria (most commonly *Streptococcus*) or viruses (typically rhinovirus), but it is difficult to distinguish bacterial from viral infections clinically.

- NSAIDs may reduce the pain of sore throat at 24 hours or less, and at 2–5 days.

  NSAIDs are associated with gastrointestinal and renal adverse effects.

- Paracetamol seems to effectively reduce the pain of acute infective sore throat after a single dose, or regular doses over 2 days.

- Antibiotics can reduce the proportion of people with symptoms associated with sore throat at 3 days.

  Reduction in symptoms seems greater for people with positive throat swabs for *Streptococcus* than for people with negative swabs.

  Antibiotics are generally associated with adverse effects such as nausea, rash, vaginitis, and headache, and widespread usage may lead to bacterial resistance.

- Antibiotics may also reduce suppurative and non-suppurative complications of group A beta haemolytic streptococcal pharyngitis, although non-suppurative complications are rare in industrialised countries.

- Corticosteroids added to antibiotics may reduce the severity of pain from sore throat in children and adults compared with antibiotics alone.

  Most studies used a single dose of corticosteroid.

  However, data from other disorders suggest that long-term use of corticosteroids is associated with serious adverse effects.

- Super-colonisation with *Streptococcus* isolated from healthy individuals apparently resistant to infections from *Streptococcus* may reduce recurrence of sore throat, although there is currently no evidence to suggest it may treat symptoms of acute sore throat.

(i) **Please visit www.clinicalevidence.bmj.com for full text and references**

What are the effects of interventions to reduce symptoms of acute infective sore throat?	
Likely To Be Beneficial	• NSAIDs
	• Paracetamol (acetaminophen)
Trade-off Between Benefits And Harms	• Antibiotics
	• Corticosteroids
Unknown Effectiveness	• Probiotics

What are the effects of interventions to prevent complications of acute infective sore throat?

Trade-off Between Benefits And Harms	• Antibiotics

Search date May 2007

DEFINITION Sore throat is an acute upper respiratory tract infection that affects the respiratory mucosa of the throat. Since infections can affect any part of the mucosa, it is often arbitrary whether an acute upper respiratory tract infection is called "sore throat" ("pharyngitis" or "tonsillitis"), "common cold", "sinusitis", "otitis media", or "bronchitis". Sometimes, all areas are affected (simultaneously or at different times) in one illness. In this review, we aim to cover people whose principal presenting symptom is sore throat. This may be associated with headache, fever, and general malaise. Suppurative complications include acute otitis media (most commonly), acute sinusitis, and peritonsillar abscess (quinsy). Non-suppurative complications include acute rheumatic fever and acute glomerulonephritis.

INCIDENCE/PREVALENCE There is little seasonal fluctuation in sore throat. About 10% of the Australian population present to primary healthcare services annually with an upper respiratory tract infection consisting predominantly of sore throat. This reflects about a fifth of the overall annual incidence. However, it is difficult to distinguish between the different types of upper respiratory tract infection. A Scottish mail survey found that 31% of adult respondents reported a severe sore throat in the previous year, for which 38% of these people visited a doctor.

AETIOLOGY/RISK FACTORS The causative organisms of sore throat may be bacteria (*Streptococcus*, most commonly group A beta haemolytic, but sometimes *Haemophilus influenzae*, *Moraxella catarrhalis*, and others) or viruses (typically rhinovirus, but also coronavirus, respiratory syncytial virus, metapneumovirus, Epstein–Barr, and others). It is difficult to distinguish bacterial from viral infections clinically. Features thought to indicate *Streptococcus* infection are: fever greater than 38.5 °C; exudate on the tonsils; anterior neck lymphadenopathy; and absence of cough. Sore throat can be caused by processes other than primary infections, including GORD, physical or chemical irritation (e.g. from nasogastric tubes, or smoke), and occasionally hay fever. However, we consider only primary infections in this review.

PROGNOSIS The untreated symptoms of sore throat disappear by 3 days in about 40% of people, and untreated fevers in about 85%. By 1 week, 85% of people are symptom free. This natural history is similar in *Streptococcus*-positive, -negative, and untested people,

Abel Wakai

KEY POINTS

- Spontaneous pneumothorax is defined as air entering the pleural space without any provoking factor, such as trauma, surgery, or diagnostic intervention.

    Incidence is 24/100,000 a year in men, and 10/100,000 in women in England and Wales, and the major contributing factor is smoking, which increases the likelihood by 22 times in men and by 8 times in women.

    While death from spontaneous pneumothorax is rare, rates of recurrence are high, with one study of men in the US finding a total recurrence rate of 35%.

- Overall, we found insufficient evidence to determine whether any intervention is more effective than no intervention for spontaneous pneumothorax.

- Chest-tube drainage appears to be a useful treatment for spontaneous pneumothorax, although the evidence is somewhat sparse.

    Small (8 French gauge) chest tubes are generally easier to insert, and may reduce the risk of subcutaneous emphysema, although successful resolution may be less likely in people with large pneumothoraces (more than 50% lung volume). We don't know whether there is a difference in duration of drainage with small tubes.

    The trials investigating the efficacy of adding suction to chest-tube drainage are too small and underpowered to detect a clinically important difference.

    We don't know whether using one-way valves on a chest tube is more effective than using drainage bottles with underwater seals. There is a suggestion, however, that one-way valves might reduce hospital admission and the need for analgesia.

- It appears that needle aspiration might be beneficial in treating people with spontaneous pneumothorax, although it is not clear whether it is more effective than chest-tube drainage.

- Pleurodesis seems to be effective in preventing recurrent spontaneous pneumothorax, although there are some adverse effects associated with the intervention.

    Chemical pleurodesis successfully reduces recurrence of spontaneous pneumothorax, although the injection has been reported to be intensely painful.

    Thorascopic surgery with talc instillation also appears to reduce recurrence of spontaneous pneumothorax, but leads to a modest increase in pain during the first 3 days.

    There is no evidence examining when pleurodesis should be given, although there is general consensus that it is warranted after the second or third episode of spontaneous pneumothorax.

(i) **Please visit www.clinicalevidence.bmj.com for full text and references**

What are the effects of treatments in people presenting with spontaneous pneumothorax?	
Likely To Be Beneficial	• Chest-tube drainage alone • Needle aspiration
Unknown Effectiveness	• Chest-tube drainage plus suction • One-way valves on chest tubes

- Small- versus standard-sized chest tubes for chest-tube drainage

What are the effects of interventions to prevent recurrence in people with previous spontaneous pneumothorax?

Trade-off Between Benefits And Harms	• Pleurodesis
Unknown Effectiveness	• Optimal timing of pleurodesis (after first, second, or subsequent episodes)

Search date April 2007

DEFINITION A pneumothorax is air in the pleural space. A **spontaneous pneumothorax** occurs when there is no provoking factor — such as trauma, surgery, or diagnostic intervention. It implies a leak of air from the lung parenchyma through the visceral pleura into the pleural space, which causes the lung to collapse and results in pain and shortness of breath. This review does not include people with **tension pneumothorax**.

INCIDENCE/PREVALENCE In a survey in Minnesota, USA, the incidence of spontaneous pneumothorax was 7/100,000 for men and 1/100,000 for women. In England and Wales, the overall rate of people consulting with pneumothorax (in both primary and secondary care combined) is 24/100,000 a year for men and 10/100,000 a year for women. The overall annual incidence of emergency hospital admissions for pneumothorax in England and Wales is 16.7/100,000 for men and 5.8/100,000 for women. Smoking increases the likelihood of spontaneous pneumothorax by 22 times for men and by 8 times for women. The incidence is directly related to the amount smoked.

AETIOLOGY/RISK FACTORS Primary spontaneous pneumothorax is thought to result from congenital abnormality of the visceral pleura, and is typically seen in young, otherwise fit people. Secondary spontaneous pneumothorax is caused by underlying lung disease, typically affecting older people with emphysema or pulmonary fibrosis.

PROGNOSIS Death from spontaneous pneumothorax is rare, with UK mortality of 1.26 per million a year for men and 0.62 per million a year for women. Published recurrence rates vary. One cohort study in Denmark found that, after a first episode of primary spontaneous pneumothorax, 23% of people suffered a recurrence within 5 years, most of them within 1 year. Recurrence rates had been thought to increase substantially after the first recurrence, but one retrospective case-control study (147 US military personnel) found that 28% of men with a first primary spontaneous pneumothorax had a recurrence; 23% of the 28% had a second recurrence; and 14% of that 23% had a third recurrence, resulting in a total recurrence rate of 35%.

502 | Asthma in adults

Rodolfo J Dennis, Ivan Solarte, and J Mark FitzGerald

KEY POINTS

- About 10% of adults have suffered an attack of asthma, and up to 5% of these have severe disease that responds poorly to treatment. These people have an increased risk of death.

- Most guidelines about the management of asthma follow stepwise protocols. This review does not endorse or follow any particular protocol, but presents the evidence about specific interventions.

- Taking short-acting beta$_2$ agonists as needed is as likely to relieve symptoms and improve lung function as a regular dosing schedule in adults with mild to moderate asthma.

- CAUTION: Long-acting beta$_2$ agonists decrease the number of exacerbations, and improve symptoms and lung function in people with mild to moderate persistent asthma that is poorly controlled with corticosteroids, but have been associated with increased asthma-related mortality, and should always be used with inhaled corticosteroids.

- Low-dose, inhaled corticosteroids improve symptoms and lung function in persistent asthma compared with placebo or regular inhaled beta$_2$ agonists.

  Leukotriene antagonists are more effective than placebo at reducing symptoms, but we don't know whether they are of benefit compared with, or in addition to, inhaled corticosteroids.

  Adding theophylline to inhaled corticosteroids may improve lung function in people with mild or moderate persistent asthma poorly controlled with inhaled corticosteroids, but we don't know if they are of benefit compared with long-acting beta$_2$ agonists, or leukotriene antagonists.

- In people with an acute attack of asthma, supplementation with 28% oxygen, systemic and inhaled corticosteroids, beta$_2$ agonists, and ipratropium bromide combined with beta$_2$ agonists all improve symptoms.

  Inhaled and oral corticosteroids may have similar effects in preventing relapse and improving lung function.

  Beta$_2$ agonists delivered from a metered-dose inhaler using a spacer are as effective at improving lung function as those given by a nebuliser, or given intravenously. Giving beta$_2$ agonists intravenously is more invasive than giving beta$_2$ agonists by nebuliser.

  In people with severe acute asthma, continuous nebulised short-acting beta$_2$ agonists may also improve lung function more than intermittent nebulised short-acting beta$_2$ agonists. Intravenous magnesium sulphate may also improve lung function in people with severe acute asthma.

  We don't know if adding nebulised magnesium to inhaled beta$_2$ agonists improves lung function in people with acute asthma.

  Mechanical ventilation may be life-saving in severe acute asthma, but is associated with high levels of morbidity.

  Specialist care of acute asthma may lead to improved outcomes compared with generalist care.

  Education to help self-manage asthma reduces admission, the number of days off work or school, and number of doctor visits.

(i) Please visit www.clinicalevidence.bmj.com for full text and references

What are the effects of treatments for chronic asthma?

Beneficial	• Adding long-acting inhaled beta$_2$ agonists in people with mild to moderate, persistent asthma

	that is poorly controlled by inhaled corticosteroids (beneficial if used with inhaled corticosteroids) • Low-dose, inhaled corticosteroids in persistent asthma • Short-acting inhaled beta$_2$ agonists as needed for symptom relief (as effective as regular use) in mild to moderate, persistent asthma
Likely To Be Beneficial	• Adding leukotriene antagonists in people with mild to moderate, persistent asthma not taking inhaled corticosteroids (likely to be better than adding no treatment, but may be less effective than adding inhaled corticosteroids) • Adding theophylline in people with mild to moderate, persistent asthma poorly controlled by inhaled corticosteroids (likely to be better than adding placebo but may be less effective than increasing dose of corticosteroids)
Unknown Effectiveness	• Adding leukotriene antagonists to inhaled corticosteroids in people with mild to moderate, persistent asthma

What are the effects of treatments for acute asthma?

Beneficial	• Controlled oxygen supplementation (28% oxygen better than 100% oxygen) • Education about acute asthma • Inhaled corticosteroids • Ipratropium bromide added to beta$_2$ agonists • Oral corticosteroids alone (as effective as combined inhaled plus oral corticosteroids) • Short courses of systemic corticosteroids (more effective than placebo) • Spacer devices for delivering beta$_2$ agonists from pressurised metered-dose inhalers (as good as nebulisers)
Likely To Be Beneficial	• Continuous nebulised short-acting beta$_2$ agonists (more effective than intermittent nebulised short-acting beta$_2$ agonists) • Magnesium sulphate (intravenous) for people with severe acute asthma (better than placebo) • Mechanical ventilation for people with severe acute asthma*

	• Specialist care (more effective than generalist care)
Unknown Effectiveness	• Adding isotonic nebulised magnesium to inhaled beta$_2$ agonists • Magnesium sulphate alone (nebulised) versus beta$_2$ agonists
Unlikely To Be Beneficial	• Helium–oxygen mixture • Intravenous short-acting beta$_2$ agonists (no more effective than nebulised short-acting beta$_2$ agonists)

Search date October 2006

*Categorisation based on consensus. Limited RCT evidence available.

DEFINITION Asthma is characterised by variable airflow obstruction and airway hyperre-sponsiveness. Symptoms include dyspnoea, cough, chest tightness, and wheezing. The normal diurnal variation of PEFR is increased in people with asthma. **Chronic asthma** is defined here as asthma requiring maintenance treatment to achieve part or total control. In a newly-diagnosed person, and when confronted with the first treatment decision, asthma should be classified by severity (intermittent, chronic mild, moderate, or severe). As further classification of disease status depends both on the severity of the disease and the response to treatment, it is now recommended that the terms "controlled", "partly controlled", and "uncontrolled" are used for people receiving treatment. **Acute asthma** is defined here as an exacerbation of underlying asthma requiring urgent treatment.

INCIDENCE/PREVALENCE The reported prevalence of asthma has been increasing worldwide, but may have currently reached a plateau. About 10% of people have suffered an attack of asthma, but epidemiological studies have also found marked variations in prevalence between and within countries.

AETIOLOGY/RISK FACTORS Most people with asthma are atopic. Exposure to certain stimuli initiates inflammation and structural changes in airways causing airway hyperre-sponsiveness and variable airflow obstruction, which in turn cause most asthma symptoms. There are many such stimuli; the more important include environmental allergens, occupational sensitising agents, and respiratory viral infections.

PROGNOSIS **Chronic asthma:** In people with mild asthma, prognosis is good, and progression to severe disease is rare. However, as a group, people with asthma lose lung function faster than those without asthma, although less quickly than people without asthma who smoke. People with chronic asthma can improve with treatment. However, some people (possibly up to 5%) have severe disease that responds poorly to treatment. These people are most at risk of morbidity and death from asthma. **Acute asthma:** About 10–20% of people presenting to the emergency department with asthma are admitted to hospital. Of these, fewer than 10% receive mechanical ventilation. Those who are ventilated are at 19-fold increased risk of ventilation for a subsequent episode. It is unusual for people to die unless they have suffered respiratory arrest before they reach hospital. One prospective study of 939 people discharged from emergency care found that 106/641 (17%, 95% CI 14% to 20%) relapsed by 2 weeks.

Nick ten Hacken, Huib Kerstjens, and Dirkje Postma

KEY POINTS

- **Bronchiectasis is characterised by irreversible widening of medium-sized airways, with inflammation, chronic bacterial infection, and destruction of bronchial walls.**

  Bronchiectasis is usually a complication of previous lower respiratory infection, and causes chronic cough and production of copious sputum, which is often purulent. Bronchiectasis may cause signs of COPD. It can also be associated with cystic fibrosis and other congenital disorders, foreign-body inhalation, and other causes of lung damage.

- **Exercise or inspiratory muscle training may improve quality of life and exercise endurance in people with bronchiectasis but without cystic fibrosis.**

- **We do not know whether bronchopulmonary hygiene physical therapy, mucolytics, inhaled hyperosmolar agents, inhaled corticosteroids, oral corticosteroids, leukotriene receptor antagonists, short-acting beta$_2$ agonists, long-acting beta$_2$ agonists, anticholinergic therapy, or surgery are beneficial, because few studies have been found.**

  Inhaled corticosteroids may reduce sputum volume compared with placebo, but have not been shown to reduce exacerbations.

  Oral methyl-xanthines and surgery are often used in bronchiectasis, but we found no good-quality studies of either treatment.

  Surgery is often considered for people with extreme damage to one or two lobes of the lung who are at risk of severe infection or bleeding.

  Prolonged-use antibiotics improve clinical response rates (according to treating physicians at follow-up), but may not reduce exacerbation rates or lung function compared with placebo.

(i) **Please visit www.clinicalevidence.bmj.com for full text and references**

What are the effects of treatments in people with bronchiectasis but without cystic fibrosis?	
Likely To Be Beneficial	• Exercise or physical training • Prolonged-use antibiotics
Unknown Effectiveness	• Anticholinergic therapy • Bronchopulmonary hygiene physical therapy • Corticosteroids (inhaled) • Corticosteroids (oral) • Hyperosmolar agents (inhaled) • Leukotriene receptor antagonists • Long-acting beta$_2$ agonists • Methyl-xanthines (oral) • Mucolytics (bromhexine or deoxyribonuclease) • Short-acting beta$_2$ agonists • Surgery

Search date July 2007

DEFINITION Bronchiectasis is defined as irreversible widening of medium-sized airways (bronchi) in the lung. It is characterised by inflammation, destruction of bronchial walls, and chronic bacterial infection. The condition may be limited to a single lobe or lung segment, or it may affect one or both lungs more diffusely. Clinically, the condition manifests as chronic cough and chronic overproduction of sputum (up to about 500 mL/day), which is often purulent. People with severe bronchiectasis may have life-threatening haemoptysis, and may develop features of chronic obstructive airways disease, such as wheezing, chronic respiratory failure, pulmonary hypertension, and right-sided heart failure.

INCIDENCE/PREVALENCE We found few reliable data. Incidence has declined over the past 50 years, and prevalence is low in higher-income countries. Prevalence is much higher in lower-income countries, and is a major cause of morbidity and mortality.

AETIOLOGY/RISK FACTORS Bronchiectasis is most commonly a long-term complication of previous lower respiratory infections, such as measles pneumonitis, pertussis, and tuberculosis. Foreign-body inhalation and allergic, autoimmune, and chemical lung damage also predispose to the condition. Underlying congenital disorders such as cystic fibrosis, cilial dysmotility syndromes, alpha$_1$ antitrypsin deficiency, and congenital immunodeficiencies may also predispose to bronchiectasis — and may be of greater aetiological importance in higher-income countries than respiratory infection. Cystic fibrosis is the most common congenital cause. This review does not deal with bronchiectasis in people with cystic fibrosis.

PROGNOSIS Bronchiectasis is a chronic condition, with frequent relapses of varying severity. Long-term prognosis is variable. Data on morbidity and mortality are sparse. Bronchiectasis frequently coexists with other respiratory disease, making it difficult to distinguish prognosis for bronchiectasis alone.

Huib Kerstjens, Dirkje Postma, and Nick ten Hacken

KEY POINTS

- The main risk factor for the development and deterioration of COPD is smoking.

- Inhaled anticholinergics and beta$_2$ agonists improve lung function and symptoms, and reduce exacerbations compared with placebo in stable COPD.

  Long-acting inhaled anticholinergic drugs may improve lung function compared with long-acting beta$_2$ agonists, but studies comparing the two classes of drug have given conflicting results.

  Combined treatment with inhaled anticholinergics and beta$_2$ agonists may improve symptoms and lung function and reduce exacerbations compared with either treatment alone, although long-term effects are unknown.

- Inhaled corticosteroids may reduce exacerbations, and oral corticosteroids may improve short-term lung function, but have serious adverse effects.

  Combined inhaled corticosteroids plus long-acting beta$_2$ agonists improve lung function and symptoms, and reduce exacerbations compared with placebo, and may be more effective than either treatment alone.

  Long-term domiciliary oxygen treatment may improve survival in people with severe daytime hypoxaemia.

  Theophyllines may improve lung function compared with placebo, but adverse effects limit their usefulness in stable COPD.

  We don't know whether mucolytic drugs, prophylactic antibiotics or alpha$_1$ antitrypsin improve outcomes in people with COPD compared with placebo.

- Combined psychosocial and pharmacological interventions for smoking cessation can slow the deterioration of lung function, but have not been shown to reduce long-term mortality compared with usual care.

  Multi-modality pulmonary rehabilitation and exercises can improve exercise capacity in people with stable COPD, but nutritional supplementation has not been shown to be beneficial.

(i) Please visit www.clinicalevidence.bmj.com for full text and references

What are the effects of maintenance drug treatment in stable COPD?

Beneficial	• Inhaled anticholinergics (improved exacerbation rate, symptoms, and FEV$_1$ compared with placebo)
	• Inhaled anticholinergics plus beta$_2$ agonists (improved FEV$_1$ compared with either drug alone)
	• Inhaled beta$_2$ agonists (improved FEV$_1$, quality of life, and exacerbation rates compared with placebo)
	• Inhaled corticosteroids plus long acting beta$_2$ agonists (improved exacerbation rate, symptoms, quality of life, FEV$_1$ compared with placebo)
Likely To Be Beneficial	• Inhaled anticholinergics compared with beta$_2$ agonists (improved FEV$_1$ compared with beta$_2$ agonists in long term)

	• Long-term domiciliary oxygen (beneficial in people with severe hypoxaemia)
Trade-off Between Benefits And Harms	• Inhaled corticosteroids (improved exacerbation rates, but may have long-term harms)
	• Theophyllines
Unknown Effectiveness	• Alpha$_1$ antitrypsin
	• Mucolytics
	• Prophylactic antibiotics
Unlikely To Be Beneficial	• Oral corticosteroids (evidence of harm but no evidence of long-term benefits)

What are the effects of non-drug interventions in stable COPD?

Beneficial	• Psychosocial plus pharmacological interventions for smoking cessation
	• Pulmonary rehabilitation
Likely To Be Beneficial	• General physical activity
	• Inspiratory muscle training
	• Peripheral muscle training
Unknown Effectiveness	• Pharmacological interventions alone for smoking cessation
	• Psychosocial interventions alone for smoking cessation
Unlikely To Be Beneficial	• Nutritional supplementation

Search date March 2005

DEFINITION Chronic obstructive pulmonary disease (COPD) is a disease state characterised by airflow limitation that is not fully reversible. The airflow limitation is usually both progressive and associated with an abnormal inflammatory response of the lungs to noxious particles or gases. Classically, it has been thought to be a combination of emphysema and chronic bronchitis, although only one of these may be present in some people with COPD. Emphysema is abnormal permanent enlargement of the air spaces distal to the terminal bronchioles, accompanied by destruction of their walls and without obvious fibrosis. Chronic bronchitis is chronic cough or mucus production for at least 3 months in at least 2 successive years when other causes of chronic cough have been excluded.

INCIDENCE/PREVALENCE COPD mainly affects middle-aged and elderly people. In 1998, the WHO estimated that COPD was the fifth most common cause of death worldwide, responsible for 4.8% of all mortality (estimated 2,745,816 deaths in 2002), and morbidity is increasing. Estimated prevalence in the USA rose by 41% between 1982 and 1994 and age-adjusted death rates rose by 71% between 1966 and 1985. All-cause age-adjusted mortality declined over the same period by 22%, and mortality from CVDs by 45%. In the UK, physician-diagnosed prevalence was 2% in men and 1% in women between 1990 and 1997.

AETIOLOGY/RISK FACTORS COPD is largely preventable. The main cause in resource-rich countries is exposure to tobacco smoke. In these countries, 85–90% of people with COPD have smoked at some point. The disease is rare in lifelong non-smokers (estimated prevalence 5% in 3 large representative US surveys of non-smokers from 1971–1984), in whom "passive" exposure to environmental tobacco smoke has been proposed as a cause. Other proposed causes include bronchial hyperresponsiveness, indoor and outdoor air pollution, and allergy.

PROGNOSIS Airway obstruction is usually progressive in those who continue to smoke, resulting in early disability and shortened survival. Smoking cessation reverts the rate of decline in lung function to that of non-smokers. Many people will need medication for the rest of their lives, with increased doses and additional drugs during exacerbations.

Lung cancer

Alan Neville

KEY POINTS

- Lung cancer is the leading cause of cancer deaths in both men and women, with 80–90% of cases caused by smoking.

  Small-cell lung cancer accounts for 20% of all cases, and is usually treated with chemotherapy. Adenocarcinoma is the main non-small-cell pathology, and is treated initially with surgery.

- In people with resectable non-small cell lung cancer, postoperative adjuvant chemotherapy may improve survival compared with surgery alone.

  Cisplatin regimens or uracil plus tegafur regimens have been shown to improve survival when given postoperatively, but increase toxicity.

  We don't know whether preoperative chemotherapy improves survival in people with resectable non-small-cell lung cancer.

- Palliative first-line chemotherapy improves survival in people with unresectable and metastatic non-small-cell lung cancer compared with supportive care, but increases the risk of adverse effects.

  First-line platinum-based regimens improve survival compared with older non-platinum agents, but we don't know whether platinum-based chemotherapy is more effective than non-platinum, third-generation chemotherapeutic agents.

  Multiple-agent first-line chemotherapy regimens are more effective than single-agent regimens, but have more adverse effects.

  We don't know whether second-line single-agent chemotherapy, or regimens with taxanes, improve survival compared with supportive care. Second-line multiple-agent chemotherapy does not increase survival, but has greater toxicity compared with single-agent regimens.

  Adding chemotherapy to thoracic irradiation may improve 2–5-year survival compared with thoracic irradiation alone, but increases adverse effects.

  We don't know how continuous hyperfractionated accelerated radiotherapy (CHART) compares with conventional radiotherapy in unresectable non-small-cell lung cancer. Non-CHART hyperfractionated radiotherapy has not been shown to increase survival compared with standard radiotherapy.

  Targeted therapy with gefitinib or erlotinib has not been shown to increase survival when used as first-line palliative therapy. We don't know whether it is beneficial as second-line therapy.

- In people with limited-stage small-cell lung cancer, adding thoracic irradiation to chemotherapy improves survival, but may increase complications.

  We don't know whether intensifying the chemotherapy dose increases survival in small-cell lung cancer, and it may increase treatment-related toxicity.

- Prophylactic cranial irradiation may improve survival in people in remission from small-cell lung cancer.

(i) **Please visit www.clinicalevidence.bmj.com for full text and references**

What are the effects of treatments for resectable non-small-cell lung cancer?

Likely To Be Beneficial	• Postoperative chemotherapy (cisplatin-based or uracil plus tegafur-based regimens) in resected stage 1–3 non-small-cell lung cancer
Unknown Effectiveness	• Preoperative chemotherapy in resectable non-small-cell lung cancer

What are the effects of treatments for unresectable non-small-cell lung cancer?

Beneficial	• First-line chemotherapy with multiple agents versus single agent
	• First-line palliative chemotherapy versus supportive care
	• Thoracic irradiation plus chemotherapy (compared with thoracic irradiation alone)
Unknown Effectiveness	• Continuous hyperfractionated accelerated radiotherapy (CHART)
	• First-line platinum-based chemotherapy versus non-platinum-based regimens
	• Second-line molecular targeted therapy with gefitinib or erlotinib for unresectable advanced non-small-cell lung cancer
	• Second-line palliative chemotherapy versus supportive care
	• Single-agent second-line chemotherapy versus each other
Unlikely To Be Beneficial	• First-line molecular targeted therapy with gefitinib or erlotinib for unresectable advanced non-small-cell lung cancer
	• Hyperfractionated radiotherapy in unresectable stage 3 non-small-cell lung cancer (excluding continuous hyperfractionated accelerated radiotherapy [CHART])
Likely To Be Ineffective Or Harmful	• Second-line chemotherapy with multiple agents versus single agent

What are the effects of treatments for small-cell lung cancer?

Beneficial	• Thoracic irradiation plus chemotherapy in limited-stage small-cell lung cancer (improves survival compared with chemotherapy alone)
Likely To Be Beneficial	• Prophylactic cranial irradiation for people in complete remission from limited or extensive-stage small-cell lung cancer
Unknown Effectiveness	• Dose intensification of chemotherapy

Search date September 2006

DEFINITION Lung cancer (bronchogenic carcinoma) is an epithelial cancer arising from the bronchial surface epithelium or bronchial mucous glands. It is broadly divided into small-cell (about 20% of all lung cancers) and non-small-cell lung cancer (about 80% of all lung cancers, of which adenocarcinoma is the most prevalent form).

INCIDENCE/PREVALENCE Lung cancer is the leading cause of cancer deaths in both men and women, annually affecting about 100,000 men and 80,000 women in the USA, and about 40,000 men and women in the UK.

AETIOLOGY/RISK FACTORS Smoking remains the major preventable risk factor, accounting for about 80–90% of all cases. Other respiratory-tract carcinogens have been identified that may enhance the carcinogenic effects of tobacco smoke, either in the workplace (e.g. asbestos and polycyclic aromatic hydrocarbons) or in the home (e.g. indoor radon).

PROGNOSIS At the time of diagnosis, 10–15% of people with lung cancer have localised disease. Of these, half will have died at 5 years despite potentially curative surgery. A similar number have locally advanced disease, and over half of people have metastatic disease at the time of diagnosis. Surgery is the treatment of choice in people with stage 1 and stage 2 non-small-cell lung cancer, unless they are not well enough to have surgery. People with stage 1A disease have an excellent overall survival rate with surgery alone. Complete resection of the cancer with or without chemotherapy and radiotherapy may be performed in some people with locally advanced stage 3 disease, but in others the disease is inoperable, and their prognosis is poorer. People with inoperable stage 3 or metastatic disease can be offered palliative chemotherapy. Chemotherapy is the mainstay of treatment in the 20% of people with small cell lung cancer, which has a high risk of metastases. About 5–10% of people with small-cell lung cancer present with central nervous system involvement, and half develop symptomatic brain metastases by 2 years. Of these, only half respond to palliative radiotherapy, and their median survival is less than 3 months.

M Riduan Joesoef and George Schmid

KEY POINTS

- Bacterial vaginosis is characterised by large numbers of anaerobic bacteria in the vagina, causing a grey, fishy-smelling discharge in half of affected women. However, the specific causative agents are unknown, and it may resolve spontaneously.

   Bacterial vaginosis is common, especially in women using IUDs, in women with new or multiple partners, and in lesbians.

   Bacterial vaginosis is associated with increased complications in pregnancy, endometritis, and increased risks of HIV infection.

- Antibiotic treatment with metronidazole and clindamycin increases cure rates compared with placebo in non-pregnant women.

   Intravaginal clindamycin may reduce systemic adverse effects, but has been associated with mild to severe colitis and vaginal candidiasis.

   We don't know which is the most effective antibiotic regimen, or what the long-term effects of treatment might be.

   More than 50% of women may have recurrence within 2 months of antibiotic treatment.

- In pregnant women with bacterial vaginosis, oral or vaginal antibiotics have not been shown overall to reduce complications of pregnancy, although studies have given conflicting results.

   Studies using higher doses of antibiotics, and where courses started earlier in pregnancy, are most likely to show a benefit.

   Treatment of women with clinically equivocal bacterial vaginosis may increase the risks of preterm birth and low birth weight.

- Treating the woman's male sexual partner with metronidazole or clindamycin does not reduce the risk of recurrence in the woman.

- In women with bacterial vaginosis who are about to undergo surgical abortion, antibiotics may reduce the risk of subsequent PID, but we don't know if they are beneficial before other procedures.

(i) **Please visit www.clinicalevidence.bmj.com for full text and references**

What are the effects of different antibacterial regimens in non-pregnant women with symptomatic bacterial vaginosis on cure rates and symptom relief?	
Beneficial	• Antibacterial treatment with metronidazole or clindamycin (short-term benefit)

What are the effects of antibacterial treatments in pregnant women to reduce adverse outcomes of pregnancy and prevent neonatal complications?	
Likely To Be Beneficial	• Antibacterial treatment (except intravaginal clindamycin) in pregnant women who have had a previous preterm birth
Unknown Effectiveness	• Antibacterial treatment (except intravaginal clindamycin) in pregnant women
Likely To Be Ineffective Or Harmful	• Intravaginal clindamycin cream

Does treating male partners prevent recurrence?

Likely To Be Ineffective Or Harmful	• Treating a woman's male sexual partner with metronidazole or clindamycin (did not reduce the woman's risk of recurrence)

What are the effects of treatment before gynaecological procedures?

Likely To Be Beneficial	• Oral or intravaginal antibacterial treatment before surgical abortion
Unknown Effectiveness	• Antibacterial treatment before gynaecological procedures other than abortion

Search date March 2004

DEFINITION Bacterial vaginosis is a microbial disease characterised by a change in the bacterial flora of the vagina from mainly *Lactobacillus* species to high concentrations of anaerobic bacteria. The condition is asymptomatic in 50% of infected women. Women with symptoms have an excessive white to grey, or malodorous vaginal discharge, or both; the odour may be particularly noticeable during sexual intercourse. Commonly practised clinical diagnosis requires three out of four features: the presence of clue cells on microscopy; a homogenous discharge adherent to the vaginal walls; pH of vaginal fluid greater than 4.5; and a "fishy" amine odour of the vaginal discharge before or after addition of 10% potassium hydroxide. Some experts prefer other methods of diagnosis, (e.g. Gram stain of vaginal secretions), particularly in a research setting. Gram stain using Nugent's criteria categorise the flora of vagina into three categories — normal, intermediate, and flora consistent with bacterial vaginosis. Abnormal vaginal flora includes intermediate flora and bacterial vaginosis.

INCIDENCE/PREVALENCE Bacterial vaginosis is the most common infectious cause of vaginitis, being about twice as common as candidiasis. Prevalences of 10–61% have been reported among unselected women from a range of settings. Data on incidence are limited but one study found that, over a 2-year period, 50% of women using an IUD had at least one episode, as did 20% of women using oral contraceptives. Bacterial vaginosis is particularly prevalent among lesbians.

AETIOLOGY/RISK FACTORS The cause of bacterial vaginosis is not fully understood. Risk factors include new or multiple sexual partners and early age of sexual intercourse, but no causative microorganism has been shown to be transmitted between partners. Use of an IUD and douching have also been reported as risk factors. Infection seems to be most common around the time of menstruation.

PROGNOSIS The course of bacterial vaginosis varies and is poorly understood. Without treatment, symptoms may persist or resolve in both pregnant and non-pregnant women. Recurrence after treatment occurs in about a third of women. A history of bacterial vaginosis is associated with increased rates of complications in pregnancy: low birthweight; preterm birth (pooled OR from 10 cohort studies: 1.8, 95% CI 1.5 to 2.6); preterm labour; premature rupture of membranes; late miscarriage; chorioamnionitis; endometritis after normal delivery (8.2% *v* 1.5%; OR 5.6, 95% CI 1.8 to 17.2); endometritis after caesarean section (55% *v* 17%; OR 5.8, 95% CI 3.0 to 10.9); and surgery to the genital tract. Women who have had a previous preterm delivery are especially at risk of complications in pregnancy, with a sevenfold increased risk of preterm birth (24/428 [5.6%] in all women *v* 10/24 [41.7%] in women with a previous preterm birth). Bacterial vaginosis can also increase the risk of HIV acquisition and transmission.

Nicola Low

KEY POINTS

- Genital chlamydia is an STD of the urethra in men, and of the endocervix or urethra (or both) in women. It is defined as uncomplicated if it has not ascended to the upper genital tract.

  It is the most commonly reported bacterial STD in resource-rich countries, with about 1300 new infections reported per 100,000 women each year in the UK, most commonly in those aged between 16 and 19 years.

  If untreated, chlamydial infection can ascend to the upper genital tract causing PID.

- Multiple-dose regimens of tetracyclines (doxycycline or tetracycline) achieve microbiological cure in at least 95% of men and non-pregnant women with genital chlamydia.

  Erythromycin also appears to be beneficial as a multiple-dose regimen, with a 2 g daily dose being more effective than 1 g.

  Ciprofloxacin seems less likely to lead to microbiological cure compared with doxycycline.

  We don't know whether multiple-dose regimens of other antibiotics (such as other macrolides, quinolones and penicillins) are effective, as few adequate studies have been found.

- A single dose of azithromycin seems as beneficial as a 7-day course of doxycycline, and produces similar rates of adverse effects.

  Single-dose treatments have the obvious advantage of improving adherence.

- In pregnant women, multiple-dose regimens of erythromycin or amoxicillin seem effective in treating chlamydial infection.

  A small study has also suggested that multiple-dose erythromycin is as effective as clindamycin in curing infection, although the size of the study makes it hard to draw definitive conclusions.

- Single-dose azithromycin may be effective in treating chlamydia in pregnant women. However, it should only be used if no adequate alternative is available.

(i) **Please visit www.clinicalevidence.bmj.com for full text and references**

What are the effects of antibiotic treatment in men and non-pregnant women with uncomplicated genital chlamydial infection?	
Beneficial	• Azithromycin (single dose)
	• Doxycycline, tetracycline (multiple-dose regimens)
Likely To Be Beneficial	• Erythromycin (multiple-dose regimens)
Unknown Effectiveness	• Multiple-dose regimens of antibiotics other than tetracycline, doxycycline, or ciprofloxacin
Unlikely To Be Beneficial	• Multiple-dose regimens of ciprofloxacin (men/non-pregnant women)

What are the effects of treatment for pregnant women with uncomplicated genital chlamydial infection?	
Likely To Be Beneficial	• Azithromycin (single dose) • Erythromycin, amoxicillin (multiple-dose regimens)
Unknown Effectiveness	• Clindamycin (multiple-dose regimens)

Search date January 2006

DEFINITION Genital chlamydia is an STD of the urethra in men, and of the endocervix or urethra (or both) in women. It is defined as **uncomplicated** if it has not ascended to the upper genital tract. Infection in women is asymptomatic in up to 80% of cases, but may cause non-specific symptoms, including vaginal discharge and intermenstrual bleeding. Infection in men causes urethral discharge and urethral irritation or dysuria, but may also be asymptomatic in up to half of cases. **Complicated** chlamydial infection includes spread to the upper genital tract (causing PID in women [see PID, p 522] and epididymo-orchitis in men) and extragenital sites, such as the eye. Interventions for complicated chlamydial infection are not included in this review.

INCIDENCE/PREVALENCE Genital chlamydia is the most commonly reported bacterial STD in resource-rich countries and reported rates increased by around 20% in the UK and USA between 2000 and 2002. In women, infection occurs most commonly between the ages of 16 and 19 years. In this age group, about 1300/100,000 new infections are reported each year in the UK, compared with 1900/100,000 in Sweden, and 2536/100,000 in the USA. The peak age group for men is 20–24 years, with about 1000/100,000 new infections a year in the UK and USA and 1200/100,000 in Sweden. Rates decline markedly with increasing age. Reported rates are highly dependent on the level of testing. The population prevalence of uncomplicated genital chlamydia in 16–24-year-olds in the UK has been estimated to be between 2% and 6% in both men and women.

AETIOLOGY/RISK FACTORS Infection is caused by the bacterium *C trachomatis* serotypes D–K. It is transmitted primarily through sexual intercourse, but also perinatally and through direct or indirect oculogenital contact.

PROGNOSIS In women, untreated chlamydial infection that ascends to the upper genital tract causes PID (see PID, p 522). Tubal infertility has been found to occur in about 11% of women after a single episode of PID, and the risk of ectopic pregnancy is increased six to sevenfold. Ascending infection in men causes epididymitis, but evidence that this causes male infertility is limited. Maternal to infant transmission can lead to neonatal conjunctivitis and pneumonitis. Chlamydia may coexist with other genital infections and may facilitate transmission and acquisition of HIV infection. Untreated chlamydial infection persists in most women for at least 60 days and for a shorter period in men. Spontaneous remission also occurs at an estimated rate of 5% a month.

Eva Jungmann

KEY POINTS

- Genital herpes is an infection with HSV-1 or HSV-2. The typical clinical features include painful shallow anogenital ulceration.

  It is among the most common STDs, with up to 23% of adults in the UK and US having antibodies to HSV-2.

- Oral antiviral treatment of someone who is seropositive for HSV seems to be effective in reducing transmission to a previously uninfected partner.

- Despite limited evidence, male-condom use is generally believed to reduce sexual transmission of herpes from infected men to uninfected sexual partners.

  We don't know how effective male-condom use is at preventing transmission from infected women to uninfected men.

  We found no evidence examining the effectiveness of female condoms in preventing transmission.

- Recombinant glycoprotein vaccines do not seem any more effective than placebo in preventing transmission to people at high risk from infection.

  We found no evidence about other vaccines.

- We found insufficient evidence to draw reliable conclusions on whether antiviral maintenance treatment in late pregnancy, or serological screening and counselling to prevent acquisition of herpes in late pregnancy are effective in preventing transmission of HSV from mother to neonate.

  Caesarean delivery in women with genital lesions at term may reduce the risk of transmission, but is associated with an increased risk of maternal morbidity and mortality.

- Oral antiviral treatments effectively decrease symptoms in people with first episodes of genital herpes, although we found insufficient evidence to establish which type was most effective.

- If herpes is recurrent, aciclovir, famciclovir, and valaciclovir are all equally beneficial in reducing duration of symptoms, lesion-healing time, and viral shedding.

  Daily maintenance treatment with oral antiviral agents effectively reduces frequency of recurrences, and improves quality of life.

  We don't know whether psychotherapy is effective in reducing recurrence.

- Oral antiviral treatments are generally believed to be useful in treating both first episodes and recurrent episodes of genital herpes in people with HIV, although evidence supporting this is sparse.

  Oral antiviral treatments are also likely to be effective in preventing recurrence of genital herpes in people with HIV.

(i) **Please visit www.clinicalevidence.bmj.com for full text and references**

What are the effects of interventions to prevent sexual transmission of HSV?	
Likely To Be Beneficial	• Antiviral treatment of infected sexual partner with valaciclovir (reduced transmission to uninfected partner) • Male-condom use to prevent sexual transmission from infected men to uninfected sexual partners*
Unknown Effectiveness	• Female condoms

	• Male-condom use to prevent sexual transmission from infected women to uninfected men
Unlikely To Be Beneficial	• Recombinant glycoprotein vaccines (gB2 plus gD2) in people at high risk of infection (no effect except in women known to be HSV-1 and HSV-2 negative before vaccination)

What are the effects of interventions to prevent transmission of HSV from mother to neonate?

Unknown Effectiveness	• Caesarean delivery in women with genital lesions at term
	• Oral antiviral maintenance treatment in late pregnancy (at least 36 weeks' gestation) in women with a history of genital herpes
	• Serological screening and counselling to prevent acquisition of HSV in late pregnancy

What are the effects of antiviral treatment in people with a first episode of genital herpes?

Beneficial	• Oral antiviral treatment with aciclovir in first episodes of genital herpes
Unknown Effectiveness	• Different types of oral antiviral treatment for first episodes of genital herpes

What are the effects of interventions to reduce the impact of recurrence?

Beneficial	• Oral antiviral maintenance treatment in people with high rates of recurrence
	• Oral antiviral treatment taken at the start of recurrence
Unknown Effectiveness	• Psychotherapy to reduce recurrence

What are the effects of treatments in people with genital herpes and HIV?

Likely To Be Beneficial	• Oral antiviral maintenance treatment with valaciclovir for preventing recurrence of genital herpes
	• Oral antiviral treatment for an acute recurrent episode of genital herpes (compared with no treatment)†

	• Oral antiviral treatment for first episode genital herpes†
Unknown Effectiveness	• Different types of oral antiviral treatment for an acute recurrent episode of genital herpes (relative benefits of different treatments unclear)

Search date August 2006

*Categorisation based on observational or non-randomised evidence.
†Categorisation based on consensus in the context of practical and ethical problems of performing RCTs.

DEFINITION Genital herpes is an infection with HSV-1 or HSV-2. The typical clinical features include painful shallow anogenital ulceration. HSV infections can be confirmed on the basis of virological and serological findings. Types of infection include **first-episode primary infection**, which is defined as HSV confirmed in a person without prior findings of HSV-1 or HSV-2 antibodies; **first-episode non-primary infection**, which is HSV-2 confirmed in a person with prior findings of HSV-1 antibodies or vice versa; **first recognised recurrence**, which is HSV-1 or HSV-2 confirmed in a person with prior findings of HSV-1 or HSV-2 antibodies; and **recurrent genital herpes**, which is caused by reactivation of latent HSV. HSV-1 can also cause gingivostomatitis and orolabial ulcers. HSV-2 can also cause other types of herpes infections, such as ocular herpes. Both virus types can cause infection of the central nervous system (e.g. encephalitis).

INCIDENCE/PREVALENCE Genital herpes infections are among the most common STDs. Seroprevalence studies showed that 22% of adults in the USA, 9% of adults in Poland, and 12% of adults in Australia had HSV-2 antibodies. The studies carried out in Poland and Australia also showed higher seroprevalence in women than in men (HSV-2 seroprevalence in Poland: 10% for women v 9% for men; P = 0.06; HSV-2 seroprevalence in Australia: 16% for women v 9% for men; RR 1.81, 95% CI 1.52 to 2.14). A UK study found that 23% of adults attending sexual health clinics, and 8% of blood donors in London, had antibodies to HSV-2. Seroprevalence of HSV-2 increased by 30.0% (95% CI 15.8% to 45.8%) between the periods 1976–1980 and 1988–1994. However, it should be noted that although antibody levels prove the existence of present or past infections, they do not differentiate between possible manifestations of HSV-2 infections (e.g. genital/ocular). Thus, the figures must be treated with caution when applied to genital herpes only.

AETIOLOGY/RISK FACTORS Both HSV-1 and HSV-2 can cause a first episode of genital infection, but HSV-2 is more likely to cause recurrent disease. Most people with HSV-2 infection have only mild symptoms and remain unaware that they have genital herpes. However, these people can still pass on the infection to sexual partners and newborns.

PROGNOSIS Sequelae of HSV infection include neonatal HSV infection, opportunistic infection in immunocompromised people, recurrent genital ulceration, and psychosocial morbidity. HSV-2 infection is associated with an increased risk of HIV transmission and acquisition. The most common neurological complications are aseptic meningitis (reported in about 25% of women during primary infection) and urinary retention (reported in up to 15% of women during primary infection). The absolute risk of neonatal infection is high (41%, 95% CI 26% to 56%) in babies born to women who acquire infection near the time of labour, and low (less than 3%) in women with established infection, even in those who have a recurrence at term. About 15% of neonatal infections result from postnatal transmission from oral lesions of relatives or hospital personnel.

Gonorrhoea

John Moran

KEY POINTS

- Gonorrhoea is caused by infection with *Neisseria gonorrhoeae*. In men, uncomplicated urethritis is the most common manifestation, while in women only about half of cases produce symptoms (such as vaginal discharge and dyspareunia).

  In the UK, diagnoses rates for gonorrhoea in 2005 were 196/100,000 for men aged 20–24 years, and 133/100,000 for women aged 16–19 years.

  Co-infection with *Chlamydia trachomatis* is reported in 10–40% of people with gonorrhoea in the USA and UK.

- Single-dose antibiotic regimens have achieved cure rates of 95% or higher in men and non-pregnant women with urogenital or rectal gonorrhoea. However, resistance to many widely available antibiotics (e.g. penicillins, tetracylines, fluoroquinolones) continues to spread, making it necessary to consider local *N gonorrhoeae* susceptibility patterns when choosing a treatment regimen.

  Single-dose antibiotics are also effective for curing gonorrhoea in pregnant women.

- In people with disseminated gonococcal infection, there is consensus that multidose regimens using injectable cephalosporins or fluoroquinolones (when the infecting organism is known to be susceptible) are the most effective treatments, although evidence supporting this is somewhat sparse.

- We found insufficient evidence to judge the best treatment for people with both gonorrhoea and chlamydia, although theory, expert opinion, and clinical experience suggest that a combination of antimicrobials active against both *N gonorrhoeae* and *C trachomatis* are effective.

 Please visit www.clinicalevidence.bmj.com for full text and references

What are the effects of treatments for uncomplicated infections in men and non-pregnant women?	
Beneficial	• Single-dose antibiotic regimens*

What are the effects of treatments for uncomplicated infections in pregnant women?	
Beneficial	• Single-dose antibiotic regimens

What are the effects of treatments for disseminated gonococcal infection?	
Likely To Be Beneficial	• Multidose antibiotic regimens†

What are the effects of dual treatment for gonorrhoea and chlamydia infection?	
Unknown Effectiveness	• Dual antibiotic treatment

Search date July 2006

*Based on results in individual arms of RCTs and observational studies.
†Based on non-RCT evidence and consensus.

DEFINITION Gonorrhoea is caused by infection with *Neisseria gonorrhoeae*. In men, uncomplicated urethritis is the most common manifestation, with dysuria and urethral discharge. Less typically, signs and symptoms are mild and indistinguishable from those of chlamydial urethritis. In women, the most common site of infection is the uterine cervix where infection results in symptoms such as vaginal discharge, lower abdominal discomfort, and dyspareunia in only half of cases. People with gonorrhoea may also have co-infection with C trachomatis.

INCIDENCE/PREVALENCE Between 1975 and 1997, the reported incidence of gonorrhoea in the USA fell by 74%, reaching a low point of 120/100,000 people. After a small increase in 1998, the rate of new gonorrhoeal infection declined steadily to an incidence of 112/100,000 people in 2004, then increased slightly to 116/100,000 in 2005. Rates are highest in younger people. In 2005, incidence was highest in women aged 15–19 years (625/100,000) and men aged 20–24 years (437/100,000). In UK genitourinary medicine clinics, diagnoses figures for 2002 were 269/100,000 for men aged 20–24 years, and 195/100,000 for women aged 16–19 years. By 2005, diagnoses of gonorrhoea had fallen to 196/100,000 for men aged 20–24 years and 133/100,000 for women aged 16–19 years. Recent studies in the USA and UK found concurrent *Chlamydia trachomatis* in 7–14% of homosexual men with gonorrhoea, in 20–30% of heterosexual men, and in 40–50% of women. Overall, co-infection with *C trachomatis* is reported in 10–40% of people with gonorrhoea.

AETIOLOGY/RISK FACTORS Most gonococcal infections result from penile–vaginal, penile–rectal, or penile–pharyngeal contact. An important minority of infections are transmitted from mother to child during birth, which can cause a sight-threatening purulent conjunctivitis (ophthalmia neonatorum). Less common are ocular infections in older children and adults as a result of sexual exposure, poor hygiene, or the medicinal use of urine.

PROGNOSIS The natural history of untreated gonococcal infection is spontaneous resolution and microbiological clearance after weeks or months of unpleasant symptoms. During this time, there is a substantial likelihood of transmission to others and of complications developing in the infected individual. In many women, the lack of readily discernible signs or symptoms of cervicitis means that infections go unrecognised and untreated. An unknown proportion of untreated infections causes local complications, including lymphangitis, periurethral abscess, bartholinitis, and urethral stricture; epididymitis in men; and in women involvement of the uterus, fallopian tubes, or ovaries causing PID (see PID, p 522). One review found N gonorrhoeae was cultured from 8–32% of women with acute PID in 11 European studies and from 27–80% of women in eight US studies. The proportion of N gonorrhoeae infections in women that lead to PID has not been well studied. However, one study of 26 women exposed to men with gonorrhoea found that 19 women were culture positive and, of these, five women had PID and another four had uterine adnexal tenderness. PID may lead to infertility (see PID, p 522). In some people, localised gonococcal infection may disseminate. A US study estimated the risk of dissemination to be 0.6–1.1% among women, whereas a European study estimated it to be 2.3–3.0%. The same European study found a lower risk in men, estimated to be 0.4–0.7%. When gonococci disseminate, they cause petechial or pustular skin lesions; asymmetrical arthropathies, tenosynovitis, or septic arthritis; and, rarely, meningitis or endocarditis.

Partner notification

Catherine Mathews and Nicol Coetzee

KEY POINTS

- Many people diagnosed with an STD do not have symptoms, and may not inform their past or current sexual partners of their diagnosis, or routinely use condoms.

- Several strategies have been used to notify and treat partners of people diagnosed with STDs, but only a limited number of RCTs of their effectiveness have been undertaken.

- Patient referral is where the index patient is encouraged to inform their past and present partners.

- Provider referral is where health professionals notify the partner without disclosing the identity of the index patient, and outreach assistance is where members of an outreach team indigenous to the community notify the partner without disclosing the identity of the index patient.

- Contract referral is where the index patient is encouraged to notify their partners, but the health professional does so if they fail to attend for treatment within an allotted time.

- Offering a choice of provider referral or patient referral may lead to more partners of people with HIV infection being notified compared with patient referral alone.

  We don't know whether contract referral or outreach assistance are beneficial in tracing partners of people with HIV.

- Contract referral may increase the proportion of partners presenting for treatment compared with patient referral in people with gonorrhoea.

  Provider referral may be beneficial in people with chlamydia.

  Contract referral strategies seem to be as effective as provider referral in the proportion of partners of people with syphilis who are notified.

- We don't know whether adding telephone reminders and contact cards, information pamphlets, or educational videos improves partner notification rates, or whether different health professionals are more effective at improving patient referral rates.

(i) **Please visit www.clinicalevidence.bmj.com for full text and references**

What are the effects of different partner notification strategies in people with different STDs?	
Likely To Be Beneficial	• Contract referral (as effective as provider referral in people with syphilis)
	• Contract referral (v patient referral) in people with gonorrhoea
	• Offering a choice between provider and patient referral (compared with offering only patient referral) in people with HIV
	• Provider referral (v patient referral) in people with non-gonococcal urethritis (mainly chlamydia)
Unknown Effectiveness	• Contract referral in people with chlamydia
	• Contract referral in people with HIV
	• Outreach assistance in people with chlamydia
	• Outreach assistance in people with gonorrhoea

- Outreach assistance in people with HIV
- Outreach assistance in people with syphilis
- Patient referral in people with syphilis
- Provider referral in people with gonorrhoea

What can be done to improve the effectiveness of patient referral in people with different STDs?	
Unknown Effectiveness	• Adding telephone reminders and contact cards to counselling
	• Counselling alone
	• Educational videos
	• Information pamphlets
	• Patient referral by different types of healthcare professionals
	• Telephone reminders alone

Search date April 2006

DEFINITION Partner notification is a process whereby the sexual partners of people with a diagnosis of STDs are informed of their exposure to infection. The main methods are patient referral, provider referral, contract referral, and outreach assistance.

INCIDENCE/PREVALENCE A large proportion of people with STDs will have neither symptoms nor signs of infection. For example, 22–68% of men with gonorrhoea who were identified through partner notification were asymptomatic. Partner notification is one of the two strategies to reach such individuals, the other strategy being screening. Managing infection in people with more than one current sexual partner is likely to have the greatest impact on the spread of STDs.

PROGNOSIS We found no studies showing that partner notification results in a health benefit, either to the partner or to future partners of infected people. Obtaining such evidence would be technically and ethically difficult. One RCT in asymptomatic women compared identifying, testing, and treating women at increased risk for cervical chlamydial infection versus usual care (women saw healthcare providers as necessary). It found that this strategy reduced incidence of PID compared with usual care (RR 0.44, 95% CI 0.20 to 0.90). This evidence suggests that partner notification, which also aims to identify and treat people who are largely unaware of infection, would provide a direct health benefit to partners who are infected.

Jonathan Ross

KEY POINTS

- PID is caused by infection of the upper female genital tract, and is often asymptomatic.

  PID is the most common gynaecological reason for admission to hospital in the USA, and is diagnosed in almost 2% of women aged 16–45 years consulting their GP in England and Wales.

  Epithelial damage from infections such as *Chlamydia trachomatis* or *Neisseria gonorrhoeae* can allow opportunistic infection from many other bacteria.

  About 20% of women with PID become infertile, 40% develop chronic pain, and 1% of women who conceive have an ectopic pregnancy.

  Spontaneous resolution of symptoms may occur in some women, but early initiation of treatment is needed to prevent impairment of fertility.

- As there are no reliable signs and symptoms of PID, empirical treatment is common.

  The positive predictive value of clinical diagnosis is 65–90% compared with laparoscopy, and observational studies suggest that delaying treatment by 3 days can impair fertility.

  The absence of infection from the lower genital tract does not exclude a diagnosis of PID.

- Oral antibiotics are likely to be beneficial, and are associated with the resolution of symptoms and signs of pelvic infection, but we don't know which antibiotic regimen is best.

  Clinical and microbiological cure rates of 88–100% have been reported after oral antibiotic treatment.

  The risks of tubal occlusion and infertility depend on severity of infection before treatment. Clinical improvement may not necessarily translate into improved fertility.

- Oral antibiotics may be as effective as parenteral antibiotics in reducing symptoms and preserving fertility, with fewer adverse effects, and outpatient treatment is as effective as inpatient treatment for uncomplicated PID. However, we don't know the optimal duration of treatment.

- Risks of PID may be increased after instrumentation of the cervix, and testing for infection before such procedures is advisable, but we don't know whether prophylactic antibiotics before IUD insertion reduce these risks.

(i) **Please visit www.clinicalevidence.bmj.com for full text and references**

What are the effects of empirical treatment in women with suspected PID compared with treatment delayed until the results of microbiological investigations are known?	
Unknown Effectiveness	• Empirical antibiotic treatment versus treatment guided by test results in women with suspected PID

How do different antimicrobial regimens compare when treating women with confirmed PID?	
Likely To Be Beneficial	• Antibiotics (for symptoms and microbiological clearance in women with confirmed PID)
	• Different durations of antibiotic treatment (no evidence as to which duration is best)

- Oral antibiotics (as effective as parenteral antibiotics)
- Outpatient (as effective as inpatient) antibiotic treatment

What are the effects of routine antibiotic prophylaxis to prevent PID before IUD insertion?

Unknown Effectiveness	• Routine antibiotic prophylaxis before IUD insertion in women at high risk
Unlikely To Be Beneficial	• Routine antibiotic prophylaxis before IUD insertion in women at low risk

Search date May 2007

DEFINITION Pelvic inflammatory disease (PID) is inflammation and infection of the upper genital tract in women, typically involving the fallopian tubes, ovaries, and surrounding structures.

INCIDENCE/PREVALENCE The exact incidence of PID is unknown, because the disease cannot be diagnosed reliably from clinical symptoms and signs. Direct visualisation of the fallopian tubes by laparoscopy is the best single diagnostic test, but it is invasive, lacks sensitivity, and is not used routinely in clinical practice. PID is the most common gynaecological reason for admission to hospital in the USA, accounting for 18/10,000 recorded hospital discharges. A diagnosis of PID is made in 1/62 (1.6%) women aged 16–45 years attending their primary-care physician in England and Wales. However, because most PID is asymptomatic, this figure underestimates the true prevalence. A crude marker of PID in resource-poor countries can be obtained from reported hospital admission rates, where it accounts for 17–40% of gynaecological admissions in sub-Saharan Africa, 15–37% in Southeast Asia, and 3–10% in India.

AETIOLOGY/RISK FACTORS Factors associated with PID mirror those for STDs — young age, reduced socioeconomic circumstances, lower educational attainment, and recent new sexual partner. Infection ascends from the cervix, and initial epithelial damage caused by bacteria (especially *Chlamydia trachomatis* and *Neisseria gonorrhoeae*) allows the opportunistic entry of other organisms. Many different microbes, including *Mycoplasma genitalium* and anaerobes, may be isolated from the upper genital tract. The spread of infection to the upper genital tract may be increased by instrumentation of the cervix, but reduced by barrier methods of contraception, levonorgestrel implants, and by oral contraceptives compared with other forms of contraception.

PROGNOSIS PID has a high morbidity; about 20% of affected women become infertile, 40% develop chronic pelvic pain, and 1% of those who conceive have an ectopic pregnancy. Uncontrolled observations suggest that clinical symptoms and signs resolve in a significant proportion of untreated women. Repeated episodes of PID are associated with a four- to sixfold increase in the risk of permanent tubal damage. One case-control study (76 cases and 367 controls) found that delaying treatment by 3 or more days is associated with impaired fertility (OR 2.6, 95% CI 1.2 to 5.9).

Henry W Buck, Jr

KEY POINTS

- **External genital warts (EGWs) are sexually transmitted benign epidermal growths on the anogenital areas of both females and males caused by HPV.**

  About 50–60% of sexually active women aged 18–49 have been exposed to HPV infection, but only 10–15% will have genital warts. Warts are more common in people with impaired immune systems, but, in people with adequate immune function, about a third can resolve spontaneously.

  Some lesions, particularly those that are pigmented, should be biopsied to rule out severe dysplasia or melanoma, but external genital warts rarely, if ever, progress to cancer.

- **Imiquimod 1% and 5% creams increase clearance of warts compared with placebo in patients without HIV, but we don't know if they are effective in people with HIV.**

  Imiquimod 5% cream may be more likely to clear warts, but increases local irritation compared with 1% imiquimod cream.

- **Topical interferon increases wart clearance at 4 weeks compared with placebo.**

  Topical interferon is preferred to systemic interferon, which has not been shown consistently to be effective, is expensive to use, and is associated with severe adverse effects.

  We don't know whether intralesional interferon is effective, although it is time consuming and expensive to use.

- **Podophyllotoxin is more effective than placebo and probably as effective as podophyllin in clearing genital warts, but may be easier to use.**

  Podophyllin may contain mutagenic compounds, and its formulation is unstandardised, so podophyllotoxin is the preferred treatment, despite the risk of local burning and bleeding.

- **There is consensus that bi- and trichloroacetic acid and cryotherapy are effective treatments for external genital warts, although we found no studies comparing them to placebo.**

- **Surgical (scissor) excision and electrosurgery may be effective at clearing genital warts at 6 months compared with no treatment, but we don't know whether laser surgery is also effective.**

- **Vaccines are effective in preventing infection and disease by HPV in young women.**

  We don't know whether vaccines are effective in people other than young women.

- **We don't know whether condom use reduces the spread of HPV infection and genital warts.**

(i) **Please visit www.clinicalevidence.bmj.com for full text and references**

What are the effects of treatments for external genital warts?	
Beneficial	• Imiquimod in people without HIV
	• Interferon (topical)
	• Podophyllotoxin
Likely To Be Beneficial	• Bi- and trichloroacetic acid*
	• Cryotherapy*

	• Electrosurgery
	• Podophyllin (probably as effective as podophyllotoxin or surgical excision)*
	• Surgical excision (as effective as podophyllin in clearing warts; more effective than podophyllin in preventing recurrence)
Unknown Effectiveness	• Imiquimod in people with HIV
	• Interferon (intralesional)
	• Laser surgery
Likely To Be Ineffective Or Harmful	• Interferon (systemic)

What are the effects of interventions to prevent transmission of external genital warts?

| **Likely To Be Beneficial** | • Vaccines |
| **Unknown Effectiveness** | • Condoms |

Search date February 2007

*No placebo-controlled RCTs found; categorisation based on consensus.

DEFINITION External genital warts (EGWs) are benign epidermal growths on the external anogenital regions. There are four morphological types: condylomatous, keratotic, papular, and flat warts. EGWs are caused by the human papilloma virus (HPV). **Diagnosis:** The majority of EGWs are diagnosed by inspection. Some clinicians apply 5% acetic acid (white vinegar) to help visualise lesions, because it produces so-called "acetowhite" change and, more importantly, defines vascular patterns characteristic for EGWs. However, the "acetowhite" change also occurs with conditions other than external genital warts, so differential diagnoses should be considered. Some lesions, particularly those that are pigmented, should be biopsied to rule out severe dysplasia or melanoma.

INCIDENCE/PREVALENCE In the USA in 2004, external genital warts accounted for more than 310,000 initial visits to private physicians' offices. In the USA, 1% of sexually active men and women aged 18–49 are estimated to have EGWs. It is believed that external and cervical lesions caused by HPV are the most prevalent STD among people aged 18–25. In the USA, 50–60% of women aged 18–25 test positive for HPV DNA, but no more than 10–15% ever have genital warts. By the age of 50, at least 80% of women will have acquired genital HPV infection. About 6.2 million Americans acquire a new genital HPV infection each year.

AETIOLOGY/RISK FACTORS External genital warts are caused by HPV, and are sexually transmitted. They are more common in people with impaired immune function. Although more than 100 types of HPV have been identified, about a third of which are found in the anogenital regions, most EGWs in immunocompetent people are caused by HPV types 6 and 11.

PROGNOSIS The ability to clear and remain free of EGWs is a function of cellular immunity. In immunocompetent people, the prognosis in terms of clearance and avoiding recurrence is good; but people with impaired cellular immunity (e.g. people with HIV and AIDS) have

(continued over)

(from previous page)

great difficulty in achieving and maintaining wart clearance. Without treatment, EGWs may remain unchanged, may increase in size or number, and about a third will clear. Clinical trials found that recurrences may happen, and may necessitate repeated treatment. EGWs rarely, if ever, progress to cancer. Recurrent respiratory papillomatosis (RRP), a rare and sometimes life-threatening condition, occurs in children of women with a history of genital warts. Its rarity makes it difficult to design studies that can evaluate whether treatment in pregnant women alters the risk.

Sarah Purdy and David DeBerker

KEY POINTS

- Acne vulgaris affects over 80% of teenagers, and persists beyond the age of 25 years in 3% of men and 12% of women.

  Typical lesions of acne include comedones, inflammatory papules and pustules. Nodules and cysts occur in more severe acne, and can cause scarring and psychological distress.

- Topical benzoyl peroxide should be considered as first-line treatment in mild acne.

  Topical benzoyl peroxide and topical azelaic acid reduce inflammatory and non-inflammatory lesions compared with placebo, but can cause itching, burning, stinging, and redness of the skin.

- Topical antibiotics such as clindamycin and erythromycin (alone or with zinc) reduce inflammatory lesions, but have not been shown to reduce non-inflammatory lesions compared with placebo. Tetracycline may reduce overall acne severity.

  Antimicrobial resistance can develop with use of topical or oral antibiotics, and their efficacy may decrease over time.

  Tetracyclines may cause skin discoloration, and should be avoided in pregnant or breastfeeding women.

  Topical preparations of tretinoin, adapalene and isotretinoin may reduce inflammatory and non-inflammatory lesions but can also cause redness, burning, dryness, and soreness of the skin.

- Oral antibiotics (doxycycline, erythromycin, lymecycline, minocycline, oxytetracycline, and tetracycline) are considered to be useful for people with more severe acne, although we don't know for sure that they are effective.

  Oral antibiotics can cause adverse effects, such as contraceptive failure.

  Minocycline has been associated with an increased risk of systemic lupus erythematosis and liver disorders.

(i) **Please visit www.clinicalevidence.bmj.com for full text and references**

What are the effects of topical treatments in people with acne vulgaris?

Beneficial	• Benzoyl peroxide
	• Clindamycin (reduced the number of inflammatory lesions)
	• Erythromycin (reduced the number of inflammatory lesions)
	• Tretinoin
Likely To Be Beneficial	• Adapalene
	• Azelaic acid
	• Erythromycin plus zinc
	• Isotretinoin
	• Tetracycline

What are the effects of oral treatments in people with acne vulgaris?

Likely To Be Beneficial	• Erythromycin
Trade-off Between Benefits And Harms	• Doxycycline • Lymecycline • Minocycline • Oxytetracycline • Tetracycline

Search date June 2006

DEFINITION Acne vulgaris is a common inflammatory pilosebaceous disease characterised by comedones, papules, pustules, inflamed nodules, superficial pus-filled cysts, and (in extreme cases) canalising and deep, inflamed, sometimes purulent sacs. Lesions are most common on the face, but the neck, chest, upper back, and shoulders may also be affected. Acne can cause scarring and considerable psychological distress. It is classified as mild, moderate, or severe. Mild acne is defined as non-inflammatory lesions (comedones), a few inflammatory (papulopustular) lesions, or both. Moderate acne is defined as more inflammatory lesions, occasional nodules, or both, and mild scarring. Severe acne is defined as widespread inflammatory lesions, nodules, or both, and scarring; moderate acne that has not settled with 6 months of treatment; or acne of any "severity" with serious psychological upset. This review does not cover acne rosacea, acne secondary to industrial occupations, and treatment of acne in people under 13 years of age.

INCIDENCE/PREVALENCE Acne is the most common skin disease of adolescence, affecting over 80% of teenagers (aged 13–18 years) at some point. Estimates of prevalence vary depending on study populations and the method of assessment used. Prevalence of acne in a community sample of 14–16-year-olds in the UK has been recorded as 50%. In a sample of adolescents from schools in New Zealand, acne was present in 91% of males and 79% of females. It has been estimated that up to 30% of teenagers have acne of sufficient severity to require medical treatment. Acne was the presenting complaint in 3.1% of people aged 13–25 years attending primary care in a UK population. Overall incidence is similar in both men and women, and peaks at 17 years of age. The number of adults with acne, including people over 25 years, is increasing; the reasons for this increase are uncertain.

AETIOLOGY/RISK FACTORS The exact cause of acne is unknown. Four factors contribute to the development of acne: increased sebum secretion rate, abnormal follicular differentiation causing obstruction of the pilosebaceous duct, bacteriology of the pilosebaceous duct, and inflammation. The anaerobic bacterium *Propionibacterium acnes* plays an important role in the pathogenesis of acne. Androgen secretion is the major trigger for adolescent acne.

PROGNOSIS In 3% of men (95% CI 1.2% to 4.8%) and 12% of women (95% CI 9% to 15%), facial acne persists after the age of 25 years, and in a few people (1% of men and 5% of women) acne persists into their 40s.

Fay Crawford

KEY POINTS

- Fungal infection of the feet can cause white and soggy skin between the toes, dry and flaky soles, or reddening and blistering of the skin all over the foot.

  Around 15–25% of people are likely to have athlete's foot at any one time.

  The infection can spread to other parts of the body and to other people.

- Topical allylamines (naftifine and terbinafine), topical azoles (clotrimazole, miconazole nitrate, tioconazole, sulconazole nitrate, bifonazole and econazole nitrate) and topical ciclopirox olamine are all more likely to cure fungal skin infections than placebo.

  We don't know if any one treatment is more effective than the others.

- We don't know whether improving foot hygiene or changing footwear can help to cure athlete's foot.

(i) **Please visit www.clinicalevidence.bmj.com for full text and references**

What are the effects of topical treatments for athlete's foot?	
Beneficial	• Topical allylamines (naftifine, terbinafine) • Topical azoles • Topical ciclopirox olamine
Unknown Effectiveness	• Improved foot hygiene, including socks, and hosiery

Search date April 2006

DEFINITION Athlete's foot is a cutaneous fungal infection caused by dermatophyte infection. It is characterised by itching, flaking, and fissuring of the skin. It may manifest in three ways: the skin between the toes may appear mascerated (white) and soggy; the soles of the feet may become dry and scaly; and the skin all over the foot may become red, and vesicular eruptions may appear. It is conventional in dermatology to refer to fungal skin infections as superficial in order to distinguish them from systemic fungal infections.

INCIDENCE/PREVALENCE Epidemiological studies have produced various estimates of the prevalence of athlete's foot. Studies are usually conducted in populations of people who attend dermatology clinics, sports centres, or swimming pools, or who are in the military. UK estimates suggest that athlete's foot is present in about 15% of the general population. Studies conducted in dermatology clinics in Italy (722 people) and China (1014 people) found prevalences of 25% and 27%, respectively. A population-based study conducted in 1148 children in Israel found the prevalence among children to be 30%.

AETIOLOGY/RISK FACTORS Swimming-pool users and industrial workers may be at increased risk of fungal foot infection. However, one survey identified fungal foot infection in only 9% of swimmers, with the highest prevalence (20%) being in men aged 16 years and older.

PROGNOSIS Fungal infections of the foot are not life threatening in people with normal immune status, but in some people they cause persistent itching and, ultimately, fissuring. Other people are apparently unaware of persistent infection. The infection can spread to other parts of the body and to other individuals.

Atopic eczema

Fiona Bath-Hextall and Hywel Williams

KEY POINTS

- Atopic eczema affects 15–20% of schoolchildren worldwide and 2–10% of adults. Only about 60% of people with eczema demonstrate atopy, with specific immunoglobulin E responses to allergens.

  Remission occurs in two thirds of children by the age of 15 years, but relapses may occur later.

- There is a consensus that emollients are effective for treating the symptoms of atopic eczema, although little high-quality research has been done to confirm this.

- Corticosteroids improve clearance of lesions and decrease relapse rates compared with placebo, although we don't know which is the most effective corticosteroid or dosing regimen.

  Topical corticosteroids seem to have few adverse effects, but may cause burning, skin thinning, and telangiectasia, especially in children.

- Pimecrolimus and tacrolimus improve clearance of lesions compared with placebo, and may have a role in people with a high risk of corticosteroid adverse effects.

- CAUTION: An association has been suggested between pimecrolimus and tacrolimus and skin cancer. They should be used only where other treatments have failed.

- We don't know whether vitamin E, pyridoxine, zinc supplementation, exclusion or elemental diets, or probiotics reduce symptoms in atopic eczema, as there are insufficient good-quality studies.

  Essential fatty acids such as evening primrose oil, blackcurrant-seed oil, or fish oil do not seem to reduce symptoms in atopic eczema.

- We don't know whether prolonged breastfeeding, reducing maternal dietary allergens, or control of house dust mites, can prevent the development of atopic eczema in children.

  Early introduction of probiotics in the last trimester of pregnancy and during breastfeeding may reduce the risk of atopic eczema in the baby.

(i) Please visit www.clinicalevidence.bmj.com for full text and references

What are the effects of self-care treatments in adults and children with established atopic eczema?	
Likely To Be Beneficial	• Emollients*

What are the effects of topical medical treatments in adults and children with established atopic eczema?	
Beneficial	• Corticosteroids
	• Pimecrolimus
	• Tacrolimus

What are the effects of dietary interventions in adults with established atopic eczema?	
Unknown Effectiveness	• Vitamin E and multivitamins

What are the effects of dietary interventions in children with established atopic eczema?

Unknown Effectiveness	• Egg and cows' milk exclusion diet • Elemental diet • Few-foods diet • Probiotics • Pyridoxine (Vitamin B6) • Zinc supplementation
Likely To Be Ineffective Or Harmful	• Essential fatty acids (evening primrose oil, blackcurrant-seed oil, fish oil)

What are the effects of primary preventive interventions in predisposed infants?

Unknown Effectiveness	• Prolonged breastfeeding by mother straight after birth

What are the effects of reducing allergens (maternal dietary restriction, control of house dust mite only)?

Likely To Be Beneficial	• Early introduction of probiotics (in last trimester or shortly after birth)
Unknown Effectiveness	• Reduction of allergens (maternal dietary restriction, control of house dust mite only)

Search date February 2005

*Based on consensus

DEFINITION Atopic eczema (also known as atopic dermatitis) is a chronic, relapsing, and itchy inflammatory skin condition. In the acute stage, eczematous lesions are characterised by poorly defined erythema with surface change (oedema, vesicles, and weeping). In the chronic stage, lesions are marked by skin thickening (lichenification). Although lesions can occur anywhere on the body, babies often have eczematous lesions on their cheeks and outer limbs before developing the more typical flexural involvement behind the knees and in the folds of the elbow and neck later in childhood. Atopy, the tendency to produce specific immunoglobulin E responses to allergens, is associated with "atopic" eczema, but up to 60% of individuals with the disease phenotype may not be atopic. This can cause confusion, for example around diagnosis, treatment, lifestyle recommendations, and genetic markers. The correct use of the term atopic eczema should therefore ideally only refer to those with a clinical picture of eczema who are also immunoglobulin E antibody high-responders. **Diagnosis:** There is no definitive "gold standard" for the diagnosis of atopic eczema, which is based on clinical features combined with a disease history. However, a UK working party developed a minimum list of reliable diagnostic criteria for atopic eczema using the Hanifin and Rajka list of clinical features as building blocks. In an independent validation study of children attending hospital dermatology outpatients, the criteria were shown to have a sensitivity of 85% and a specificity of 96% when compared with a dermatologist's diagnosis. There are several severity scoring systems, used mainly in clinical trials, including the SCORing Atopic Dermatitis (SCORAD) and the six-area,

(continued over)

(from previous page)

six-sign atopic dermatitis severity score (SASSAD) indexes. Quantitative scales used for measuring atopic eczema severity in clinical trials are too complex and difficult to interpret in clinical practice. The division of atopic eczema into mild, moderate, and severe mainly depends on the intensity of itching symptoms (e.g. resulting in sleep loss), the extent of involvement, and course of disease. **Population:** For the purposes of this review, we included all adults and children defined as having established atopic eczema. Where either adults or children are considered separately, this is highlighted in the text. We also included studies assessing primary prevention in those at risk of developing atopic eczema for specific interventions: prolonged breastfeeding, maternal dietary restriction, house dust mite restriction, and early introduction of probiotics.

INCIDENCE/PREVALENCE Atopic eczema affects 15–20% of school-age children at some stage, and 2–10% of adults in the UK. Prevalence data for the symptoms of atopic eczema were collected in the global International Study of Asthma and Allergies in Childhood (ISAAC). The results of the study suggest that atopic eczema is a worldwide problem affecting 5–20% of children. One UK-based population study showed that 2% of children under the age of 5 years have severe disease, and 84% have mild disease. Around 2% of adults have atopic eczema, and many of these have a more chronic and severe form.

AETIOLOGY/RISK FACTORS The causes of eczema are not well understood and are probably due to a combination of genetic and environmental factors. In recent years, research has pointed to the possible role of environmental agents, such as house dust mites, pollution, and prenatal or early exposure to infections. The world allergy association's revised nomenclature for allergy also states that what is commonly called atopic eczema is not one specific disease, but encompasses a spectrum of allergic mechanisms.

PROGNOSIS Remission occurs by the age of 15 years in 60–70% of cases, although some relapse may occur later. Although no treatments are currently known to alter the natural history of atopic eczema, several interventions can help to control symptoms. Development and puberty may be delayed in the more severely affected child.

Sanjay Rajpara and Anthony Ormerod

KEY POINTS

- Basal cell carcinoma (BCC) is the most common form of skin cancer, predominantly affecting the head and neck, and can be diagnosed clinically in most cases.

  Metastasis of BCC is rare, but localised tissue invasion and destruction can lead to morbidity.

  Risk factors for BCC include tendency to freckle, degree of sun exposure, excessive sun-bed use, and smoking.

  Incidence of BCC increases markedly after the age of 40 years, but incidence in younger people is rising, possibly as a result of increased sun exposure.

- Excisional surgery is considered likely to be effective in treating BCC.

  Similar treatment-response rates at 1 year after treatment have been reported for excisional surgery compared with curettage plus cryotherapy and photodynamic therapy.

  Excisional surgery is associated with fewer adverse effects compared with photodynamic therapy and curettage plus cryotherapy, and seems to be associated with improved cosmetic results compared with curettage plus cryotherapy 1 year after treatment.

  We can't compare the effectiveness of surgical excision with Moh's micrographic surgery in treating recurrent BCC, but excisional surgery seems to be associated with more adverse effects compared with Moh's micrographic surgery.

- Cryotherapy, with or without curettage, photodynamic therapy , and curettage and cautery/electrodesiccation may be effective treatments for BCC in the short term (up to 1 year after treatment).

  Cryotherapy alone seems to be as effective as photodynamic therapy for superficial and nodular BCCs, but photodynamic therapy may produce better cosmetic results compared with cryotherapy alone.

  We don't know how cryotherapy with curettage compares with photodynamic therapy or cryotherapy alone.

  Twofold treatments with photodynamic therapy performed a week apart with delta-aminolaevulinic acid (ALA-PDT) may be more effective than single treatments in the short term.

  There seems to be no difference in effectiveness between ALA-PDT using a broadband halogen light source and ALA-PDT using a laser light source.

- Imiquimod 5% cream may be beneficial for the treatment of superficial and nodular BCCs compared with placebo in the short term (within 6 months after starting treatment).

  It seems that more-frequent application of imiquimod 5% improves response rates compared with lower-frequency regimens, but is also associated with increased frequency of adverse effects

- We don't know whether fluorouracil is effective in the short-term treatment of BCC.

- Excisional surgery, cryotherapy alone, photodynamic therapy, and curettage and cautery/electrodesiccation are thought to be beneficial in preventing long-term recurrence of BCC.

- We don't know whether imiquimod 5% and fluorouracil are effective in preventing BCC recurrence in the longer term (at or beyond 2 years' treatment).

Please visit www.clinicalevidence.bmj.com for full text and references

What are the effects of interventions on treatment response/recurrence (within 1 year of therapy) in people with basal cell carcinoma?

Likely To Be Beneficial	• Cryotherapy/cryosurgery (as effective as photodynamic therapy; in combination with curettage seems to be as effective as excisional surgery)
	• Curettage and cautery/electrodesiccation (likely to be beneficial for low-risk BCC)*
	• Imiquimod 5% cream (better than placebo at 6 months, insufficient evidence to compare with other treatments)
	• Photodynamic therapy
	• Surgery (excisional or Moh's micrographic surgery)*
Unknown Effectiveness	• Fluorouracil

What are the effects of interventions on long-term recurrence (a minimum of 2 years after treatment) in people with basal cell carcinoma?

Likely To Be Beneficial	• Cryotherapy/cryosurgery*
	• Curettage and cautery/electrodesiccation*
	• Photodynamic therapy*
	• Surgery (conventional or Moh's micrographic surgery)†
Unknown Effectiveness	• Fluorouracil
	• Imiquimod 5% cream

Search date February 2007

*Categorisation is based on consensus and expert opinion.
†Categorisation is based on consensus and observational data.

DEFINITION Basal cell carcinoma (BCC) is the most common cancer found in humans. It is a slow-growing, locally invasive, malignant epidermal skin tumour which mainly affects white people. Although metastasis is rare, BCC can cause morbidity by local tissue invasion and destruction, particularly on the head and neck. The clinical appearances and morphology are diverse, including nodular, cystic, ulcerated ("rodent ulcer"), superficial, morphoeic (sclerosing), keratotic, and pigmented variants. Most BCCs (85%) develop on the head and neck. **Diagnosis:** The diagnosis of BCC is made clinically in most cases. A biopsy is performed for histological diagnosis when there is doubt about clinical diagnosis, and when people are referred for specialised forms of treatment.

INCIDENCE/PREVALENCE The reported incidence of BCC varies in the literature. The incidence was reported to be 788 per 100,000 population a year in 1995 in Australia, and 146 per 100,000 population a year in 1990 in the USA. A Dutch study reported an incidence of 200 per 100,000 population a year, whereas the incidence in the UK is reported to be lower, at about 100 cases per 100,000 population a year. Because of incomplete registration of cases, some of these estimates may be low. The incidence of BCC increases markedly after the age of 40 years, and the incidence in younger people is increasing, possibly as a result of increased sun exposure.

AETIOLOGY/RISK FACTORS The reported risk factors for developing BCC include fair skin, tendency to freckle, degree of sun exposure, excessive sun-bed use, smoking, radiotherapy, phototherapy, male gender, and a genetic predisposition. Although cumulative lifetime sunlight exposure is a major risk factor for the development of BCC, it does not accurately predict the frequency of BCC development at a particular site on its own. Other contributory factors are skin phenotype (e.g. Fitzpatrick I and II), number of lifetime visits to tanning beds, number of pack years of smoking, and number of blistering sunburns. Immunosuppressed patients are also at increased risk for non-melanoma skin cancer, including BCC. The risk increases with duration of immunosuppression, and about 16% of people with renal transplants develop BCC — a 10-fold increased risk compared with the general population. An autosomal dominant condition, naevoid BCC syndrome (Gorlin's syndrome) is characterised by the occurrence of multiple BCCs and developmental abnormalities.

PROGNOSIS The following factors can affect prognosis: tumour size, site, type, growth pattern/histological subtype, failure of previous treatment (recurrence), and immunosuppression. BCCs in close proximity to important body structures can potentially increase morbidity as a result of local tissue invasion or recurrence, and so BCCs can be categorised based on their location as: high risk (nose, nasal-labial fold, eyelids and periorbital areas, lips, chin, and ears); medium risk (scalp, forehead, pre- and post-auricular areas, and malar areas); and low risk (neck, trunk, and extremities). Histologically, micronodular, infiltrative, morphoeic, and basosquamous types of BCC are classed as high risk. Distant metastases are rare. Although some BCCs tend to infiltrate tissues in a three-dimensional manner, growth is usually localised to the area of origin. However, if left untreated, BCC can cause extensive tissue destruction with infiltration in deeper tissues, such as bone and brain. BCCs may remain small for years with little tendency to grow, grow rapidly, or proceed by successive spurts of extension of tumour and partial regression. Therefore, the clinical course of BCC is unpredictable.

538 | Cellulitis and erysipelas

Andrew D Morris

KEY POINTS

- Cellulitis is a common problem caused by spreading bacterial inflammation of the skin, with redness, pain, and lymphangitis. Up to 40% of people have systemic illness.

  Erysipelas is a form of cellulitis with marked superficial inflammation, typically affecting the lower limbs and the face.

  Risk factors include lymphoedema, leg ulcer, toe-web intertrigo, and traumatic wounds.

  The most common pathogens in adults are streptococci and *Staphylococcus aureus*.

  Cellulitis and erysipelas can result in local necrosis and abscess formation. Around a quarter of people have more than one episode of cellulitis within 3 years.

- Antibiotics cure 50–100% of infections, but we don't know which antibiotic regimen is most successful.

  We don't know whether antibiotics are as effective when given orally as when given intravenously, or whether intramuscular administration is more effective than intravenous.

  A 5-day course of antibiotics may be as effective as a 10-day course at curing the infection and preventing early recurrence.

- Although there is consensus that treatment of predisposing factors can prevent recurrence of cellulitis or erysipelas, we found no studies that assessed the benefits of this approach.

(i) **Please visit www.clinicalevidence.bmj.com for full text and references**

What are the effects of treatments for cellulitis and erysipelas?	
Unknown Effectiveness	• Comparative effects of different antibiotics
	• Comparative effects of different routes of administration of antibiotics
	• Duration of antibiotics

What are the effects of treatments to prevent recurrence of cellulitis and erysipelas?	
Likely To Be Beneficial	• Antibiotics (prophylactic) to prevent recurrence of cellulitis and erysipelas
Unknown Effectiveness	• Treatment of predisposing factors

Search date May 2007

DEFINITION **Cellulitis** is a spreading bacterial infection of the dermis and subcutaneous tissues. It causes local signs of inflammation, such as warmth, erythema, pain, lymphangitis, and frequently systemic upset with fever and raised white blood cell count. **Erysipelas** is a form of cellulitis and is characterised by pronounced superficial inflammation. The term erysipelas is commonly used when the face is affected. The lower limbs are by far the most common sites affected by cellulitis and erysipelas, but any area, such as the ears, trunk, fingers, and toes, can be affected.

INCIDENCE/PREVALENCE We found no validated recent data on the incidence of cellulitis or erysipelas worldwide. UK hospital incidence data reported 69,576 episodes of cellulitis and 516 episodes of erysipelas in 2004–2005. Cellulitis infections of the limb accounted for most of these infections (58,824 episodes).

AETIOLOGY/RISK FACTORS The most common infective organisms for cellulitis and erysipelas in adults are streptococci (particularly *Streptococcus pyogenes*) and *Staphylococcus aureus*. In children, *Haemophilus influenzae* was a frequent cause before the introduction of the *Haemophilus influenzae* type B vaccination. Several risk factors for cellulitis and erysipelas have been identified in a case-control study (167 cases and 294 controls): lymphoedema (OR 71.2, 95% CI 5.6 to 908.0), leg ulcer (OR 62.5, 95% CI 7.0 to 556.0), toe web intertrigo (OR 13.9, 95% CI 7.2 to 27.0), and traumatic wounds (OR 10.7, 95% CI 4.8 to 23.8).

PROGNOSIS Cellulitis can spread through the bloodstream and lymphatic system. A retrospective case study of people admitted to hospital with cellulitis found that systemic symptoms, such as fever and raised white blood cell count, were present in up to 42% of cases at presentation. Lymphatic involvement can lead to obstruction and damage of the lymphatic system that predisposes to recurrent cellulitis. Recurrence can occur rapidly, or after months or years. One prospective cohort study found that 29% of people with erysipelas had a recurrent episode within 3 years. Local necrosis and abscess formation can also occur. It is not known whether the prognosis of erysipelas differs from cellulitis. We found no evidence about factors that predict recurrence, or a better or worse outcome. We found no good evidence on the prognosis of untreated cellulitis.

Fungal toenail infections

Fay Crawford and Jill Ferrari

KEY POINTS

- Fungal toenail infection (onychomycosis) is characterised as infection of part or all of the toenail unit, which includes the nail plate, the nail bed, and the nail matrix. Over time, the infection causes discoloration and distortion of part or all of the nail unit.

  Fungal infections are reported to cause 23% of foot diseases and 50% of nail conditions in people seen by dermatologists, but are less common in the general population, affecting 3–5% of people.

  Infection can cause discomfort in walking, pain, or limitation of activities.

- People taking oral antifungal drugs reported greater satisfaction and fewer onychomycoses-related problems, such as embarrassment, self-consciousness, and being perceived as unclean by others, compared with people using topical antifungals.

  Oral antifungals have general adverse effects which include gastrointestinal complaints (such as diarrhoea), rash, and respiratory complaints. It was rare for people to withdraw from an RCT because of adverse effects.

- Both oral itraconazole and oral terbinafine effectively increase cure rates of fungal toenail infection, with terbinafine appearing to be slightly more effective.

  Adverse effects unique to terbinafine include sensory loss, such as taste, smell, or hearing disturbance.

- Alternative oral antifungal treatments include fluconazole, which seems to modestly improve cure rates, and ketoconazole and griseofulvin, which may be effective; but the evidence is insufficient to allow us to know for certain.

- Topical ciclopirox seems to modestly improve symptoms of fungal toenail infection compared with placebo.

  We found no evidence examining the effectiveness of other topical agents such as ketoconazole, fluconazole, amorolfine, terbinafine, tioconazole, or butenafine.

  We don't know whether mechanical debridement has any effect on fungal toenail infection, as we found no adequate studies.

Please visit www.clinicalevidence.bmj.com for full text and references

What are the effects of oral treatments for fungal toenail infections?	
Beneficial	• Oral itraconazole (more effective than placebo, but probably less effective than terbinafine) • Oral terbinafine
Likely To Be Beneficial	• Oral fluconazole (although benefits are modest, even after long-term treatment)
Unknown Effectiveness	• Oral griseofulvin • Oral ketoconazole

What are the effects of topical treatments for fungal toenail infections?

Likely To Be Beneficial	• Topical ciclopirox (although benefits are modest, even after long-term treatment)
Unknown Effectiveness	• Mechanical debridement • Topical amorolfine • Topical butenafine • Topical fluconazole • Topical ketoconazole • Topical terbinafine • Topical tioconazole

Search date June 2006

DEFINITION Fungal toenail infection (onychomycosis) is characterised as infection of part or all of the nail unit, which includes the nail plate, the nail bed, and the nail matrix. Over time, the infection causes discoloration and distortion of part or all of the nail unit. The tissue under and around the nail may also thicken. This review deals exclusively with dermatophyte toenail infections (see aetiology) and excludes candidal or yeast infections.

INCIDENCE/PREVALENCE Fungal infections are reported to cause 23% of foot diseases and 50% of nail conditions in people seen by dermatologists, but are less common in the general population, affecting 3–5% of people. The prevalence varies among populations, which may be because of differences in screening techniques. In a large European project (13,695 people with a range of foot conditions), 35% had a fungal infection diagnosed by microscopy/culture. One prospective study in Spain (1000 adults aged over 20 years old) reported a prevalence of fungal toenail infection of 2.7% (infection defined as clinically abnormal nails with positive microscopy and culture). In Denmark, one study (5755 adults aged over 18 years old) reported the prevalence of fungal toenail infection as 4.0% (determined by positive fungal cultures). The incidence of mycotic nail infections may have increased over the past few years, perhaps because of increasing use of systemic antibiotics, immunosuppressive treatment, more advanced surgical techniques, and the increasing incidence of HIV infection. However, this was contradicted by a study in an outpatient department in Eastern Croatia, which compared the prevalence of fungal infections between two time periods (1986–1988, 47,832 people; 1997–2001, 75,691 people). It found that the prevalence of fungal infection overall had increased greatly over the 10 years, but the percentage of fungal infections affecting the nail had decreased by 1% (fungal infections overall: 0.26% in 1986–1988 v 0.73% in 1997–2001; nail: 10.31% in 1986–1988 v 9.31% in 1997–2001).

AETIOLOGY/RISK FACTORS Fungal nail infections are most commonly caused by anthropophilic fungi called dermatophytes. The genera *Trichophyton*, *Epidermophyton*, and *Microsporum* are typically involved, specifically *T rubrum*, *T mentagrophytes* var *interdigitale*, and *E floccosum*. Other fungi, moulds, or yeasts may be isolated, such as *Scopulariopsis brevicaulis*, *Aspergillus*, *Fusarium*, and *Candida albicans*. *T rubrum* is now regarded as the most common cause of onychomycosis in the world. Several factors that increase the risk of developing a fungal nail infection have been identified. One survey found that 26% of people with diabetes had onychomycosis and that diabetes increased the risk of infection, but the type and severity of diabetes was not correlated with infection (OR 2.77, 95% CI 2.15 to 3.57). Another survey found that PVD (OR 1.78, 95% CI 1.68 to 1.88) and immunosuppression (OR 1.19, 95% CI 1.01 to 1.40) increased the risk of infection. These factors may explain the general increase in prevalence of onychomycosis in the elderly population. Environmental exposures, such as occlusive footwear or warm, damp conditions, have been cited as risk factors, as has trauma. Fungal skin infection has been

(continued over)

(from previous page)

proposed as a risk factor. However, one large observational study, which included 5413 people with positive mycology, found that only a small proportion (21.3%) had both skin and toenail infections.

PROGNOSIS Onychomycosis does not have serious consequences in otherwise healthy people. However, the Achilles project (846 people with fungal toenail infection) found that many people complain of discomfort in walking (51%), pain (33%), or limitation of their work or other activities (13%). Gross distortion and dystrophy of the nail may cause trauma to the adjacent skin, and may lead to secondary bacterial infection. In immunocompromised people, there is a risk that this infection will disseminate. Quality-of-life measures that are specific to onychomycosis have recently been developed. Studies using these indicators suggest that onychomycosis has negative physical and psychosocial effects.

Ian Burgess

KEY POINTS

- Head lice can only be diagnosed by finding live lice, as eggs take 7 days to hatch and may appear viable for weeks after death of the egg.

  Infestation may be more likely in school children, with risks increased in children with more siblings, longer hair, and of lower socioeconomic group.

- Malathion lotion may increase lice eradication compared with phenothrin or permethrin. Current best practice is to treat with two applications 7 days apart, and to check for cure at 14 days.

  Studies comparing malathion or permethrin with wet combing have given conflicting results, possibly because of varying insecticide resistance.

- Permethrin may be more effective at eradicating lice compared with lindane.

  Eradication may be increased by adding co-trimoxazole to topical permethrin, although this increases adverse effects.

- We don't know whether combinations of insecticides are beneficial compared with single agents or other treatments.

- We don't know whether dimeticone or pyrethrum are beneficial compared with other insecticides.

- CAUTION: Lindane has been associated with central nervous system toxicity.

- We don't know whether herbal and essential oils eradicate lice compared with other treatments.

ⓘ **Please visit www.clinicalevidence.bmj.com for full text and references**

What are the effects of treatments for head lice?	
Likely To Be Beneficial	• Malathion • Permethrin
Trade-off Between Benefits And Harms	• Oral co-trimoxazole (trimethoprim plus sulfamethoxazole)
Unknown Effectiveness	• Combinations of insecticides • Dimeticone • Herbal and essential oils • Lindane • Mechanical removal of lice or viable eggs by combing • Phenothrin • Pyrethrum

Search date October 2006

DEFINITION Head lice are obligate ectoparasites of socially active humans. They infest the scalp and attach their eggs to the hair shafts. Itching, resulting from multiple bites, is not diagnostic but may increase the index of suspicion. Eggs glued to hairs, whether hatched (nits) or unhatched, are not proof of active infection, because eggs may retain a viable appearance for weeks after death. A conclusive diagnosis can only be made by finding live lice. One observational study compared two groups of children with louse eggs but no lice

(continued over)

(from previous page)

at initial assessment. Over 14 days, more children with five or more eggs within 6 mm of the scalp developed infestations compared with those with fewer than five eggs. Adequate follow-up examinations using detection combing are more likely to be productive than nit removal to prevent reinfestation. Infestations are not self-limiting.

INCIDENCE/PREVALENCE We found no studies on incidence and few recently published studies of prevalence in resource-rich countries. Anecdotal reports suggest that prevalence has increased in the past few years in most communities in Europe, the Americas, and Australasia. A recent cross-sectional study from Belgium (6169 children, aged 2.5–12.0 years) found a prevalence of 8.9%. An earlier pilot study (677 children, aged 3–11 years) showed that in individual schools the prevalence was as high as 19.5%. One cross-sectional study from Belgium found that head lice were significantly more common in children from families with lower socioeconomic status (OR 1.25, 95% CI 1.04 to 1.47); in children with more siblings (OR 1.2, 95% CI 1.1 to 1.3); and in children with longer hair (OR 1.20, 95% CI 1.02 to 1.43), although hair length may influence the ability to detect infestation. The socioeconomic status of the family was also a significant influence on the ability to treat infestations successfully; the lower the socioeconomic status the greater the risk of treatment failure (OR 1.70, 95% CI 1.05 to 2.70).

AETIOLOGY/RISK FACTORS Observational studies indicate that infestations occur most frequently in school children, although there is no evidence of a link with school attendance. We found no evidence that lice prefer clean hair to dirty hair.

PROGNOSIS The infestation is almost harmless. Sensitisation reactions to louse saliva and faeces may result in localised irritation and erythema. Secondary infection of scratches may occur. Lice have been identified as primary mechanical vectors of scalp pyoderma caused by streptococci and staphylococci usually found on the skin.

Graham Worrall

KEY POINTS

- HSV-1 infection usually causes a mild, self-limiting, painful blistering around the mouth, with 20-40% of adults affected at some time.

  Primary infection usually occurs in childhood, after which the virus is thought to remain latent in the trigeminal ganglion.

  Recurrence may be triggered by factors such as exposure to bright light, stress, and fatigue.

- Oral antiviral agents such as aciclovir may reduce the duration of pain and time to healing for a first attack of herpes labialis compared with placebo, but we don't know for sure.

  We don't know whether topical antiviral agents can reduce pain or time to healing in a first attack.

- Prophylactic oral antiviral agents may reduce the frequency and severity of attacks compared with placebo, but we don't know the best timing and duration of treatment.

  We don't know whether topical antiviral treatments are beneficial as prophylaxis against recurrent attacks.

  Ultraviolet sunscreen may reduce recurrent attacks, but we don't know for sure.

- Oral and topical antiviral agents may reduce the duration of pain and the time to heal in recurrent attacks of herpes labialis.

  Oral aciclovir and valaciclovir may marginally reduce healing time if taken early in a recurrent attack, but valaciclovir may cause headache.

  A 1-day course of valaciclovir may be as effective as a 2-day course.

  Topical aciclovir and penciclovir slightly reduce healing time, and penciclovir may reduce duration of pain, compared with placebo.

- We don't know whether topical anaesthetic agents or zinc oxide cream reduce healing time. Zinc oxide cream may increase skin irritation.

(i) **Please visit www.clinicalevidence.bmj.com for full text and references**

What are the effects of antiviral treatments for the first attack of herpes labialis?

Likely To Be Beneficial	• Oral antiviral agents (aciclovir)
Unknown Effectiveness	• Topical antiviral agents

What are the effects of interventions aimed at preventing recurrent attacks of herpes labialis?

Likely To Be Beneficial	• Oral antiviral agents (aciclovir)
	• Sunscreen
Unknown Effectiveness	• Topical antiviral agents

What are the effects of treatments for recurrent attacks of herpes labialis?

Likely To Be Beneficial	• Oral antiviral agents (aciclovir and valaciclovir)
Unknown Effectiveness	• Topical anaesthetic agents • Topical antiviral agents (slightly reduced healing time with aciclovir or penciclovir and limited effect on duration of pain) • Zinc oxide cream

Search date April 2006

DEFINITION Herpes labialis is a mild, self-limiting infection with HSV-1. It causes pain and blistering on the lips and perioral area (cold sores); fever and constitutional symptoms are rare. Most people have no warning of an attack, but some experience a recognisable prodrome.

INCIDENCE/PREVALENCE Herpes labialis accounts for about 1% of primary care consultations in the UK each year; 20–40% of people have experienced cold sores at some time.

AETIOLOGY/RISK FACTORS Herpes labialis is caused by HSV-1. After the primary infection, which usually occurs in childhood, the virus is thought to remain latent in the trigeminal ganglion. A variety of factors, including exposure to bright sunlight, fatigue, or psychological stress, can precipitate a recurrence.

PROGNOSIS In most people, herpes labialis is a mild, self-limiting illness. Recurrences are usually shorter and less severe than the initial attack. Healing is usually complete in 7–10 days without scarring. Rates of reactivation are unknown. Herpes labialis can cause serious illness in immunocompromised people.

James Larkin and Martin Gore

KEY POINTS

- There are 8100 new cases of malignant melanoma and 1800 deaths a year in the UK, largely as a result of metastatic disease.

  The median survival of people with metastatic melanoma is 6–9 months after diagnosis, with 10% of people alive at 5 years.

  Chemotherapy is given with palliative rather than curative intent for metastatic disease.

- Consensus is that it is reasonable to give chemotherapy to people with metastatic melanoma.

  Chemotherapy for metastatic melanoma has been associated with serious adverse effects. However, these tend to be manageable, and it is reasonable to give chemotherapy to people with metastatic melanoma, although there are no good-quality studies to support this view, and only a small proportion of people may benefit.

- Dacarbazine or temozolomide are the standard first-line chemotherapy.

  Both dacarbazine and temozolomide are associated with similar progression-free survival and fewer adverse effects compared with other single-agent or combined chemotherapy.

  Combined chemotherapy is no more effective at increasing overall survival compared with single-agent chemotherapy. Combined chemotherapy is associated with more adverse effects compared with single-agent chemotherapy.

- Immunotherapy (interferon alfa or interferon alfa plus interleukin-2) is unlikely to increase survival when added to chemotherapy, and is associated with influenza-like symptoms and myelosuppression.

(i) **Please visit www.clinicalevidence.bmj.com for full text and references**

What are the effects of chemotherapy for metastatic melanoma?	
Trade-off Between Benefits And Harms	• Chemotherapy plus supportive palliative care versus supportive palliative care alone* • Dacarbazine or temozolomide (both associated with similar progression-free survival and fewer adverse effects compared with other single-agent or combined chemotherapy)
Unlikely To Be Beneficial	• Combined chemotherapy (no more effective at increasing overall survival than single-agent and associated with serious adverse effects)

What are the effects of immunotherapy for metastatic melanoma?	
Unlikely To Be Beneficial	• Adding interferon alfa plus interleukin-2 to chemotherapy (increased adverse effects and no benefit in overall survival compared with chemotherapy alone)

> • Adding interferon alfa to chemotherapy (increased adverse effects and no benefit in overall survival compared with chemotherapy alone)

Search date September 2006

*Categorisation based on consensus.

DEFINITION Malignant melanoma is a tumour derived from melanocytes in the basal layer of the epidermis. The systemic treatment of malignant melanoma with distant metastases is reviewed here. For the purposes of this review, we will cover only cutaneous melanoma with distant metastases. Non-metastatic malignant melanoma is covered in a separate review (see malignant melanoma [non-metastatic], p 547).

INCIDENCE/PREVALENCE There are 8100 new cases of malignant melanoma and 1800 deaths a year in the UK. Malignant melanoma accounts for 10% of all skin cancers and is the primary cause of death from skin cancer. It occurs more frequently on exposed skin, such as the backs of men, and the lower legs of women.

AETIOLOGY/RISK FACTORS Environmental factors such as exposure to ultraviolet light (especially episodes of severe sunburn in childhood), and genetic factors such as a family history of the disease are known to be risk factors for the development of melanoma. In addition, skin colour and the number of moles a person has correlate closely with the risk of developing malignant melanoma.

PROGNOSIS The median survival of people with metastatic melanoma is 6–9 months after diagnosis, with 10% of people alive at 5 years. Chemotherapy is given with palliative rather than curative intent in metastatic disease.

Philip Savage

KEY POINTS

- The incidence of malignant melanoma has increased over the past 25 years in the UK, but death rates have remained fairly constant. Five-year survival ranges from 20–95% depending on disease stage.

  Risks are greater in white populations and in people with higher numbers of skin naevi.

  Prognosis depends on depth of tumour, ulceration, and number of lymph nodes involved. Survival may be better in women compared with men, and for lesions on the limbs compared with the trunk.

  Lesions can recur after 5–10 years, so long-term surveillance may be required.

- Sunscreens have not been shown to reduce the risk of malignant melanoma, but sunscreen use does not necessarily correlate with reduced total ultraviolet light exposure.

- Wide (3 cm) excision of lesions leads to reduced local recurrence compared with narrow (1 cm) excision in people with tumours greater than 2 mm Breslow thickness.

  Wide (3–5 cm) excision is unlikely to be more beneficial than narrow (1–2 cm) excision in people with tumours of less than 2 mm Breslow thickness, and may increase the need for skin grafts.

- Elective lymph-node dissection is unlikely to increase survival in people without clinically detectable lymph-node metastases.

  We don't know whether sentinel lymph-node biopsy is beneficial.

- We don't know whether adjuvant treatment with vaccines, high-dose interferon alfa, or surveillance for early treatment of recurrence improve survival.

  Low- and intermediate-dose interferon are unlikely to improve relapse rates or survival compared with no adjuvant treatment.

  High-dose interferon alfa may increase the time until relapse compared with no adjuvant treatment, but overall survival seems to be unchanged.

  Severe adverse effects occur in 10–75% of people receiving interferon alfa treatment.

(i) **Please visit www.clinicalevidence.bmj.com for full text and references**

What are the effects of interventions to prevent malignant melanoma?

Unknown Effectiveness	• Sunscreens

Is there an optimal surgical margin for the primary excision of melanoma?

Likely To Be Beneficial	• Wide (3 cm) excision in tumours greater than 2 mm Breslow depth (less local recurrence than narrow 1 cm excision)
Unlikely To Be Beneficial	• Wide (3–5 cm) excision in tumours less than 2 mm Breslow depth (no better than narrow 1–2 cm excision)

What are the effects of elective lymph-node dissection in people with malignant melanoma with clinically uninvolved lymph nodes?	
Unlikely To Be Beneficial	• Elective lymph-node dissection

What are the effects of sentinel lymph-node biopsy in people with malignant melanoma with clinically uninvolved lymph nodes?	
Unknown Effectiveness	• Sentinel lymph-node biopsy

What are the effects of adjuvant treatment for malignant melanoma?	
Unknown Effectiveness	• Adjuvant vaccines in people with malignant melanoma • High-dose adjuvant interferon alfa • Surveillance for early treatment of recurrence
Unlikely To Be Beneficial	• Low- and intermediate-dose adjuvant interferon alfa

Search date October 2006

DEFINITION Malignant melanoma is a tumour derived from melanocytes in the basal layer of the epidermis. After malignant transformation, the cancer cells become invasive and penetrate into and beyond the dermis. Malignant melanoma is described by stages (I–IV), which relate to the depth of dermal invasion and the presence of ulceration. Metastatic spread can occur to the regional lymph nodes or to distant sites, particularly the lungs, liver, and central nervous system.

INCIDENCE/PREVALENCE The incidence of melanoma varies widely in different populations and is about 10–20 times higher in white than non-white populations. Estimates suggest that the number of cases of melanoma in the UK has increased about fourfold over the past 25 years. Despite this rising incidence, death rates have changed more modestly, and in some populations are now beginning to fall. The increased early diagnosis of thin, good prognosis melanoma and melanoma *in situ* are the main reasons for the divergent findings on incidence and death rates.

AETIOLOGY/RISK FACTORS The risk factors for the development of melanoma can be divided into genetic and environmental. Alongside the genetic risk factors of skin type and hair colour, the number of naevi a person has correlates closely with the risk of developing malignant melanoma. Although the risk of developing malignant melanoma is higher in fair-skinned populations living in areas of high sun exposure, the exact relationship between sun exposure, sunscreen use, skin type, and risk is not clear. High total lifetime exposure to excessive sunlight, and episodes of severe sunburn in childhood, are both associated with an increased risk of developing malignant melanoma in adult life. However, people do not necessarily develop malignancy at the sites of maximum exposure to the sun.

PROGNOSIS The prognosis of early-stage malignant melanoma, which is clinically limited to the primary skin site (stages I–II), is predominantly related to the depth of dermal invasion and the presence of ulceration. In stage III disease, where disease is present in the regional lymph nodes, the prognosis becomes worse with the increasing number of nodes involved. For example, a person with a thin lesion (Breslow thickness below 1.0 mm) without lymph node involvement has a 95% chance of surviving 5 years. However, if the regional lymph nodes are macroscopically involved, the overall survival at 5 years is only 20–50%. In addition to tumour thickness and lymph node involvement, several studies have shown a better prognosis in women and in people with lesions on the limbs compared with those with lesions on the trunk. Lesions can recur after after 5–10 years, so long-term surveillance may be required.

Psoriasis (chronic plaque)

Luigi Naldi and Berthold Rzany

KEY POINTS

- Psoriasis affects 1–3% of the population, in some people causing changes to the nails and joints in addition to skin lesions.

- We don't know whether treatments that might affect possible triggers, such as acupuncture, balneotherapy, fish oil supplementation, or psychotherapy, improve symptoms of psoriasis, as few studies have been found.

- There is consensus that topical emollients and salicylic acid are effective as initial and adjunctive treatment for people with chronic plaque psoriasis, but we don't know whether tars are effective.

  Dithranol may improve lesions compared with placebo, but it may be less effective than topical vitamin D derivatives such as calcipotriol.

  Topical potent corticosteroids may improve psoriasis compared with placebo, and efficacy may be increased by adding tazarotene, oral retinoids, or vitamin D and derivatives, or by wrapping in occlusive dressings.

  We don't know whether tars are more effective than placebo, ultraviolet light, or vitamin D derivatives in people with chronic plaque psoriasis.

- CAUTION: Tazarotene, vitamin D and derivatives, and oral retinoids are potentially teratogenic, and are contraindicated in women who may be pregnant.

- PUVA, heliotherapy, and ultraviolet B may improve lesions and reduce relapse, but increase the risk of photoaging, and of skin cancer.

- There is consensus that heliotherapy and ultraviolet B are beneficial.

- Methotrexate and ciclosporin seem to have similar efficacy at clearing lesions and maintaining remission, but both can cause serious adverse effects.

- Oral retinoids may improve clearance of lesions, alone or with ultraviolet light, but may be less effective than ciclosporin.

- Cytokine inhibitors (etanercept and infliximab) and T-cell-targeted therapies (alefacept, efalizumab) may improve lesions, but long-term effects are unknown.

- We don't know whether leflunomide improves psoriasis.

- The Ingram regimen is considered to be effective, but we don't know whether Goeckerman treatment or other combined treatments are beneficial.

ⓘ **Please visit www.clinicalevidence.bmj.com for full text and references**

What are the effects of non-drug treatments (other than ultraviolet light) for chronic plaque psoriasis?

Unknown Effectiveness	• Acupuncture
	• Balneotherapy
	• Fish oil supplementation
	• Psychotherapy

What are the effects of topical drug treatments for chronic plaque psoriasis?

Beneficial	• Tazarotene
	• Vitamin D derivatives (topical)
Likely To Be Beneficial	• Dithranol
	• Emollients*
	• Keratolytics (salicylic acid, urea) (as an adjunct to other treatments)*
Trade-off Between Benefits And Harms	• Corticosteroids (topical)
Unknown Effectiveness	• Tars

What are the effects of ultraviolet light treatments for chronic plaque psoriasis?

Likely To Be Beneficial	• Heliotherapy*
	• PUVA*
	• Ultraviolet B*
Unknown Effectiveness	• Phototherapy plus balneotherapy
	• Ultraviolet A

What are the effects of systemic drug treatments for chronic plaque psoriasis?

Trade-off Between Benefits And Harms	• Alefacept
	• Ciclosporin
	• Efalizumab
	• Etanercept
	• Fumaric acid derivatives
	• Infliximab
	• Methotrexate
	• Retinoids (oral etretinate, acitretin)
Unknown Effectiveness	• Leflunomide
	• Pimecrolimus (oral)

What are the effects of combined treatment with drugs plus ultraviolet light on chronic plaque psoriasis?

| Likely To Be Beneficial | • Ingram regimen* |
| **Trade-off Between Benefits And Harms** | • Adding oral retinoids to PUVA |

	• Ultraviolet B plus oral retinoids (combination better than either treatment alone)
Unknown Effectiveness	• Adding calcipotriol (topical) to PUVA or PUVB • Goeckerman treatment • Ultraviolet B light plus emollients

What are the effects of combined systemic plus topical drug treatments for chronic plaque psoriasis?

Trade-off Between Benefits And Harms	• Retinoids (oral) plus topical corticosteroids (more effective than either treatment alone)
Unknown Effectiveness	• Systemic drug treatment plus topical vitamin D derivatives

Search date July 2006

*Based on consensus.

DEFINITION Chronic plaque psoriasis, or psoriasis vulgaris, is a chronic inflammatory skin disease characterised by well demarcated erythematous scaly plaques on the extensor surfaces of the body and scalp. The lesions may occasionally itch or sting, and may bleed when injured. Dystrophic nail changes or nail pitting are found in more than a third of people with chronic plaque psoriasis, and psoriatic arthropathy occurs in 1% to more than 10%. The condition waxes and wanes, with wide variations in course and severity among individuals. Other varieties of psoriasis include guttate, inverse, pustular, and erythrodermic psoriasis. This review deals only with treatments for chronic plaque psoriasis and does not cover nail involvement or scalp psoriasis.

INCIDENCE/PREVALENCE Psoriasis affects 1–3% of the general population. It is believed to be less frequent in people from Africa and Asia, but we found no reliable epidemiological data to support this.

AETIOLOGY/RISK FACTORS About a third of people with psoriasis have a family history of the disease, but physical trauma, acute infection, and some medications (e.g. lithium and beta-blockers) are believed to trigger the condition. A few observational studies have linked the onset or relapse of psoriasis with stressful life events, and personal habits, including cigarette smoking and, less consistently, alcohol consumption. Others have found an association between psoriasis and BMI, and with a diet low in fruit and vegetables.

PROGNOSIS We found no long-term prognostic studies. With the exceptions of erythrodermic and acute generalised pustular psoriasis (severe conditions which affect less than 1% of people with psoriasis and require intensive hospital care), psoriasis is not known to affect mortality. Psoriasis may substantially affect quality of life, by influencing a negative body image and self-image, and limiting daily activities, social contacts, and work. One systematic review (search date 2000, 17 cohort studies) suggested that severe psoriasis may be associated with lower levels of quality of life than mild psoriasis. At present, there is no cure for psoriasis. However, in many people it can be well controlled with treatment, at least in the short term.

Paul Johnstone and Mark Strong

KEY POINTS

- Scabies is an infestation of the skin by the mite *Sarcoptes scabiei*. In adults, the most common sites of infestation are the fingers and the wrists, although infection may manifest in elderly people as a diffuse truncal eruption.

  Scabies is a common public health problem, with an estimated prevalence of 300 million cases worldwide, the majority of which are in resource-poor countries.

- Permethrin is highly effective at increasing clinical and parasitic cure of scabies within 28 days.

  Lindane is also effective in treating scabies, although it has now been withdrawn from the UK market.

  Both lindane and permethrin may be more likely to be related to rare severe adverse effects, such as convulsions or death, than other treatments such as benzyl benzoate, crotamiton, or malathion.

- Crotamiton successfully produces clinical or parasitic cure after 28 days, although it is less effective than permethrin.

- We found insufficient evidence to judge the effectiveness of benzyl benzoate, malathion, or sulphur compounds for treating scabies.

- As a systemic treatment, oral ivermectin appears to be beneficial in increasing clinical cure rates compared with placebo.

  Oral ivermectin may be effective when included in the treatment of hyperkeratotic crusted scabies and in people with concomitant HIV disease.

(i) **Please visit www.clinicalevidence.bmj.com for full text and references**

What are the effects of topical treatments for scabies?	
Beneficial	• Crotamiton (as effective as lindane but less effective than permethrin) • Permethrin
Trade-off Between Benefits And Harms	• Lindane
Unknown Effectiveness	• Benzyl benzoate • Malathion • Sulphur compounds

What are the effects of systemic treatments for scabies?	
Likely To Be Beneficial	• Oral ivermectin

Search date March 2006

DEFINITION Scabies is an infestation of the skin by the mite *Sarcoptes scabiei*. Typical sites of infestation are skin folds and flexor surfaces. In adults, the most common sites are between the fingers and on the wrists, although infection may manifest in elderly people as

(continued over)

(from previous page)

a diffuse truncal eruption. In infants and children, the face, scalp, palms, and soles are also often affected. Infection with the scabies mite causes discomfort and intense itching of the skin, particularly at night, with irritating papular or vesicular eruptions. The discomfort and itching can be especially debilitating among immunocompromised people, such as those with HIV/AIDS.

INCIDENCE/PREVALENCE Scabies is a common public health problem with an estimated prevalence of 300 million cases worldwide, mostly affecting people in resource-poor countries, where prevalence can exceed 50%. In industrialised countries it is most common in institutionalised communities. Case studies suggest that epidemic cycles occur every 7–15 years, and that these partly reflect the population's immune status.

AETIOLOGY/RISK FACTORS Scabies is particularly common where there is social disruption, overcrowding with close body contact, and limited access to water. Young children, immobilised elderly people, people with HIV/AIDS, and other medically and immunologically compromised people are predisposed to infestation and have particularly high mite counts.

PROGNOSIS Scabies is not life threatening, but the severe, persistent itch and secondary infections may be debilitating. Occasionally, crusted scabies develops. This form of the disease is resistant to routine treatment and can be a source of continued reinfestation and spread to others.

Seborrhoeic dermatitis | 557

Juan Jorge Manriquez and Pablo Uribe

KEY POINTS

- Seborrhoeic dermatitis affects at least 1–3% of the population and causes red patches with greasy scales on the face, chest, skin flexures, and scalp.

  The cause of seborrhoeic dermatitis is unknown. *Malassezia* yeasts are considered to have an important role producing an inflammatory reaction involving T cells and complement.

  Known risk factors include immunodeficiency, neurological or cardiac disease, and alcoholic pancreatitis. In this review, however, we deal with treatment in immunocompetent adults who have no known predisposing conditions.

  Seborrhoeic dermatitis tends to relapse after treatment.

- In adults with seborrhoeic dermatitis of the scalp, antifungal preparations containing ketoconazole improve symptoms compared with placebo.

  Bifonazole and selenium sulphide are also likely to be effective, but we don't know whether terbinafine is beneficial as no studies have been found.

  There is consensus that topical corticosteroids are effective in treating seborrhoeic dermatitis of the scalp in adults, although no studies have been found.

  Tar shampoo may reduce scalp dandruff and redness compared with placebo.

- In adults with seborrhoeic dermatitis of the face and body, short courses of topical corticosteroids are considered to be effective if used episodically, although no studies have been found that assessed this.

  Ketoconazole cream or gel and bifonazole cream may improve skin symptoms compared with placebo.

  We don't know whether terbinafine or selenium sulphide are also beneficial as no studies have been found.

  We don't know whether emollients or topical lithium succinate improve lesions compared with no treatment.

(i) **Please visit www.clinicalevidence.bmj.com for full text and references**

What are the effects of topical treatments for seborrhoeic dermatitis of the scalp in adults?

Beneficial	• Ketoconazole
Likely To Be Beneficial	• Bifonazole
	• Corticosteroids (topical) (hydrocortisone, betamethasone valerate, clobetasone butyrate, mometasone furoate, clobetasol propionate)*
	• Selenium sulphide
	• Tar shampoo
Unknown Effectiveness	• Terbinafine

What are the effects of topical treatments for seborrhoeic dermatitis of the face and body in adults?	
Beneficial	• Ketoconazole
Likely To Be Beneficial	• Bifonazole • Corticosteroids (topical) (hydrocortisone, betamethasone valerate, clobetasone butyrate, mometasone furoate, clobetasol propionate; short-term episodic treatment in adults)*
Unknown Effectiveness	• Emollients • Lithium succinate • Selenium sulphide • Terbinafine

Search date February 2007

*Based on consensus.

DEFINITION Seborrhoeic dermatitis occurs in areas of the skin with a rich supply of sebaceous glands, and manifests as red, sharply marginated lesions with greasy looking scales. On the face it mainly affects the medial aspect of the eyebrows, the area between the eyebrows, and the nasolabial folds. It may also affect the skin on the chest (commonly presternal) and the flexures. On the scalp it manifests as dry, flaking desquamation (dandruff) or yellow, greasy scaling with erythema. Dandruff is a lay term commonly used in the context of mild seborrhoeic dermatitis of the scalp. However, any scalp condition that produces scales could be labelled as dandruff. There is also an infantile variant, commonly affecting the scalp, flexures, and genital area, but this infantile variant seems to have a different pathogenesis than adult seborrhoeic dermatitis. Common differential diagnoses for seborrhoeic dermatitis of the scalp are psoriasis, eczema (see review on atopic eczema, p 532), and tinea capitis.

INCIDENCE/PREVALENCE Seborrhoeic dermatitis is estimated to affect around 1–3% of the general population. However, this is likely to be an underestimate because people do not tend to seek medical advice for mild dandruff.

AETIOLOGY/RISK FACTORS The cause of seborrhoeic dermatitis is unknown and seems to be a multifactorial disease. *Malassezia* yeasts, a genus classified in seven species, are considered to have an important role in seborrhoeic dermatitis producing an inflammatory reaction involving T cells and complement. Conditions that have been reported to predispose to seborrhoeic dermatitis include HIV, neurological conditions such as Parkinson's disease, neuronal damage such as facial nerve palsy, spinal injury, ischaemic heart disease, and alcoholic pancreatitis. In this review, we deal with treatment in immunocompetent adults who have no known predisposing conditions.

PROGNOSIS Seborrhoeic dermatitis is a chronic condition that tends to flare and remit spontaneously, and is prone to recurrence after treatment.

Squamous cell carcinoma of the skin (non-metastatic) | 559

Adèle Green and Alvin H Chong.

KEY POINTS

- Cutaneous squamous cell carcinoma is a malignant tumour of keratinocytes arising in the epidermis, with histological evidence of dermal invasion.

  Incidence varies by country and skin colour, and is as high as 1/100 in white residents of tropical Australia.

  People with fair skin colour who sunburn easily without tanning, people with xeroderma pigmentosum, and people who are immunosuppressed are most susceptible to squamous cell carcinoma.

- Daily use of sunscreen to the head, neck, arms, and hands seems to reduce the incidence of squamous cell carcinoma more than discretionary use.

  Daily sunscreen to the head, neck, arms, and hands also seems to reduce the rate of acquisition of solar keratoses more than discretionary use, and to reduce the incidence of new solar keratoses in people who had previous solar keratoses.

- With regard to surgery, we found no evidence to assess the optimal primary excision margin required to prevent recurrence of squamous cell carcinoma.

  We also found no evidence examining whether micrographically controlled surgery is more beneficial than primary excision, although it is generally considered more tissue sparing because of its specificity in determining the amount of normal surrounding tissue removed.

- We do not know whether radiotherapy after surgery reduces local recurrence compared with surgery alone.

Please visit www.clinicalevidence.bmj.com for full text and references

Does the use of sunscreen help to prevent cutaneous squamous cell carcinoma?	
Likely To Be Beneficial	• Daily use of sunscreens in preventing development of new solar keratoses • Daily use of sunscreens in prevention of squamous cell carcinoma

What is the optimal margin for primary excision of cutaneous squamous cell carcinoma?	
Unknown Effectiveness	• Optimal primary excision margin

Does micrographically controlled surgery result in lower rates of local recurrence than standard primary excision?	
Unknown Effectiveness	• Micrographically controlled surgery versus primary excision

Does radiotherapy after surgery affect local recurrence of cutaneous squamous cell carcinoma?	
Unknown Effectiveness	• Radiotherapy after surgery (compared with surgery alone)

Search date January 2007

DEFINITION Cutaneous squamous cell carcinoma is a malignant tumour of keratinocytes arising in the epidermis, showing histological evidence of dermal invasion.

INCIDENCE/PREVALENCE Incidence rates are often derived from surveys, because few cancer registries routinely collect notifications of squamous cell carcinoma of the skin. Incidence rates on exposed skin vary markedly around the world according to skin colour and latitude, and range from negligible rates in black populations and in white populations living at high latitudes, to rates of about 1/100 in white residents of tropical Australia.

AETIOLOGY/RISK FACTORS People with fair skin colour who sunburn easily without tanning, people with xeroderma pigmentosum, and those who are immunosuppressed are susceptible to squamous cell carcinoma. The strongest environmental risk factor for squamous cell carcinoma is chronic sun exposure. Cohort and case control studies have found that the risk of squamous cell carcinoma is three times greater in people with fair skin colour, a propensity to burn on initial exposure to sunlight, or a history of multiple sunburns. Clinical signs of chronic skin damage, especially solar keratoses, are also risk factors for cutaneous squamous cell carcinoma. In people with multiple solar keratoses (greater than 15), the risk of squamous cell carcinoma is 10–15 times greater than in people with no solar keratoses.

PROGNOSIS Prognosis is related to the location and size of tumour, histological pattern, depth of invasion, perineural involvement, and immunosuppression. A worldwide review of 95 case series, each consisting of at least 20 people, found that the overall metastasis rate for squamous cell carcinoma on the ear was 11% and on the lip 14%, compared with an average for all sites of 5%. A review of 71 case series found that lesions less than 2 cm in diameter have less than half the local recurrence rate compared with lesions greater than 2 cm (7% v 15%), and less than a third of the rate of metastasis (9% v 30%).

Rubeta Matin

KEY POINTS

- Vitiligo is an acquired skin disorder characterised by white (depigmented) patches in the skin, due to the loss of functioning melanocytes.

  Vitiligo patches can appear anywhere on the skin, but common sites are usually around the orifices, the genitals, or sun-exposed areas such as the face and hands.

  The extent and distribution of vitiligo often changes during the course of a person's lifetime, and its progression is unpredictable.

- Limited courses of potent topical corticosteroids are a safe and effective therapy for localised vitiligo, and are often the first-choice treatment for this.

  The consensus is that adverse effects of oral corticosteroids outweigh the benefits in vitiligo. There is currently insufficient evidence available to assess their effectiveness.

- Narrowband UVB is considered a safe and effective therapy for moderate to severe generalised vitiligo and is often the first-choice treatment for this.

- Tacrolimus requires further evaluation but is well tolerated in children and adults without the long-term adverse effects of topical corticosteroids.

  There is currently insufficient evidence available to assess other immunomodulators in vitiligo.

- Vitiligo patches in certain body areas, like acral, palms and soles, lips, mucosa, nipple, and segmental forms in any area are relatively resistant to all conventional treatment modalities.

  In these cases counselling and cosmetic camouflage become a priority, and often no therapies are advocated.

- There is insufficient evidence to assess topical vitamin D analogues, levamisole, and broadband UVB in vitiligo.

- General consensus is that oral PUVA is effective for the treatment of vitiligo in adults, whereas topical PUVA is unlikely to be effective. However, topical PUVA has fewer adverse effects than oral PUVA. PUVA is likely to be harmful in children.

Please visit www.clinicalevidence.bmj.com for full text and references

What are the effects of medical treatments for vitiligo in adults?	
Beneficial	• Corticosteroids (topical)
Unknown Effectiveness	• Immunomodulators (topical)
	• Levamisole (oral)
	• Vitamin D analogues (topical)
Likely To Be Ineffective Or Harmful	• Corticosteroids (oral)*

What are the effects of ultraviolet light treatments for vitiligo in adults?

Likely To Be Beneficial	• Oral PUVA* • Ultraviolet B (narrowband)
Unknown Effectiveness	• Ultraviolet B (broadband)
Unlikely To Be Beneficial	• Topical PUVA

What are the effects of medical treatments for vitiligo in children?

Beneficial	• Corticosteroids (topical)
Likely To Be Beneficial	• Immunomodulators (topical)
Unknown Effectiveness	• Vitamin D analogues (topical)
Likely To Be Ineffective Or Harmful	• Corticosteroids (oral)*

What are the effects of ultraviolet light treatments for vitiligo in children?

Likely To Be Beneficial	• Ultraviolet B (narrowband)*
Likely To Be Ineffective Or Harmful	• Oral or topical PUVA*

Search date March 2006

*Categorisation based on consensus.

DEFINITION Vitiligo is an acquired skin disorder characterised by white (depigmented) patches in the skin, due to the loss of functioning melanocytes. The hair and, rarely, the eyes may also lose colour. Vitiligo patches can appear anywhere on the skin, but common sites are usually around the orifices, the genitals, or sun-exposed areas such as the face and hands. The disease is classified according to its extent and distribution, and can be subdivided into generalised or localised. In practice, there is considerable overlap between these types, and people often have vitiligo that cannot be categorised or will change during the course of their lifetime. Therefore, for the purposes of this review, we have included all people diagnosed with vitiligo of any type. Children were defined as people aged 15 years and below.

INCIDENCE/PREVALENCE Vitiligo is estimated to affect 1% of the world population, regardless of age, gender, and skin colour. Anyone of any age can develop vitiligo, but it is rarely reported to be present at birth. In a Dutch study, 50% of people reported that the disease appeared before the age of 20 years.

AETIOLOGY/RISK FACTORS The aetiology of vitiligo is uncertain, although genetic, immunological, and neurogenic factors seem to play a role. In about a third of people affected, there is a family history of vitiligo, but there are few epidemiological studies to confirm this. Current research focuses on finding the genes responsible; however, certain triggers (e.g. trauma to the skin, hormonal changes, and stress) may be necessary for the disease to become apparent. Autoimmune mechanisms are thought to be responsible in the pathogenesis of vitiligo (especially in generalised or focal non-dermatomal vitiligo). This is supported by an increased incidence of antibodies found in people with vitiligo. Furthermore, vitiligo is often associated with autoimmune diseases, such as thyroid diseases, pernicious anaemia, and diabetes mellitus; also, melanocyte antibodies, the incidence of which correlates with disease activity, have been found in people with vitiligo. Involvement of cellular immunity has been considered because T lymphocytes and macrophages in perilesional skin have also been frequently reported. Regarding segmental vitiligo, the neural hypothesis suggests that it is due to an accumulation of a neurochemical substance, which decreases melanin production.

PROGNOSIS Vitiligo is not life threatening, and is mostly asymptomatic (although it does increase the risk of sunburn of the affected areas). The association of vitiligo and skin cancer remains an area of controversy. The occurrence of skin cancer in long-lasting vitiligo is rare, although studies have demonstrated increased PUVA-associated skin cancers. A Swedish study, which followed up people treated with PUVA over 21 years, demonstrated an increased risk of squamous cell carcinomas. Furthermore, the risk of malignant melanoma increases among people treated with PUVA approximately 15 years after the first treatment. The effects of vitiligo can be both cosmetically and psychologically devastating, resulting in low self-esteem and poor body image. The anxieties regarding the disease tend to occur in view of a lack of understanding of the aetiology and unpredictability of the course. **Progression:** The course of generalised vitiligo is unpredictable; lesions may remain stable for years, or, more commonly, may progress while alternating with phases of stabilisation, or, less commonly, slowly progress for several years to cover the entire body surface. In some instances, people may undergo rapid, complete depigmentation within 1 or 2 years. In segmental vitiligo, lesions tend to spread rapidly at onset and show a more stable course thereafter. **Predicting treatment responsiveness:** There are certain disease characteristics that help to predict the outcome of therapy. Besides age, duration of disease, localisation, and extent of depigmentation, current disease activity should also be taken into consideration during clinical decision making. This is essential in people with vitiligo vulgaris, when the disease activity may fluctuate at a given time. Medical therapies and ultraviolet light treatments may be equally effective in active and stable disease, but this may not be true for other treatments (e.g. surgery). An associated skin manifestation is the phenomenon of "koebnerization", which plays an important role in the appearance of new lesions in vitiligo. It occurs in most people with vitiligo. This knowledge is important, because elimination of frictional trauma in the form of occlusive garments, wrist bands, and necklaces prevents occurrence of new lesions in the cosmetically important areas in a case of progressive vitiligo. Furthermore, it has been reported that the presence of positive experimentally induced Koebner phenomenon is associated with active disease, but not necessarily more severe disease – that is, in terms of the extent of depigmentation. The presence of Koebner phenomenon may be a valuable clinical factor to assess disease activity, and may predict responsiveness to certain treatments. A case series reported that people who were Koebner phenomenon positive (induced experimentally) were significantly more responsive to topical fluticasone propionate combined with ultraviolet A therapy, but for narrowband ultraviolet B treatment, there was no difference in response, suggesting that people in active and stable stages of the disease may respond equally well to ultraviolet B.

Nai Ming Luk and Yuk Ming Tang

KEY POINTS

- Warts are caused by HPV, of which there are over 100 types, which probably infects the skin via areas of minimal trauma.

  Risk factors include use of communal showers, occupational handling of meat, and immunosuppression.

  In immunocompetent people, warts are harmless and resolve as a result of natural immunity within months or years.

- Topical salicylic acid increases complete wart clearance compared with placebo.

  Cryotherapy may be as effective at increasing wart clearance as topical salicylic acid, but studies have been small, and have given inconclusive results.

  Photodynamic treatment increases the proportion of warts cured compared with placebo, and may be more effective than cryotherapy, but increases pain or discomfort.

- Contact immunotherapy with dinitrochlorobenzene may increase wart clearance compared with placebo, but can cause inflammation.

  We don't know whether intralesional bleomycin speeds up clearance of warts compared with placebo, as studies have given conflicting results.

  We don't know whether cimetidine, formaldehyde, glutaraldehyde, homeopathy, occlusive treatment with duct tape, pulsed dye laser, surgery, or oral zinc sulphate increase cure rates compared with placebo, as few high-quality studies have been found.

- For what is such a common condition, there are few large high-quality RCTs available to inform clinical practice.

(i) **Please visit www.clinicalevidence.bmj.com for full text and references**

What are the effects of treatments for warts (non-genital)?	
Beneficial	• Salicylic acid (topical)
Likely To Be Beneficial	• Contact immunotherapy (dinitrochlorobenzene) • Cryotherapy (limited evidence that may be as effective as salicylic acid) • Photodynamic treatment
Unknown Effectiveness	• Bleomycin (intralesional) • Cimetidine • Duct-tape occlusion • Formaldehyde • Glutaraldehyde • Homeopathy • Pulsed dye laser • Surgical procedures • Zinc sulphate (oral)

Search date November 2006

DEFINITION Non-genital warts (verrucas) are an extremely common, benign, and usually self-limited skin disease. Infection of epidermal cells with HPV results in cell proliferation and a thickened, warty papule on the skin. There are over 100 different types of HPV. The appearance of warts is determined by the type of virus and the location of the infection. Any area of skin can be infected, but the most common sites are the hands and feet. Genital warts are not covered in this review (see review on genital warts, p 526). **Common warts** are most often seen on the hands and present as skin coloured papules with a rough "verrucous" surface. **Flat warts** are most often seen on the backs of the hands and on the legs. They appear as slightly elevated, small plaques that are skin coloured or light brown. **Plantar warts** occur on the soles of the feet and look like very thick callouses.

INCIDENCE/PREVALENCE There are few reliable, population-based data on the incidence and prevalence of non-genital warts. Prevalence probably varies widely between different age groups, populations, and periods of time. Two large population-based studies found prevalence rates of 0.84% in the USA and 12.9% in Russia. Prevalence is highest in children and young adults, and two studies in school populations have shown prevalence rates of 12% in 4–6 year olds in the UK and 24% in 16–18 year olds in Australia.

AETIOLOGY/RISK FACTORS Warts are caused by HPV, of which there are over 100 different types. They are most common at sites of trauma, such as the hands and feet, and probably result from inoculation of virus into minimally damaged areas of epithelium. Warts on the feet can be acquired from walking barefoot in areas where other people walk barefoot. One observational study (146 adolescents) found that the prevalence of warts on the feet was 27% in those that used a communal shower room and 1.3% in those that used the locker (changing) room. Warts on the hand are also an occupational risk for butchers and meat handlers. One cross-sectional survey (1086 people) found that the prevalence of warts on the hand was 33% in abattoir workers, 34% in retail butchers, 20% in engineering fitters, and 15% in office workers. Immunosuppression is another important risk factor. One observational study in immunosuppressed renal transplant recipients found that, at 5 years or longer after transplantation, 90% had warts.

PROGNOSIS Non-genital warts in immunocompetent people are harmless and usually resolve spontaneously as a result of natural immunity within months or years. The rate of resolution is highly variable and probably depends on several factors, including host immunity, age, HPV type, and site of infection. One cohort study (1000 children in long-stay accommodation) found that two thirds of warts resolved without treatment within a 2-year period. One systematic review (search date 2000, 17 RCTs) comparing local treatments versus placebo found that about 30% of people using placebo (range 0–73%) had no warts after about 10 weeks (range 4–24 weeks).

566 Wrinkles

Miny Samuel, Rebecca Brooke, and Christopher Griffiths

KEY POINTS

- Skin disorders associated with photodamage from ultraviolet light include wrinkles, hyperpigmentation, tactile roughness, and telangiectasia, and are more common in people with white compared with other skin types.

  Wrinkles are also associated with aging, hormonal status, smoking, and intercurrent disease.

- We don't know whether sunscreens or topical vitamins C or E prevent wrinkles, as no studies have been found.

- Exposure to ultraviolet light may be associated with photodamage to the skin. Guidelines suggest that avoiding direct sunlight, either by staying indoors or in the shade, or by wearing protective clothing, is the most effective measure for reducing exposure to ultraviolet light.

- We don't know whether topical vitamins C or E improve the appearance of wrinkles, as studies have been small. They may cause stinging and erythema.

- Topical tretinoin improves fine wrinkles compared with placebo cream in people with mild to moderate photodamage, but its effect on coarse wrinkles is unclear.

  Topical tretinoin may cause itching, burning, erythema, and skin peeling.

  Isotretinoin cream improves fine and coarse wrinkles compared with vehicle cream in people with mild to severe photodamage, but causes severe irritation of the face in 5–10% of people.

  Tazarotene may be more effective than tretinoin at improving fine and coarse wrinkles in people with moderate photodamage, although studies have given inconclusive results. It can cause burning of the skin.

- We don't know whether retinyl esters, topical or oral natural cartilage polysaccharides, alpha or beta hyaroxyl acids, or chemical peel are beneficial.

- We don't know whether dermabrasion is more effective at improving wrinkles compared with carbon dioxide laser, as studies have given inconclusive results, but adverse effects are common with both treatments, especially erythema.

  We don't know whether variable pulse erbium:YAG laser or facelifts improve wrinkles, as few studies have been found.

(i) Please visit www.clinicalevidence.bmj.com for full text and references

What are the effects of interventions to prevent skin wrinkles?	
Unknown Effectiveness	• Sunscreens • Vitamin C or E (topical)

What are the effects of treatments for skin wrinkles?	
Beneficial	• Tazarotene (improved fine wrinkles) • Tretinoin (improved fine wrinkles)
Trade-off Between Benefits And Harms	• Isotretinoin
Unknown Effectiveness	• Carbon dioxide laser • Chemical peel

- Dermabrasion
- Facelift
- Glycolic acid or lactic acid (topical)
- Oral natural cartilage polysaccharides
- Retinyl esters
- Topical natural cartilage polysaccharides
- Variable pulse erbium:YAG laser
- Vitamin C or E (topical)

Search date December 2005

DEFINITION Wrinkles, also known as rhytides, are visible creases or folds in the skin. Wrinkles less than 1 mm in width and depth are defined as fine wrinkles, and those greater than 1 mm as coarse wrinkles. Most RCTs have studied wrinkles on the face, forearms, and hands.

INCIDENCE/PREVALENCE We found no information on the incidence of wrinkles alone, but only on the incidence of skin photodamage — which includes a spectrum of features such as wrinkles, hyperpigmentation, tactile roughness, and telangiectasia. The incidence of skin disorders associated with ultraviolet light increases with age and develops over several decades. One Australian study (1539 people, aged 20–55 years living in Queensland) found moderate to severe photodamage in 72% of men and 47% of women under 30 years of age. Severity of photodamage was significantly greater with increasing age, and was independently associated with solar keratoses (P less than 0.01) and skin cancer (P less than 0.05). Wrinkling was more common in people with white skin (especially skin phototypes I and II). We found few reports of photodamage in black skin (phototypes V and VI). One study reported that the incidence of photodamage in European and North American populations with Fitzpatrick skin types I, II, and III is about 80–90%. As Asian skin is more pigmented (Fitzpatrick skin types III–V), wrinkling is not readily apparent until the age of about 50 years, with wrinkles being less severe than in white skin of similar age. A prospective study (85 white women living in North America, and 70 Japanese women living in Tokyo, aged 20–69 years) that compared age-related changes in wrinkles in eight areas of the facial skin (forehead, glabella, upper eyelid, corner of the eye, lower eyelid, nasolabial groove, cheek, and corner of the mouth) and sagging in the subzygomatic area, found more wrinkle formation in all areas of the face in younger age groups of white women than in Japanese women (aged 20–29 years: P less than 0.05 for all comparisons of wrinkling of facial areas). Another prospective study (160 Chinese women and 160 French women, aged 20–60 years) found that wrinkle onset was delayed by about 10 years in Chinese women compared with French women.

AETIOLOGY/RISK FACTORS Wrinkles may be caused by intrinsic factors (e.g. aging, hormonal status, and intercurrent diseases) and by extrinsic factors (e.g. exposure to ultraviolet radiation, and cigarette smoke). These factors contribute to epidermal thinning, loss of elasticity, skin fragility, and creases and lines in the skin. The severity of photodamage varies with skin type, which includes skin colour, and the capacity to tan. It is becoming increasingly clear that brief incidental sun exposures that occur during the activities of daily living add significantly to the average individual's daily exposure to ultraviolet light. One review of five observational studies found that facial wrinkles in men and women were more common in smokers than in non-smokers. It also found that the risk of moderate to severe wrinkles in lifelong smokers was more than twice that in current smokers (RR 2.57, 95% CI 1.83 to 3.06). The effects of pregnancy and menopause on facial wrinkling have also been investigated by some researchers. In postmenopausal women, oestrogen deficiency is thought to be an important contributory factor for development of wrinkles. One observational study (186 Korean women, aged 20–89 years) found that facial wrinkling increased significantly with an increase in the number of full-term pregnancies (OR 1.84, 95% CI 1.02 to 3.31) and the number of years since menopause

(continued over)

(from previous page)

(OR 3.91, 95% CI 1.07 to 14.28). However, postmenopausal women who had HRT had significantly less facial wrinkling compared with postmenopausal women who had no history of HRT (OR 0.22, 95% CI 0.05 to 0.95).

PROGNOSIS Wrinkles cannot be considered a medical illness requiring intervention, but concerns about changes in physical appearance brought on by aging can have a detrimental effect on quality of life. In some cases, concerns about physical appearance can affect personal interactions, occupational functioning, and self-esteem. Geographical differences, culture, and personal values potentially influence a person's anxieties about aging. In societies in which the maintenance of a youthful appearance is valued, the demand for interventions that ameliorate visible signs of aging grows as aging populations expand.

Paul Montgomery and Jane Lilly

KEY POINTS

- Up to 40% of adults have insomnia, with difficulty getting to sleep, early waking, or feeling unrefreshed on waking.

  The prevalence of insomnia increases with age. Other risk factors include psychological factors, stress, daytime napping, and hyperarousal.

  Primary insomnia is a chronic and relapsing condition that may increase the risks of accidents, and is associated with dementia, depression, and falls.

- We don't know whether CBT, exercise programmes, or timed exposure to bright light can improve sleep quality compared with no treatment.

- Zaleplon, zolpidem, and zopiclone may improve sleep latency in elderly people, although long-term effects are unknown, and they are likely to cause adverse effects.

  Zolpidem and zopiclone may also increase sleep duration and improve sleep quality compared with placebo in the short term.

  Zaleplon has not been shown to improve sleep duration, number of awakenings, or sleep quality, and may cause rebound insomnia after discontinuation of treatment.

- Benzodiazepines may improve sleep outcomes compared with placebo or other treatments, but are likely to cause adverse effects.

  We don't know what the long-term effects of benzodiazepines are.

  Benzodiazepines can cause impairment of memory, cognitive and psychological function, and rebound insomnia. They may increase the risks of accidents, falls, and hip fractures in elderly people.

- We don't know whether diphenhydramine improves sleep quality in elderly people.

(i) Please visit www.clinicalevidence.bmj.com for full text and references

What are the effects of non-drug treatments for insomnia in elderly people?	
Unknown Effectiveness	• CBT
	• Exercise programmes
	• Timed exposure to bright light

What are the effects of drug treatments for insomnia in elderly people?	
Trade-off Between Benefits And Harms	• Benzodiazepines (quazepam, flurazepam, brotizolam, nitrazepam, loprazolam, midazolam, temazepam, and triazolam)
	• Zaleplon (improved sleep latency but increased rebound insomnia compared with placebo)
	• Zolpidem (may improve short-term sleep outcomes compared with placebo, but also increased rebound insomnia and adverse effects)

	• Zopiclone (may be as effective at improving sleep quality as benzodiazepines but with similar adverse effects)
Unknown Effectiveness	• Diphenhydramine

Search date October 2006

DEFINITION Insomnia is defined by the *International Classification of Sleep Disorders-2* (ICSD-2) as repeated difficulty with sleep initiation, duration, consolidation, or quality, occurring despite adequate time and opportunity for sleep, and results in some form of daytime impairment. **Chronic insomnia** is defined as insomnia occurring for at least three nights a week for 1 month or more. **Primary insomnia** is defined as chronic insomnia without specific underlying medical, psychiatric, or other sleep disorders, such as sleep apnoea, depression, dementia, periodic limb movement disorder, or circadian rhythm sleep disorder. This review only covers primary insomnia in people aged 60 years and over.

INCIDENCE/PREVALENCE One population survey in Sweden found that across all adult age groups, up to 40% of people have insomnia. A US survey in people aged 18–79 years found that insomnia affected 35% of all adults during the course of one year, and that prevalence increased with age, with estimates ranging from 31–38% in people aged 18–64 years, to 45% in people aged 65–79 years. One US prospective cohort study in people aged over 65 years old found that between 23–34% had insomnia, and between 7–15% had chronic insomnia. It also reported a higher incidence of insomnia in women than in men.

AETIOLOGY/RISK FACTORS The cause of insomnia is uncertain. The risk of primary insomnia increases with age and may be related to changes in circadian rhythms associated with age, or the onset of chronic conditions and poorer health as a result of aging. Psychological factors and lifestyle changes may exacerbate perceived effects of changes in sleep patterns associated with age, leading to reduced satisfaction with sleep. Other possible risk factors in all age groups include hyperarousal, chronic stress, and daytime napping.

PROGNOSIS We found few reliable data on long-term morbidity and mortality in people with primary insomnia. Primary insomnia is a chronic and relapsing condition. Likely consequences include reduced quality of life and increased risk of accidents owing to daytime sleepiness. People with primary insomnia may be at greater risk of dependence on hypnotic medication, depression, dementia, and falls, and may be more likely to require residential care.

Andrew Herxheimer

KEY POINTS

- Jet lag is a syndrome associated with rapid long-haul flights across several time zones, characterised by sleep disturbances, daytime fatigue, reduced performance, gastrointestinal problems, and generalised malaise.

  It is caused by a disruption of the 'body clock', which gradually adapts under the influence of light and dark, mediated by melatonin secreted by the pineal gland: darkness switches on melatonin secretion, exposure to strong light switches it off.

  The incidence and severity of jet lag increases with the number of time zones crossed; it tends to be worse on eastward than on westward flights.

- Melatonin reduces subjective ratings of jet lag on eastward and on westward flights compared with placebo.

  The adverse effects of melatonin have not been systematically studied, but people with epilepsy and people taking an oral anticoagulant should probably not use it without medical supervision.

- Hypnotics (zopiclone or zolpidem), taken before bedtime on the first few nights after flying, may reduce the effects of jet lag by improving sleep quality and duration, but not other components of jet lag.

  However, they are associated with a various adverse effects, including headache, dizziness, nausea, confusion, and amnesia, which may outweigh any short-term benefits.

- We found no studies that examined the effectiveness of lifestyle or environmental adaptations (such as eating, avoiding alcohol or caffeine, sleeping, daylight exposure or arousal).

  It is generally agreed that, after a westward flight, it is worth staying awake while it is daylight at the destination and trying to sleep when it gets dark. After an eastward flight, one should stay awake but avoid bright light in the morning, and be outdoors as much as possible in the afternoon. This will help adjust the body clock and turn on the body's own melatonin secretion at the right time.

(i) Please visit www.clinicalevidence.bmj.com for full text and references

What are the effects of interventions to prevent or minimise jet lag?

Likely To Be Beneficial	• Melatonin*
Trade-off Between Benefits And Harms	• Hypnotics
Unknown Effectiveness	• Lifestyle and environmental adaptations (eating, avoiding alcohol or caffeine, sleeping, daylight exposure, arousal)

Search date November 2006

*The adverse effects of melatonin have not yet been adequately investigated.

DEFINITION Jet lag is a syndrome associated with rapid long-haul flights across several time zones, characterised by sleep disturbances, daytime fatigue, reduced performance,

(continued over)

(from previous page)

gastrointestinal problems, and generalised malaise. As with most syndromes, not all of the components must be present in any one case. It is caused by the "body clock" continuing to function in the day–night rhythm of the place of departure. The rhythm adapts gradually under the influence of light and dark, mediated by melatonin secreted by the pineal gland: darkness switches on melatonin secretion, exposure to strong light switches it off.

INCIDENCE/PREVALENCE Jet lag affects most air travellers crossing five or more time zones. The incidence and severity of jet lag increases with the number of time zones crossed.

AETIOLOGY/RISK FACTORS Someone who has previously experienced jet lag is liable to do so again. Jet lag worsens with the more time zones crossed in one flight, or series of flights, within a few days. Westward travel generally causes less disruption than eastward travel as it is easier to lengthen, rather than to shorten, the natural circadian cycle.

PROGNOSIS Jet lag is worst immediately after travel and gradually resolves over 4–6 days as the person adjusts to the new local time. The more time zones crossed, the longer it takes to wear off.

Sleep apnoea

Michael Hensley and Cheryl Ray

KEY POINTS

- Sleep apnoea is the popular term for OSAHS. OSAHS is abnormal breathing during sleep that causes recurrent arousals, sleep fragmentation, daytime sleepiness, and nocturnal hypoxaemia.

  Apnoea may be "central", in which there is cessation of inspiratory effort, or "obstructive", in which inspiratory efforts continue but are ineffective because of upper airway obstruction.

  It affects up to 24% of men and 9% of women in the US, with obesity being a major determinant.

- In people with severe OSAHS, nasal CPAP has been shown to reduce daytime sleepiness compared with control treatments.

  Although effective, it can be difficult to get people to comply with the prescribed CPAP regimen. There is some evidence that educational or psychological interventions may improve compliance with CPAP.

  Compliance does not seem any better with alternative treatments, such as automatically titrated CPAP, bi-level positive airway pressure, patient-titrated CPAP, or CPAP plus humidification.

- Oral appliances that produce anterior advancement of the mandible seem to be effective in improving sleep-disordered breathing in people with OSAHS.

  Oral appliances are probably not as effective as CPAP, and we don't know how well they work in the long term.

- We found insufficient evidence to judge the effectiveness of weight loss on OSAHS (either severe or non-severe), although there is consensus that advice about weight reduction is an important component of management of OSAHS.

- It seems that nasal CPAP will also be beneficial to people suffering from non-severe OSAHS.

  Nasal CPAP is less acceptable to people with non-severe OSAHS, and we don't know whether measures aimed at improving compliance effectively increase usage.

Please visit www.clinicalevidence.bmj.com for full text and references

What are the effects of treatment for severe OSAHS?	
Beneficial	• Nasal CPAP (severe OSAHS)
Likely To Be Beneficial	• Oral appliances (severe OSAHS)
Unknown Effectiveness	• Measures aimed at improving compliance with nasal CPAP (severe OSAHS)
	• Weight loss (severe OSAHS)

What are the effects of treatment for non-severe OSAHS?	
Likely To Be Beneficial	• Nasal CPAP (non-severe OSAHS)

	• Oral appliances (non-severe OSAHS; more effective than no treatment, control appliance, or placebo but less effective than nasal CPAP)
Unknown Effectiveness	• Measures aimed at improving compliance with nasal CPAP (non-severe OSAHS) • Weight loss (non-severe OSAHS)

Search date May 2006

DEFINITION Sleep apnoea is the popular term for obstructive sleep apnoea-hypopnoea syndrome (OSAHS). OSAHS is abnormal breathing during sleep that causes recurrent arousals, sleep fragmentation, and nocturnal hypoxaemia. The syndrome includes daytime sleepiness, impaired vigilance and cognitive functioning, and reduced quality of life. Apnoea is the absence of airflow at the nose and mouth for at least 10 seconds, and hypopnoea is a major reduction (over 50%) in airflow also for at least 10 seconds. Apnoeas may be "central", in which there is cessation of inspiratory effort, or "obstructive", in which inspiratory efforts continue, but are ineffective because of upper airway obstruction. The diagnosis of OSAHS is made when a person with daytime symptoms has significant sleep-disordered breathing revealed by polysomnography (study of sleep state, breathing, and oxygenation) or by more limited studies (e.g. measurement of oxygen saturation overnight). Criteria for the diagnosis of significant sleep-disordered breathing have not been rigorously assessed, but they have been set by consensus and convention. Diagnostic criteria have variable sensitivity and specificity. For example, an apnoea/hypopnoea index (AHI) of fewer than five episodes of apnoea or hypopnoea per hour of sleep is considered normal. However, people with upper airway resistance syndrome have an index below five episodes an hour, and many healthy elderly people have an index greater than five episodes an hour. In an effort to achieve international consensus, new criteria have been proposed and are becoming more widely used. The severity of OSAHS can be classified by the severity of two factors: daytime sleepiness and AHI. Severe OSAHS is defined as severe sleep-disordered breathing (AHI more than 30 episodes per hour) plus symptoms of excessive daytime sleepiness (such as Epworth Sleepiness Scale more than 10 or Multiple Sleep Latency Test less than 5 minutes). Central sleep apnoea and sleep-associated hypoventilation syndromes are not covered in this review.

INCIDENCE/PREVALENCE The Wisconsin Sleep Cohort Study (more than 1000 people; mean age 47 years) in North America found prevalence rates for an AHI of more than five episodes an hour of 24% in men and 9% in women, and for OSAHS with an index greater than five episodes an hour plus excessive sleepiness of 4% in men and 2% in women. There are international differences in the occurrence of OSAHS, of which obesity is considered to be an important determinant. Ethnic differences in prevalence have also been found after adjustment for other risk factors. Little is known about the incidence in resource-poor countries.

AETIOLOGY/RISK FACTORS The site of upper airway obstruction in OSAHS is around the level of the tongue, soft palate, or epiglottis. Disorders that predispose to either narrowing of the upper airway or reduction in its stability (e.g. obesity, certain craniofacial abnormalities, vocal cord abnormalities, enlarged tonsils, and enlarged tongue) have been associated with an increased risk of OSAHS. It has been estimated that a 1 kg/m^2 increase in BMI (3.2 kg for a person 1.8 m tall) leads to a 30% increase (95% CI 13% to 50%) in the relative risk of developing abnormal sleep-disordered breathing (AHI at least 5 episodes/hour) over a period of 4 years. Other strong associated risk factors include increasing age, and sex (male to female ratio 2:1). Weaker associations include menopause, family history, smoking, and night-time nasal congestion.

PROGNOSIS The long-term prognosis of people with untreated severe OSAHS is poor with respect to quality of life, likelihood of motor vehicle accidents, hypertension, and possibly CVD and premature mortality. Unfortunately, the prognosis of treated OSAHS is also unclear. The limitations in the evidence include bias in the selection of participants, short duration of follow-up, and variation in the measurement of confounders (e.g. smoking, alcohol use, and other cardiovascular risk factors). Treatment is widespread, making it difficult to find evidence on prognosis for untreated OSAHS. Observational studies support a causal association between OSAHS and systemic hypertension, which increases with the severity of OSAHS (OR 1.21 for non-severe OSAHS to 3.07 for severe OSAHS). OSAHS increases the risk of motor vehicle accidents three- to sevenfold. It is associated with increased risk of premature mortality, CVD, and impaired neurocognitive functioning.

Sam H Ahmedzai and Jason Boland

KEY POINTS

- Constipation is reported in 52% of people with advanced malignancy. This figure rises to 87% in people who are terminally ill and taking opioids. Constipation may be the most common adverse effect of opioids. There is no reason to believe that people with chronic non-malignant disease who take opioids will be any less troubled by this adverse effect.

- There is some RCT evidence, supported by consensus, that the oral laxatives lactulose, macrogol/electrolyte solutions, and senna are probably of similar efficacy in people with opioid-induced constipation.

  Macrogol/electrolyte solutions may have a better adverse-effect profile than the other oral laxatives.

  We found no good-quality studies on other oral laxatives such as ispaghula husk and liquid paraffin. Liquid paraffin is associated with severe adverse effects, and is not recommended for long-term use.

- We found no RCT evidence assessing rectally applied agents (arachis oil enema, glycerol suppository, phosphate enema, sodium citrate micro-enema).

- There is consensus that the opioid antagonists alvimopan, methylnaltrexone, and naloxone, can reverse not only the constipation, but also potentially the other gastrointestinal symptoms induced by opioids.

  Naloxone may provoke reversal of opioid analgesia, but this is less likely with alvimopan or methylnaltrexone. Naloxone may also cause mild degrees of opioid withdrawal, but this has not been reported with methylnaltrexone or alvimopan.

- Further RCTs assessing all the currently available treatments are needed.

(i) **Please visit www.clinicalevidence.bmj.com for full text and references**

What are the effects of oral laxatives for constipation in people prescribed opioids?	
Beneficial	• Lactulose * • Macrogols (polyethylene glycols) plus electrolyte solutions* • Senna *
Unknown Effectiveness	• Bisacodyl • Co-danthrusate/co-danthramer • Docusate • Ispaghula husk • Magnesium salts • Methylcellulose • Sodium picosulfate

What are the effects of rectally applied medications in people for constipation in people prescribed opioids?	
Unknown Effectiveness	• Arachis oil enema • Glycerol suppository

- Liquid paraffin
- Phosphate enema
- Sodium citrate micro-enema

What are the effects of opioid antagonists for constipation in people prescribed opioids?

Likely To Be Beneficial	• Opioid antagonists (alvimopan, methylnaltrexone, naloxone) *

Search date August 2006

* Based on limited RCT evidence supported by clinical consensus.

DEFINITION Constipation is infrequent defecation with increased difficulty or discomfort, and with reduced number of bowel movements, which may or may not be abnormally hard. It can have many causes, one of which is opioid use. Opioid-induced bowel dysfunction (OBD) encompasses a wide range of associated symptoms, including abdominal distension and pain, gastric fullness, nausea, vomiting, anorexia, confusion, and overflow diarrhoea. These symptoms may also be associated with constipation because of other causes. This review focuses only on constipation in people prescribed opioids. For the purposes of this review, we have used the NICE definition of supportive care as follows: supportive care "helps the patient and their family to cope with cancer and treatment of it — from pre-diagnosis, through the process of diagnosis and treatment, to cure, continuing illness or death and into bereavement. It helps the patient to maximise the benefits of treatment and to live as well as possible with the effects of the disease. It is given equal priority alongside diagnosis and treatment". This definition was written in relation to people with cancer, but is applicable to all people with chronic or terminal illness, for example heart failure or lung disease. We have used the WHO definition of palliative care as follows: "Palliative care is an approach that improves the quality of life of patients and their families facing the problem associated with life-threatening illness, through the prevention and relief of suffering by means of early identification and impeccable assessment and treatment of pain and other problems, physical, psychosocial and spiritual". Although this definition of palliative care does not specify incurable or terminal illness, there is consensus that palliative care applies to people approaching the end of life; that is, people with a prognosis of less than a year. Thus, both supportive and palliative care embrace the same priorities of maximising quality of life, but supportive care aims to do this in people who may live longer, become cured, or who are living in remission from their disease.

INCIDENCE/PREVALENCE In one prospective cohort study (1000 people with advanced cancer), constipation was reported to occur in 52%. In another prospective cohort study (498 people in hospice with advanced cancer) this figure rose to 87% in people who were terminally ill and taking opioids. A survey (76 people) carried out by the American Pain Society found that in people with chronic pain of non-cancer origin treated with opioids, the incidence of constipation was five times higher than in another US survey of 10,018 US controls (health status of controls not defined). Fifty-eight per cent of people who took opioids regularly required more than two types of treatment for constipation. The prevalence of constipation is not the same with all opioids. One systematic review (search date 2004, 6 RCTs, 1220 people, 657 with cancer, 563 with chronic painful diseases taking opioids for 28 days or more) found that significantly more people had constipation when taking modified-release oral morphine than taking transdermal fentanyl (16% with transdermal fentanyl v 37% with modified-release oral morphine; P less than 0.001). One RCT (212 people with cancer), assessing people who were taking opioids for 14 days or less, found that significantly more people taking modified-release oral morphine than taking transdermal fentanyl had constipation (27.2% with transdermal fentanyl v 44.5% with modified-release oral morphine; P less than 0.001).

AETIOLOGY/RISK FACTORS The constipating effect of opioids is through their action on mu-opioid receptors in the submucosal plexus of the gastrointestinal tract. This decreases

(continued over)

(from previous page)

gastrointestinal motility by decreasing propulsive peristalsis (while increasing circular contractions), decreases secretions (pancreatic and biliary), and increases intestinal fluid absorption. There is also a central descending opioid-mediated effect, so that even spinally administered opioids cause decreased gastric emptying and prolonged oral–caecal transit time. The opioid-induced increase in circular muscle contractions causes colicky pain. There is good evidence from RCTs and animal studies that, compared with water-soluble opioids such as morphine and oxycodone, the more lipid soluble opioids such as fentanyl and buprenorphine are less likely to cause constipation while maintaining the same degree of analgesic effect. This is probably caused by their much-reduced time in the systemic circulation. Other risk factors for constipation and bowel dysfunction in people taking opioids for advanced cancer include hypercalcaemia, reduced mobility, reduced fluid and food intake, dehydration, anal fissures, and mechanical obstruction. Lack of privacy for defecation may also play a part for people in hospital. Drugs that can cause or exacerbate constipation include anticholinergics. In the treatment of cancer, thalidomide, vinca alkaloids, and $5HT_3$ antagonists can all cause constipation. Additionally there is an increased risk of constipation in people with autonomic neuropathy caused by diabetes mellitus, for example, and in people with neuromuscular problems, such as spinal cord compression.

PROGNOSIS One single-centre observational study (50 people) found a correlation between persistent constipation and poorer performance status (94% of people with Eastern Cooperative Oncology Group [ECOG] score 3 or 4 were constipated). This study failed to show a correlation between total opioid dose and degree of constipation.

KEY POINTS

- Delirium is common in the last weeks of life, occurring in 26–44% of people with advanced cancer in hospital, and in up to 88% of people with terminal illness in the last days of life.

  Delirium is part of a wide range of organic mental disorders which includes dementia, organic mood disorder, and organic anxiety disorder. Delirium, like dementia, is marked by a general cognitive impairment whereas, in other organic mental disorders, impairment is more selective. Delirium is distinguished from dementia in that it is deemed to be, at least potentially, reversible.

- This systematic review focuses on people with delirium secondary to underlying terminal illness, who are being treated in the supportive and palliative care setting.

- We found little RCT evidence in people with delirium caused by underlying terminal illness. It would be unethical to perform a placebo-controlled trial, and it should be acknowledged that undertaking any form of clinical trial in this particularly vulnerable group of people is difficult.

  There is consensus based on observational evidence and experience that haloperidol, and other butyrophenones, such as droperidol, are effective for the management of delirium, and they are widely used. However, few RCTs assessing their effects have been undertaken.

  Although benzodiazepines, especially midazolam, are used extensively in people with delirium who are terminally ill, we found no evidence from well-conducted trials that they are beneficial.

  We also don't know whether haloperidol, barbiturates, phenothiazines, or propofol are effective in people with delirium caused by underlying disease. All of these drugs are associated with serious adverse effects and some, such as barbiturates, may in fact cause confusion and agitation. We also don't know if artificial hydration is effective in people with delirium.

- We don't know whether switching opioids is helpful in people who have developed opioid-induced delirium.

ⓘ **Please visit www.clinicalevidence.bmj.com for full text and references**

What are the effects of interventions at the end of life in people with delirium caused by underlying terminal illness?	
Likely To Be Beneficial	• Haloperidol*
Unknown Effectiveness	• Artificial hydration
	• Barbiturates
	• Benzodiazepines
	• Opioid switching
	• Phenothiazines
	• Propofol

Search date July 2006

---

* Based on consensus.

DEFINITION Delirium is defined as a non-specific, global cerebral dysfunction with concurrent disturbances of consciousness, attention, thinking, perception, memory, psychomotor behaviour, emotion, and the sleep–wake cycle. In assessing clinical research, there is some difficulty in that the terms delirium and cognitive failure are at times used interchangeably. Cognitive failure encompasses both delirium (which is common in people with advanced disease in the last weeks of life) and dementia, and amnesic disorders (which are relatively rare in this population). This systematic review covers only people with delirium secondary to underlying terminal illness, who are being treated in the palliative care setting. For the purposes of this review, we have used the NICE definition of supportive care as follows: supportive care "helps the patient and their family to cope with cancer and treatment of it — from prediagnosis, through the process of diagnosis and treatment, to cure, continuing illness or death and into bereavement. It helps the patient to maximise the benefits of treatment and to live as well as possible with the effects of the disease. It is given equal priority alongside diagnosis and treatment." This definition was written in relation to people with cancer, but is applicable to all people with terminal illness. We have used the WHO definition of palliative care as follows: "Palliative care is an approach that improves the quality of life of patients and their families facing the problem associated with life-threatening illness, through the prevention and relief of suffering by means of early identification and impeccable assessment and treatment of pain and other problems, physical, psychosocial and spiritual." Although this definition of palliative care does not specify incurable or terminal illness, there is consensus that palliative care applies to people approaching the end of life, that is, people with prognosis of less than a year. Thus, both supportive and palliative care embrace the same priorities of maximising quality of life; but supportive care aims to do this in people who may live longer, become cured, or who are in remission from their disease.

INCIDENCE/PREVALENCE Delirium is common in the last weeks of life, occurring in 26–44% of people with advanced cancer in hospital, and in up to 88% of people with a terminal illness in the last days of life. A key difficulty in assessing the prevalence and incidence of delirium in a population with advanced disease relates to the variety of screening instruments, scales, and terminology used (cognitive failure, delirium, agitation, and restlessness).

AETIOLOGY/RISK FACTORS Delirium is part of a wide range of organic mental disorders which includes dementia, organic mood disorder, and organic anxiety disorder. Delirium, like dementia, is marked by a general cognitive impairment whereas, in other organic mental disorders, impairment is more selective. Delirium is distinguished from dementia in that delirium is deemed to be, at least potentially, reversible. In a palliative-care population (47 people with terminal cancer who died in hospital in whom there were 66 episodes of cognitive failure over 3 days), it was possible to attribute a cause for the delirium in less than 50% of people. These causes included drugs, sepsis, brain metastasis, organ failure, hypercalcaemia, and hyponatraemia. The list of potential causes of delirium is extensive, but in end-stage disease can be subdivided as follows: **Central nervous system causes:** primary brain tumours; metastatic spread to the central nervous system; **Metabolic causes:** organ failure (e.g. hyperbilirubinaemia and uraemia); electrolyte disturbance (e.g. hyponatraemia and hypercalcaemia); hypoxia; **Treatment effects:** cytotoxic chemotherapy; radiotherapy (especially cranial irradiation); **Other drug effects:** commonly: corticosteroids; opioids; and anticholinergics; **Other causes:** anaemia; nutritional deficiencies (e.g. vitamin B_{12} deficiency); and paraneoplastic syndromes.

PROGNOSIS The prognosis of terminal illness is worsened by delirium. In one systematic review, six of seven prospective studies found a significant association with decreased survival in people with delirium and end-stage cancer.

Paul Keeley

KEY POINTS

- Nausea and vomiting occur in 40–70% of people with cancer, and are also common in other chronic conditions such as hepatitis C and inflammatory bowel disease. Nausea and vomiting become more common as disease progresses.

- Nausea and vomiting may occur as a result of the disease or its treatment.

- The evidence base for treatment-related causes of nausea and vomiting (chemotherapy and radiotherapy) is much greater and more robust than for disease-related causes.

- Metoclopramide is likely to be effective for reducing episodes of vomiting in people having chemotherapy.

  Dexamethasone, in combination with other anti-emetics, reduces acute and delayed emesis compared with placebo in people receiving emetogenic chemotherapy, and it may be more effective than metoclopramide in this population.

  $5HT_3$ antagonists also reduce acute vomiting in people having chemotherapy compared with metoclopramide-based regimens, and this benefit is enhanced by the addition of dexamethasone.

  There is consensus that haloperidol, phenothiazines, and venting gastrostomy are effective for controlling nausea and vomiting in people with cancer.

- Cannabinoids are effective for nausea and vomiting in people receiving chemotherapy, but they may be associated with a high and often unacceptable burden of adverse effects.

- We don't know whether antihistamines, antimuscarinics, antipsychotics, benzodiazepines, or NK1 antagonists are effective in people with cancer-related nausea and vomiting.

- Despite the lack of robust RCT evidence, there is a consensus based on clinical experience that antihistamines have a place in the management of nausea and vomiting, especially that related to motion sickness, mechanical bowel obstruction, and raised intracranial pressure.

  We don't know whether any other interventions are effective for controlling nausea and vomiting in people with chronic conditions other than cancer.

(i) **Please visit www.clinicalevidence.bmj.com for full text and references**

What are the effects of treatments for nausea and vomiting occurring either as a result of the disease or its treatment in adults with cancer?

Beneficial	• $5HT_3$ antagonists for the control of chemotherapy-related nausea and vomiting
	• Dexamethasone for the control of chemotherapy-related nausea and vomiting
Likely To Be Beneficial	• Aprepitant (enhances effects of a conventional antiemetic regimen)
	• Haloperidol for the control of nausea and vomiting in people with cancer*
	• Metoclopramide for the control of chemotherapy-related nausea and vomiting

	• Phenothiazines for the control of nausea and vomiting in people with cancer*
	• Venting gastrostomy for the control of nausea and vomiting in people with cancer*
Trade-off Between Benefits And Harms	• Cannabinoids for the control of chemotherapy-related nausea and vomiting
Unknown Effectiveness	• 5HT$_3$ antagonists for the control of radiotherapy-related nausea and vomiting
	• Antihistamines for the control of nausea and vomiting in people with cancer
	• Antimuscarinics for the control of nausea and vomiting in people with cancer
	• Antipsychotics (atypical) for the control of nausea and vomiting in people with cancer
	• Benzodiazepines for the control of chemotherapy-related nausea and vomiting

What are the effects of treatments for nausea and vomiting occurring either as a result of the disease or its treatment in adults with chronic diseases other than cancer?

Likely To Be Beneficial	• Antihistamines for the control of nausea and vomiting in chronic diseases other than cancer *
Unknown Effectiveness	• 5HT$_3$ antagonists for the control of nausea and vomiting in chronic diseases other than cancer
	• Antimuscarinics for the control of nausea and vomiting in chronic diseases other than cancer
	• Antipsychotics (atypical) for the control of nausea and vomiting in chronic diseases other than cancer
	• Benzodiazepines for the control of nausea and vomiting in chronic diseases other than cancer
	• Butyrophenones for the control of nausea and vomiting in chronic diseases other than cancer
	• Cannabinoids for the control of nausea and vomiting in chronic diseases other than cancer
	• Corticosteroids for the control of nausea and vomiting in chronic diseases other than cancer
	• NK1 antagonists for the control of nausea and vomiting in chronic diseases other than cancer
	• Phenothiazines for the control of nausea and vomiting in chronic diseases other than cancer
	• Prokinetics for the control of nausea and vomiting in chronic diseases other than cancer

● Venting gastrostomy for the control of nausea and vomiting in chronic diseases other than cancer

Search date December 2005

*Based on consensus; RCTs unlikely to be conducted.

DEFINITION Nausea and vomiting (emesis) are common in people with cancer and other chronic diseases. They may occur because of several factors, which can be most easily thought of as disease related and treatment related. The evidence base for treatment-related causes of nausea and vomiting (chemotherapy and radiotherapy) is much greater and more robust than for disease-related causes. This review focuses on the management of nausea and vomiting in people with cancer or other chronic conditions; it does not include people with postoperative nausea and vomiting. For the purposes of this review, we have used the NICE definition of supportive care as follows: supportive care "helps the patient and their family to cope with cancer and treatment of it – from pre-diagnosis, through the process of diagnosis and treatment, to cure, continuing illness or death and into bereavement. It helps the patient to maximise the benefits of treatment and to live as well as possible with the effects of the disease. It is given equal priority alongside diagnosis and treatment". This definition was written in relation to people with cancer but is applicable to all people with chronic or terminal illness, for example heart failure or lung disease. We have used the WHO definition of palliative care as follows: "Palliative care is an approach that improves the quality of life of patients and their families facing the problem associated with life-threatening illness, through the prevention and relief of suffering by means of early identification and impeccable assessment and treatment of pain and other problems, physical, psychosocial and spiritual". Although this definition of palliative care does not specify incurable or terminal illness, there is consensus that palliative care applies to people approaching the end of life; that is, people with a prognosis of less than a year. Thus both supportive and palliative care embrace the same priorities of maximising quality of life, but supportive care aims to do this in people who may live longer, become cured, or who are living in remission from their disease.

INCIDENCE/PREVALENCE Nausea and vomiting occur in 40–70% of people with cancer and are also common in other chronic conditions such as hepatitis C and inflammatory bowel disease. Nausea and vomiting become more common as disease progresses.

AETIOLOGY/RISK FACTORS Nausea and vomiting are complex neurological and physical phenomena involving a range of areas of the central nervous system and gastrointestinal tract. In palliative and supportive care, nausea may be because of chemotherapy, especially platinum-based chemotherapy, other drugs (opiates, antibiotics), or radiotherapy. It may also have disease-related causes, for example metabolic (hypercalcaemia, uraemia), cranial (raised intracranial pressure, VIIIth nerve tumours), gastrointestinal (gastric outflow obstruction, hepatomegaly constipation, bowel obstruction, or ileus), or psychogenic (anticipatory nausea and vomiting, anxiety, or fear).

PROGNOSIS In many cases, nausea will respond to treatment of the underlying cause, for example nausea resulting from metabolic disturbance such as hypercalcaemia. Nausea resulting from emetogenic drugs such as opioids may resolve if the opioid is switched.

Justin Stebbing, Sarah Slater, and Maurice Slevin

KEY POINTS

- Median survival from metastatic breast cancer is 12 months without treatment, but young people can survive up to 20 years with the disease, whereas in other metastatic cancers this would be considered unusual.

- Antioestrogens (tamoxifen) result in tumour responses in about a third of women with oestrogen receptor-positive metastatic breast cancer when used as first-line treatment, but most women eventually develop resistant disease.

  Progestins and ovarian ablation may be as effective as tamoxifen, while adding tamoxifen to gonadorelin analogues increases survival and response rates.

  Selective aromatase inhibitors may be as effective as tamoxifen, and more effective than progestins in delaying disease progression as first- or second-line treatment in postmenopausal women, with similar overall survival. The benefit may be greatest in oestrogen receptor-positive women.

- Hormonal treatment using tamoxifen or progestins may be preferable to chemotherapy as first-line treatment in women with oestrogen receptor-positive disease.

- First-line chemotherapy is associated with an objective tumour response in 40–60% of women, of median duration of 6–12 months. Complete remission may occur in some women, whereas others show little or no response at all.

  Classical non-taxane combination chemotherapy, especially those containing anthracyclines, may be more effective than modified regimens and as effective as hormonal treatments in prolonging survival.

  The optimum duration of chemotherapy is unknown. Increasing the dose may increase serious adverse effects without prolonging survival.

  Taxane-based chemotherapy may increase tumour response and survival compared with some non-taxane regimens as second-line treatment. No clear benefit has been found in first-line treatment.

- Adding trastuzumab to standard chemotherapy increases response rates and overall survival in women with *HER2/neu* overexpression, but risks of cardiac function are increased in women also receiving anthracyclines.

- Bisphosphonates reduce skeletal complications from bone metastases, while radiotherapy may reduce pain and complications from bone metastases, cranial nerve or spinal cord compression, and in brain or choroidal metastases.

(i) **Please visit www.clinicalevidence.bmj.com for full text and references**

What are the effects of first-line hormonal treatment?

Beneficial	• Hormonal treatment with antioestrogens (tamoxifen) or progestins (no significant difference in survival compared with non-taxane combination chemotherapy so may be preferable in women with oestrogen receptor-positive disease)
	• Selective aromatase inhibitors in postmenopausal women (at least as effective as tamoxifen in delaying disease progression)

	• Tamoxifen in oestrogen receptor-positive women
Likely To Be Beneficial	• Combined gonadorelin analogues plus tamoxifen in premenopausal women
Trade-off Between Benefits And Harms	• Ovarian ablation in premenopausal women (no significant difference in response rates or survival compared with tamoxifen but associated with substantial adverse effects) • Progestins (beneficial in women with bone metastases or anorexia compared with tamoxifen; higher doses associated with adverse effects)

What are the effects of second-line hormonal treatment in women who have not responded to tamoxifen?

Beneficial	• Selective aromatase inhibitors in postmenopausal women (prolonged survival compared with progestins, no significant difference in time to progression compared with antioestrogens)
Likely To Be Ineffective Or Harmful	• Progestins (less effective in prolonging survival than selective aromatase inhibitors and have more adverse effects)

What are the effects of first-line chemotherapy?

Beneficial	• Anthracycline-based non-taxane combination chemotherapy regimens (CAF) containing doxorubicin (delayed progression, increased response rates and survival compared with non-anthracycline-based regimens); Classical non-taxane combination chemotherapy (CMF) (increases response rates and survival compared with modified CMF)
Trade-off Between Benefits And Harms	• Taxane-based combination chemotherapy (may increase response rates compared with non-taxane combination chemotherapy but with increased adverse effects)
Likely To Be Ineffective Or Harmful	• High-dose chemotherapy (no significant difference in overall survival compared with standard chemotherapy and increased adverse effects)

What are the effects of first-line chemotherapy in combination with a monoclonal antibody?

Beneficial	• Chemotherapy plus monoclonal antibody (trastuzumab) in women with overexpressed *HER2/neu* oncogene

What are the effects of second-line chemotherapy?

Likely To Be Beneficial	• Taxane-based combination chemotherapy (increases response rate in women with anthracycline-resistant disease compared with non-taxane combination chemotherapy)
Unknown Effectiveness	• Capecitabine for anthracycline-resistant disease • Semisynthetic vinca alkaloids for anthracycline-resistant disease

What are the effects of treatments for bone metastases?

Beneficial	• Radiotherapy plus appropriate analgesia*
Likely To Be Beneficial	• Bisphosphonates

What are the effects of treatments for spinal cord metastases?

Beneficial	• Radiotherapy* • Radiotherapy plus high-dose corticosteroids in women with spinal cord compression

What are the effects of treatments for cerebral metastases?

Likely To Be Beneficial	• Radiotherapy*
Unknown Effectiveness	• Intrathecal chemotherapy • Radiation sensitisers • Surgical resection

What are the effects of treatments for choroidal metastases?

Likely To Be Beneficial	• Radiotherapy*

Search date June 2006

*Not based on RCT evidence.

DEFINITION Metastatic or advanced breast cancer is the presence of disease at distant sites such as the bone, liver, or lung. Symptoms may include pain from bone metastases, breathlessness from spread to the lungs, and nausea or abdominal discomfort from liver involvement.

INCIDENCE/PREVALENCE Breast cancer is the second most frequent cancer in the world, and is by far the most common malignant disease in women (22% of all new cancer cases). Worldwide, the ratio of mortality to incidence is about 36%. It ranks fifth as a cause of death from cancer overall (although it is the leading cause of cancer mortality in women —

the 370,000 annual deaths represent 13.9% of cancer deaths in women). In the USA, metastatic breast cancer causes 46,000 deaths annually, and in the UK causes 15,000 deaths annually. It is the most prevalent cancer in the world today and there are an estimated 3.9 million women alive who have had breast cancer diagnosed in the past 5 years (compared, for example, with lung cancer, where there are 1.4 million alive). The true prevalence of metastatic disease is high because some women live with the disease for many years. Since 1990, there has been an overall increase in incidence rates of about 1.5% annually.

AETIOLOGY/RISK FACTORS The risk of metastatic disease relates to known adverse prognostic factors in the original primary tumour. These factors include oestrogen receptor-negative disease, primary tumours 3 cm or more in diameter, and axillary node involvement — recurrence occurred within 10 years of adjuvant chemotherapy for early breast cancer in 60–70% of node-positive women and 25–30% of node-negative women in one large systematic review.

PROGNOSIS Metastatic breast cancer is not treatable by primary surgery and is currently considered incurable. Prognosis depends on age, extent of disease, and oestrogen receptor status. There is also evidence that overexpression of the product of the *HER2/neu* oncogene, which occurs in about a third of women with metastatic breast cancer, is associated with a worse prognosis. A short disease-free interval (e.g. less than 1 year) between surgery for early breast cancer and developing metastases suggests that the recurrent disease is likely to be resistant to adjuvant treatment. In women who receive no treatment for metastatic disease, the median survival from diagnosis of metastases is 12 months. However, young people with good performance status may survive for 15–20 years (whereas in other metastatic cancers, this would be considered very unusual). The choice of first-line treatment (hormonal or chemotherapy) is based on a variety of clinical factors. In many countries, such as the USA, Canada, and some European countries, there is evidence of a decrease in death rates in recent years. This probably reflects improvements in treatment (and therefore improved survival) as well as earlier diagnosis.

Justin Stebbing, Geoff Delaney, and Alastair Thompson

KEY POINTS

- Breast cancer affects at least 1 in 10 women in the UK, but most present with primary operable disease, which has an 80% 5-year survival rate overall.

- In women with ductal carcinoma *in situ,* radiotherapy reduces local recurrence and invasive carcinoma after breast-conserving surgery, but may not improve survival.

- In women with primary operable breast cancer, survival may be increased by full surgical excision, tamoxifen, chemotherapy, radiotherapy, ovarian ablation, or trastuzumab (in women who overexpress *HER2/neu* oncogene).

  Incomplete excision may increase the risk of local recurrence, but less-extensive mastectomy that excises all local disease is as effective as radical mastectomy at prolonging survival, with better cosmetic results.

  Axillary clearance (removal of all axillary lymph nodes) achieves local disease control, but has not been shown to increase survival, and can cause arm lymphoedema.

  Sentinel lymph node biopsy or 4-node sampling may adequately stage the axilla with less morbidity compared with axillary clearance.

  Adjuvant tamoxifen reduces the risk of recurrence and death in women with oestrogen-positive tumours, but adverse effects begin to outweigh benefit after 5 years of treatment.

  Primary chemotherapy may facilitate successful breast-conserving surgery instead of mastectomy. Adjuvant combination chemotherapy improves survival compared with no chemotherapy, with greatest benefit likely with anthracycline-based regimens at standard doses for 4–6 months.

  Radiotherapy decreases recurrence and mortality after breast-conserving surgery. Post-mastectomy radiotherapy for women who are node-positive or at high risk of recurrence decreases recurrence and mortality, but may increase mortality in node-negative women.

  Adjuvant aromatase inhibitors improve disease-free survival compared with tamoxifen, but their effect on overall survival is unclear. Adjuvant taxoid regimens may improve disease-free survival over standard anthracycline-based therapy.

- In women with locally advanced breast cancer, radiotherapy may be as effective as surgery or tamoxifen at increasing survival and local disease control.

  Adding tamoxifen or ovarian ablation to radiotherapy increases survival compared with radiotherapy alone, but adding chemotherapy may not reduce recurrence or mortality compared with radiotherapy alone.

  Chemotherapy alone, while widely used, does not improve survival in women with locally advanced breast cancer.

(i) **Please visit www.clinicalevidence.bmj.com for full text and references**

What are the effects of interventions after breast-conserving surgery for ductal carcinoma *in situ*?	
Likely To Be Beneficial	• Radiotherapy (reduced recurrence)
Unknown Effectiveness	• Tamoxifen plus radiotherapy (reduced recurrence in women with oestrogen receptor-positive tumours)

What are the effects of treatments for primary operable breast cancer?

Beneficial	• Adjuvant aromatase inhibitors
	• Adjuvant combination chemotherapy (better than no chemotherapy)
	• Adjuvant tamoxifen (in women with oestrogen receptor-positive tumours)
	• Anthracycline regimens as adjuvant chemotherapy (better than standard CMF [cyclophosphamide, methotrexate, and fluorouracil] regimens)
	• Chemotherapy plus monoclonal antibody (trastuzumab) in women with overexpressed *HER2/neu* oncogene
	• Less-extensive mastectomy (similar survival to more extensive surgery, and better cosmetic outcome)
	• Ovarian ablation in premenopausal women
	• Radiotherapy after breast-conserving surgery (reduced local recurrence and breast cancer mortality compared with breast-conserving surgery alone)
	• Radiotherapy after mastectomy in women at high risk of local recurrence
Likely To Be Beneficial	• Adjuvant taxanes
	• Primary chemotherapy (reduced mastectomy rates and had similar survival rates to adjuvant chemotherapy)
	• Radiotherapy plus tamoxifen after breast-conserving surgery (reduced local recurrence rates)
	• Total nodal radiotherapy
Trade-off Between Benefits And Harms	• Axillary clearance
	• Axillary radiotherapy
	• Axillary sampling
	• Radiotherapy after mastectomy in women not at high risk of local recurrence
Unknown Effectiveness	• Different primary chemotherapy regimens (insufficient evidence regarding which regimen is most effective)
	• Less than whole-breast radiotherapy plus breast-conserving surgery
	• Radiotherapy to the internal mammary chain

	• Radiotherapy to the ipsilateral supraclavicular fossa • Sentinel node biopsy (versus axillary dissection plus sentinel node dissection)
Unlikely To Be Beneficial	• Enhanced dose regimens of adjuvant combination chemotherapy • Prolonged adjuvant combination chemotherapy (8–12 months v 4–6 months)
Likely To Be Ineffective Or Harmful	• High-dose chemotherapy plus autologous stem cell transplantation

What are the effects of interventions in locally advanced breast cancer (stage III B)?

Likely To Be Beneficial	• Adding hormonal treatment to radiotherapy (improves survival compared with radiotherapy alone) • Postoperative radiotherapy (in women also receiving postoperative systemic treatment) • Radiotherapy (similar effectiveness to surgery) • Surgery (similar effectiveness to radiotherapy)
Unknown Effectiveness	• Adding chemotherapy (cyclophosphamide/methotrexate/fluorouracil or anthracycline-based regimens) to radiotherapy • Radiotherapy (low-dose versus tamoxifen)
Unlikely To Be Beneficial	• Hormonal treatment versus multimodal treatment

Search date January 2007

DEFINITION This review examines the effects of treatment for non-metastatic, primary breast cancer. **Ductal carcinoma *in situ*** is a non-invasive tumour characterised by the presence of malignant cells in the breast ducts, but with no evidence that they breach the basement membrane and invade into periductal connective tissues. **Invasive breast cancer** occurs when cancer cells spread beyond the basement membrane, which covers the underlying connective tissue in the breast. This tissue is rich in blood vessels and lymphatic channels capable of carrying cancer cells beyond the breast. Invasive breast cancer can be separated into three main groups: early invasive breast cancer, locally advanced breast cancer, and metastatic breast cancer (see review on breast cancer [metastatic], p 584). **Operable breast cancer** is apparently restricted to the breast and to local lymph nodes, and can be removed surgically. Although women do not have overt metastases at the time of staging, they remain at risk of local recurrence, and of metastatic spread. They can be divided into those with tumours greater than 4 cm or with multifocal cancers that are usually treated by mastectomy, and those with tumours less than 4 cm cancers that can be treated by breast-conserving surgery. **Locally advanced breast cancer** is defined according to the TNM staging system of the UICC as stage IIIB (includes T4 a–d; N2 disease, but absence of metastases). It is a disease presentation with clinical or histopathological evidence of skin and/or chest-wall involvement, and/or axillary nodes matted together by tumour extension. **Metastatic breast cancer** is presented in a separate review (see review on breast cancer [metastatic], p 584).

INCIDENCE/PREVALENCE Breast cancer affects 1/10–1/11 women in the UK and causes about 21,000 deaths a year. Prevalence is about five times higher, with over 100,000 women in the UK living with breast cancer at any one time. Of the 36,000 new cases of breast cancer each year in England and Wales, most will present with primary operable disease.

AETIOLOGY/RISK FACTORS The risk of breast cancer increases with age, doubling every 10 years up to the menopause. Risk factors include an early age at menarche, older age at menopause, older age at birth of first child, family history, atypical hyperplasia, excess alcohol intake, radiation exposure to developing breast tissue, oral contraceptive use, postmenopausal HRT, and postmenopausal obesity. Risk in different countries varies fivefold. The cause of breast cancer in most women is unknown. About 5% of breast cancers can be attributed to mutations in the genes *BRCA1* and *BRCA2*, but the contribution to inherited breast cancer of other genes, including *Chk2*, *ATM*, *p53*, and *PTEN*, is currently less well established.

PROGNOSIS Non-metastatic carcinoma of the breast is potentially curable. The risk of relapse depends on various clinicopathological features, of which axillary node involvement, tumour grade, tumour size, and oestrogen receptor status are the most prognostically important. Of women with operable disease, 80% are alive 5 years after diagnosis and treatment (adjuvant treatment is given to most women after surgery). Risk of recurrence is highest during the first 5 years, but the risk remains even 15–20 years after surgery. Recurrence at 10 years, according to one large systematic review, is 60–70% in node-positive women, and 25–30% in node-negative women. The prognosis for disease-free survival at 5 years is worse for stage IIIB (33%) than that for stage IIIA (71%). Overall survival at 5 years is 44% for stage IIIB and 84% for stage IIIA. Poor survival and high rates of local recurrence characterise locally advanced breast cancer.

Nigel Bundred

KEY POINTS

- Breast pain may be cyclical (worse before a period) or non-cyclical, originating from the breast or the chest wall, and occurs at some time in 70% of women.

   Cyclical breast pain resolves spontaneously in 20–30% of women, but tends to recur in 60% of women.

   Non-cyclical pain responds poorly to treatment but tends to resolve spontaneously in half of women.

- There is a consensus that topical NSAIDs are effective and well tolerated in relieving breast pain.

- Danazol, tamoxifen, toremifene, gonadorelin analogues, and gestrinone may reduce breast pain but can all cause adverse effects.

   Danazol can cause weight gain, deepening of the voice, menorrhagia, and muscle cramps, and has androgenic effects on the fetus.

   Tamoxifen and toremifene may increase the risk of venous thromboembolism and are not licensed for breast pain in the UK or USA.

   Bromocriptine reduces breast pain compared with placebo, but its licence for this indication has been withdrawn in the USA because of frequent and intolerable adverse effects.

   Breast pain may be made worse by HRT, which is also associated with increased risks of breast cancer, venous thromboembolism, and gall bladder disease.

- Evening primrose oil has not been shown to improve breast pain and has had its licence withdrawn for this indication in the UK owing to lack of efficacy.

   We don't know whether a low-fat, high-carbohydrate diet, lisuride, tibolone, progestogens, pyridoxine, diuretics, antibiotics, or vitamin E reduce breast pain, as few studies have been found.

Please visit www.clinicalevidence.bmj.com for full text and references

What are the effects of treatments for breast pain?	
Likely To Be Beneficial	• Topical NSAIDs
Trade-off Between Benefits And Harms	• Danazol • Gestrinone • Gonadorelin analogues (LHRH analogues) • Tamoxifen • Toremifene
Unknown Effectiveness	• Antibiotics • Diet (low fat, high carbohydrate) • Diuretics • Lisuride • Progestogens • Pyridoxine • Tibolone

	• Vitamin E
Unlikely To Be Beneficial	• Danazol compared with tamoxifen (pain relief may be greater with tamoxifen but adverse effects common with both interventions)
	• HRT (oestrogen; use associated with increased risk of breast pain)
Likely To Be Ineffective Or Harmful	• Bromocriptine
	• Evening primrose oil

Search date January 2006

DEFINITION Breast pain can be differentiated into cyclical mastalgia (worse before a menstrual period) or non-cyclical mastalgia (unrelated to the menstrual cycle). Cyclical pain is often bilateral, usually most severe in the upper outer quadrants of the breast, and may be referred to the medial aspect of the upper arm. Non-cyclical pain may be caused by true breast pain or chest wall pain located over the costal cartilages. Specific breast pathology and referred pain unrelated to the breasts are not included in this review.

INCIDENCE/PREVALENCE Up to 70% of women develop breast pain in their lifetime. Of 1171 US women attending a gynaecology clinic for any reason, 69% suffered regular discomfort, which was judged as severe in 11% of women, and 36% had consulted a doctor about breast pain.

AETIOLOGY/RISK FACTORS Breast pain is most common in women aged 30–50 years.

PROGNOSIS Cyclical breast pain resolves spontaneously within 3 months of onset in 20–30% of women. The pain tends to relapse and remit, and up to 60% of women develop recurrent symptoms 2 years after treatment. Non-cyclical pain responds poorly to treatment but may resolve spontaneously in about 50% of women.

Des Spence

KEY POINTS

- Vulvovaginal candidiasis is characterised by vulval itching and abnormal 'cheese-like' or watery vaginal discharge.

  Vulvovaginal candidiasis is estimated to be the second most common cause of vaginitis after bacterial vaginosis. *Candida albicans* accounts for 85–90% of cases.

  Risk factors include pregnancy, diabetes mellitus, and systemic antibiotics. Incidence increases with the onset of sexual activity but associations with different types of contraceptives are unclear.

  Recurrent symptoms are common but are caused by candidiasis in only a third of cases.

- Intravaginal imidazoles reduce symptoms of acute vulvovaginal candidiasis in non-pregnant women.

  Intravaginal imidazoles (butoconazole, clotrimazole, miconazole) reduce symptoms compared to placebo and all seem to have similar efficacy compared with each other. RCTs suggest that single-dose regimens may be as effective as multiple-dose regimens.

  Intravaginal imidazoles seem as effective as oral fluconazole or itraconazole in treating acute attacks.

- Intravaginal nystatin reduces symptoms, but we don't know how it compares with intravaginal imidazoles.

- The benefits of other intravaginal treatments remain unclear, and some may be associated with serious adverse effects.

  We found no evidence assessing intravaginal boric acid or tea tree oil.

  We found no evidence assessing garlic or yoghurt.

  We found no evidence on efficacy of douching, but it is associated with serious adverse effects, such as PID and infections, endometritis, and ectopic pregnancy.

  Oral fluconazole and itraconazole are likely to be beneficial in preventing recurrence of infection.

  Treating the woman's male sexual partner does not reduce symptoms or prevent recurrence in the woman.

ⓘ **Please visit www.clinicalevidence.bmj.com for full text and references**

What are the effects of drug treatments for acute vulvovaginal candidiasis in non-pregnant symptomatic women?	
Beneficial	• Intravaginal imidazoles for acute infection • Oral fluconazole for acute infection • Oral itraconazole for acute infection
Likely To Be Beneficial	• Intravaginal nystatin for acute infection

What are the effects of alternative or complementary treatments for acute vulvovaginal candidiasis in non-pregnant symptomatic women?	
Unknown Effectiveness	• Douching for acute infection • Garlic for acute infection

- Intravaginal boric acid for acute infection

- Intravaginal tea tree oil for acute infection

- Yoghurt containing *Lactobacillus acidophilus* (oral or vaginal) for acute infection

What are the effects of treating a male sexual partner to resolve symptoms and prevent recurrence in non-pregnant women with symptomatic acute vulvovaginal candidiasis?

Unlikely To Be Beneficial	• Treating a male sexual partner to resolve symptoms and prevent symptomatic recurrence in women with symptomatic acute vulvovaginal candidiasis

What are the effects of drug treatments for recurrent vulvovaginal candidiasis in non-pregnant symptomatic women?

Likely To Be Beneficial	• Oral fluconazole to prevent recurrence
	• Oral itraconazole to prevent recurrence
Unknown Effectiveness	• Intravaginal imidazoles to prevent recurrence

What are the effects of alternative or complementary treatments for symptomatic recurrent vulvovaginal candidiasis in non-pregnant women?

Unknown Effectiveness	• Douching to prevent recurrence
	• Garlic to prevent recurrence
	• Intravaginal boric acid to prevent recurrence
	• Intravaginal tea tree oil to prevent recurrence
	• Yoghurt containing *Lactobacillus acidophilus* (oral or vaginal) to prevent recurrence

What are the effects of treating a male sexual partner in non-pregnant women with symptomatic recurrent vulvovaginal candidiasis?

Unknown Effectiveness	• Treating a male sexual partner to resolve symptoms and prevent recurrence in women with symptomatic recurrent vulvovaginal candidiasis

What are the effects of treating asymptomatic non-pregnant women with a positive swab for candidiasis?

Unknown Effectiveness	• Alternative or complementary treatments for asymptomatic women

• Drug treatments for asymptomatic women

Search date October 2006

DEFINITION **Vulvovaginal candidiasis** is defined as symptomatic vaginitis (inflammation of the vagina), which often involves the vulva, caused by infection with a *Candida* yeast. Predominant symptoms are vulval itching and abnormal vaginal discharge (which may be minimal, a "cheese-like" material, or a watery secretion). Differentiation from other forms of vaginitis requires the presence of yeast on microscopy of vaginal fluid. **Recurrent vulvovaginal candidiasis** is commonly defined as four or more symptomatic episodes a year.

INCIDENCE/PREVALENCE Vulvovaginal candidiasis is estimated to be the second most common cause of vaginitis after bacterial vaginosis. Estimates of its incidence are limited and often derived from women who attend hospital clinics. Asymptomatic prevalence has been reported in 10% of women and self-reported history of at least one episode of vulvovaginal candidiasis has been as high as 72%. Recurrent symptoms are common but are caused by candidiasis in only a third of cases.

AETIOLOGY/RISK FACTORS *Candida albicans* accounts for 85–90% of cases of vulvovaginal candidiasis. Development of symptomatic vulvovaginal candidiasis probably represents increased growth of yeast that previously colonised the vagina without causing symptoms. Risk factors for vulvovaginal candidiasis include pregnancy, diabetes mellitus, and systemic antibiotics. The evidence that different types of contraceptives are associated with risk factors is contradictory. The incidence of vulvovaginal candidiasis rises with initiation of sexual activity, but we found no direct evidence that vulvovaginal candidiasis is transmitted sexually.

PROGNOSIS We found few descriptions of the natural history of untreated vulvovaginal candidiasis. Discomfort is the main complication and can include pain while passing urine or during sexual intercourse. Balanitis in male partners of women with vulvovaginal candidiasis can occur, but it is rare.

Cervical cancer

Sudha Sundar, Amanda Horne, and Sean Kehoe

KEY POINTS

- Worldwide, cervical cancer is the second most common cancer in women.

  In the UK, incidence fell after the introduction of the cervical screening programme to the current level of approximately 3200 cases and 1000 deaths a year.

  About 80% of tumours are squamous type, and staging is based on the FIGO classification.

  Survival ranges from almost 100% 5-year disease-free survival for treated stage Ia disease to 5–15% in stage IV disease. Survival is also influenced by tumour bulk, age, and comorbid conditions.

  Development of cervical cancer is strongly associated with HPV infection, acquired mainly by sexual intercourse.

  The peak prevalence of infection is 20–30% in women aged 20–30 years, but in 80% of cases the infection resolves within 12–18 months.

  Other risk factors for cervical cancer include early onset of sexual activity, multiple sexual partners, long-term use of oral contraceptives, tobacco smoking, low socioeconomic status, immunosuppressive therapy, and micronutrient deficiency.

- Vaccination against HPV is effective in preventing certain types of HPV infection, and at reducing rates of cervical intraepithelial neoplasia, but there has been insufficient long-term follow-up to assess effects on cervical cancer rates.

- Conisation with adequate excision margins is considered effective for microinvasive carcinoma, and can preserve fertility; however, it is associated with an increased risk of preterm delivery and low birthweight.

  Conisation is often performed for stage Ia1 disease, but evidence for its benefit is from observational studies only.

- Radical trachelectomy plus lymphadenectomy can lead to similar long-term survival rates as radical hysterectomy, but with preserved fertility.

  Limited evidence shows that radical trachelectomy plus lymphadenectomy results in similar disease-free survival in women with early-stage cervical cancer compared with radical hysterectomy, but has higher intraoperative complications, and up to 8% recurrence of carcinoma.

- Limited evidence shows that radiotherapy is as effective as surgery in early-stage disease.

  Overall and disease-free survival are similar after radiotherapy or radical hysterectomy plus lymphadenectomy, but radiotherapy is less likely to cause severe adverse effects.

- Chemoradiotherapy improves survival compared with radiotherapy in women with bulky early-stage cervical cancer.

  Combined chemoradiotherapy improves overall and progression-free survival when used either before or after hysterectomy, but is associated with more haematological and gastrointestinal toxicity compared with radiotherapy alone.

- The benefits of neoadjuvant chemotherapy plus surgery compared with radiotherapy alone are unknown.

Please visit www.clinicalevidence.bmj.com for full text and references

What are the effects of interventions to manage early-stage cervical cancer?

Likely To Be Beneficial	• Conisation of the cervix for microinvasive carcinoma (stage Ia1)*

	• Radiotherapy versus surgery (consensus that both likely to be beneficial but unclear how they compare)*
Unknown Effectiveness	• Radical trachelectomy plus lymphadenectomy (preserved fertility compared with hysterectomy)

What are the effects of interventions to prevent cervical cancer?

Unknown Effectiveness	• HPV vaccine (reduces rates of HPV infection and CIN but effects on rates of cervical cancer unclear)

What are the effects of interventions to manage bulky early-stage cervical cancer?

Beneficial	• Chemoradiotherapy (increased survival compared with radiotherapy alone)
Unknown Effectiveness	• Neoadjuvant chemotherapy

Search date November 2006

*Based on consensus

DEFINITION Cervical cancer is a malignant neoplasm arising from the uterine cervix. About 80% of cervical cancers are of the squamous type; the remainder are adenocarcinomas, adenosquamous carcinomas, and other rare types. Staging of cervical cancer is based on clinical evaluation. Management is determined by tumour bulk and stage. **Population:** This review deals with treatments for early-stage cancer (defined as FIGO stage Ia1, Ia2, Ib1, and small IIa tumours) and bulky early-stage disease (defined as FIGO stage Ib2 and larger IIa tumours).

INCIDENCE/PREVALENCE Cervical cancer is the second most common cancer in women, with about 450,000 new cases diagnosed worldwide each year. Most (80%) cases occur in resource-poor countries that have no effective screening programmes. The incidence of cervical cancer in the UK and Europe has greatly reduced since the introduction of a screening programme for detecting precancerous cervical intraepithelial neoplasia. Cervical cancer incidence fell by 42% between 1988 and 1997 in England and Wales. This fall has been reported to be related to the cervical screening programme. In England and Wales, cervical cancer has an annual incidence of 3200 women, and causes about 1000 deaths each year.

AETIOLOGY/RISK FACTORS Risk factors for cervical cancer include sexual intercourse at an early age, multiple sexual partners, tobacco smoking, long-term oral contraceptive use, low socioeconomic status, immunosuppressive therapy, and micronutrient deficiency. Persistent infection by oncogenic, high-risk strains of HPV is strongly associated with the development of cervical cancer. HPV strains 16 and 18 cause about 70% of cervical cancer and high-grade cervical intraepithelial neoplasia. The virus is acquired mainly by sexual intercourse, and has a peak prevalence of 20–30% in women aged 20–30 years, although in 80% of cases the infection is transient and resolves within 12–18 months.

PROGNOSIS Overall, 5-year disease-free survival is 50–70% for stages Ib2 and IIb, 30–50% for stage III, and 5–15% for stage IV. In women who receive treatment, 5-year survival in stage Ia approaches 100%, falling to 70–85% for stage Ib1 and smaller IIa tumours. Survival in women with more locally advanced tumours is influenced by tumour bulk, the person's age, and coexistent medical conditions. Untreated mortality in locally advanced disease is high.

Michelle L Proctor and Cynthia M Farquhar

KEY POINTS

- Dysmenorrhoea may begin soon after the menarche, in which case it often improves with age, or it may originate later in life after the onset of an underlying causative condition.

  Dysmenorrhoea is common, and in up to 20% of women it may be severe enough to interfere with daily activities.

  Dysmenorrhoea is more likely in women who smoke, in those with an earlier age at menarche, or with longer duration of menstruation.

- NSAIDs, reduce moderate to severe pain in women with primary dysmenorrhoea compared with placebo, but we don't know whether any one NSAID is superior.

  Aspirin, paracetamol, and compound analgesics may reduce pain in the short term, although few studies have been of good quality.

  The herbal remedy toki-shakuyaku-san may reduce pain after 6 months compared with placebo, but we don't know whether any other herbal remedy is beneficial.

  Thiamine and vitamin E may reduce pain compared with placebo in women with primary dysmenorrhoea.

- We don't know whether combined oral contraceptives reduce the pain of dysmenorrhoea, as studies have been small and have used products that are no longer available.

- Topical heat (about 39 °C) may be as effective as ibuprofen and more effective than paracetamol at reducing pain.

  High-frequency TENS may reduce pain compared with sham TENS, but seems less effective than ibuprofen.

  Acupressure may be more effective than sham acupressure at relieving dysmenorrhoea, and may be as effective as ibuprofen at relieving pain.

  Spinal manipulation seems to be no more effective than placebo at reducing pain after 1 month in women with primary dysmenorrhoea.

  We don't know whether acupuncture, relaxation or aerobic exercise, fish oil, magnesium, vitamin B12, surgical interruption of pelvic nerve pathways, or magnets reduce dysmenorrhoea, as few studies have been found.

ⓘ Please visit www.clinicalevidence.bmj.com for full text and references

What are the effects of treatments for dysmenorrhoea?	
Beneficial	• NSAIDs (other than aspirin)
Likely To Be Beneficial	• Acupressure
	• Aspirin, paracetamol, and compound analgesics
	• TENS (high-frequency stimulation only; effects of low-frequency stimulation remain unclear)
	• Thiamine
	• Toki-shakuyaku-san (herbal remedy)
	• Topical heat (about 39 °C)

	• Vitamin E
Unknown Effectiveness	• Acupuncture
	• Behavioural interventions
	• Combined oral contraceptives
	• Fish oil
	• Herbal remedies other than toki-shakuyaku-san
	• Magnesium
	• Magnets
	• Surgical interruption of pelvic nerve pathways
	• Vitamin B_{12}
Unlikely To Be Beneficial	• Spinal manipulation

Search date July 2006

DEFINITION Dysmenorrhoea is painful menstrual cramps of uterine origin. It is commonly divided into primary dysmenorrhoea (pain without organic pathology) and secondary dysmenorrhoea (pelvic pain associated with an identifiable pathological condition, such as endometriosis [see endometriosis, p 599] or ovarian cysts). The initial onset of primary dysmenorrhoea is usually shortly after menarche (6–12 months), when ovulatory cycles are established. Pain duration is commonly 8–72 hours and is usually associated with the onset of menstrual flow. Secondary dysmenorrhoea can also occur at any time after menarche, but may arise as a new symptom during a woman's fourth and fifth decades, after the onset of an underlying causative condition. This review deals with both primary and secondary dysmenorrhoea; however, it should be noted that most RCTs are in women with primary dysmenorrhoea. Endometriosis, which can cause secondary dysmenorrhoea, is covered in a separate review (see endometriosis, p 599).

INCIDENCE/PREVALENCE Variations in the definition of dysmenorrhoea make it difficult to determine prevalence precisely. Studies tend to report on prevalence in adolescent girls, and the type of dysmenorrhoea is not always specified. Adolescent girls tend to have a higher prevalence of primary dysmenorrhoea than older women, as primary dysmenorrhoea can improve with age (see prognosis). Secondary dysmenorrhoea rates may be lower in adolescents, as onset of causative conditions may not yet have occurred. Therefore, the results from prevalence studies of adolescents may not always be extrapolated to older women, or be accurate estimates of the prevalence of secondary dysmenorrhoea. However, various types of studies have found a consistently high prevalence in women of different ages and nationalities. One systematic review (search date 1996) of the prevalence of chronic pelvic pain, summarising both community and hospital surveys from developed countries, estimated prevalence to be 45–95%. A second systematic review of studies in resource-poor countries (search date 2002) found that 25–50% of adult women and about 75% of adolescents experienced pain with menstruation, with 5–20% reporting severe dysmenorrhoea or pain that prevents them from participating in their usual activities.

AETIOLOGY/RISK FACTORS A longitudinal study of a representative sample of women born in 1962, residing in Göteborg, Sweden, found that the severity of dysmenorrhoea was significantly associated with the duration of menstrual flow (average duration of menstrual flow was 5.0 days for women with no dysmenorrhoea and 5.8 days for women with severe dysmenorrhoea, where severe dysmenorrhoea was defined as pain that did not respond well to analgesics and clearly inhibited daily activity; P less than 0.001; WMD −0.80, 95% CI −1.36 to −0.24); younger age at menarche (13.1 years in women without dysmenorrhoea v 12.6 years in women with severe dysmenorrhoea; P less than 0.01; WMD 0.50, 95% CI 0.09 to 0.91); and cigarette smoking (41% of smokers and 26% of non-smokers experienced moderate or severe dysmenorrhoea). There is also some evidence of a dose–response relationship between exposure to environmental tobacco smoke and increased incidence of dysmenorrhoea.

PROGNOSIS Primary dysmenorrhoea is a chronic recurring condition that affects most young women. Studies of the natural history of this condition are sparse. One longitudinal study in Scandinavia found that primary dysmenorrhoea often improves in the third decade of a woman's reproductive life, and is also reduced after childbirth. We found no studies that reliably examined the relationship between the prognosis of secondary dysmenorrhoea and the severity of the underlying pathology, such as endometriosis.

Neil Johnson and Cynthia M. Farquhar

KEY POINTS

- Ectopic endometrial tissue is found in up to 20% of asymptomatic women, up to 60% of those with dysmenorrhoea, and up to 30% of women with subfertility, with a peak incidence at around 40 years of age. However, symptoms may not correlate with laparoscopic findings.

   Without treatment, endometrial deposits may resolve spontaneously in up to a third of women, deteriorate in nearly half, and remain unchanged in the remainder.

   Oral contraceptives reduce the risk of endometriosis, whereas an early menarche and late menopause increase the risk.

- Hormonal treatments (oral contraceptives, danazol, gestrinone, gonadorelin analogues, and medroxyprogesterone acetate) can reduce the pain attributed to endometriosis when given at diagnosis, but adverse effects are common.

   Combined oral contraceptives may be less effective than gonadorelin analogues, but are less likely to reduce bone-mineral density or to cause other adverse effects, such as hot flushes and vaginal dryness.

   We do not know whether hormonal treatment given before surgery makes it easier to perform surgery, or reduces subsequent pain.

- Laparoscopic removal of endometrial deposits reduces pain and improves quality of life compared with no removal, but it can be complicated by adhesions and damage to other pelvic structures.

   Combining laparoscopic removal of deposits with uterine nerve ablation may improve pain relief compared with diagnostic laparoscopy alone, but we do not know whether uterine nerve ablation alone is of any benefit in reducing symptoms.

   Laparoscopic excision of endometrial cysts in the ovary may reduce pelvic pain and recurrence of cysts compared with laparoscopic drainage and cyst wall electrosurgical ablation, with similar risks of adverse effects.

- The hormonal treatments danazol, medroxyprogesterone acetate, and gonadorelin analogues may reduce pain and other symptoms when given for 6 months after conservative surgery, although studies of other hormonal treatments have given conflicting results.

- We do not know whether HRT prevents or promotes recurrence of endometriosis in women who have had oophorectomy.

(i) **Please visit www.clinicalevidence.bmj.com for full text and references**

What are the effects of hormonal treatments given at diagnosis of endometriosis?	
Beneficial	• Combined oral contraceptives at diagnosis
	• Progestogens (other than dydrogesterone) at diagnosis
Trade-off Between Benefits And Harms	• Danazol, gestrinone, or gonadorelin analogues at diagnosis
Unknown Effectiveness	• Dydrogesterone at diagnosis

What are the effects of hormonal treatments before surgery for endometriosis?

Unknown Effectiveness	• Hormonal treatment before surgery

What are the effects of non-hormonal medical treatments for endometriosis?

Unknown Effectiveness	• NSAIDs

What are the effects of surgical treatments for endometriosis?

Likely To Be Beneficial	• Laparoscopic removal of endometriotic deposits alone • Laparoscopic removal of endometriotic deposits plus uterine nerve ablation
Unknown Effectiveness	• Laparoscopic removal plus presacral neurectomy • Laparoscopic uterine nerve ablation alone • Presacral neurectomy alone

What are the effects of hormonal treatment after conservative surgery for endometriosis?

Likely To Be Beneficial	• Hormonal treatment after conservative surgery

What are the effects of hormonal treatment after oophorectomy (with or without hysterectomy) for endometriosis?

Unknown Effectiveness	• Hormonal treatment after oophorectomy

What are the effects of treatments for ovarian endometrioma?

Likely To Be Beneficial	• Laparoscopic cystectomy for ovarian endometrioma (reduces pain compared with drainage and cyst wall electrosurgical ablation)

Search date April 2006

DEFINITION Endometriosis is characterised by ectopic endometrial tissue, which can cause dysmenorrhoea, dyspareunia, non-cyclical pelvic pain, and subfertility. Diagnosis is made by laparoscopy. Most endometrial deposits are found in the pelvis (ovaries, peritoneum, uterosacral ligaments, pouch of Douglas, and rectovaginal septum). Extrapelvic deposits, including those in the umbilicus and diaphragm, are rare. Severity of endometriosis is

(continued over)

(from previous page)

defined by the American Fertility Society: this review uses the terms mild (stage I and II), moderate (stage III), and severe (stage IV). Endometriomas are cysts of endometriosis within the ovary. This review assesses dysmenorrhoea, dyspareunia (painful sexual intercourse), dyschezia (painful defecation), and non-cyclical pelvic pain associated with endometriosis. For infertility associated with endometriosis, see female infertility, p 602.

INCIDENCE/PREVALENCE In asymptomatic women, the prevalence of endometriosis is 2–22%. Variations in estimates of prevalence are thought to be mostly because of differences in diagnostic thresholds and criteria between studies, and in variations in childbearing age between populations, rather than underlying genetic differences. In women with dysmenorrhoea, the incidence of endometriosis is 40–60%, and in women with subfertility it is 20–30%. The severity of symptoms and the probability of diagnosis increase with age. Incidence peaks at about 40 years of age. Symptoms and laparoscopic appearance do not always correlate.

AETIOLOGY/RISK FACTORS The cause of endometriosis is unknown. Risk factors include early menarche and late menopause. Embryonic cells may give rise to deposits in the umbilicus, whereas retrograde menstruation may deposit endometrial cells in the diaphragm. Use of oral contraceptives reduces the risk of endometriosis, and this protective effect persists for up to 1 year after their discontinuation.

PROGNOSIS We found two RCTs in which laparoscopy was repeated after treatment in women given placebo. Over 6–12 months, endometrial deposits resolved spontaneously in up to a third of women, deteriorated in nearly half, and were unchanged in the remainder.

Hesham Al-Inany

KEY POINTS

- About 17% of couples in industrialised countries seek help for infertility, which may be caused by ovulatory failure, tubal damage or endometriosis, or a low sperm count.

- In women with infertility, in vitro fertilisation may be as likely to lead to pregnancy as intracytoplasmic sperm injection, but increases the risks of multiple pregnancy.

  GnRH agonists also increase pregnancy rates, but GnRH antagonists may be less effective.

  Intrauterine insemination plus controlled ovarian stimulation is considered beneficial in women with unexplained infertility or cervical hostility.

- In women with ovulatory disorders, clomifene and tamoxifen increase ovulation and pregnancy rates, and metformin increases ovulation rates.

  Gonadotrophins may increase pregnancy rates, but may increase the risk of ovarian cancer, ovarian hyperstimulation syndrome, and multiple pregnancy.

  Laparoscopic ovarian drilling may be as effective as gonadotrophins.

  We don't know whether cyclofenil, pulsed GnRG, gonadotrophin priming of oocytes before in vitro maturation, or ovarian wedge biopsy increase pregnancy rates compared with no treatment.

- In women with tubal infertility, tubal flushing increases pregnancy rates, with oil soluble media possibly more effective than water-soluble media.

  Tubal surgery before in vitro fertilisation may increase pregnancy rates compared with no treatment in women with hydrosalpinges, but we don't know whether selective salpingography plus tubal catheterisation is beneficial.

- In women with endometriosis, adding gonadotrophins to intrauterine insemination increases live birth rates compared with intrauterine insemination alone.

  Laparoscopic ablation of endometrial deposits may increase live birth rates compared with diagnostic laparoscopy.

  Drugs to induce ovarian suppression may not increase pregnancy rates.

Please visit www.clinicalevidence.bmj.com for full text and references

What are the effects of treatments for infertility caused by ovulation disorders?	
Likely To Be Beneficial	• Clomifene • In vitro fertilisation in ovulation disorders* • Metformin
Trade-off Between Benefits And Harms	• Gonadotrophins
Unknown Effectiveness	• Cyclofenil • Gonadotrophin priming of oocytes before in vitro maturation • GnRH agonists plus gonadotrophins • GnRH antagonists

- Intrauterine insemination plus controlled ovarian stimulation

- Laparoscopic ovarian drilling

- Ovarian wedge biopsy

- Pulsatile GnRH

- Tamoxifen

What are the effects of treatments for tubal infertility?

Beneficial	• In vitro fertilisation in tubal obstruction*
Likely To Be Beneficial	• Tubal flushing with oil soluble media
	• Tubal surgery before in vitro fertilisation
Unknown Effectiveness	• Selective salpingography plus tubal catheterisation
	• Tubal flushing with water soluble media

What are the effects of treatments for infertility associated with endometriosis?

Likely To Be Beneficial	• Intrauterine insemination plus gonadotrophins
	• In vitro fertilisation in endometriosis*
	• Laparoscopic ablation of endometrial deposits
Likely To Be Ineffective Or Harmful	• Drug-induced ovarian suppression

Search date April 2004

*No RCTs, but strong observational evidence that in vitro fertilisation increases live birth rates.

DEFINITION This review focuses on infertility related to factors associated with the woman rather than the man. Normal fertility has been defined as achieving a pregnancy within 2 years by regular unprotected sexual intercourse. However, many define infertility as the failure to conceive after 1 year of unprotected intercourse. Infertility can be primary, in women who have never conceived, or secondary, in women who have previously conceived. This review will deal with infertility owing to endometriosis, ovulation disorders, and tubal infertility. Endometriosis is a progressive disease which occurs when the endometrial tissue lining the uterus grows outside the uterus and attaches to the ovaries, fallopian tubes, or other organs in the abdominal cavity (See endometriosis, p 602). Ovulation disorders are defined by the failure of an ovum to be expelled because of a malfunction in the ovary, and are a major cause of infertility. Tubal infertility is the inability to conceive owing to a blockage in one or both fallopian tubes, and is a common cause of infertility.

INCIDENCE/PREVALENCE Although there is no evidence of a major change in the prevalence of female infertility, many more couples are seeking help than previously. Currently, about 1/6 (17%) couples in industrialised countries will seek medical advice for infertility. Rates of primary infertility vary widely between countries, ranging from less than

6% in China, Malawi, Tanzania, and Zambia; 9% in the Philippines; more than 10% in Finland, Sweden, and Canada; and 18% in Switzerland. Reported rates of secondary infertility are less reliable.

AETIOLOGY/RISK FACTORS In the UK, about 10–20% of infertility cases are unexplained. The rest are caused by ovulatory failure (27%), tubal damage (14%), endometriosis (5%), low sperm count or quality (19%), and other causes (5%).

PROGNOSIS In resource-rich countries, 80–90% of couples attempting to conceive are successful after 1 year and 95% after 2 years. The chances of becoming pregnant vary with the cause and duration of infertility, the woman's age, the woman's previous pregnancy history, and the availability of different treatment options. For the first 2–3 years of unexplained infertility, cumulative conception rates remain high (27–46%) but decrease with increasing age of the woman and duration of infertility. The background rates of spontaneous pregnancy in infertile couples can be calculated from longitudinal studies of infertile couples who have been observed without treatment.

Anne Lethaby and Beverley Vollenhoven

KEY POINTS

- Between 5–77% of women may have fibroids, depending on the method of diagnosis used. Fibroids may be asymptomatic, or may present with menorrhagia, pain, infertility, or recurrent pregnancy loss.

  Risk factors for fibroids include obesity, having no children, and no long-term use of the oral contraceptive pill. Fibroids tend to shrink or fibrose after the menopause.

- Gonadorelin analogues (GnRHa) reduce bleeding compared with placebo, but can cause menopausal symptoms and bone loss, which may limit their long-term use.

  Adding progesterone, tibolone, or raloxifene to GnRHa may prevent these adverse effects, but their addition doesn't produce any greater effect on fibroid symptoms compared with GnRHa alone.

- We don't know whether NSAIDs or the levonorgestrel intrauterine system improve symptoms of fibroids.

- GnRHa given before fibroid surgery reduce bleeding, and increase the likelihood of having a vaginal rather than abdominal hysterectomy, but increase anti-oestrogenic adverse effects (such as hot flushes, change in breast size, vaginal symptoms).

- Total abdominal hysterectomy is considered to be beneficial in reducing fibroid-related symptoms, but total vaginal hysterectomy and total laparoscopic hysterectomy may have lower risks of complications, and shorter recovery times.

  Laparoscopically assisted vaginal hysterectomy may increase operative times and blood loss compared with total vaginal hysterectomy.

- Myomectomy maintains fertility, but we don't know whether it is better at reducing fibroid symptoms compared with hysterectomy.

  Laparoscopic myomectomy reduces complications and recovery time compared with abdominal myomectomy.

  We don't know whether thermal myolysis with laser, hysteroscopic resection, thermal balloon ablation, or rollerball ablation, or magnetic resonance-guided focused ultrasound surgery are beneficial in women with fibroids compared with hysterectomy, as we found no studies.

(i) Please visit www.clinicalevidence.bmj.com for full text and references

What are the effects of medical treatment alone in women with fibroids?

Likely To Be Beneficial	• GnRHa plus progestogen (no significant difference in heavy bleeding compared with GnRHa alone, but adding progestogen reduces vasomotor symptoms and hot flushes associated with GnRHa
	• GnRHa plus raloxifene (reduces fibroid size and bone mineral density loss, no significant difference in fibroid related symptoms, cognitive measures, mood, quality of life, and hot flushes)
	• GnRHa plus tibolone (no significant difference in fibroid symptoms compared with GnRHa alone, but

	adding tibolone reduces hot flushes and prevents loss in bone mineral density associated with GnRHa).
Trade-off Between Benefits And Harms	● GnRHa alone
Unknown Effectiveness	● GnRHa plus combined oestrogen–progestogen (insufficient evidence on effects compared with GnRHa plus progestogen) ● GnRHa plus tibolone (similar reductions in bone mineral density compared with hysterectomy plus oophorectomy) ● Levonorgestrel intrauterine system ● NSAIDs

In women scheduled for fibroid surgery, what are the effects of preoperative medical treatments?

Likely To Be Beneficial	● GnRHa

What are the effects of surgical treatments in women with fibroids?

Beneficial	● Laparoscopic myomectomy (maintains fertility compared with hysterectomy; reduces recovery time and postoperative pain compared with abdominal myomectomy)
Likely To Be Beneficial	● Laparoscopically assisted vaginal hysterectomy (reduces recovery time and postoperative pain compared with total abdominal hysterectomy, but increases operating time and blood loss compared with total vaginal hysterectomy) ● Total abdominal hysterectomy (reduces fibroid related symptoms compared with no treatment)* ● Total abdominal myomectomy (maintains fertility compared with hysterectomy but increases recovery time and postoperative pain compared with laparoscopic myomectomy) ● Total laparoscopic hysterectomy (reduces postoperative fever, hospital stay, and recovery time compared with total abdominal hysterectomy) ● Total vaginal hysterectomy (reduces operation time, blood loss, pain, fever, and hospital stay compared with total abdominal hysterectomy, and increases satisfaction with operation)
Unknown Effectiveness	● Hysteroscopic resection

- Magnetic resonance-guided focused ultrasound (magnetic resonance imaging-guided focused ultrasound surgery)
- Rollerball endometrial ablation
- Thermal balloon ablation
- Thermal myolysis with laser

Search date November 2006

*Based on consensus; RCTs unlikely to be conducted.

DEFINITION Fibroids (uterine leiomyomas) are benign tumours of the smooth muscle cells of the uterus. Women with fibroids can be asymptomatic, or may present with menorrhagia (30%), pelvic pain with or without dysmenorrhoea or pressure symptoms (34%), infertility (27%), and recurrent pregnancy loss (3%). Much of the data describing the relationship between the presence of fibroids and symptoms are based on uncontrolled studies that have assessed the effect of myomectomy on the presenting symptoms. One observational study (142 women) undertaken in the USA suggested that the prevalence of fibroids in infertile women can be as high as 13%, but no direct causal relationship between fibroids and infertility has been established.

INCIDENCE/PREVALENCE The reported incidence of fibroids varies from 5.4–77.0%, depending on the method of diagnosis used (the gold standard is histological evidence). It is not possible to state the actual incidence of fibroids, because some women with fibroids will not have symptoms, and will therefore not be tested for fibroids. Observational evidence suggests that, in premenopausal women, the incidence of fibroids increases with age, reducing during menopause. Based on postmortem examination, 50% of women were found to have these tumours. Gross serial sectioning at 2 mm intervals of 100 consecutive hysterectomy specimens revealed the presence of fibroids in 50/68 (73%) premenopausal women and 27/32 (84%) postmenopausal women. These women were having hysterectomies for reasons other than fibroids. The incidence of fibroids in black women is three times greater than that in white women, based on ultrasound or hysterectomy diagnosis. Submucosal fibroids have been diagnosed in 6–34% of women having a hysteroscopy for abnormal bleeding, and in 2–7% of women having infertility investigations.

AETIOLOGY/RISK FACTORS The cause of fibroids is unknown. Each fibroid is of monoclonal origin and arises independently. Factors thought to be involved include the sex steroid hormones oestrogen and progesterone, as well as the insulin-like growth factors, epidermal growth factor, and transforming growth factor. Risk factors for fibroid growth include nulliparity, and obesity. Risk also reduces consistently with increasing number of term pregnancies; women with five term pregnancies have a quarter of the risk of nulliparous women (P less than 0.001). Obesity increases the risk of fibroid development by 21% with each 10 kg weight gain (P = 0.008). The combined oral contraceptive pill also reduces the risk of fibroids with increasing duration of use (women who have taken oral contraceptives for 4–6 years compared with women who have never taken oral contraceptives: OR 0.8, 95% CI 0.5 to 1.2; women who have taken oral contraceptives for at least 7 years compared with women who have never taken oral contraceptives: OR 0.5, 95% CI 0.3 to 0.9). Women who have had injections containing 150 mg depot medroxyprogesterone acetate also have a reduced incidence compared with women who have never had injections of this drug (OR 0.44, 95% CI 0.36 to 0.55).

PROGNOSIS There are few data on the long-term untreated prognosis of these tumours, particularly in women asymptomatic at diagnosis. One small case control study reported that, in a group of 106 women treated with observation alone over 1 year, there was no significant change in symptoms and quality of life over that time. Fibroids tend to shrink or fibrose after the menopause.

Joseph Loze Onwude

KEY POINTS

- Prolapse of the uterus or vagina is usually the result of loss of pelvic muscle support, and causes mainly non-specific symptoms. It may affect over half of women aged 50–59 years, but spontaneous regression may occur.

  Risks of genital prolapse increase with advancing parity and age, increasing weight of the largest baby delivered, and hysterectomy.

- We don't know whether pelvic floor muscle exercises or vaginal oestrogen improve symptoms in women with genital prolapse, as we found no studies of adequate quality.

  The consensus is that vaginal pessaries are effective for relief of symptoms in women waiting for surgery, or in whom surgery is contraindicated, but we don't know this for sure.

- In women with upper vaginal-wall prolapse, abdominal sacral colpopexy reduces the risk of recurrent prolapse, dyspareunia, and stress incontinence compared with sacrospinous colpopexy.

  Posterior intravaginal slingplasty may be as effective as vaginal sacrospinous colpopexy at preventing recurrent prolapse.

  Abdominal sacrohysteropexy may reduce the recurrence of prolapse, but be less effective at reducing symptoms, compared with vaginal hysterectomy and repair.

- In women with anterior vaginal-wall prolapse, anterior vaginal wall repair may be more effective than Burch colposuspension, and recurrence can be further reduced by adding mesh reinforcement to anterior colporrhaphy.

  In women with posterior vaginal-wall prolapse, posterior colporrhaphy is more likely to prevent recurrence than transanal repair of rectocoele or enterocoele.

  We don't know whether adding mesh reinforcement improves success rates in women having posterior colporrhaphy.

- We don't know how surgical treatment compares with non-surgical treatment in women with prolapse of the upper, anterior, or posterior vaginal wall.

(i) Please visit www.clinicalevidence.bmj.com for full text and references

What are the effects of non-surgical treatments in women with genital prolapse?

Likely To Be Beneficial	• Vaginal pessaries*
Unknown Effectiveness	• Pelvic-floor muscle exercises • Vaginal oestrogen

What are the effects of surgical treatments in women with genital prolapse?

Beneficial	• Abdominal sacral colpopexy versus sacrospinous colpopexy (vaginal sacral colpopexy) for upper vaginal-wall vault prolapse • Anterior colporrhaphy with mesh reinforcement versus traditional anterior colporrhaphy in women with anterior vaginal-wall prolapse

	• Posterior colporrhaphy versus transanal repair in women with posterior vaginal-wall prolapse
	• Traditional anterior colporrhaphy versus abdominal Burch colposuspension in women with anterior vaginal-wall prolapse
Likely To Be Beneficial	• Abdominal sacrohysteropexy versus vaginal hysterectomy and repair for upper vaginal-wall prolapse
	• Posterior colporrhaphy with mesh versus posterior colporrhaphy without mesh reinforcement in women with posterior vaginal-wall prolapse
	• Posterior intravaginal slingplasty (infracoccygeal sacropexy) versus vaginal sacrospinous colpopexy for upper vaginal-wall prolapse
	• Ultralateral anterior colporrhaphy versus traditional anterior colporrhaphy
Unknown Effectiveness	• Different types of suture versus each other
	• Mesh or synthetic grafts versus native (autologous) tissue
	• Open abdominal surgery versus laparoscopic surgery
	• Surgical versus non-surgical treatment in women with anterior vaginal-wall prolapse
	• Surgical versus non-surgical treatment in women with posterior vaginal-wall prolapse
	• Surgical versus non-surgical treatment in women with upper vaginal-wall prolapse
Unlikely To Be Beneficial	• Ultralateral anterior colporrhaphy with cadaveric fascia patch versus ultralateral anterior colporrhaphy alone in women with anterior vaginal-wall prolapse

Search date August 2006

*Consensus regards vaginal pessaries as effective.

DEFINITION Genital prolapse (also known as pelvic organ prolapse) refers to uterine, uterovaginal, or vaginal prolapse. Genital prolapse has several causes but occurs primarily from loss of muscle support in the pelvic region. For ease of understanding, in this review we have attempted to use the most common and descriptive terminology. In uterine prolapse the uterus descends into the vaginal canal with the cervix at its leading edge; this may, in turn, pull down the vagina, in which case it may be referred to as uterovaginal prolapse. In the case of vaginal prolapse, one or more regions of the vaginal wall protrude into the vaginal canal. Vaginal prolapse is classified according to the region of the vaginal wall that is affected: a cystocoele involves the upper anterior vaginal wall, urethrocoele the lower anterior vaginal wall, rectocoele the lower posterior vaginal wall, and enterocoele the upper posterior vaginal wall. After hysterectomy, the apex of the vagina may prolapse as a vault prolapse. This usually pulls down the anterior and posterior vaginal walls as well. The two main systems for grading the severity of genital prolapse are the Baden–Walker halfway system and the Pelvic Organ Prolapse Quantification (POPQ) system. Mild genital prolapse may be asymptomatic. Symptoms of genital prolapse are mainly non-specific. Common symptoms include pelvic heaviness, genital bulge, and difficulties during sexual intercourse, such as pain or loss of vaginal sensation. Symptoms that may be more commonly associated with specific forms of prolapse include urinary incontinence, which is associated with cystocoele; incomplete urinary emptying, which is associated with cystocoele or uterine prolapse, or both; and need to apply digital pressure to the perineum or posterior vaginal wall for defaecation, which is associated with rectocoele.

INCIDENCE/PREVALENCE Prevalence estimates vary widely, depending on the population and the way in which women were recruited into studies. One study conducted in the USA (497 women aged 18–82 years attending a routine general gynaecology clinic) found that 93.6% had some degree of genital prolapse (43.3% POPQ stage 1, 47.7% POPQ stage 2, 2.6% POPQ stage 3, and 0% POPQ stage 4). In that study the incidence of clinically relevant prolapse (POPQ stage 2 or above) was found to increase with advancing parity: non-parous, 14.6%; one to three births, 48.0%; and more than three births, 71.2%. One Swedish study (487 women) found that 30.8% of women between the ages of 20 and 59 years had some degree of genital prolapse on clinical assessment. The prevalence of genital prolapse increased with age, from 6.6% in women aged 20–29 years to 55.6% in women aged 50–59 years. A cross-sectional study (241 perimenopausal women aged 45–55 years seeking to enter a trial of HRT) found that 23% had POPQ stage 1 genital prolapse, 4% had POPQ stage 2 prolapse, and no women had POPQ stage 3 or 4 prolapse. One cross-sectional study conducted in the UK (285 perimenopausal and postmenopausal women attending a menopause clinic with climacteric symptoms) found that 20% had some degree of uterovaginal or vault prolapse, 51% some degree of anterior wall vaginal prolapse, and 27% some degree of posterior wall vaginal prolapse. Severe prolapse (equivalent to POPQ stage 3 or 4) was found in 6% of women. One prospective study (412 postmenopausal women aged 50–79 years) found that the baseline prevalence of cystocoele was 24.6% (prevalence for grade 1 was 14.4%, 2 was 9.5%, and 3 was 0.7%), the baseline prevalence of rectocoele was 12.9% (prevalence for grade 1 was 7.8% and 2 was 5.1%), and the baseline prevalence of uterine prolapse was 3.8% (prevalence for grade 1 was 3.3% and 2 was 0.6%). Among women who entered the study, the annual incidence of cystocoele was 9%, rectocoele was 6%, and uterine prolapse was 2%.

AETIOLOGY/RISK FACTORS The strongest risk factor for pelvic organ prolapse is parity, because childbirth can cause damage to the pudendal nerves, fascia, and supporting structures, as well as muscle. A Swedish population-based study found that the prevalence of genital prolapse was higher in parous women (44%) than in non-parous women (5.8%). In addition, it found an association with pelvic floor muscle tone and genital prolapse. One case control study found that other strong risk factors for severe (POPQ stages 3 or 4) genital prolapse are increasing age (OR 1.12 for each additional year, 95% CI 1.09 to 1.15), increasing weight of largest baby delivered vaginally (OR 1.24 for each additional 1 lb [450 g], 95% CI 1.06 to 1.44), previous hysterectomy (OR 2.37, 95% CI 1.16 to 4.86), and previous surgery for genital prolapse (OR 5.09, 95% CI 1.49 to 17.26). The study did not find a significant association between severe genital prolapse and chronic medical conditions such as obesity, hypertension, or COPD.

PROGNOSIS We found no reliable information about the natural history of untreated mild genital prolapse (POPQ stages 1 and 2, Baden–Walker grades 1 and 2). We found one prospective study on the progression of genital prolapse in women who were treated or untreated with HRT (oestrogen plus progesterone). However, the results were not reported separately by treatment group and therefore they may not apply to untreated women. In addition, the investigators used an examination technique whose reliability, reproducibility, and ability to discriminate between absence of prolapse and mild prolapse was not known. It found that, over 1 year, cystocoeles progressed from grade 1 to grades 2–3 in 9% of cases, regressed from grades 2–3 to grade 0 in 9%, and regressed from grade 1 to grade 0 in 23%. Rectocoeles progressed from grade 1 to grades 2–3 in 1%, but regressed from grades 2–3 to grade 0 in 3%, and from grade 1 to grade 0 in 2%. Uterine prolapse regressed from grade 1 to grade 0 in 48%. The incidence of morbidity associated with genital prolapse is also difficult to estimate. The annual incidence of hospital admission for prolapse in the UK has been estimated at 2.04/1000 women under the age of 60 years. Genital prolapse is also a major cause of gynaecological surgery.

Intimate partner violence towards women

Joanne Klevens and Laura Sadowski

KEY POINTS

- Between 10–70% of women may have been physically or sexually assaulted by a partner at some stage, with reported assault rates against men about a quarter the rate against women. In at least half of people studied, the problem lasts for five years or more.

  Intimate partner violence (IPV) has been associated with socioeconomic and personality factors, marital discord, exposure to violence in family of origin, and partner's drug or alcohol abuse.

  Women reporting IPV are more likely than other women to complain of poor physical or mental health and disability.

- Advocacy may reduce revictimisation rates compared with no treatment, but may have low levels of acceptability.

- Cognitive trauma therapy may reduce post-traumatic stress disorder and depression compared with no treatment.

- Peer support groups may improve psychological distress and decrease use of healthcare services compared with no intervention.

- Cognitive behavioural counselling may reduce minor physical or sexual IPV, both minor and severe psychological IPV, and depression compared with no counselling.

- Career counselling plus critical consciousness awareness may increase a woman's confidence and awareness of the impact of IPV on her life compared with career counselling alone.

  We don't know whether other types of counselling are effective compared with no counselling. Although empowerment counselling appears to reduce trait anxiety, it does not appear to reduce current anxiety or depression or improve self-esteem.

  We don't know how different types of counselling compare with each other.

- Safety planning may reduce the rate of subsequent abuse in the short term, but longer-term benefit is unknown.

- We don't know whether the use of shelters reduces revictimisation, as little research has been done.

- Nurse support and guidance is probably unlikely to be beneficial in IPV.

Please visit www.clinicalevidence.bmj.com for full text and references

What are the effects of interventions initiated by healthcare professionals aimed at female victims of intimate partner violence?

Likely To Be Beneficial	• Advocacy
	• Career counselling plus critical consciousness awareness (more effective than career counselling alone)
	• Cognitive behavioural counselling versus no counselling
	• Cognitive trauma therapy versus no treatment
	• Peer support groups

	• Safety planning
Unknown Effectiveness	• Counselling (various types) versus no counselling
	• Different types of counselling versus each other (relative benefits unclear)
	• Shelters
Unlikely To Be Beneficial	• Nurse support and guidance

Search date December 2006

DEFINITION Intimate partner violence (IPV) is actual or threatened physical or sexual violence, or emotional or psychological abuse (including coercive tactics), by a current or former spouse or dating partner (including same-sex partners). Other terms commonly used to describe IPV include domestic violence, domestic abuse, spouse abuse, marital violence, and battering.

INCIDENCE/PREVALENCE Between 10% and 69% of women participating in population-based surveys in 48 countries reported being physically assaulted by a partner during their lifetime. Rates of reported assault by a partner are 4.3 times higher among women than men. Nearly 25% of surveyed women in the USA reported being physically or sexually assaulted or both by a current or former partner at some time, and 1.5% were victimised during the previous 12 months. Rates of violence against pregnant women range from 0.9% to 20%. Between 11.7% and 24.5% of women in prenatal clinics and 5.5% and 17.0% of women in primary or ambulatory care reported being abused by a partner in the past year.

AETIOLOGY/RISK FACTORS Two systematic reviews found that physical IPV toward women is associated with lower levels of education and unemployment, low family income, and marital discord, and partner's lower level of occupation, childhood experiences of abuse, witnessing interparental violence, higher levels of anger, depression, stress, heavy or problem drinking, drug use, jealousy, and lack of assertiveness with spouse. A similar review of research on psychological aggression found that the few demographic and psychological variables assessed were either inconsistently associated with psychological IPV or were found to be associated with psychological IPV in studies with serious methodological limitations.

PROGNOSIS A large longitudinal study of couples suggests that IPV tends to disappear over time within most relationships; however, couples reporting frequent or severe IPV are more likely to remain violent. For all ethnic groups, half of those reporting moderate IPV did not report occurrences of IPV at 5-year follow-up; but, for people of black or Hispanic origin reporting severe IPV, only a third did not report occurrences of domestic violence at 5-year follow-up. A case control study conducted in middle-class working women found that, compared with non-abused women, women abused by their partners during the previous 9 years were significantly more likely to have or report headaches (48% v 35%), back pain (40% v 25%), STDs (6% v 2%), vaginal bleeding (17% v 6%), vaginal infections (30% v 21%), pelvic pain (17% v 9%), painful intercourse (13% v 7%), UTIs (22% v 12%), appetite loss (9% v 3%), digestive problems (35% v 19%), abdominal pain (22% v 11%), and facial injuries (8% v 1%). After adjusting for age, race, insurance status, and cigarette smoking, a cross-sectional survey found that women experiencing psychological abuse are also more likely to report poor physical and mental health, disability preventing work, arthritis, chronic pain, migraine and other frequent headaches, STDs, chronic pelvic pain, stomach ulcers, spastic colon, frequent indigestion, diarrhoea, and constipation.

Edward Morris and Janice Rymer

KEY POINTS

- In the UK, the median age for onset of menopausal symptoms is 45.5–47.5 years.

    Symptoms associated with the menopause include vasomotor symptoms, sleeplessness, mood changes, reduced energy levels, loss of libido, vaginal dryness, and urinary symptoms.

    Many symptoms, such as hot flushes, are temporary, but those resulting from reduced hormone levels, such as genital atrophy, may be permanent.

- Progestogens are beneficial in reducing menopausal vasomotor symptoms compared with placebo. However, the clinical usefulness of progestogens given alone for menopausal symptoms is limited by the unwanted adverse effects of the relatively high doses need to achieve relief of menopausal symptoms.

    Progestogens used alone or with oestrogens reduce vasomotor symptoms in perimenopausal women.

- Oestrogens reduce vasomotor and sexual symptoms, but increase the risk of serious adverse effects.

    Oestrogens, used alone or with progestogens, reduce vasomotor, urogenital, and psychological symptoms, and improve quality of life compared with placebo over 3–6 months.

    However, oestrogens increase the risk of breast cancer, endometrial cancer, stroke, and venous thromboembolism.

    Phyto-oestrogens, such as in soy flour, have not been shown consistently to improve symptoms, and may increase the risk of endometrial hyperplasia in perimenopausal women.

- Tibolone reduces vasomotor symptoms in postmenopausal women compared with placebo.

    Tibolone may improve sexual function compared with placebo, or with combined oestrogens plus progestogens.

    However, tibolone may be less effective in reducing vasomotor symptoms than oestrogens and progestogen combined treatment.

- Testosterone reduces sexual symptoms in postmenopausal women, but does not seem to reduce vasomotor symptoms, compared with oestrogen HRT alone.

- We don't know whether antidepressants reduce vasomotor symptoms in postmenopausal women.

- We don't know whether clonidine, black cohosh, and agnus castus reduce menopausal symptoms.

- CAUTION: Women who have an intact uterus and who are prescribed oestrogen replacement therapy should also take continuous or cyclical progestogens.

(i) **Please visit www.clinicalevidence.bmj.com for full text and references**

What are the effects of medical treatments for menopausal symptoms?

Beneficial	• Tibolone
Trade-off Between Benefits And Harms	• Oestrogens alone (improved menopausal symptoms but increased risk of breast cancer,

	endometrial cancer, stroke, and venous thromboembolism after long-term use)
	• Oestrogens plus progestogens (improved menopausal symptoms but increased risk of breast cancer, stroke, and venous thromboembolism after long-term use)
	• Progestogens alone
Unknown Effectiveness	• Antidepressants
	• Clonidine
	• Testosterone

What are the effects of non-prescribed treatments for menopausal symptoms?

Unknown Effectiveness	• Agnus castus
	• Black cohosh
	• Phyto-oestrogens

Search date December 2006

DEFINITION Menopause is defined as the end of the last menstrual period. A woman is deemed to be postmenopausal 1 year after her last period. For practical purposes, most women are diagnosed as menopausal after 1 year of amenorrhoea. Menopausal symptoms often begin in the perimenopausal years. The complex of menopausal symptomatology includes vasomotor symptoms (hot flushes), sleeplessness, mood changes, reduction in energy levels, loss of libido, vaginal dryness, and urinary symptoms.

INCIDENCE/PREVALENCE In the UK, the mean age for the start of the menopause is 50 years and 9 months. The median onset of the perimenopause is 45.5–47.5 years. One Scottish survey (6096 women aged 45–54 years) found that 84% of women had experienced at least one of the classic menopausal symptoms, with 45% finding one or more symptoms to be a problem.

AETIOLOGY/RISK FACTORS Urogenital symptoms of menopause are caused by decreased oestrogen concentrations, but the cause of vasomotor symptoms and psychological effects is complex and remains unclear.

PROGNOSIS Menopause is a physiological event. Timing of the natural menopause in healthy women may be determined genetically. Although endocrine changes are permanent, menopausal symptoms such as hot flushes, which are experienced by about 70% of women, usually resolve with time but, in some women, can persist for decades. However, some symptoms, such as genital atrophy, may remain the same or worsen.

Menorrhagia

Kirsten Duckitt and Sally Collins

KEY POINTS

- Menorrhagia limits normal activities, and causes anaemia in two thirds of women with objective menorrhagia (blood loss of more than 80 mL blood per cycle).

  Prostaglandin disorders may be associated with idiopathic menorrhagia, and with heavy bleeding caused by fibroids, adenomyosis, or use of IUDs.

  Fibroids have been found in 10% of women with menorrhagia overall, and in 40% of women with severe menorrhagia; but half of women having a hysterectomy for menorrhagia are found to have a normal uterus.

- NSAIDs, tranexamic acid, and danazol all reduce blood loss compared with placebo.

  Tranexamic acid and danazol may be more effective in reducing blood loss than NSAIDs, tamsylate, and oral progestogens, but any benefits of danazol have to be weighed against the high risk of adverse effects.

  NSAIDs reduce dysmenorrhoea, and may be as effective at reducing menstrual blood loss as oral progestogens given in the luteal phase, but we don't know how they compare with etamsylate, combined oral contraceptives, intrauterine progestogens, or gonadorelin analogues.

  We don't know whether combined oral contraceptives, levonorgestrel-releasing IUDs, or GnRHa are effective at reducing menorrhagia, as few studies have been found.

- Hysterectomy reduces blood loss and reduces the need for further surgery compared with medical treatments or endometrial destruction, but can lead to complications in up to a third of women.

  Endometrial destruction is more effective at reducing menorrhagia compared with medical treatment, but complications can include infection, haemorrhage, and uterine perforation.

  We don't know whether any one type of endometrial destruction is superior compared with the other types, or whether dilatation and curettage has any effect on menstrual blood loss.

- Preoperative GnRHa reduces long-term postoperative moderate or heavy blood loss, and increase amenorrhoea compared with placebo, but we don't know whether oral progestogens or danazol are also beneficial when used preoperatively.

(i) Please visit www.clinicalevidence.bmj.com for full text and references

What are the effects of medical treatments for menorrhagia?

Beneficial	• NSAIDs
	• Tranexamic acid
Trade-off Between Benefits And Harms	• Danazol
Unknown Effectiveness	• Contraceptives (combined oral)
	• Etamsylate
	• GnRHa

	• Intrauterine progestogens
Unlikely To Be Beneficial	• Progestogens (oral) for longer cycle
Likely To Be Ineffective Or Harmful	• Progestogens (oral) in luteal phase only

What are the effects of surgical treatments for menorrhagia?

Beneficial	• Hysterectomy (reduces menstrual blood loss compared with intrauterine progestogens or endometrial destruction; also reduces need for further surgery compared with endometrial destruction)
Likely To Be Beneficial	• Endometrial destruction (reduces menstrual blood loss compared with medical treatment)
Unknown Effectiveness	• Dilatation and curettage

What are the effects of endometrial thinning before endometrial destruction in treating menorrhagia?

Beneficial	• GnRHa
Unknown Effectiveness	• Danazol • Progestogens (oral)

Search date September 2006

DEFINITION Menorrhagia is defined as heavy but regular menstrual bleeding. **Idiopathic ovulatory menorrhagia** is regular heavy bleeding in the absence of recognisable pelvic pathology or a general bleeding disorder. **Objective menorrhagia** is taken to be a total menstrual blood loss of 80 mL or more in each menstruation. Subjectively, menorrhagia may be defined as a complaint of regular excessive menstrual blood loss occurring over several consecutive cycles in a woman of reproductive years.

INCIDENCE/PREVALENCE In the UK, 5% of women aged 30–49 years consult their general practitioner each year with menorrhagia. In New Zealand, 2–4% of primary care consultations by premenopausal women are for menstrual problems.

AETIOLOGY/RISK FACTORS Idiopathic ovulatory menorrhagia is thought to be caused by disordered prostaglandin production within the endometrium. Prostaglandins may also be implicated in menorrhagia associated with uterine fibroids, adenomyosis, or the presence of an IUD. Fibroids have been reported in 10% of women with menorrhagia (80–100 mL/cycle) and 40% of those with severe menorrhagia (200 mL/cycle or more).

PROGNOSIS Menorrhagia limits normal activities and causes iron deficiency anaemia in two thirds of women proven to have objective menorrhagia. One in five women in the UK and one in three in the USA have a hysterectomy before the age of 60 years; menorrhagia is the main presenting problem in at least 50% of these women. About 50% of women who have a hysterectomy for menorrhagia are found to have an anatomically normal uterus.

Sean Kehoe and Jo Morrison

KEY POINTS

- Ovarian cancer is the fourth most common cause of cancer deaths in the UK.

  Incidence rises with age, and peaks in the seventh and eighth decades of life.

  Risk factors include family history of ovarian cancer, increasing age, and low parity. Risks are reduced by using the oral contraceptive pill for more than 5 years, tubal ligation, hysterectomy, breastfeeding, increased age at menarche, decreased age at menopause, and use of NSAIDs.

  In the UK, the 5-year relative survival rate at diagnosis for women aged 15–39 years is nearly 70%. In comparison, it is only 12% for women diagnosed over 80 years of age.

- Standard treatment for advanced ovarian cancer is surgical debulking, followed by chemotherapy.

  Evidence from case series suggests that maximal surgical cytoreduction is strongly associated with improved survival in advanced ovarian cancer.

  Subsequent debulking or second-look surgery seem unlikely to improve survival, especially if initial surgery achieved optimal cytoreduction.

- Platinum-based regimens are now standard first-line chemotherapy and have been shown to be beneficial in prolonging survival compared with non-platinum-based regimens.

  Platinum compounds seem to be the main beneficial agent, with little additional survival benefit from adding non-platinum (excluding taxanes) chemotherapeutic agents to platinum.

  Carboplatin is as effective in prolonging survival as cisplatin, but with less-severe adverse effects.

- Taxanes may increase survival if added to platinum chemotherapy compared with platinum-based regimens alone, but studies have given conflicting results.

  One randomised trial suggests paclitaxel is as effective at prolonging survival as docetaxel when combined with a platinum drug.

(i) **Please visit www.clinicalevidence.bmj.com for full text and references**

What are the effects of surgical treatments for ovarian cancer that is advanced at first presentation?	
Unknown Effectiveness	• Primary surgery
Unlikely To Be Beneficial	• Interval debulking in women who have residual tumours after primary surgery • Second-look surgery versus watchful waiting

What are the effects of platinum-based chemotherapy for ovarian cancer that is advanced at first presentation?	
Likely To Be Beneficial	• Carboplatin plus taxane versus cisplatin plus taxane
Unlikely To Be Beneficial	• Combination platinum-based chemotherapy versus single-agent platinum chemotherapy

> (cisplatin or carboplatin alone may be as effective as platinum plus non-platinum [excluding taxanes] combination regimens)

What are the effects of taxane-based chemotherapy for ovarian cancer that is advanced at first presentation?

Unknown Effectiveness	• Adding a taxane to a platinum-based compound
	• Paclitaxel versus docetaxel

Search date September 2007

DEFINITION Ovarian tumours are classified according to the assumed cell type of origin (surface epithelium, stroma, or germ cells). Epithelial tumours account for over 90% of ovarian cancers. These can be further grouped into histological types (serous, mucinous, endometroid, and clear cell). Epithelial ovarian cancer is staged using the FIGO classification. This review is limited to first-line treatment in women with advanced (FIGO stage 2–4) invasive epithelial ovarian cancer at first presentation.

INCIDENCE/PREVALENCE The worldwide incidence of ovarian cancer according to the GLOBOCAN database was 204,499 cases in 2002. There is a worldwide variation with highest rates in Lithuania, Denmark, and Estonia, and lowest rates in Egypt, Malawi, and Mali. This may be because of variation in reproductive practice, use of the oral contraceptive pill, breastfeeding habits, and age of menarche and menopause. The incidence of ovarian cancer rises steadily with increasing age and peaks in the seventh and eighth decades of life. In the UK, it is the fourth most common cause of cancer deaths, with about 6900 new cases diagnosed annually and 4600 deaths from the disease each year. The incidence of ovarian cancer seems to be stabilising in some other countries, and in some resource rich countries (Finland, Denmark, New Zealand, and the USA) rates are declining.

AETIOLOGY/RISK FACTORS Risk factors include family history of ovarian cancer, increasing age, and low parity. More controversial are subfertility and use of fertility drugs. Use of the oral contraceptive pill for more than 5 years reduces the risk by 30–40%. Other factors associated with risk reduction are tubal ligation, hysterectomy, breastfeeding, increasing age of menarche, decreasing age of menopause, and use of NSAIDs.

PROGNOSIS Survival rates vary according to the age of the woman, stage of the disease, and residual tumour after surgery. The most important determinant of survival seems to be the stage of disease at diagnosis. Diagnosis at an early stage has a 5-year survival rate of greater than 70%, but for those diagnosed with advanced stage disease it is about 15%. Younger women survive longer than older women, even after adjustments for general life expectancy. In the UK, the 5-year relative survival rate at diagnosis for women aged 15–39 years is nearly 70%. In comparison, it is only 12% for women diagnosed over 80 years of age.

Hesham Al-Inany

KEY POINTS

- PCOS is characterised by an accumulation of incompletely developed follicles in the ovaries due to anovulation, associated with increased ovarian androgen production.

  PCOS is diagnosed in up to 10% of women attending gynaecology clinics, but the prevalence in the population as a whole is unclear.

  PCOS has been associated with hirsutism, infertility, acne, weight gain, type 2 diabetes, CVD, and endometrial hyperplasia.

- Metformin may improve menstrual pattern and oligomenorrhoea compared with placebo, and may reduce hirsutism compared with placebo or cyproterone acetate-ethinylestradiol.

  Cyproterone acetate-ethinylestradiol (co-cyprindiol) may reduce hirsutism but increases the risk of venous thromboembolism compared with placebo.

  Finasteride may reduce hirsutism compared with placebo, and seems to be as effective as spironolactone or cyproterone acetate-ethinylestradiol.

  Flutamide may be more effective at reducing hirsutism compared with finasteride, but studies have given conflicting results.

  Combined treatment with flutamide plus cyproterone acetate-ethinylestradiol may reduce the number of women with oligomenorrhoea compared with flutamide alone.

- We don't know whether interventions to achieve weight loss improve clinical outcomes in women with PCOS.

  We don't know whether ketoconazole or mechanical hair removal reduce hirsutism compared with other treatments.

(i) **Please visit www.clinicalevidence.bmj.com for full text and references**

What are the effects of treatments?

Likely To Be Beneficial	• Finasteride (may be similarly effective in reducing hirsutism compared with spironolactone, and cyproterone acetate–ethinylestradiol) • Flutamide (may be similarly effective in reducing hirsutism compared with finasteride and spironolactone) • Metformin (improved menstrual pattern compared with placebo; reduced hirsutism compared with cyproterone acetate–ethinylestradiol) • Spironolactone (may be similarly effective for reducing hirsutism as flutamide and finasteride)
Trade-off Between Benefits And Harms	• Cyproterone acetate–ethinylestradiol (co-cyprindiol; reduced hirsutism but increased risk of venous thromboembolism)
Unknown Effectiveness	• Interventions to achieve weight loss • Ketoconazole • Mechanical hair removal

Search date October 2005

DEFINITION Polycystic ovary syndrome (PCOS; Stein–Leventhal syndrome, sclerocystic ovarian disease) is defined as an accumulation of many incompletely developed follicles in the ovaries owing to chronic anovulation with an increase in ovarian androgen production.

INCIDENCE/PREVALENCE PCOS is diagnosed in 4–10% of women attending gynaecology clinics in resource-rich countries, but this figure may not reflect the true prevalence, because there have been no specific population-based studies, and the criteria used for diagnosis are varied. Most women present in their thirties.

AETIOLOGY/RISK FACTORS The aetiology is unknown. Genetic factors may play a part, but the exact mechanisms are unclear. Two studies found some evidence of familial aggregation of hyperandrogenaemia (with or without oligomenorrhoea) in first-degree relatives of women with PCOS. In the first study, 22% of sisters of women with PCOS fulfilled diagnostic criteria for PCOS. In the second study, of the 78 mothers and 50 sisters evaluated clinically, 19 (24%) mothers and 16 (32%) sisters had PCOS.

PROGNOSIS There is some evidence that women with PCOS are at increased risk of developing type 2 diabetes and cardiovascular disorders secondary to hyperlipidaemia compared with women who do not have PCOS. Oligomenorrhoeic and amenorrhoeic women are at increased risk of developing endometrial hyperplasia and, later, endometrial carcinoma.

Premenstrual syndrome

Irene Kwan and Joseph Loze Onwude

KEY POINTS

- A woman has premenstrual syndrome (PMS) if she complains of recurrent psychological and/or physical symptoms occurring during the luteal phase of the menstrual cycle, and often resolving by the end of menstruation. Symptom severity can vary between women.

  Premenstrual symptoms occur in 95% of all women of reproductive age. Severe, debilitating symptoms (PMS) occur in about 5% of those women.

  There is no consensus on how symptom severity should be assessed, which has led to a wide variety of symptoms scales, making it difficult to synthesise data on treatment efficacy. The cyclical nature of the condition also makes it difficult to conduct RCTs.

  There is little good evidence for any of the wide range of treatments available, and the selection of treatment is mainly governed by personal choice. The clinician plays a key role in facilitating this choice, and in reassuring women with PMS without co-existing gynaecological problems that there is nothing seriously wrong.

- Drug treatments can be effective at reducing premenstrual symptoms, but some are associated with significant adverse effects.

  There is good evidence that spironolactone improves mood and somatic symptoms in women with PMS.

  Alprazolam (during the luteal phase), metolazone, and NSAIDs (such as mefanamic acid, and napoxen sodium) may also be effective in treating the main physical and psychological symptoms of PMS.

  Buspirone (luteal or continuous), and gonadorelin analogues seem to improve overall self-rated symptoms. Gonadorelin is effective in improving symptoms, but is associated with serious risks of osteoporosis when used for more than 6 months.

  Other drug treatments, such as clomipramine, danazol, and SSRIs, may improve psychological symptoms, but are associated with serious adverse effects.

- Progesterone and progesterone-like drugs reduce premenstrual symptoms, but are associated with several adverse effects.

  We don't know whether other hormonal treatments such as oestrogen and tibolone are effective in reducing symptoms of PMS.

  Oral contraceptives (24/4 schedule [24 out of 28 days]) are likely to be effective in reducing symptoms of PMS.

- There is insufficient evidence to assess the efficacy of CBT in treating the psychological symptoms of PMS.

- We also don't know how effective physical therapy techniques (bright light therapy, chiropractic manipulation, exercise, reflexology, relaxation, and acupuncture) are in relieving symptoms of PMS.

- We found good evidence that pyridoxine (vitamin B6) reduces the overall symptoms of PMS. Calcium supplements may also be effective.

  We don't know whether other supplements, such as evening primrose oil or magnesium supplements, are a useful treatment for PMS.

- Surgery is indicated only if there are coexisting gynaecological problems.

  There is a consensus that hysterectomy with bilateral oophorectomy or laparoscopic bilateral oophorectomy almost completely eradicate the symptoms of PMS, although we could not find any RCTs that examined this.

  We don't know whether endometrial ablation has the same effect.

(i) **Please visit www.clinicalevidence.bmj.com for full text and references**

What are the effects of drug treatments in women with premenstrual syndrome?

Beneficial	• Spironolactone
Likely To Be Beneficial	• Alprazolam
	• Buspirone
	• Gonadorelin analogues for less than 6 months
	• Metolazone
	• NSAIDs
Trade-off Between Benefits And Harms	• Clomipramine
	• Danazol
	• SSRIs

What are the effects of hormonal treatments in women with premenstrual syndrome?

Likely To Be Beneficial	• Contraceptives (oral)
Trade-off Between Benefits And Harms	• Progesterone
	• Progestogens
Unknown Effectiveness	• Oestrogens
	• Tibolone

What are the effects of psychological interventions in women with premenstrual syndrome?

Unknown Effectiveness	• CBT

What are the effects of physical therapy in women with premenstrual syndrome?

Unknown Effectiveness	• Acupuncture
	• Bright light therapy
	• Chiropractic manipulation
	• Exercise
	• Reflexology
	• Relaxation

What are the effects of dietary supplements in women with premenstrual syndrome?

Beneficial	• Pyridoxine
Likely To Be Beneficial	• Calcium supplements
Unknown Effectiveness	• Evening primrose oil • Magnesium supplements

What are the effects of surgical treatments in women with premenstrual syndrome?

Likely To Be Beneficial	• Hysterectomy alone or plus bilateral oophorectomy* • Laparoscopic bilateral oophorectomy*
Unknown Effectiveness	• Endometrial ablation

Search date November 2006

*No RCTs but consensus that effective and an RCT unlikely to be performed.

DEFINITION A woman has premenstrual syndrome (PMS) if she complains of recurrent psychological and/or physical symptoms occurring specifically during the luteal phase of the menstrual cycle, and often resolving by the end of menstruation. The symptoms can also persist during the bleeding phase. **Severe premenstrual syndrome:** The definition of severe PMS varies among RCTs, but in recent studies standardised criteria have been used to diagnose one variant of severe PMS — premenstrual dysphoric disorder. This criteria is based on at least five symptoms, including one of four core psychological symptoms (from a list of 17 physical and psychological symptoms), being severe before menstruation starts and mild or absent after menstruation. The 17 symptoms are depression, feeling hopeless or guilty, anxiety/tension, mood swings, irritability/persistent anger, decreased interest, poor concentration, fatigue, food craving or increased appetite, sleep disturbance, feeling out of control or overwhelmed, poor coordination, headache, aches, swelling/bloating/weight gain, cramps, and breast tenderness.

INCIDENCE/PREVALENCE Premenstrual symptoms occur in 95% of all women of reproductive age; severe, debilitating symptoms (PMS) occur in about 5% of those women.

AETIOLOGY/RISK FACTORS The cause is unknown, but hormonal and other factors (possibly neuroendocrine) probably contribute.

PROGNOSIS Except after oophorectomy, symptoms of PMS usually recur when treatment is stopped.

Ignacio Neumann, M Fernanda Rojas, and Philippa Moore

KEY POINTS

- Pyelonephritis is usually caused by ascent of bacteria from the bladder, most often *Escherichia coli*, and is more likely in people with structural or functional urinary tract abnormalities.

  The prognosis is good if pyelonephritis is treated appropriately, but complications include renal abscess, renal impairment, and septic shock.

- Consensus is that oral antibiotics, given in the outpatient setting, are effective in non-pregnant women with uncomplicated pyelonephritis, although no placebo-controlled studies have been found.

  We don't know whether any one treatment regimen is more effective, or what the optimum duration of treatment is, although it may be sensible to continue treatment for at least 10 days.

  Broader spectrum antibiotics, such as quinolones, may be more effective compared with narrower spectrum antibiotics, such as ampicillin, amoxicillin, or co-trimoxazole, in areas where resistance to these is common.

  In the outpatient setting, we don't know whether intravenous antibiotics are more effective in non-pregnant women with uncomplicated pyelonephritis compared with oral regimens.

- Intravenous antibiotics are considered effective in women admitted to hospital with uncomplicated pyelonephritis.

  We don't know which is the most effective intravenous antibiotic regimen, or the optimum duration of treatment.

  Combining intravenous plus oral antibiotics may be no more effective that oral antibiotics alone, but the evidence is weak.

- We don't know whether inpatient treatment improves outcomes compared with outpatient treatment.

- We found no evidence that simple analgesics, NSAIDs, or urinary analgesics reduce pain from uncomplicated pyelonephritis.

  NSAIDs may worsen renal function and should be used in caution in women with pyelonephritis.

Please visit www.clinicalevidence.bmj.com for full text and references

What are the effects of oral antibiotic treatments for acute pyelonephritis in women with uncomplicated infection?

Likely To Be Beneficial	• Antibiotics (oral) versus placebo*
Unknown Effectiveness	• Antibiotics (oral) versus each other • Oral versus intravenous antibiotics

What are the effects of antibiotic treatments for acute pyelonephritis in women admitted to hospital with uncomplicated infection?

Likely To Be Beneficial	• Antibiotics (intravenous) versus placebo*
Unknown Effectiveness	• Antibiotics (intravenous) versus each other

- Intravenous antibiotics plus oral antibiotics (unclear which combinations are more effective or if combination is more effective than oral alone)

- Intravenous versus oral antibiotics

What is the effect of inpatient versus outpatient management for acute pyelonephritis in women with uncomplicated infection?

Unknown Effectiveness	• Relative effectiveness of inpatient versus outpatient management

What are the effects of analgesia in women with uncomplicated acute pyelonephritis?

Unknown Effectiveness	• NSAIDs
	• Simple systemic analgesics (non-opioids)
	• Urinary analgesics

Search date February 2007

*Categorisation is not based on placebo-controlled RCTs. Such studies are likely to be considered unethical.

DEFINITION Acute pyelonephritis, or upper UTI, is an infection of the kidney characterised by pain when passing urine, fever, chills, flank pain, nausea, and vomiting. White blood cells are almost always present in the urine. White blood cell casts are occasionally seen on urine microscopy. There is no consensus on the definitions for grades of severity. However, in practice, people with acute pyelonephritis may be divided into people who are able to take oral antibiotics, who do not have signs of sepsis, and may be managed at home, and those who require intravenous antibiotics in hospital. Some consider the absolute indications for hospitalisation to be persistent vomiting, progression of uncomplicated UTI, suspected sepsis, or urinary tract obstruction. Pyelonephritis is considered uncomplicated if caused by a typical pathogen in an immunocompetent person who has normal renal anatomy and renal function. There is little difference in the treatment of men and non-pregnant women. **Diagnosis:** Women presenting with fever and back pain suggest a possible diagnosis of acute pyelonephritis. Urinalysis and urine culture should be performed to confirm the diagnosis. Pyuria is present in almost all patients and can be detected rapidly with leukocyte esterase test (S: 74% to 95% and E: 94% to 98%) or the nitrite test (S: 92% to 100% and E: 35% to 85%). Bacterial growth of 104-10-5 is 10.000-100.000 colony-forming units on urine culture of a mid-stream specimen will confirm bacteriological diagnosis.

INCIDENCE/PREVALENCE The estimated annual incidence per 10,000 people is 27.6 cases in the USA and 35.7 cases in South Korea. Worldwide prevalence and incidence are unknown. The highest incidence of pyelonephritis occurs during the summer months. Women are approximately five times more likely than men to be hospitalised with acute pyelonephritin.

AETIOLOGY/RISK FACTORS Pyelonephritis is most commonly caused when bacteria in the bladder ascend the ureters and invade the kidneys. In some cases, this may result in bacteria entering and multiplying in the bloodstream. The most frequently isolated organism is *Escherichia coli* (56–85%); others include *Enterococcus faecalis*, *Klebsiella pneumoniae*, and *Proteus mirabilis*. In eldery people, *E.coli* is less common (60%), whereas people who have diabetes mellitus tend to have infections caused by Klebsiella, Enterobacter, Clostridium, or Candida. People with structural or functional urinary tract abnormalities are more prone to pyelonephritis that is refractory to oral therapy or complicated by bacteraemia. Risk factors associated with pyelonephritis in healthy women are sexual intercourse, use of spermicide, UTI in the previous 12 months, a mother with a history of UTI, diabetes, and urinary incontinence. The most important risk factor for complicated UTI is obstruction of the urinary tract. The incidence of drug-resistant microorganisms varies in different geographical areas. Recent hospitalisation, recent use of antibiotics, immunosuppression, recurrent pyelonephritis, and nephrolithiasis increase the risk of drug resistance.

PROGNOSIS Prognosis is good if uncomplicated pyelonephritis is treated appropriately. Complications include renal abscess, septic shock, and renal impairment, including acute renal failure. Short-term independent risk factors for mortality include age above 65 years, septic shock, being bedridden, and immunosuppression. Conditions such as underlying renal disease, diabetes mellitus, and immunosuppression may worsen prognosis, but we found no good long-term evidence about rates of sepsis or death among people with such conditions.

Recurrent cystitis in non-pregnant women

Ayan Sen

KEY POINTS

- Cystitis is a bacterial infection of the lower urinary tract which causes pain when passing urine and causes frequency, urgency, haematuria, and suprapubic pain not associated with passing urine.

  Recurrent cystitis is usually defined as three episodes of UTI in the past 12 months or two episodes in the past 6 months.

  It is common in healthy young women, with one study finding 27% of women developing a second infection within 6 months of the first, and 2.7% having a second recurrence during this period.

- Continuous antibiotic prophylaxis lasting 6–12 months reduces the rate of recurrence, although there is no consensus about when to start the treatment, nor how long it should last.

  Trimethoprim, co-trimoxazole, nitrofurantoin, cefaclor, and quinolones seem equally effective at reducing recurrence rates.

- Postcoital antibiotics (taken within 2 hours of intercourse) reduce the rate of clinical recurrence of cystitis as effectively as continuous treatment.

- We don't know whether single-dose self-administered co-trimoxazole or continuous prophylaxis with methenamine hippurate are effective in preventing recurrence of cystitis, as the studies were too small to be able to detect any clinically relevant differences.

- Cranberry products (either juice or capsules) seem to significantly reduce the recurrence of symptomatic cystitis.

  There is no clear evidence as to the amount and concentration of cranberry juice that needs to be consumed, or the length of time for the treatment to be most effective.

- There is no evidence examining whether passing urine after intercourse is effective at preventing UTI.

(i) **Please visit www.clinicalevidence.bmj.com for full text and references**

Which interventions prevent further recurrence of cystitis in women experiencing at least two infections per year?	
Beneficial	• Continuous antibiotic prophylaxis (trimethoprim, co-trimoxazole, nitrofurantoin, cefaclor, or a quinolone) • Postcoital antibiotic prophylaxis (co-trimoxazole, nitrofurantoin, or a quinolone)
Likely To Be Beneficial	• Cranberry juice and cranberry products
Unknown Effectiveness	• Continuous prophylaxis with methenamine hippurate • Passing urine after intercourse • Single-dose self-administered co-trimoxazole

Search date May 2005

DEFINITION In most cases, cystitis is a bacterial infection of the lower urinary tract which causes pain when passing urine and causes frequency, urgency, haematuria, and suprapubic pain not associated with passing urine. White blood cells and bacteria are almost always present in the urine. A recurrent UTI is a symptomatic UTI that follows clinical resolution of an earlier infection generally, but not necessarily, after treatment. Recurrent cystitis is usually defined in the literature as three episodes of UTI in the past 12 months or two episodes in the past 6 months. Recurrent UTIs cause serious discomfort to women, and have a high impact on ambulatory healthcare costs as a result of outpatient visits, diagnostic tests, and prescriptions.

INCIDENCE/PREVALENCE Recurrent cystitis is common among young healthy women, even though they generally have anatomically and physiologically normal urinary tracts. One study found that nearly half of the women whose uncomplicated UTIs resolved spontaneously developed a recurrent UTI within the first year. In a study of college women with their first UTI, 27% experienced at least one culture-confirmed recurrence within the 6 months of the initial infection, and 2.7% had a second recurrence over this time period. In a Finnish study of women aged 17–82 years who had *Escherichia Coli* cystitis, 44% had a recurrence within 1 year, 53% in women older than 55 years, 36% in younger women. No large population-based studies have been performed yet to determine what proportion of women with UTI develops a pattern of high-frequency recurrence. Occasionally, recurrences are due to a persistent focus of infection, but the vast majority is thought to represent reinfection. A recurrence is defined clinically as a relapse if it is caused by the same species as that causing the original UTI, and if it occurs within 2 weeks after treatment. It is considered reinfection if it occurs more than 2 weeks after treatment of the original infection. Most women are able to diagnose their own episodes of recurrent cystitis from symptoms (positive predictive value in one RCT 92%).

AETIOLOGY/RISK FACTORS Cystitis is caused by uropathogenic bacteria in the faecal flora that colonise the vaginal and periurethral openings, and ascend the urethra into the bladder. Sexual intercourse, diaphragm–spermicide use, and a history of recurrent UTI have been shown to be strong and independent risk factors for cystitis. Use of spermicide-coated condoms may also increase the risk of UTI. Antimicrobial use has been shown to adversely affect the vaginal flora in animals and humans, and recent use of antibiotics is strongly associated with risk of cystitis. however, risk factors specific to women with recurrent cystitis have received little study. In a large, case controlled study of women, comprising 229 cases and 253 controls, with and without a history of recurrent UTI, the strongest risk factor for recurrence in a multivariate analysis was the frequency of sexual intercourse. Other risk factors included spermicide use in the past year, new sex partner during the past year, having a first UTI at or before age 15 years, and having a mother with history of UTIs. Urine-voiding disorders, such as those associated with prolapse, multiple sclerosis, bladder cancer, or bladder stones are also associated with increased risk. An association has been found between pre- and postcoital voiding, frequency of urination, delayed voiding habits, douching, and BMI. A possible association between smoking (which is strongly associated with bladder cancer) and recurrent cystitis has not been assessed. These behavioural patterns have never been evaluated in prospective, randomised trials. Data suggest that pelvic anatomical differences may have a role in predisposing some young women to recurrent UTI, especially those who do not have other risk factors. In postmenopausal women, reduced oestrogen levels seem to contribute to recurrent cystitis in healthy women. The vagina, bladder, and urethra respond to oestrogen, and when the hormonal level in the body is reduced, the tissues of these organs become thinner, weaker, and dry. The changes in the tissues of the bladder and urethra and the associated loss of protection against infection-causing germs may cause an increased risk of UTI in postmenopausal women. Cystitis is also more common during pregnancy because of changes in the urinary tract. As the uterus grows, its increased weight can block the drainage of urine from the bladder, causing an infection. Women are at increased risk for recurrent cystitis from weeks 6–24 of pregnancy.

PROGNOSIS We found little evidence on the long-term effects of untreated cystitis. One study found that progression to pyelonephritis was infrequent, and that most cases of cystitis regressed spontaneously, although symptoms sometimes persisted for several months. However, bacteriuria in pregnant women carries a much greater risk of progressing to pyelonephritis than in non-pregnant women (28% v 1%) and is associated with serious risks.

Joseph L Onwude

KEY POINTS

- Stress incontinence, involving involuntary leaking of urine on effort, exertion, sneezing, or coughing, affects 17–45% of adult women.

    Risk factors include pregnancy (especially with vaginal delivery), smoking, and obesity.

- Pelvic floor muscle exercises improve symptoms and reduce incontinence episodes compared with no treatment. Pelvic floor electrical stimulation and vaginal cones are also effective compared with no treatment.

    Pelvic floor electrical stimulation can cause tenderness and vaginal bleeding, whereas vaginal cones can cause vaginitis and abdominal pain. Pelvic floor muscle exercises can cause discomfort.

- Oestrogen supplements increase cure rates compared with placebo, but there are risks associated with their long-term use. They can be less effective at reducing incontinence compared with pelvic floor muscle exercises.

- SRIs (duloxetine 80 mg/day) reduce stress incontinence compared with placebo at 4–12 weeks, or compared with pelvic floor muscle exercises, but increase the risk of adverse effects, such as headache and gastric problems.

- We do not know whether adrenergic agonists improve incontinence compared with placebo or with other treatments, but they can cause insomnia, restlessness, and vasomotor stimulation. Phenylpropanolamine has been withdrawn from the US market because of an increased risk of haemorrhagic stroke.

- Open retropubic colposuspension may be more likely to cure stress incontinence than anterior vaginal repair or needle suspension at 1–5 years. Complication rates are similar to those with other surgical procedures, but are higher than with non-surgical treatments.

    Suburethral slings, including tension-free vaginal tape, are as effective as open retropubic colposuspension in curing stress incontinence over 5 years. Complications of tension-free vaginal tape include bladder perforation.

    Transobturator foramen procedures may be as effective as tension-free vaginal tape.

- Laparoscopic colposuspension seems to be as effective over 2–5 years as open retropubic colposuspension or tension-free vaginal tape.

(i) **Please visit www.clinicalevidence.bmj.com for full text and references**

What are the effects of non-surgical treatments for women with stress incontinence?

Beneficial	• SRIs (duloxetine)
Likely To Be Beneficial	• Pelvic floor electrical stimulation • Pelvic floor muscle exercises • Vaginal cones
Trade-off Between Benefits And Harms	• Oestrogen supplements
Unknown Effectiveness	• Adrenoceptor agonists

What are the effects of surgical treatments for women with stress incontinence?

Beneficial	• Laparoscopic colposuspension (similar cure rates to open retropubic colposuspension and tension-free vaginal tape) • Open retropubic colposuspension (higher cure rates than non-surgical treatment, anterior vaginal repair, or needle suspension, but more adverse effects than non-surgical treatment)
Likely To Be Beneficial	• Suburethral slings other than tension-free vaginal tape (similar cure rates to open retropubic colposuspension and needle suspension, but more perioperative complications than needle suspension)
Trade-off Between Benefits And Harms	• Tension-free vaginal tape (similar cure rates to open retropubic colposuspension, but associated with bladder perforation)
Unknown Effectiveness	• Transobturator foramen procedures (limited evidence of similar cure rates to tension-free vaginal tape)
Unlikely To Be Beneficial	• Anterior vaginal repair (lower cure rates than open retropubic colposuspension) • Needle suspension (lower cure rates and more surgical complications than open retropubic colposuspension)

Search date December 2006

DEFINITION Stress incontinence is involuntary leakage of urine on effort or exertion, or on sneezing or coughing. Stress incontinence predominantly affects women, and can cause social and hygiene problems. Typically, there is no anticipatory feeling of needing to pass urine. Under urodynamic testing, urodynamic stress incontinence is confirmed by demonstrating loss of urine when intravesical pressure exceeds maximum urethral pressure, in the absence of a detrusor contraction. A confirmed diagnosis of urodynamic stress incontinence is particularly important before surgical treatment, given that the symptoms of stress incontinence can occur in people with detrusor overactivity, which is confirmed by the demonstration of uninhibited bladder contractions. This review deals with stress incontinence in general.

INCIDENCE/PREVALENCE Stress incontinence is a common problem. Prevalence has been estimated at 17–45% of adult women in resource-rich countries. One cross-sectional study (15,308 women in Norway, aged under 65 years) found that the prevalence of stress incontinence was 4.7% in women who had not borne a child, 6.9% in women who had had caesarean deliveries only, and 12.2% in women who had had vaginal deliveries only.

AETIOLOGY/RISK FACTORS Aetiological factors include pregnancy, vaginal or caesarean delivery, cigarette smoking, and obesity. One cross-sectional study (15,308 women in Norway) found that, when compared with women who have not borne a child, the risk of stress incontinence was increased in women who have delivered by caesarean section (age-adjusted OR 1.4, 95% CI 1.0 to 2.0) or by vaginal delivery (age-adjusted OR 3.0, 95%

(continued over)

(from previous page)

CI 2.5 to 3.5). The risk of stress incontinence was also increased in women who had a vaginal delivery compared with women who had a caesarean section (adjusted OR 2.4, 95% CI 1.7 to 3.2). One case control study (606 women) found that the risk of "genuine", now called "urodynamic", stress incontinence, was increased in former smokers (adjusted OR 2.20, 95% CI 1.18 to 4.11) and in current smokers (adjusted OR 2.48, 95% CI 1.60 to 3.84). We found no reliable data measuring the risks associated with obesity.

PROGNOSIS We found no reliable data about the natural history of stress incontinence. Untreated stress incontinence is believed to be a persistent, lifelong condition.

David Jerrard

KEY POINTS

- Mammalian bites are usually caused by dogs, cats, or humans, and are more prevalent in children (especially boys) than in adults.

  Animal bites are usually caused by the person's pet and, in children, frequently involve the face.

  Human bites tend to occur in children as a result of playing or fighting, while in adults they are usually the result of physical or sexual abuse.

  Mixed aerobe and anaerobe infection is the most common type of infection, and can occur in up to half of human bites.

- Few strategies to prevent mammalian bites have been adequately researched.

  Educating schoolchildren may make them more cautious around dogs compared with no education.

- There is consensus that tetanus immunisation should be given routinely as part of wound care of mammalian bites, but no studies have assessed the benefit of this strategy.

  Immunisation does not need to be performed if there is a record of a tetanus shot having been given in the previous 5 years.

- Antibiotics may prevent infection in high-risk bites to the hand, but we don't know if it is worth giving prophylactic antibiotics after other types of mammalian bites.

  High-risk bites are those with deep puncture or crushing, with much devitalised tissue, or those which are dirty.

  Bites that occurred more than 24 hours previously, or those with only simple epidermal stripping, scratches and abrasions, are unlikely to benefit from antibiotic treatment.

- There is consensus that wound debridement, irrigation, decontamination, and primary wound closure are beneficial in reducing infection, but we don't know this for sure.

- There is consensus that antibiotics help to cure infected bite wounds although few studies have been done.

  Selection of appropriate antibiotics depends on the likely mouth flora of the biting animal, and the skin flora of the recipient.

(i) **Please visit www.clinicalevidence.bmj.com for full text and references**

What are the effects of interventions to prevent mammalian bites?

Likely To Be Beneficial	• Education progammes in school children
Unknown Effectiveness	• Education in specific occupational groups

What are the effects of measures to prevent complications from mammalian bites?

Likely To Be Beneficial	• Antibiotic prophylaxis for human bites
	• Debridement, irrigation, and decontamination*

	• Primary wound closure • Tetanus immunisation after mammalian bites*
Unknown Effectiveness	• Antibiotic prophylaxis for non-human mammalian bites

What are the effects of treatments for infected mammalian bites?

Likely To Be Beneficial	• Antibiotics for treating infected bites
Unknown Effectiveness	• Comparative effectiveness of different antibiotics

Search date August 2005

*No RCT evidence, but there is consensus that treatment is likely to be beneficial.

DEFINITION Bite wounds are mainly caused by humans, dogs, or cats. They include superficial abrasions (30–43%), lacerations (31–45%), and puncture wounds (13–34%).

INCIDENCE/PREVALENCE Bite wounds account for about 1–2% of all emergency department visits annually in the USA, costing over US $100 million annually. In the USA, an estimated 3.5–4.7 million dog bites occur each year. About one in five people bitten by a dog seek medical attention, and 1% of those require admission to hospital. Between a third and half of all mammalian bites occur in children. Human bites are the most prevalent mammalian bites after those of dogs and cats, accounting for up to 2–3% of mammalian bites.

AETIOLOGY/RISK FACTORS In over 70% of cases, people are bitten by their own pets or by an animal known to them. Males are more likely to be bitten than females, and are more likely to be bitten by dogs, whereas females are more likely to be bitten by cats. One study found that children under 5 years old were significantly more likely than older children to provoke animals before being bitten. One study of infected dog and cat bites found that the most commonly isolated bacteria was *Pasteurella*, followed by *Streptococci*, *Staphylococci*, *Moraxella*, *Corynebacterium*, and *Neisseria*. Mixed aerobic and anaerobic infection was more common than anaerobic infection alone. Human bites commonly occur in children as a result of fighting or playing. In adults, bites commonly occur during physical or sexual abuse. Tooth abrasions to the knuckles (or "clenched-fist injuries") can occur during fist fighting.

PROGNOSIS In the USA, dog bites cause about 20 deaths a year. In children, dog bites frequently involve the face, potentially resulting in severe lacerations and scarring. Rabies, a life-threatening viral encephalitis, may be contracted as a consequence of being bitten or scratched by a rabid animal. More than 99% of human rabies occurs in resource-poor countries where canine rabies is endemic. Transmission of rabies from domestic animals such as dogs and cats to humans is extremely rare in the USA, Europe, and Canada. The incidence of rabies transmission in dog bites sustained in Africa, Southeast Asia, and India is significantly higher. Human bites, particularly those to the hand, are often complicated by infection. One study reported infection in 48% of untreated bites to the hand.

Jason Wasiak and Heather Cleland

KEY POINTS

- Superficial burns that affect the epidermis and upper dermis only are characterised by redness of the skin which blanches on pressure, pain, and hypersensitivity. The skin blisters within hours and usually heals with minimal scarring within 2–3 weeks if no infection is present.

  Most minor burns occur in the home, with less than 5% requiring hospital treatment.

  Cooling the burn for 20–30 minutes with cold tap water within 3 hours of the injury reduces pain and wound oedema, but prolonged cooling or use of iced water may worsen tissue damage, or cause hypothermia.

- We don't know whether alginate dressings, antibiotics, chlorhexidine-impregnated paraffin gauze dressing, foam dressing, hydrocolloid dressing, hydrogel dressing, paraffin gauze dressing, polyurethane film, or silicone-coated nylon dressing are effective in treating minor burns.

  Topical antibacterial substances such as chlorhexidine may be toxic to regenerating epithelial cells and their use may delay healing in wounds that are not infected.

- Silver sulfadiazine cream may prolong healing times and increase pain compared with other treatments.

(i) Please visit www.clinicalevidence.bmj.com for full text and references

What are the effects of treatments for minor thermal burns?	
Unknown Effectiveness	• Alginate dressing
	• Antibiotics
	• Chlorhexidine-impregnated paraffin gauze dressing
	• Foam dressing
	• Hydrocolloid dressing
	• Hydrogel dressing
	• Paraffin gauze dressing
	• Polyurethane film
	• Silicone-coated nylon dressing
Likely To Be Ineffective Or Harmful	• Silver sulfadiazine cream

Search date January 2006

DEFINITION Burn depth is classified as erythema (first degree) involving the epidermis only, superficial partial thickness (second degree) involving the epidermis and upper dermis, deep partial thickness (second degree) involving the epidermis and dermis, and full-thickness burns (third degree) involving the epidermis, dermis, and damage to appendages. This review deals with minor thermal burns — that is, superficial partial-thickness burns that do not involve the hands or face. Superficial partial-thickness burns are caused by exposure to heat sufficient to cause damage to the epidermis and papillary dermis of the skin. They are characterised by pain and hypersensitivity. The skin seems moist and pink or

(continued over)

(from previous page)

red, and is perfused, as demonstrated by blanching on pressure. This type of injury will blister within hours and heal within 2–3 weeks with minimal scarring if no infection is present. The severity of a superficial partial-thickness burn is usually judged by the percentage of total body surface area involved: less than 15% total body surface area for adults and 10% total body surface area for children.

INCIDENCE/PREVALENCE The incidence of minor thermal burns is difficult to estimate. Generally, less than 5% of all burn injuries requiring treatment will necessitate admission to hospital. Worldwide estimates surrounding all thermal burn injuries suggest that about two million people are burned, up to 80,000 are hospitalised, and 6500 die of burn wounds every year.

AETIOLOGY/RISK FACTORS The pattern of injury varies among different age groups. Males aged 18–25 years seem more susceptible to injury owing to a variety of causes — mainly flame, electrical, and, to a lesser extent, chemicals. Many burn injuries in this age group are due to the inappropriate use of flammable agents such as petrol. However, most burns occur in the home. Thermal burns, in particular scalds, are common among the young as well as the elderly. The kitchen is reported to be the most common place of injury for children, as is the bathroom for the elderly. Those with concomitant conditions or complicating factors such as motor or neurological impairment are at greater risk.

PROGNOSIS Superficial partial thickness burns will heal spontaneously with minimal hypertrophic scarring within 2–3 weeks if the wound remains free of infection. The capacity to heal is also dependent on the health and age of the individual, with the elderly and those with concomitant medical conditions prone to delayed healing. Cooling the burn, as part of the initial emergency treatment, significantly reduces pain and wound oedema if started within 3 hours of injury. The optimal time to cool a wound may vary from 20–30 minutes using tap water (at a temperature of 5–25 °C). Use of iced water or prolonged periods of cooling can deepen tissue injury, induce hypothermia, and are best avoided. Cleaning solutions and dressings aim to prevent wound infection. The ideal dressing will establish an optimum microenvironment for wound healing. It will maintain the wound temperature and moisture level, permit respiration, allow epithelial migration, and exclude environmental bacteria.

Nicky Cullum and Emily Petherick

KEY POINTS

- Unrelieved pressure or friction of the skin, particularly over bony prominences, can lead to pressure ulcers, which affect up to a third of people in hospitals or community care, and a fifth of nursing-home residents.

  Pressure ulcers are more likely in people with reduced mobility and poor skin condition, such as older people or those with vascular disease.

- Alternative foam mattresses (such as viscoelastic foam) reduce the incidence of pressure ulcers in people at risk compared with standard hospital foam mattresses, although we don't know which is the best alternative to use.

  Low-air-loss beds may reduce the risk of pressure ulcers compared with standard intensive-care beds, but we don't know whether pressure-relieving overlays on operating tables are also beneficial compared with other pressure-relieving surfaces.

  Medical sheepskin overlays may reduce the risk of pressure ulcers compared with standard care.

- Hydrocellular heel supports may decrease the risk of pressure ulcers compared with orthopaedic wool padding, but air-filled vinyl boots with foot cradles and low-air-loss hydrotherapy beds may increase the risk of ulcers compared with other pressure-relieving surfaces.

  We don't know if other physical interventions, such as alternating-pressure surfaces, seat cushions, electric profiling beds, low-tech constant low-pressure supports, repositioning, or topical lotions and dressings are effective for preventing pressure ulcers. We also don't know whether pressure ulcers can be prevented by use of nutritional interventions.

- In people with pressure ulcers, air-fluidised supports may improve healing compared with standard care, although they can make it harder for people to get in and out of bed independently.

- Hydrocolloid dressings may also improve healing rates compared with standard dressings.

- We don't know whether healing is improved in people with pressure ulcers by use of other treatments such as alternating-pressure surfaces, debriding agents, low-tech constant low pressure supports, low-air-loss beds, seat cushions, dressings other than hydrocolloid, topical phenytoin, surgery, electrotherapy, ultrasound, low level laser therapy, topical negative pressure, or nutritional interventions.

(i) **Please visit www.clinicalevidence.bmj.com for full text and references**

What are the effects of preventive interventions in people at risk of developing pressure ulcers?	
Beneficial	• Foam alternatives (compared with standard foam mattresses)
Likely To Be Beneficial	• Low-air-loss beds in intensive care (more effective than standard beds; effects relative to alternating-pressure mattresses unclear) • Medical sheepskin overlays (compared with standard care)
Unknown Effectiveness	• Alternating pressure surfaces (compared with standard foam mattress or constant low-pressure supports)

	• Different seat cushions
	• Electric profiling beds
	• Hydrocellular heel supports (compared with orthopaedic wool padding)
	• Low-tech constant low pressure supports
	• Nutritional supplements
	• Pressure-relieving overlays on operating tables (compared with standard tables)
	• Repositioning (including regular "turning")
	• Topical lotions and dressings
Unlikely To Be Beneficial	• Air-filled vinyl boots
	• Low-air-loss hydrotherapy beds (compared with other pressure-relieving surfaces)

What are the effects of treatments in people with pressure ulcers?

Likely To Be Beneficial	• Air-fluidised supports (more effective than standard care)
	• Hydrocolloid dressings (compared with standard dressings)
Unknown Effectiveness	• Alternating-pressure surfaces
	• Debridement
	• Dressings other than hydrocolloid
	• Electrotherapy
	• Low-air-loss beds
	• Low level laser treatment
	• Low-tech constant low pressure supports
	• Nutritional supplements
	• Seat cushions
	• Surgery
	• Therapeutic ultrasound
	• Topical negative pressure
	• Topical phenytoin

Search date February 2007

DEFINITION Pressure ulcers (also known as pressure sores, bed sores, and decubitus ulcers) may present as persistently hyperaemic, blistered, broken, or necrotic skin, and may extend to underlying structures, including muscle and bone. Pressure ulcers are usually graded on a scale of 1 to 4, with a higher grade indicating greater ulcer severity.

INCIDENCE/PREVALENCE Reported prevalence rates range from 4.7–32.1% for hospital populations, 4.4–33.0% for community-care populations, and 4.6–20.7% for nursing-home populations.

AETIOLOGY/RISK FACTORS Pressure ulcers are caused by unrelieved pressure, shear, or friction. They are most common below the waist and at bony prominences, such as the sacrum, heels, and hips. They occur in all healthcare settings. Increased age, reduced mobility, impaired nutrition, vascular disease, faecal incontinence, and skin condition at baseline consistently emerge as risk factors. However, the relative importance of these and other factors is uncertain.

PROGNOSIS There are little data on prognosis of untreated pressure ulcers. The presence of pressure ulcers has been associated with a two- to fourfold increased risk of death in elderly people and people in intensive care. However, pressure ulcers are a marker for underlying disease severity and other comorbidities, rather than an independent predictor of mortality.

E Andrea Nelson and June Jones

KEY POINTS

- Leg ulcers are usually secondary to venous reflux or obstruction, but 20% of people with leg ulcers have arterial disease, with or without venous disorders.

- Compression bandages and stockings heal more ulcers compared with no compression, but we don't know which bandaging technique is most effective.

   Compression is used for people with ulcers caused by venous disease, who have an adequate arterial supply to the foot, and who don't have diabetes or rheumatoid arthritis.

   The effectiveness of compression bandages depends on the skill of the person applying them.

   We don't know whether intermittent pneumatic compression is beneficial compared with compression bandages or stockings.

- Occlusive (hydrocolloid) dressings are no more effective than simple low-adherent dressings in people treated with compression, but we don't know whether semi-occlusive dressings are beneficial.

- Peri-ulcer injections of granulocyte-macrophage colony stimulating factor may increase healing, but we don't know whether other locally applied agents, or therapeutic ultrasound are beneficial, as few studies have been found.

- Oral pentoxifylline increases ulcer healing in people receiving compression, and oral flavonoids, sulodexide, and mesoglycan may also be effective.

   We don't know whether oral aspirin, rutosides, thromboxane alpha$_2$ antagonists, zinc, debriding agents, intravenous prostaglandin E1, superficial vein surgery, skin grafting, leg ulcer clinics, larval therapy, or laser treatment increase healing of ulcers in people treated with compression.

- Compression bandages and stockings reduce recurrence of ulcers compared with no compression, and should ideally be worn for life.

   Superficial vein surgery may also reduce recurrence, but we don't know whether systemic drug treatment is effective.

(i) **Please visit www.clinicalevidence.bmj.com for full text and references**

What are the effects of standard treatments for venous leg ulcers?

Beneficial	• Compression bandages and stockings (more effective than no compression)
	• Compression stockings versus short-stretch bandages (both beneficial, but insufficient evidence to compare treatments)
	• Different types of multilayer elastomeric high-compression regimens (equally effective in increasing healing rates)
	• Multilayer elastomeric high-compression bandages (more effective in increasing healing rates than single-layer bandages)
	• Multilayer elastomeric high-compression bandages versus short-stretch bandages or Unna's boot (both beneficial in increasing healing rates, but unclear how they compare with each other)

	• Multilayer elastomeric versus non-elastomeric high-compression bandages (both beneficial, but unclear how they compare with each other)
	• Single-layer non-elastic system versus multilayer elastic system (both beneficial, but insufficient evidence to compare treatments)
	• Single-layer non-elastic system versus multilayer non-elastic system (both beneficial, but insufficient evidence to compare treatments)
Likely To Be Beneficial	• Peri-ulcer injection of granulocyte-macrophage colony-stimulating factor
Unknown Effectiveness	• Compression bandages or stockings versus intermittent pneumatic compression (insufficient evidence to compare)
	• Debriding agents
	• Foam, film, hyaluronic acid-derived dressings, collagen, cellulose, or alginate (semi-occlusive) dressings
	• Intermittent pneumatic compression
	• Topical antimicrobial agents
	• Topical calcitonin gene-related peptide plus vasoactive intestinal polypeptide
	• Topically applied platelet derived growth factor
	• Topical mesoglycan
	• Topical negative pressure
	• Topical recombinant keratinocyte growth factor 2
Unlikely To Be Beneficial	• Hydrocolloid (occlusive) dressings in the presence of compression
	• Topically applied autologous platelet lysate
	• Topically applied freeze-dried keratinocyte lysate

What are the effects of adjuvant treatments for venous leg ulcers?

Beneficial	• Oral pentoxifylline
Likely To Be Beneficial	• Cultured allogenic bilayer skin replacement
	• Oral flavonoids
	• Oral sulodexide
	• Systemic mesoglycan
Unknown Effectiveness	• Cultured allogenic single-layer dermal replacement
	• Intravenous prostaglandin E1

- Larval therapy
- Laser treatment (low level)
- Oral aspirin
- Oral rutosides
- Oral thromboxane alpha$_2$ antagonists
- Oral zinc
- Skin grafting
- Superficial vein surgery
- Therapeutic ultrasound

What are the effects of organisational interventions for venous leg ulcers?

Unknown Effectiveness	• Leg ulcer clinics

What are the effects of interventions to prevent recurrence of venous leg ulcers?

Beneficial	• Compression stockings
Likely To Be Beneficial	• Superficial vein surgery
Unknown Effectiveness	• Oral rutoside • Oral stanozolol

Search date July 2006

DEFINITION Definitions of leg ulcers vary, but the following is widely used: loss of skin on the leg or foot that takes more than 6 weeks to heal. Some definitions exclude ulcers confined to the foot, whereas others include ulcers on the whole of the lower limb. This review deals with ulcers of venous origin in people without concurrent diabetes mellitus, arterial insufficiency, or rheumatoid arthritis.

INCIDENCE/PREVALENCE Between 1.5 and 3.0/1000 people have active leg ulcers. Prevalence increases with age to about 20/1000 in people aged over 80 years. Most leg ulcers are secondary to venous disease; other causes include arterial insufficiency, diabetes, and rheumatoid arthritis. The annual cost to the NHS in the UK has been estimated at £300 million. This does not include the loss of productivity due to illness.

AETIOLOGY/RISK FACTORS Leg ulceration is strongly associated with venous disease. However, about a fifth of people with leg ulceration have arterial disease, either alone or in combination with venous problems, which may require specialist referral. Venous ulcers (also known as varicose or stasis ulcers) are caused by venous reflux or obstruction, both of which lead to poor venous return and venous hypertension.

PROGNOSIS People with leg ulcers have a poorer quality of life than age-matched controls because of pain, odour, and reduced mobility. In the UK, audits have found wide variation in the types of care (hospital inpatient care, hospital clinics, outpatient clinics, home visits), in the treatments used (topical agents, dressings, bandages, stockings), and in healing rates and recurrence rates (26–69% in 1 year).

NOTE
When looking up a class of drug, the reader is advised to also look up specific examples of that class of drug where additional entries may be found. The reverse situation also applies.

Index

Refeeding, anorexia nervosa, 328
Reflexology, premenstrual syndrome, 624, 625
Rehabilitation
  cardiac, 45, 46
  chronic obstructive pulmonary disease (COPD), 507, 508
  hip fracture, 381, 383
  multiple sclerosis, 436, 438
  Parkinson's disease, 439, 440–1
  shoulder pain, 409
  stroke, 48
  vestibular, 194
Rehydration therapy
  see also Fluid therapy; Hydration
  diarrhoea, 263, 264, 265
  gastroenteritis, 94
  sickle cell disease, 13
Relationship development intervention, autism, 71, 72
Relaxation therapy
  dysmenorrhoea, 599
  epilepsy, 427
  generalised anxiety disorder, 349, 350
  panic disorder, 356
  premenstrual syndrome, 624, 625
  tension-type headache, 431, 432
Reminiscence therapy, dementia, 340, 341
Renal failure
  see also End-stage renal disease
  acute, 299–302
    prevention, 299, 300
    treatments for critically ill people, 299, 300–1
  chronic, 303–6
    drug treatments, 303
    lifestyle interventions, 303, 304
Renal replacement therapy, 299, 300, 301
Renal scarring, children, 125, 126, 127–8
Repaglinide, diabetes, 134, 135
Resins, CVD prevention, 37, 38
Respiratory syncytial virus immunoglobulin, bronchiolitis, 77, 78
Rest
  see also Bed rest
  chronic fatigue syndrome, 372, 373
Resuscitation
  cardiorespiratory arrest, 80, 81
  perinatal asphyxia, 118, 119
Retinal detachment, 232–4
  prevention of progression, 232
  proliferative vitreoretinopathy treatment, 232–3
  surgical interventions, 232
Retinoids, psoriasis, 552, 553, 554
Retinyl esters, wrinkles, 566, 567
Revascularisation
  angina, 21, 22
  cardiogenic shock, 16, 17
  CVD prevention, 45, 47

Rhegmatogenous retinal detachment (RRD)
  see Retinal detachment
Rheumatoid arthritis, 405–7
  drug treatments, 405–6
Ribavirin
  bronchiolitis, 78
  hepatitis C, 270, 271
Rice-based oral rehydration solution, diarrhoea, 263, 265
Rifabutin
  M avium complex (MAC) disease, 245, 246
  P carinii pneumonia, 245
  tuberculosis, 250, 251
Rifampicin
  leprosy, 277
  MRSA, 291, 292
  tuberculosis, 250, 251, 296, 297
Rifaximin, colonic diverticular disease, 160
Rimantadine, influenza, 273, 274
Rimonabant, obesity, 213
Risedronate, fracture prevention in postmenopausal women, 374
Risperidone
  autism, 71, 72
  bipolar disorder, 331
  dementia, 340, 341
  post-traumatic stress disorder, 359, 360
  schizophrenia, 362, 363
Rituximab, non-Hodgkin's lymphoma (NHL), 10
Rivastigmine, dementia, 340, 341
Rizatriptan, migraine, 104
Rollerball endometrial ablation, fibroids, 608, 610
Rubber band ligation, haemorrhoids, 175
Rubella, 100–3
  vaccination, 100–3
Rupatadine, seasonal allergic rhinitis, 201
Rutosides
  haemorrhoids in pregnancy, 464, 465
  venous leg ulcers, 642, 644
Rye grass pollen extract, benign prostatic hyperplasia, 313, 314
Sacrohysteropexy, genital prolapse, 611, 612
Safety planning, intimate partner violence, 614, 615
St John's wort, depression, 88, 89, 343, 344
  postnatal depression, 475
Salbutamol
  asthma, 68, 69
  bronchiolitis, 77
Salicylic acid
  psoriasis, 552, 553
  warts, 564
Saline
  conjunctivitis, 220, 221
  nasal washes, sinusitis, 203, 204
Salmeterol, asthma, 68